Thyroid Ablation

Roberto Valcavi • Erivelto Volpi
Juan Pablo Dueñas • Gregory W. Randolph
Editors

Thyroid Ablation

An International Guide

Springer

Editors
Roberto Valcavi
Department of Endocrinology
The Endocrine & Thyroid Clinic
Reggio Emilia, Italy

Juan Pablo Dueñas
Integral Endocrine Surgery Clinic
Medellín, Colombia

Erivelto Volpi
Department of Head and Neck Surgery
Oswaldo Cruz German Hospital
São Paulo, Brazil

Gregory W. Randolph
Division of Thyroid and Parathyroid
Surgery, Department of Otolaryngology
Massachusetts Eye and Ear,
Harvard Medical School
Boston, MA, USA

ISBN 978-3-031-88228-9 ISBN 978-3-031-88229-6 (eBook)
https://doi.org/10.1007/978-3-031-88229-6

This Springer imprint is published by the registered company Springer Nature Switzerland AG
The registered company address is: Gewerbestrasse 11, 6330 Cham, Switzerland

To my wife, Benedetta, for her invaluable help and infinite patience.

Roberto Valcavi

To my wife, Mari, and my son, Leonardo, for their endless love, and to our patients, the primary reason for this book.

Erivelto Volpi

I dedicate this book to my wife, Lorraine Randolph, and to our patients.

Gregory W. Randolph

I dedicate this book to my wife, Virginia; my children Leticia, Emilio and Juan Santiago; and my family for their unwavering support and encouragement, and to all our patients for their trust.

Juan Pablo Dueñas

Preface

For many years, a total thyroidectomy had long been considered the only safe and effective surgical option for patients diagnosed with thyroid nodules. However, as a major operation, thyroid surgery requires a lengthy hospitalisation and recovery period. Furthermore, because the entire thyroid gland is removed, a lifelong thyroid hormone replacement therapy is necessary in order to control certain metabolic processes, and other supplements may be required to balance calcium levels.

Today, however, patients diagnosed with thyroid nodules have an array of alternative medical options besides a total thyroidectomy. These include ethanol ablation (EA), radiofrequency ablation (RFA), laser ablation (LA), microwave ablation (MWA) and high-intensity focused ultrasound (HI-FU) ablation which, with the exception of ethanol ablation, all apply heat to the nodule causing thermal tissue necrosis, leading to nodule shrinkage of up to 80% in some cases.

Given that these are all minimally invasive percutaneous treatments, there are several advantages over a total thyroidectomy such as no hospital admission, no need for incisions, hence absence of scars, no intubation for general anaesthesia, no drainage tubes, fewer post-operative complications, minimal side effects and faster recovery to normal daily routines as well as an overall better quality of life in the long run.

This book outlines in great detail these ablation techniques by explaining how each one is performed and emphasising what precautions should be taken when performing them, evaluating their advantages and disadvantages, assessing side effects and complications and measuring post-procedural results and expected patient outcomes.

Many other related topics such as surgical and radiologic neck anatomy, TIRADS and artificial intelligence, fine needle aspiration biopsy (FNAB) and core needle biopsy (CNB), active nodular surveillance, thyroid nodular pathology, molecular testing of thyroid nodules, learning curve and training and future developments in thermal ablation are also discussed in this book.

As the title suggests, the compiling of this book has been an international effort with over 40 authors of various medical and technical backgrounds coming from more than 15 different countries. Coordinating this endeavour has been fairly challenging but at the same time rather rewarding and quite enjoyable. The following 27 chapters represent the state of the art of thyroid ablation techniques presented by the leading authorities in this medical field and should be illuminating for endocrinologists and interventional endocrinologists, head and neck and endocrine surgeons, interventional radiologists, nuclear medicine technologists and other specialists.

Reggio Emilia, Italy — Roberto Valcavi
Boston, MA, USA — Gregory W. Randolph
Medellín, Colombia — Juan Pablo Dueñas
São Paulo, Brazil — Erivelto Volpi

Contents

Contributors

Devaprabu Abraham Division of Endocrinology, Department of Internal Medicine, University of Utah Health, Salt Lake City, UT, USA

Nikita R. Abraham Molecular Medicine Program (U2M2), Office of Research Integrity and Compliance, University of Utah, Salt Lake City, UT, USA

Jules Aljammal American Diplomat of Endocrinology and Metabolism, The Thyroid Clinic Utah, Salt Lake City, UT, USA

Tejas S. Athni Division of Thyroid and Parathyroid Endocrine Surgery, Department of Otolaryngology-Head and Neck Surgery, Massachusetts Eye and Ear Infirmary, Harvard Medical School, Boston, MA, USA

Ahmed Said Badr Radiology Department, National Hepatology and Tropical Medicine Research Institute, Cairo, Egypt

Chelsey K. Baldwin Department of Endocrinology, School of Medicine and Health Sciences, The George Washington University, Washington, DC, USA

Fernando Diego Choque Chavez Hospital Clinic Barcelona, Barcelona, Spain

Xavier Serres Créixams Radiology Unit, Vall d'Hebron Hospital Universitari, Barcelona, Spain

Mary Elizabeth Cunnane Department of Radiology, Massachusetts Eye and Ear, Boston, MA, USA

Orlandi Davide Department of Radiology, Ospedale Evangelico Internazionale, Genoa, Italy

Louise Davies Department of Surgery, Geisel School of Medicine at Dartmouth, Hanover, NH, USA

Juan Pablo Dueñas Integral Endocrine Surgery Clinic, Medellín, Colombia

Cosimo Durante Department of Translational and Precision Medicine, SAPIENZA University of Rome, Rome, Italy

Alaa Eid Elbanna Radiology Department, National Hepatology and Tropical Medicine Research Institute, Cairo, Egypt

Leslie Eldeiry Department of Endocrinology, Harvard Vanguard Medical Associates/Atrius Health, Boston, MA, USA

Safaa ElMandouh Radiology Department, National Hepatology and Tropical Medicine Research Institute, Cairo, Egypt

Mohamed Fawzi Radiology Department, National Hepatology and Tropical Medicine Research Institute, Cairo, Egypt

José Miguel Escudero Fernández Radiology Unit, Vall d'Hebron Hospital Universitari, Barcelona, Spain

Tatiana Ferraro Department of Surgery, School of Medicine and Health Sciences, The George Washington University, Washington, DC, USA

Andrea Frasoldati Endocrinology Unit, Arcispedale S. Maria Nuova, Azienda USL-IRCCS di Reggio Emilia, Reggio Emilia, Italy

Hossein Gharib Endocrinology Division, Mayo Clinic College of Medicine, Rochester, MN, USA

Caterina Giannitto Department of Diagnostic Radiology, IRCCS Humanitas Research Hospital, Milan, Italy
Department of Biomedical Sciences, Humanitas University, Milan, Italy

Turtulici Giovanni Ospedale Evangelico, Genoa, Italy
Department of Radiology, Ospedale Evangelico Internazionale, Genoa, Italy

Yasuhiro Ito Department of Surgery, Kuma Hospital, Kobe, Hyogo, Japan

Antonio Rahal Junior Department of Interventional Radiology, University of Sao Paulo, Sao Paulo, Brazil
Thyroid Imaging and Intervention Center, Hospital Israelita Albert Einstein, Sao Paulo, Brazil

Amanda Silver Karcioglu, MD, FACS Division of Otolaryngology-Head and Neck Surgery, Department of Surgery, Endeavor Health - Teaching Affiliate of the University of Chicago, Chicago, IL, USA
Pritzker School of Medicine, University of Chicago, Chicago, IL, USA

Jennifer H. Kuo The Columbia Thyroid Center, Section of Endocrine Surgery, Columbia University, New York, NY, USA

Giovanni Mauri European Institute of Oncology, Milan, Italy

Creteanu Mihai Arcadia Hospital, Iasi, Romania

Akira Miyauchi Department of Surgery, Kuma Hospital, Kobe, Hyogo, Japan

Hervé Monpeyssen Thyroid Unit, American Hospital of Paris, Neuilly-sur-Seine, France

Micheal Ezzat Narouz Radiology Department, National Hepatology and Tropical Medicine Research Institute, Cairo, Egypt

Roberto Negro Department of Experimental Medicine, University of Salento, Lecce, Italy
Division of Endocrinology, "V. Fazzi" Hospital, Lecce, Italy

Julia E. Noel Division of Otolaryngology Head & Neck Surgery, Santa Clara Valley Medical Center, Santa Clara, CA, USA
Department of Otolaryngology-Head & Neck Surgery, Stanford University School of Medicine, Stanford, CA, USA

Salem I. Noureldine Department of Surgery, School of Medicine and Health Sciences, The George Washington University, Washington, DC, USA

Roberto Novizio Volunteer Consultant Endocrinologist, A. Cardarelli Hospital, Naples, Italy

Lisa A. Orloff Department of Otolaryngology-Head & Neck Surgery, Stanford University School of Medicine, Stanford, CA, USA

Simonetta Piana Pathology Unit, Arcispedale S. Maria Nuova, Azienda USL-IRCCS di Reggio Emilia, Reggio Emilia, Italy

Ping Liang Chinese People's Liberation Army General Hospital, Beijing, China

Lin Zheng Chinese People's Liberation Army General Hospital, Beijing, China

Kharisa N. Rachmasari Division of Endocrinology, Diabetes and Nutrition, Mayo Clinic, Rochester, MN, USA

Gregory W. Randolph Division of Thyroid and Parathyroid Surgery, Department of Otolaryngology, Massachusetts Eye and Ear, Harvard Medical School, Boston, MA, USA
Division of Surgical Oncology, Endocrine Surgery Service, Department of Surgery, Massachusetts General Hospital, Harvard Medical School, Boston, MA, USA

Yujie Ren Jiangsu Province Hospital on Integration of Traditional Chinese and Western Medicine, Nanjing, China

Gilles Russ Endocrinology Unit, Ospedale Regionale di Lugano, Ente Ospedaliero Cantonale (EOC), Lugano, Switzerland

Marika D. Russell Department of Otolaryngology-Head & Neck Surgery, Massachusetts Eye and Ear, Boston, MA, USA
Division of Thyroid and Parathyroid Endocrine Surgery, Department of Otolaryngology-Head and Neck Surgery, Massachusetts Eye and Ear Infirmary, Harvard Medical School, Boston, MA, USA

Catherine F. Sinclair Department of Surgery, Monash University, Melbourne, VIC, Australia
Icahn School of Medicine at Mount Sinai, New York, NY, USA

Marialuisa Sponziello Department of Translational and Precision Medicine, SAPIENZA University of Rome, Rome, Italy

Mattia Squarcia Hospital Clinic Barcelona, Barcelona, Spain

Marius N. Stan Division of Endocrinology, Diabetes and Nutrition, Mayo Clinic, Rochester, MN, USA

Jose Higino Steck Campinas State University, Sao Paulo, Brazil

Elisavietta Tenuta Department of Diagnostic Radiology, IRCCS Humanitas Research Hospital, Milan, Italy
Department of Biomedical Sciences, Humanitas University, Milan, Italy

Roberto Valcavi, MD Department of Endocrinology, The Endocrine & Thyroid Clinic, Reggio Emilia, Italy

Evandro C. G. Vasconcelos Endocrine Neck Surgery, Nossa Senhora das Graças Hospital, Curitiba, Parana, Brazil

Erivelto Volpi Department of Head and Neck Surgery, Oswaldo Cruz German Hospital, São Paulo, Brazil

Shuhang Xu Jiangsu Province Hospital on Integration of Traditional Chinese and Western Medicine, Nanjing, China

Jie Yu Chinese People Liberation Army General Hospital, Beijing, China

1 Neck Surgical Anatomy

Erivelto Volpi and Evandro C. G. Vasconcelos

1.1 Introduction

The neck is a vital conduit connecting the Central Nervous System to the rest of the body. Every primary sense, including sight, hearing, and taste, traverses the neck through specific cervical regions occupied by cranial nerves. Additionally, many essential neural functions, such as swallowing and proprioception, pass through this crucial anatomical area.

The lymphatic and vascular systems navigate through the deep and superficial cervical fascial layers, where the surrounding muscular structures protect them. In this densely packed yet safeguarded environment lies the visceral compartment, where the thyroid and parathyroid glands are situated adjacent to the tracheoesophageal complex. Radiofrequency ablation (RFA) has gained recognition as a minimally invasive therapeutic technique for treating benign thyroid nodules and small, localized thyroid cancers. By utilizing thermal energy, RFA effectively reduces the volume of the targeted tissue while preserving the thyroid's normal tissue. However, the success and safety of this procedure heavily depend on a thorough understanding of the complex neck anatomy. This includes knowledge of the vascular, neural, and musculoskeletal structures surrounding the thyroid gland. In this text, we will explore the significance of anatomical knowledge in enhancing the safety and efficacy of thyroid RFA. While RFA is effective, healthcare professionals must possess a profound understanding of neck anatomy to avoid complications that may arise during the procedure. This includes potential damage to vital structures such as the recurrent laryngeal nerve, blood vessels, and the trachea.

To facilitate the understanding of the importance of the structures related to the thyroid gland in RFA, we divide the chapter into two topics: *thyroid anatomy* and *surrounding structures*.

1.2 Thyroid Anatomy

Anatomical position—The thyroid gland is situated in the lower anterior part of the neck, extending across the trachea and thyroid cartilage. It lies inferior to the larynx and anterior to the trachea, extending from about the level of the fifth to the sixth cervical vertebra [1, 2]. The gland's typical location allows for easy accessibility during surgical procedures. Still, it also places it in proximity to critical structures such as the recurrent laryngeal nerve and major blood vessels.

Shape and Size—The thyroid gland resembles a butterfly or an "H"-shaped structure with two distinct lobes connected by a narrow isthmus.

E. Volpi (✉)
Department of Head and Neck Surgery, Oswaldo Cruz German Hospital, São Paulo, Brazil

E. C. G. Vasconcelos
Endocrine Neck Surgery, Nossa Senhora das Graças Hospital, Curitiba, Parana, Brazil

R. Valcavi et al. (eds.), *Thyroid Ablation*, https://doi.org/10.1007/978-3-031-88229-6_1

Each lobe generally measures 4–6 cm in length and 1.5–2 cm in width, but size can vary widely among individuals [2–4]. The isthmus typically spans about 1–2 cm in width and lies anterior to the second and third tracheal rings. The lobes of the thyroid gland may exhibit asymmetry, with the right lobe often being slightly larger than the left lobe in many individuals [2, 5, 6].

Gross Anatomy—When viewed from the front, the thyroid gland is a vital structure with various surface features, including lobes. The right and left lobes are typically symmetrical but may vary in size; each lobe usually measures 4–6 cm long and is connected by the isthmus, which is about 1–2 cm wide. The lobes typically extend from the level of the fifth cervical vertebra (C5) to the sixth tracheal ring [2, 6, 7]. Because of their rich blood supply, the surface of the lobes may appear smooth and reddish-brown [5, 8, 9] (Fig. 1.1).

Blood Supply—Understanding the blood supply to the thyroid gland is vital for those involved in thermal ablations. The thyroid gland is highly vascularized and receives its blood supply primarily from two main arteries and some minor contributors.

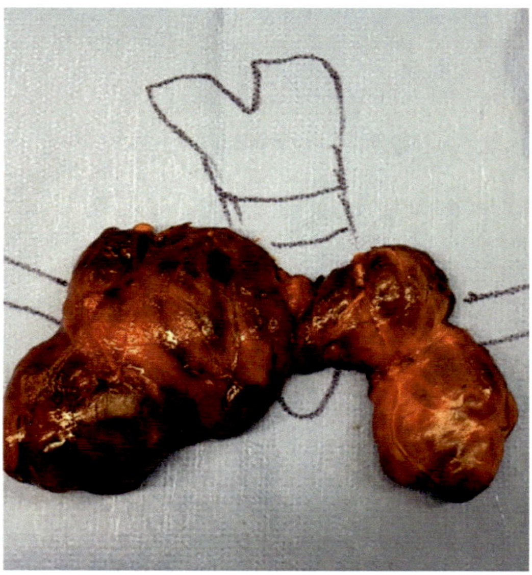

Fig. 1.1 A considerable goiter growing to the superior mediastinum, causing tracheal deviation

Major Arteries

1. *Superior Thyroid Artery*
   - Origin: The superior thyroid artery arises from the external carotid artery, typically at the level of the thyroid cartilage.
   - Course: This artery descends to the thyroid gland and runs medial to the sternocleidomastoid muscle (SCM). As it approaches the gland, it typically bifurcates into anterior and posterior branches [6, 9, 10].
   - Branches and Supply:
     - The anterior branch supplies the upper portion of the thyroid lobes and isthmus.
     - The posterior branch often gives off small perforating branches that supply the larynx and far-cervical structures [6, 9–11].
2. *Inferior Thyroid Artery*
   - Origin: The inferior thyroid artery usually originates from the thyrocervical trunk, a branch of the subclavian artery.
   - Course: This artery ascends toward the thyroid gland, typically running posterior to the carotid sheath, which contains the common carotid artery, internal jugular vein, and vagus nerve.
   - Branches and Supply:
     - The inferior thyroid artery primarily supplies the lower portions of the thyroid lobes and isthmus and may also branch off to the parathyroid glands located on the posterior aspect of the thyroid gland [5, 6, 10].
     - It often leads to ascending branches that pass closely to the trachea, further enhancing its supply [5, 6, 10].
3. *Thyroid Ima Artery* (Variable)
   - Origin: Although not present in all individuals, the thyroid IMA artery can originate from the aorta, brachiocephalic trunk, or subclavian artery.
   - Course: This artery ascends vertically to supply the isthmus or lower parts of the thyroid lobes, and when present, it contributes significantly to the gland's vascular supply [6, 7, 10].

Venous Drainage—The thyroid gland's venous drainage is accomplished through several veins that correspond closely to the arterial supply.

1. *Superior Thyroid Vein*
   - Course: The superior thyroid vein, which drains the upper portions of the thyroid gland, typically empties into the internal jugular vein. There may be multiple branches contributing to this drainage.
2. *Middle Thyroid Vein*
   - Course: The middle thyroid vein collects blood from the middle portion of the thyroid lobes and drains directly into the internal jugular vein.
3. *Inferior Thyroid Vein*
   - Course: The inferior thyroid vein, which drains the lower parts of the thyroid gland, empties into the brachiocephalic vein. It may have several branches draining into the left and right brachiocephalic veins [6, 9, 10, 12] Table 1.1.

Table 1.1 Summarizes the arterial supply and venous drainage of the thyroid gland

Arterial supply	–	**Superior Thyroid Artery**: Branch of the external carotid artery, supplies the upper part of the thyroid gland
	–	**Inferior Thyroid Artery**: Branch of the thyrocervical trunk (which is a branch of the subclavian artery), supplies the lower part of the thyroid gland
	–	**Thyroid Ima Artery**: Present in some individuals, it arises from the brachiocephalic trunk or aortic arch, supplying the isthmus of the thyroid
Venous drainage	–	**Superior Thyroid Vein**: Drains into the internal jugular vein, collecting blood from the upper part of the thyroid
	–	**Middle Thyroid Vein**: Also drains into the internal jugular vein, collecting blood from the middle part of the thyroid
	–	**Inferior Thyroid Veins**: Drains into the brachiocephalic veins, collecting blood from the lower part of the thyroid gland

Lymphatic Drainage of the Thyroid—The thyroid gland's lymphatic drainage is primarily through a network of lymphatic vessels that carry lymph to regional lymph nodes. The significant pathways for lymphatic drainage include the pretracheal, paratracheal, and lateral cervical lymph nodes. Lymph vessels drain laterally from the thyroid to the jugular chain and deep cervical lymph nodes. The pretracheal lymph nodes located anterior to the trachea and paratracheal lymph nodes along the trachea's lateral aspects receive lymphatic drainage directly from the thyroid gland [1, 13–15]. In cases of thyroid malignancy, these nodes are often the first sites of metastasis and are critical in assessing the disease's extent during surgical procedures. From the paratracheal nodes, lymph flows to the lateral cervical lymph nodes, including those in the jugular chain (levels II–IV) and level V, which contains the posterior triangle group of lymph nodes, which may also be involved in lateral drainage. This pathway is particularly significant in the presence of thyroid malignancies, where the lateral spread of cancer to these nodes indicates a higher stage of cancer [13–15]. A rigorous evaluation of the lymph nodes before thermal ablation for malignancies is paramount to avoid the wrong indication of this therapy.

The thyroid bed—The region where the thyroid gland is located is termed the thyroid bed, which encompasses the central neck lymph node compartment. This anatomical space is defined laterally by the common carotid arteries, inferiorly by the sternal notch, and superiorly by the hyoid bone [1–3, 5, 14, 15]. The trachea, esophagus, parathyroid glands, laryngeal nerves, and several essential lymph node chains within this region, including the paratracheal and pretracheal lymph nodes, are situated [1, 7, 14, 15]. Nonsurgical management of posterior lymph nodes and parathyroids is seldom reported and may be a future frontier to be endeavored by ablation techniques. Therefore, with deep knowledge of anatomical aspects of such sensitive and vital structures, the most careful approach to deploying protective techniques (such as hydrodissection) must be used in the thyroid bed (Fig. 1.2).

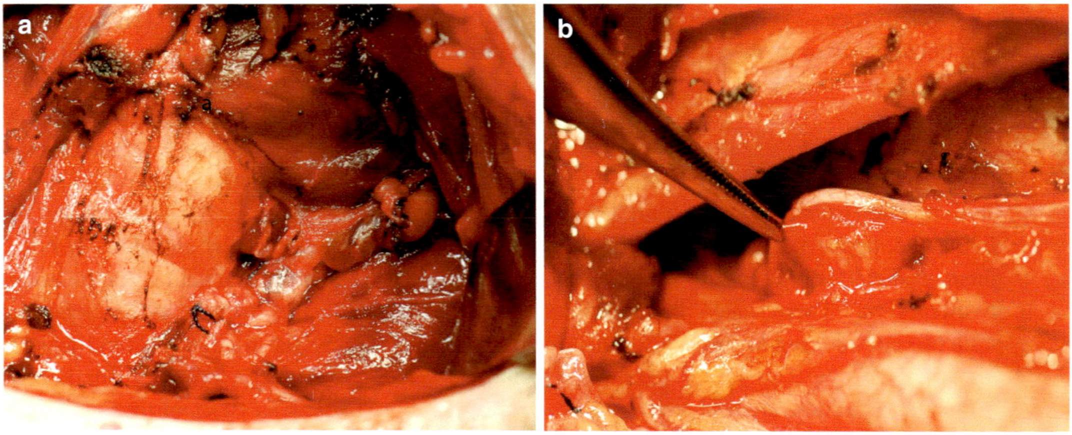

Fig. 1.2 (**a**) After a total thyroidectomy, the thyroid bed showed trachea, the superior parathyroid gland, the left recurrent laryngeal nerve, and lymph node metastasis in the central compartment with close relation to the recurrent laryngeal nerve. (**b**) A lymph node metastasis under the recurrent laryngeal nerve (courtesy of Dr. Higino Steck)

1.3 Surrounding Structures

The cervical fascia is a crucial structural component of the neck, serving as a protective sheath that envelops vital anatomical structures, including muscles, blood vessels, nerves, and organs. It comprises multilayered planes with distinct roles and relationships to surrounding tissues, facilitating their functions. The cervical fascia consists primarily of three layers: the superficial cervical fascia, the deep cervical fascia, and the pretracheal fascia. Understanding the organization of these fascial layers and their relationship with the thyroid gland is essential for interventions in the neck, including surgical procedures [1].

1.4 Layers of Cervical Fascia

1. *Superficial Cervical Fascia*: The superficial layer lies beneath the skin and contains subcutaneous fat, cutaneous nerves, and the platysma muscle. It has limited relevance to the thyroid gland but protects underlying structures and assists in the movement of the skin during head and neck motion [15].
2. *Deep Cervical Fascia*: This layer is more complex and organized into three main divisions: the investing, pretracheal, and prevertebral.
   - *Investing Layer:* This outermost layer encases the sternocleidomastoid and trapezius muscles and the submandibular and parotid glands. The investing layer also forms a sheath for the thyroid gland, anchoring it and providing some degree of mobility within the neck [15, 16].
   - *Pretracheal Layer*: This layer is particularly significant regarding the thyroid gland, as it surrounds both the thyroid gland and the trachea. The pretracheal fascia creates a protective environment for these structures as they perform their essential functions in metabolism and respiration [15–17]. This layer extends from the hyoid bone to the thorax, enveloping the thyroid gland laterally and posteriorly.
   - *Prevertebral Layer*: Located deep in the pretracheal and investing layers, this fascia surrounds the cervical vertebrae and associated muscles. While it does not directly interact with the thyroid gland, it forms the deep boundary of the neck and provides support and stability to the surrounding structures [15–17].

Trachea and Esophagus—Anatomically, the thyroid gland is anterior to the trachea and inferior to the larynx. The two lobes of the thyroid typically extend from the level of the sixth cervical vertebra to the second or third tracheal ring [2, 5, 6]. The isthmus of the thyroid connects the two lobes across the trachea at the level of the second and third tracheal rings, thereby contributing to the thyroid's close association with the trachea. This proximity is clinically significant as it increases the risk of injury to the trachea during thermal ablation procedures and surgeries and affects the management of thyroid malignancies that may invade surrounding tissues [8, 18]. The esophagus is located posterior to the trachea at the level of the thyroid gland and generally runs from the cervical region down into the thorax. This proximity means that enlargements of the thyroid, such as in cases of goiter or thyroid neoplasms, can lead to compression of the esophagus, resulting in swallowing difficulties [19, 20]. The esophagus is typically flanked by the recurrent laryngeal nerve, which innervates the vocal cords and runs closely to the trachea. These anatomical relationships are critical in thyroid surgery to avoid nerve injury [1, 3, 21]. Furthermore, the anatomical configuration of the thyroid gland can vary among individuals, with potential variations in the positions of the trachea and esophagus, as well as the presence of ectopic thyroid tissue. Such variations may necessitate careful preoperative imaging and thorough knowledge of individual anatomy to avoid complications [21, 22] (Fig. 1.3).

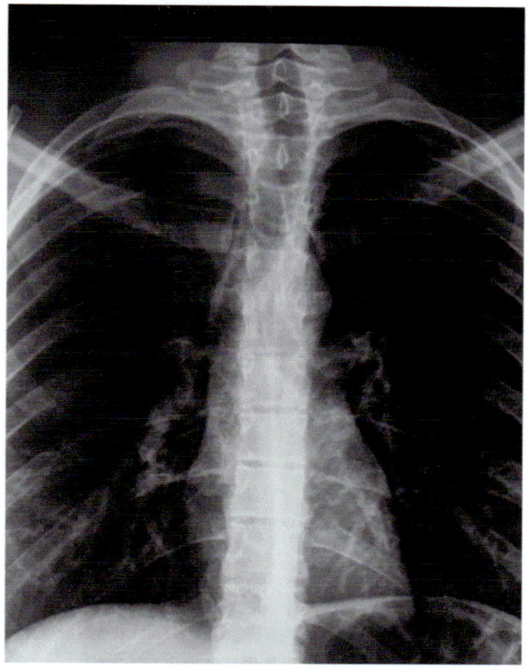

Fig. 1.3 The X-ray of the same patient in Fig. 1.1 shows a significant tracheal deviation

Recurrent Laryngeal Nerve (RLN)—As in surgeries, the jeopardization of the RLN is one of the feared complications of thermal ablations. The RLN has a unique pathway that varies between the right and left sides of the body. On the right side, the nerve branches off the vagus nerve and loops around the right subclavian artery before ascending between the trachea and esophagus to reach the larynx. The left RLN, on the other hand, loops around the aortic arch before traversing upward between the trachea and esophagus to innervate the larynx [2]. This anatomical distinction must be noted, as it can significantly influence strategies, approaches, and outcomes in surgeries and minimally invasive treatments. *Relationship to the Thyroid Gland:* Both the right and left recurrent laryngeal nerves run in close proximity to the thyroid gland, often just posteriorly to its lobes. This anatomical relationship is crucial during thermal therapies as the RLN may risk injury or damage [2, 3, 8, 9, 21–23]. In most individuals, the thyroid gland lies medial to the RLN. Studies have revealed that anatomical variations can be as high as 20%, underscoring the importance of preoperative imaging and careful intraoperative exploration [21–23]. The knowledge of the anatomical relationship between the thyroid gland and the recurrent laryngeal nerve is complex and vital for safe thermal ablation treatments. A clear understanding of this relationship, including the unique pathways of the RLN and the potential for anatomical variations, is essential for those who perform these treatments (Fig. 1.4).

External Branch of the Superior Laryngeal Nerve (EBSLN)—The EBSLN plays a

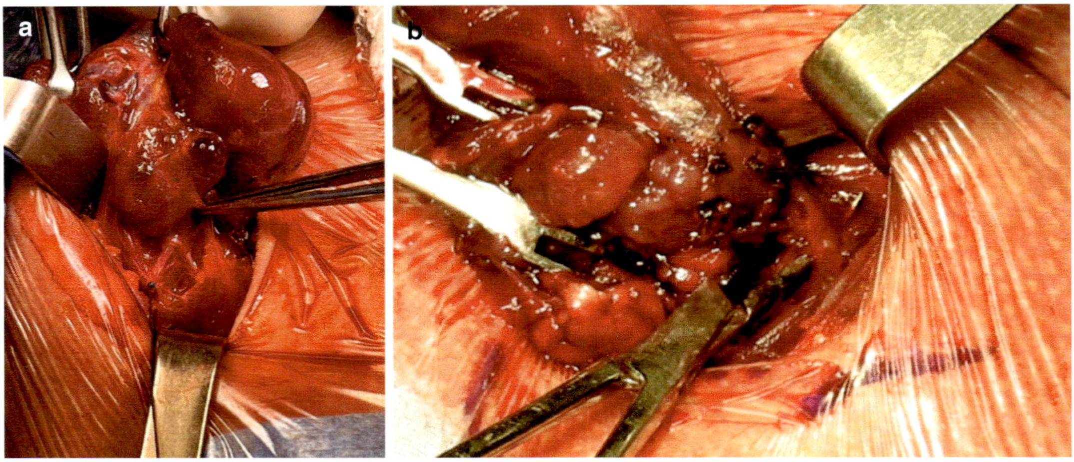

Fig. 1.4 Two variations of the relationship of the recurrent laryngeal nerve and the inferior thyroid artery. (**a**) The RLN over the ITA. (**b**) The RLN under the ITA

significant role in laryngeal function and voice modulation. It innervates the cricothyroid muscle, essential for tense voice production and pitch regulation. The relationship between the EBSLN and the thyroid gland is crucial for understanding surgical anatomy, particularly in thyroid surgery, where the risk of nerve injury can lead to debilitating vocal changes; the superior laryngeal nerve branches off from the neck's vagus nerve (cranial nerve X). The external branch runs along the lateral surface of the thyroid gland and is closely associated with the upper pole of the gland [9, 24, 25]. As it descends, the EBSLN typically courses near the superior thyroid artery, making its path variable and subject to anatomical variations. This proximity to the thyroid gland's upper pole is anatomically significant; due to its location, the external branch is at risk for injury during thyroid surgeries, especially lobectomies or total thyroidectomies [24, 25]. The anatomical variations in the path of the EBSLN can lead to misidentification or unintentional damage during dissection, underscoring the importance of thorough anatomical knowledge for surgeons [3, 24, 25]. Even though the potential for harm to this nerve in thermal ablations is minimal when ablating nodules in the upper pole of the thyroid gland, we recommend hydrodissection of the region to minimize the risk of injury over this nerve.

Parathyroid Glands—The parathyroid glands are small, endocrine glands in the neck, typically on the posterior surface of the thyroid gland. Their primary function is to regulate calcium levels in the blood through parathyroid hormone (PTH) secretion. Understanding the anatomy of the parathyroid glands is crucial for clinicians, especially surgeons, as these glands are often incidental findings during thyroid surgeries, and their preservation is essential to avoid postoperative complications, such as hypoparathyroidism. Typically, there are four parathyroid glands although the number can vary among individuals. They are usually found on the posterior surface of the thyroid lobes, with two glands on each lobe. The superior parathyroid glands are typically found at the level of the cricoid cartilage. In contrast, the inferior parathyroid glands are often located at the level where the thyroid gland's inferior pole meets the trachea [4–6]. Also, ectopic parathyroid glands may exist; these can be found in various locations, including the mediastinum, thymus, and carotid arteries [4–7, 9]. The vascularization of the parathyroid glands is primarily provided by branches of the inferior thyroid artery, with additional contributions from the superior thyroid artery [4, 9, 10]. The rich vascular supply is essential for the glands' function as they require a steady blood flow to effectively secrete PTH and respond to changes in calcium levels in the bloodstream. The anatomy of the parathyroid glands is particularly significant in surgical procedures involving the thyroid or parathyroid glands. During thyroidectomy, for example, there is a risk of inadvertently damaging or removing surrounding parathyroid tissues, which can lead to hypoparathyroidism and associated complications like hypocalcemia [3–5, 10]. Comprehensive knowledge of parathyroid anatomy, variations, and surgical techniques to preserve these glands is crucial for minimizing surgical complications [3–7, 9, 10]. Since there are no reports of hypocalcemia following thermal ablation of thyroid nodules, we can state that the risk of this complication is virtually zero; however, the knowledge of parathyroid anatomy and its relationship with surrounding structures, especially the RLN is crucial when considering treating parathyroid adenomas.

1.5 Muscles Related to the Thyroid Gland: Sternocleidomastoid Muscle (SCM)

The SCM is a prominent muscle extending along the neck's sides. It originates from the manubrium of the sternum (medial head) and the clavicle (lateral head) and inserts at the mastoid process of the temporal bone [26].

Strap Muscles—The strap muscles, also called the infrahyoid muscles, include four pairs: the sternohyoid, sternothyroid, omohyoid, and thyrohyoid. These muscles are organized into two layers: a superficial layer consisting of the sternohyoid and omohyoid muscles and a deeper layer made up of the sternothyroid and thyrohyoid muscles (X). The sternothyroid muscle forms part of the lateral surface of the thyroid gland, attaching to the thyroid cartilage and supporting the superior pole of the gland. The superior belly of the omohyoid and sternohyoid muscles borders the thyroid gland anteriorly, while the anterior aspect of the sternocleidomastoid muscle overlaps these two structures. An avascular fascia connects the sternothyroid and sternohyoid muscles at the midline, and this fascia is often incised during thyroid surgery. The infrahyoid muscles play a vital role in swallowing and phonation by facilitating the movement and positioning of the larynx. Furthermore, the SCM rotates the head to the same side (ipsilateral) and turns the shoulder toward the opposite side (contralateral) [15, 27].

Carotid Artery—The carotid artery's close anatomical relationship with the thyroid gland necessitates careful consideration during surgical procedures such as thyroidectomy. Potential hemorrhage is a possible complication from procedures jeopardizing the carotid artery, like thermal ablations, and special care with this crucial structure is of paramount importance in these procedures. Overview and Branches: the carotid arteries consist of the common carotid artery (CCA) and its bifurcation into the internal carotid artery (ICA) and external carotid artery (ECA).

- Common Carotid Artery: This artery typically arises from the aorta on the left side and the brachiocephalic trunk on the right side. It ascends in the neck, traveling within the carotid sheath with the internal jugular vein and vagus nerve. The common carotid artery bifurcates at the level of the upper border of the thyroid cartilage (corresponding to C4–C5 vertebrae) into the ICA and ECA.
- Internal Carotid Artery: This artery supplies blood to the brain, forehead, eyes, and face parts. It enters the skull through the carotid canal.
- External Carotid Artery: The ECA supplies blood to the face and neck through several branches, including the superior thyroid artery, which is crucial for vascularizing the thyroid gland [28, 29] (Fig. 1.5).

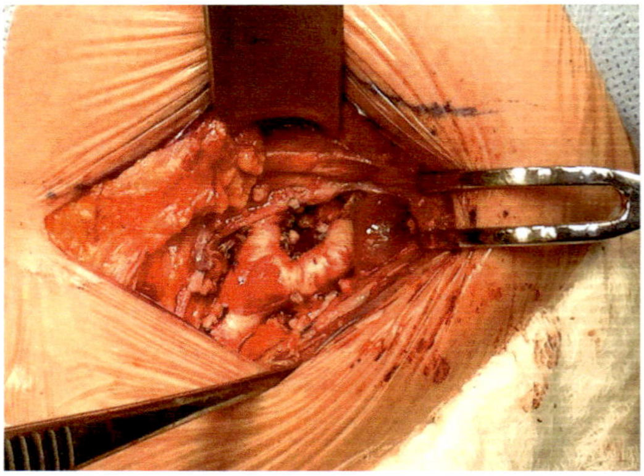

Fig. 1.5 In neck dissection of recurrent thyroid cancer, where it is possible to see the bifurcation of the common carotid artery into the external carotid artery and internal carotid artery; additionally, it is possible to see the Accessory Nerve (Cranial Nerve XI), running superficially to the internal carotid artery

Jugular Veins—The jugular veins are responsible for draining blood from the head and neck regions, and there are three primary types:

- Internal Jugular Vein (IJV): This vein collects venous blood from the brain, face, neck, and skull. It runs lateral to the carotid artery in the carotid sheath, receiving blood from the superior thyroid vein, middle thyroid vein, and various venous sinuses of the skull.
- External Jugular Vein (EJV)**:** This vein drains blood from the superficial parts of the face and neck. It runs across the SCM muscle and usually empties into the subclavian vein.
- Anterior Jugular Vein**:** This vein drains the anterior part of the neck and may connect with the EJV [30–32].

The proximity of the carotid artery and internal jugular vein to the thyroid influences surgical approaches, imaging techniques, and clinical outcomes in patients with thyroid disorders. A comprehensive understanding of the anatomy and relationship of the thyroid gland to the carotid artery and jugular vein allows healthcare professionals to execute procedures more safely and manage potential complications effectively.

1.6 Conclusions

Unique anatomical variations may exist in the thyroid gland and surrounding structures, which can significantly influence RFA outcomes. For example, an aberrant course of the recurrent laryngeal nerve may increase the risk of injury. Assessment of individual patient anatomy through imaging studies before RFA can inform procedural strategies, maximizing safety and efficacy. The anatomy of the neck is better understood as a folder cabinet subdivided into regions of interest. In each of them, the location of the most sensitive and essential anatomic structures should be detailed to the ablation operator for the appropriate care and best results. Therefore, establishing safe roads is a safety approach pattern recommended from the least to the most experienced to avoid complications and achieve the best results.

References

1. Carlson GW. Surgical anatomy of the neck. Surg Clin North Am. 1993;73(4):837–52. https://doi.org/10.1016/S0039-6109(16)46087-1.
2. Joshi SD, Joshi SS, Daimi SR, Athavale SA. The thyroid gland and its variations: a cadaveric study. Folia Morphol (Warsz). 2010;69(1):47–50. PMID: 20235050.
3. Bliss RD, Gauger PG, Delbridge LW. Surgeon's approach to the thyroid gland: surgical anatomy and the importance of technique. World J Surg. 2000;24(8):891–7. https://doi.org/10.1007/s002680010173. PMID: 10865032.
4. Miller FR. Surgical anatomy of the thyroid and parathyroid glands. Otolaryngol Clin North Am. 2003;36(1):1–7, vii. PMID: 12803005. https://doi.org/10.1016/s0030-6665(02)00132-9.
5. Mansberger AR Jr, Wei JP. Surgical embryology and anatomy of the thyroid and parathyroid glands. Surg Clin North Am. 1993;73(4):727–46. https://doi.org/10.1016/s0039-6109(16)46082-2. PMID: 8378818.
6. Policeni BA, Smoker WR, Reede DL. Anatomy and embryology of the thyroid and parathyroid glands. Semin Ultrasound CT MR. 2012;33(2):104–14. https://doi.org/10.1053/j.sult.2011.12.005. PMID: 22410358.
7. Fancy T, Gallagher D, Hornig JD. Surgical anatomy of the thyroid and parathyroid glands. Otolaryngol

Clin North Am. 2010;43(2):221–7. https://doi.org/10.1016/j.otc.2010.01.001.
8. Loré JM Jr. Practical anatomical considerations in thyroid tumor surgery. Arch Otolaryngol. 1983;109(9):568–74. PMID: 6882263.
9. Dozois RR, Beahrs OH. Surgical anatomy and technique of thyroid and parathyroid surgery. Surg Clin North Am. 1977;57(4):647–61. https://doi.org/10.1016/s0039-6109(16)41280-6. PMID: 897961.
10. Branca JJV, Lascialfari Bruschi A, Pilia AM, Carrino D, Guarnieri G, Gulisano M, Pacini A, Paternostro F. The thyroid gland: a revision study on its vascularization and surgical implications. Medicina (Kaunas). 2022;58(1):137. https://doi.org/10.3390/medicina58010137. PMID: 35056445; PMCID: PMC8779193.
11. Tzortzis AS, Antonopoulos I, Pechlivanidou E, Chrysikos D, Pappas N, Troupis T. Anatomical variations of the superior thyroid artery: a systematic review. Morphology. 2023;107(358):100597. https://doi.org/10.1016/j.morpho.2023.03.002. Epub 2023 Apr 13. PMID: 37061377.
12. Wafae N, Hirose K, Franco C, Wafae GC, Ruiz CR, Daher L, Person OC. The anatomy of the human thyroid veins and its surgical application. Folia Morphol (Warsz). 2008;67(4):221–5. PMID: 19085858.
13. Likhterov I, Reis LL, Urken ML. Central compartment management in patients with papillary thyroid cancer presenting with metastatic disease to the lateral neck: anatomic pathways of lymphatic spread. Head Neck. 2017;39(5):853–9. https://doi.org/10.1002/hed.24568. Epub 2017 Mar 2. PMID: 28252836.
14. Sturgeon C, Yang A, Elaraj D. Surgical management of lymph node compartments in papillary thyroid cancer. Surg Oncol Clin N Am. 2016;25(1):17–40. https://doi.org/10.1016/j.soc.2015.08.013. PMID: 26610772.
15. Norris CD, Anzai Y. Anatomy of neck muscles, spaces, and lymph nodes. Neuroimaging Clin N Am. 2022;32(4):831–49. https://doi.org/10.1016/j.nic.2022.07.027. Epub 2022 Sep 21. PMID: 36244726.
16. Sutcliffe P, Lasrado S. Anatomy, head and neck, deep cervical neck fascia. 2023. In: StatPearls [Internet]. Treasure Island: StatPearls Publishing; 2024. PMID: 31082135.
17. Warshafsky D, Goldenberg D, Kanekar SG. Imaging anatomy of deep neck spaces. Otolaryngol Clin North Am. 2012;45(6):1203–21. https://doi.org/10.1016/j.otc.2012.08.001. PMID: 23153745.
18. Ha EJ, Baek JH, Lee JH. The efficacy and complications of radiofrequency ablation of thyroid nodules. Curr Opin Endocrinol Diabetes Obes. 2011;18(5):310–4. https://doi.org/10.1097/MED.0b013e32834a9168. PMID: 21841482.
19. Olson SE, Starling J, Chen H. Symptomatic benign multinodular goiter: unilateral or bilateral thyroidectomy? Surgery. 2007;142(4):458–61; discussion 461–2. PMID: 17950336. https://doi.org/10.1016/j.surg.2007.07.003.
20. Rodrigues MG, de Araujo Filho VJF, de Matos LL, Hojaij FC, Simões CA, de Araujo Neto VJF, Ramos DM, Mahmoud RL, de Moraes Mosca L, Manta GB, Brandão EMVLG, Cernea CR. Substernal goiter and laryngopharyngeal reflux. Arch Endocrinol Metab. 2017;61(4):348–53. https://doi.org/10.1590/2359-3997000000266. Epub 2017 Jun 26. PMID: 28658344; PMCID: PMC10118925.
21. Liddy W, Wu CW, Dionigi G, Donatini G, Giles Senyurek Y, Kamani D, Iwata A, Wang B, Okose O, Cheung A, Saito Y, Casella C, Aygun N, Uludag M, Brauckhoff K, Carnaille B, Tunca F, Barczyński M, Kim HY, Favero E, Innaro N, Vamvakidis K, Serpell J, Romanchishen AF, Takami H, Chiang FY, Schneider R, Dralle H, Shin JJ, Abdelhamid Ahmed AH, Randolph GW. Varied recurrent laryngeal nerve course is associated with increased risk of nerve dysfunction during thyroidectomy: results of the surgical anatomy of the recurrent laryngeal nerve in thyroid surgery study, an international multicenter prospective anatomic and electrophysiologic study of 1000 monitored nerves at risk from the International Neural Monitoring Study Group. Thyroid. 2021;31(11):1730–40. https://doi.org/10.1089/thy.2021.0155. PMID: 34541890.
22. Ngo Nyeki AR, Njock LR, Miloundja J, Evehe Vokwely JE, Bengono G. Recurrent laryngeal nerve landmarks during thyroidectomy. Eur Ann Otorhinolaryngol Head Neck Dis. 2015;132(5):265–9. https://doi.org/10.1016/j.anorl.2015.08.002. Epub 2015 Aug 31. PMID: 26338514.
23. Ling XY, Smoll NR. A systematic review of variations of the recurrent laryngeal nerve. Clin Anat. 2016;29(1):104–10. https://doi.org/10.1002/ca.22613. Epub 2015 Oct 5. PMID: 26297484.
24. Sakorafas GH, Kokoropoulos P, Lappas C, Sampanis D, Smyrniotis V. External branch of the superior laryngeal nerve: applied surgical anatomy and implications in thyroid surgery. Am Surg. 2012;78(9):986–91. PMID: 22964209.
25. Morton RP, Whitfield P, Al-Ali S. Anatomical and surgical considerations of the external branch of the superior laryngeal nerve: a systematic review. Clin Otolaryngol. 2006;31(5):368–74. https://doi.org/10.1111/j.1749-4486.2006.01266.x. Erratum in: Clin Otolaryngol. 2007 Feb;32(1):78. PMID: 17014444.
26. Silawal S, Schulze-Tanzil G. The sternocleidomastoid muscle variations: a mini literature review. Folia Morphol (Warsz). 2023;82(3):507–12. https://doi.org/10.5603/FM.a2022.0045. Epub 2022 May 24. PMID: 35607877.
27. Kohan EJ, Wirth GA. Anatomy of the neck. Clin Plast Surg. 2014;41(1):1–6. https://doi.org/10.1016/j.cps.2013.09.016. PMID: 24295343.

28. Dungan DH, Heiserman JE. The carotid artery: embryology, normal anatomy, and physiology. Neuroimaging Clin N Am. 1996;6(4):789–99. PMID: 8824131.
29. Hayashi N, Hori E, Ohtani Y, Ohtani O, Kuwayama N, Endo S. Surgical anatomy of the cervical carotid artery for carotid endarterectomy. Neurol Med Chir (Tokyo). 2005;45(1):25–9; discussion 30. PMID: 15699617. https://doi.org/10.2176/nmc.45.25.
30. Mumtaz S, Singh M. Surgical review of the anatomical variations of the internal jugular vein: an update for head and neck surgeons. Ann R Coll Surg Engl. 2019;101(1):2–6. https://doi.org/10.1308/rcsann.2018.0185. Epub 2018 Oct 16. PMID: 30322289; PMCID: PMC6303832.
31. Rusu MC, Tudose RC, Vrapciu AD, Toader C, Popescu ȘA. Anatomical variations of the external jugular vein: a pictorial and critical review. Medicina (Kaunas). 2023;59(3):622. https://doi.org/10.3390/medicina59030622. PMID: 36984623; PMCID: PMC10052824.
32. Lee DH, Cho YS, Jung WH, Lim SC, Nam KI. Anatomical characteristics of the anterior jugular vein and its clinical relevance. J Craniofac Surg. 2022;33(5):1385–7. https://doi.org/10.1097/SCS.0000000000008594. Epub 2022 Feb 25. PMID: 35220348.

2 Neck Ultrasound and Radiologic Anatomy

Caterina Giannitto and Elisavietta Tenuta

2.1 Introduction

Knowledge of ultrasound (US)-based thyroid anatomy and surrounding structures may help in the early detection, prevention, and proper management of complications during US-guided interventions of the thyroid gland [1]. Optimal US requires appropriate equipment with high-resolution small-parts transducers that make use of high US frequencies between 5 and 20 MHz (most commonly 7.5–10 MHz). Typically, the position entails gentle hyperextension of the neck with a soft pillow for support beneath the shoulders. For a safe ablation, operators need to identify anatomic landmarks, and under US monitoring, the spinal needle is inserted into the target thyroid lesion, in most cases along its longest axis. The fiber tip should be positioned at a minimum safety distance of 5–10 mm from the critical structures of the neck. In case of lesions close to the carotid vessels or the trachea wall, a preliminary hydro-dissection with saline solution may be performed to separate the target from the vital structure [2]. The knowledge of cross-sectional head and neck anatomy will facilitate head and neck US performance [3]. Therefore, the purposes of this chapter will be to describe US-based anatomy of the neck with specific attention to the thyroid and its surroundings in the infrahyoid region of the neck, describing the anatomy and the US features of the structures located in the visceral, carotid, retropharyngeal, perivertebral, and posterior cervical spaces (Fig. 2.1).

C. Giannitto (✉) · E. Tenuta
Department of Diagnostic Radiology, IRCCS Humanitas Research Hospital, Milan, Italy

Department of Biomedical Sciences, Humanitas University, Milan, Italy
e-mail: caterina.giannitto@hunimed.eu; elisavietta.tenuta@humanitas.it

R. Valcavi et al. (eds.), *Thyroid Ablation*, https://doi.org/10.1007/978-3-031-88229-6_2

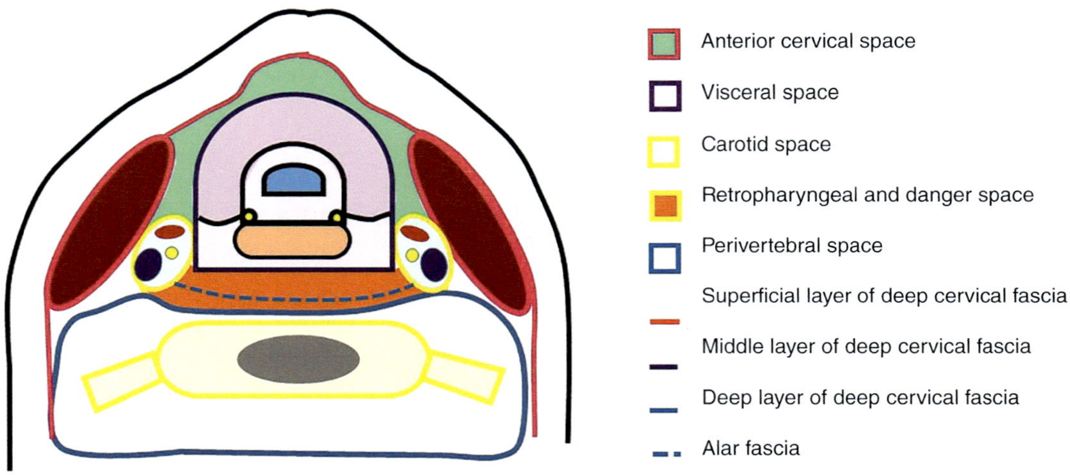

Fig. 2.1 Schematic diagram of infrahyoid deep neck spaces. The visceral space contains thyroid and parathyroid glands, trachea, esophagus, recurrent laryngeal nerves, and pretracheal and paratracheal nodes. The carotid space contains the cranial nerves IX–XII, internal jugular vein, and the internal carotid artery. The retropharyngeal space (RPS) is anterior to the vertebral column. The infrahyoid RPS contains fat only. The danger space is a potential space in the posterior RPS, separated from the anterior RPS by the alar fascia. The perivertebral space (PVS) includes the prevertebral PVS and the paraspinal PVS. The prevertebral PVS contains brachial plexus and phrenic nerve, vertebral body, veins, arteries, and prevertebral and scalene muscles within. The paraspinal PVS contains only posterior vertebra elements and paraspinal muscles

2.2 Visceral Space and Perithyroidal Anatomic Landmarks

The visceral space is a cylindrical space bounded by the middle layer of the deep cervical fascia, which extends from the hyoid bone to the upper mediastinum. It is delimited anterolaterally by the anterior cervical space, posterolaterally by the carotid space, and posteriorly by the retropharyngeal space [4–6]. It includes the thyroid and parathyroid glands, the larynx, the hypopharynx, the cervical segments of the trachea and esophagus, and the recurrent laryngeal nerve (RLN).

2.2.1 Thyroid and Normal Anatomic Landmarks on US

The thyroid gland is a butterfly-shaped organ located in the midline within the visceral space, anterior to the prevertebral space. Anteriorly, the gland is covered by the superficial fascia and platysma, and, posteriorly, the condensation of the deep cervical fascia forms the suspensory ligament of Berry affixing the thyroid to the first two tracheal rings and to the inferior margin of the cornu of the cricoid cartilage [7]. It consists of two lateral lobes which are united by isthmus located anterior to the trachea. Despite these general features, the thyroid gland is known to have many morphological variations. The pyramidal lobe may branch from the right or left lobe, the isthmus, or from only one lobe with the absence of the isthmus. The incidence of this lobe was found to be 55% in a postmortem study [8]. The thyroid gland surrounds the trachea and lies posterior to the infrahyoid strap muscles (sternohyoid and sternothyroid). Its posteromedial border is near the tracheoesophageal groove, which contains the RLN, the parathyroid glands, and lymph nodes (Figs. 2.1 and 2.2).

At US, the most superficial structures encountered are the skin and subcutaneous tissue. The dermis is the most superficial layer with a thickness of 1–2 mm and has a similar echogenicity to the thyroid gland. Just deep to it is a layer of subcutaneous fat that is brighter than the dermis and

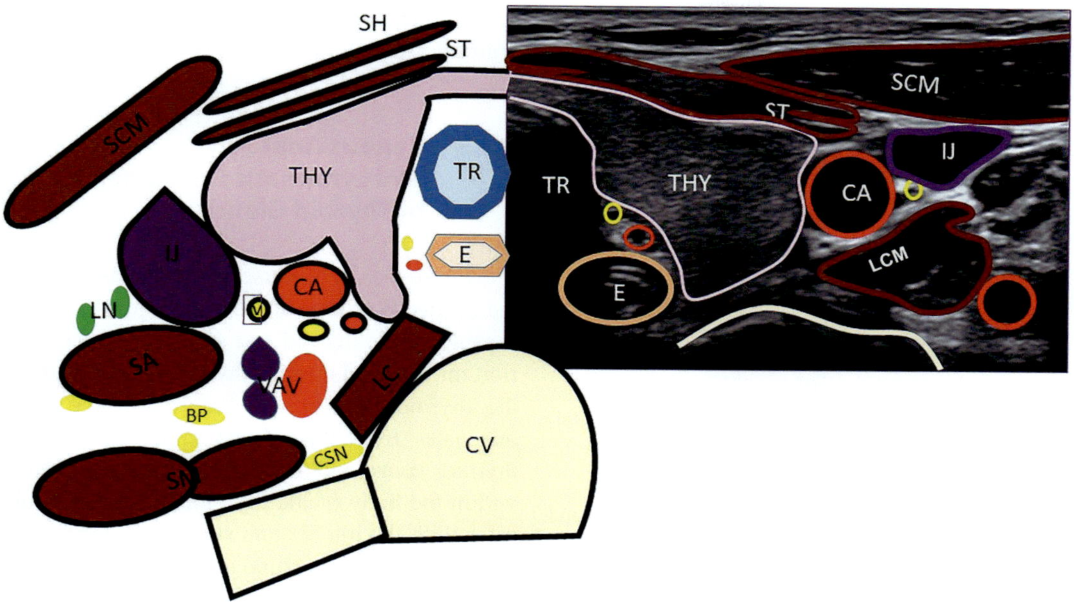

Fig. 2.2 Normal Thyroid Appearance and Anatomic Landmarks in Neck Ultrasound. Schematic diagram represents anatomic landmarks of thyroid and its surroundings, highlighted on trasverse US on the right. *SH* Sternohyoid muscle, *ST* Sternothyroid muscle, *SCM* Sternocleidomastoid muscle, *THY* Thyroid, *IJ* Internal Jugular Vein, *CA* Carotid Artery, *VAV* Vertebral artery and vein, *TR* trachea, *E* Esophagus, *SA and SM* Anterior and Middle scalene muscle, *LCM* Longus Colli Muscle, *V* Vagus nerve, *BP* brachial plexus, *CNS* cervical spine nerve, *CV* Cervical Vertebra, *LN* Lymph Nodes

is starkly contrasted with the muscle layers that lie beneath it. To either side of the midline, just below the subcutaneous fat, lie the strap muscles, specifically the sternohyoid more superficially and medial and the sternothyroid, deeper and more lateral. They are quite hypoechoic relative to the overlying fat and underlying thyroid, and each is enveloped by a fine white line [3, 9]. Normal thyroid tissue appears hyperechoic as compared to the overlying strap muscles, homogeneously echogenic with a uniform echotexture. The thyroid lobes are normally 4–6 cm in craniocaudal length and 1.3–1.8 cm in their anteroposterior and transverse dimensions; the isthmus normally has an anteroposterior thickness of up to 3 mm. Each lobe is located between the trachea medially and the carotid artery laterally. The tracheal cartilages can also be seen as very bright hyperechoic stripes surrounding the black lumen. Lateral to the thyroid, the common carotid artery and more laterally, the internal jugular vein can be found. Sometimes, the vagal nerve becomes visible next to the blood vessels. In the depth, the thyroid adjoins the scalene muscles and the vertebral column. The upper esophagus can commonly be seen under the left thyroid lobe, next to the vertebral column. Sometimes it could be covered by the acoustic shadow of the trachea. The esophagus is characterized by an onion-like pattern. Especially in the sagittal plane, swallowing of saliva can be observed. Sometimes, the esophagus also can be seen under the right thyroid lobe (Fig. 2.2). The cricoid and thyroid cartilages can be seen cranial to the thyroid [10].

2.2.2 Arterial Supply of Thyroid Gland

The superior thyroid artery is most commonly described as the first branch of the external carotid artery arising close to the carotid bifurca-

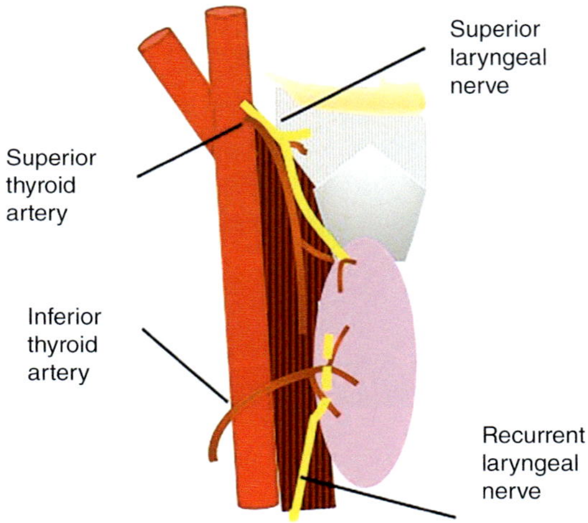

Fig. 2.3 Schematic diagrams of thyroid arteries and nerves

tion. It travels on the external surface of the inferior constrictor muscles of the larynx, along with the superior thyroid vein, entering the gland posteromedially just below the highest point of the upper lobe [11] (Fig. 2.3). At this point, it lies superficial to the external branch of the superior laryngeal nerve [12]. Although the common carotid artery usually has no branches, on occasion, the superior thyroid artery may arise from the common carotid artery proximal to the bifurcation [13, 14].

The inferior thyroid artery is a branch of the thyrocervical trunk that originates from the subclavian artery. It courses superiorly along the anterior scalene muscle and then it turns medially traveling behind the carotid sheath with variable relationship to the sympathetic chain. It then turns sharply and descends on the posterior surface of the lateral lobes where it forms two branches before entering the inferior pole (Fig. 2.3).

Thyroidea ima artery has a variable origin and may arise from the aortic arch, subclavian, brachiocephalic trunk, common carotid artery, or the internal thoracic arteries [15]. Although this is a small vessel, on occasion, it may replace the inferior thyroid artery and become a major arterial supply to the gland. It courses superiorly anterior to the trachea to supply the gland near the midline, and for this reason, it is in danger of injury during US interventions.

2.2.3 Venous Anatomy and Lymphatic Drainage of Thyroid Gland

The dense plexus of vessels as they pass through the connective tissue of the lobules join under the capsule of the thyroid and give rise to the superior, middle, and inferior thyroid veins. The middle thyroid vein in the majority of the cases originates from the middle third. The inferior thyroid veins and their tributaries arise from within the body of the thyroid, and it communicates with the middle and superior thyroid veins and forms a plexus behind the sternothyroid muscle in front of the trachea [16, 17]. It could be a source of massive hemorrhage during US procedures.

Lymphatic drainage occurs through the prelaryngeal, pretracheal, and paratracheal lymph nodes (level 6).

2.2.4 Nervous System of Thyroid

The vagus nerve originates from the medulla oblongata and exits the skull through the pars nervosa of the jugular foramen. The superior ganglion (jugular ganglion) of the vagus nerve is located within the jugular foramen. Just below this ganglion is the takeoff point of the superior laryngeal nerves (SLN). In about 1.5 cm inferiorly, the SLN divides into the internal and external branches [18]. The external branch of the superior laryngeal nerve (EBSLN) courses anteriorly and inferiorly with variable course along the inferior pharyngeal constrictor muscles and the branches of superior thyroid artery [19]. It curves anteriorly and medially close to the lower edge of the thyroid cartilage before innervating of the cricothyroid muscle (Fig. 2.3). The EBSLN approaches the larynx within the sternothyrolaryngeal (Joll's) triangle. The limits of this triangle are the inferior laryngeal constrictor and cricothyroid muscle medially, sternothyroid muscle anteriorly, and superior thyroid pole anteriorly [20]. Different types of relationship between the EBSLN and the upper pole of the thyroid and superior thyroid artery was noted. EBSLN can cross superior thyroid artery more than 1 cm above the upper pole of the thyroid, or within 1 cm of the upper pole and under the cover of the upper pole or immediately above the upper pole of the thyroid gland [21, 22]. The internal branch of the superior laryngeal nerve pierces the thyrohyoid membrane in association with the superior thyroid artery [23] (Fig. 2.3). After giving rise to SLN, the vagus descends in the carotid sheath in the neck initially at a location medial to the internal jugular and subsequently at a posterior position between the internal jugular vein and internal carotid artery inferiorly [20]. The RLN arises as the vagus courses anteriorly to the aortic arches. On the right side, the nerve recurs around the right subclavian artery, while on the left, the nerve recurs around the ligamentum arteriosum. They ascend superiorly and medially toward the tracheoesophageal groove giving rise to the tracheal and esophageal branches. The RLN enters the larynx deep to the inferior constrictor muscle and posterior to the cricothyroid joint (Figs. 2.3 and 2.4). When the right subclavian artery arises from a left aortic arch, the innominate artery is absent under which the right RLN loops to ascend in the neck. Therefore, the right RLN arises from the vagus in the cervical region [20]. Depending on its point of origin, the non-RLN courses inferiorly along the vagus usually passing behind the common carotid artery. It can arise at the level of the thyroid cartilage or the superior thyroid pole and pass directly to the larynx. It is also reported to arise at the level of the inferior thyroid artery, passing to the tracheoesophageal groove at the level of the inferior pole of the thyroid gland and then following the normal course of the RLN. On the left side, nonrecurrent laryngeal nerve is associated with situs inversus when there is a right aortic arch. Preoperative identification of an aberrant right subclavian artery or "arteria lusoria" by US and computed tomography could be beneficial [24–26].

Normal peripheral nerves can usually be demonstrated with high-resolution US; with 10–17 MHz frequency probes. On longitudinal scans, the nerve is seen as a striated pattern with several parallel echogenic lines of its internal structures [1, 27–29]. The cervical course of the vagus nerve can be easily visualized on US as a 2-mm to 3-mm diameter structure located within the carotid sheath (Fig. 2.4), posterolateral to the common carotid artery and posteromedial to the internal jugular vein [1]. The anterior variation in which the nerve passes in front of the common carotid artery is relatively common with a reported prevalence of up to 18.9%; whereas medial or posterior variation has a lower prevalence. The RLN and SLN are not directly visualized on US due to their small diameter. Therefore, knowledge of their expected course and variation is essential to prevent complications [1].

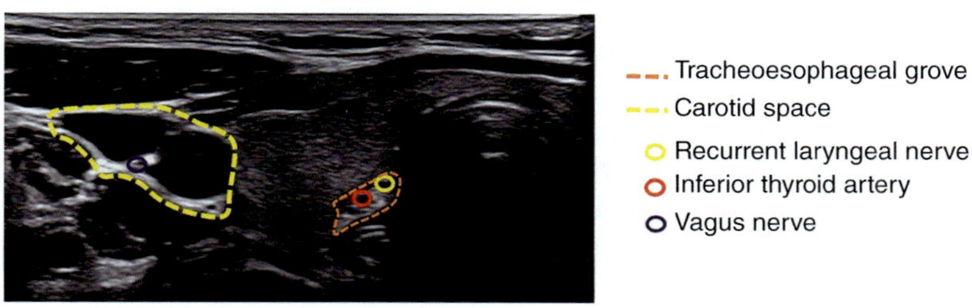

Fig. 2.4 Tracheoesophageal groove and carotid space. In this transverse US image at the level of the thyroid, orange dotted line indicates the tracheoesophageal groove, that represents a potential location of the RLN (yellow circle) and inferior thyroid artery (red circle). Yellow dotted line indicates the carotid space with CA, IJ and V (purple circle)

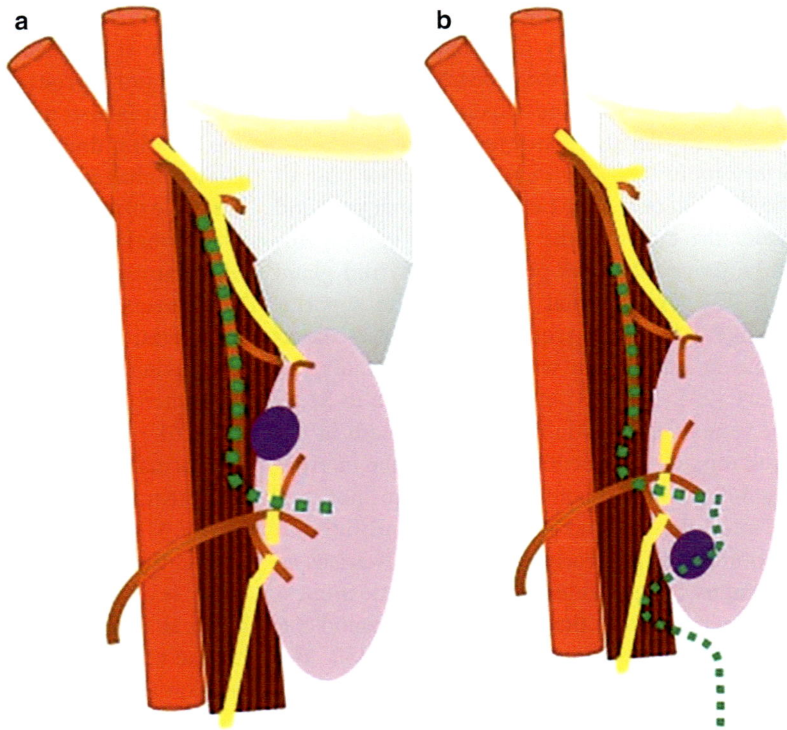

Fig. 2.5 Schematic diagrams of area of distribution (green dotted lines) of ectopic superior (**a**) and inferior (**b**) parathyroid glands (purple circles)

2.2.5 Parathyroid Glands

There are usually four parathyroid glands, two upper and two lower, located in the visceral space posterior to the thyroid, adjacent to the tracheo-esophageal groove. **Superior parathyroid glands** are located near the posterolateral aspect of the superior pole of the thyroid, 1 cm superior to the junction of the RLN, and the inferior thyroid artery, deep to the plane of the recurrent laryngeal nerve. **Inferior parathyroid glands** are located near the inferior poles of the thyroid glands, within 1–2 cm of the insertion of the inferior thyroid artery into the inferior pole of the thyroid, superficial to the plane of the RLN. Parathyroid glands could be supernumerary and ectopic. Fewer than 2% of the ectopic glands are superior parathyroids; they are located behind the pharynx or esophagus. Approximately 50% are inferior parathyroids, and 15% of these are located within 1 cm from the lower pole of the thyroid. In 35% of the cases, the ectopic gland is located anywhere from the angle of the jaw to the anterior mediastinum. The most common sites are right below the lower pole of the thyroid or thymus. Figure 2.5 shows the area of distribution of ectopic parathyroid glands. The parathyroid glands cannot be assessed by US in normal condition [5, 6, 30].

2.3 Carotid Space

The carotid space consists of two cylindrical areas that extend from the base of the skull to the aortic arch. It is delimited by the deep cervical fascia (superficial, medial, and deep layer). It contains the internal carotid artery, internal jugular vein, sympathetic plexus, cranial nerves (IX–XII), supra- and infrahyoid cervical lymph nodes, the common carotid artery, and the vagus [31]. It is surrounded by the anterior cervical space, anteriorly, by the visceral and retropharyngeal spaces medially, and by the perivertebral and posterior cervical spaces, posteriorly (Figs. 2.1, 2.2, and 2.4). The common carotids run behind the sternocleidomastoid muscles and medial to the internal jugular veins. The vagus nerves run behind the two vessels. The internal jugular veins descend within the neck laterally to the common carotid, and finally merge with the subclavian veins, forming the brachiocephalic venous trunks.

2.4 Retropharyngeal and Danger Spaces

The retropharyngeal space is a midline space extending from the skull base to the upper mediastinum. It is located posterior to the pharynx and cervical esophagus. The alar fascia separates it from the danger space which is located anterior to the perivertebral space. The suprahyoid part of retropharyngeal space contains fat and lymph nodes, these are absent in the infrahyoid portion of this space [32]. The danger space extends further inferiorly into the posterior mediastinum, and it cannot be distinguished from retropharyngeal space on imaging in a healthy patient.

2.5 Perivertebral Space

The perivertebral space extends from the skull base to the clavicles and includes prevertebral and paraspinal portions. The prevertebral space is located posterior to the pharynx and cervical esophagus, and medial to the carotid space and to the anterior portion of the posterior cervical space. It contains the prevertebral muscles, the scalene muscles (anterior, middle, and posterior), the roots of the brachial plexus, the phrenic nerve, the vertebral arteries and veins, and the bodies and pedicles of the vertebrae. The paraspinal space lies posterior to the transverse processes and lateral to the posterior arches and the spinous processes of the cervical vertebrae. It is located medial to the posterior cervical space, and it contains the paraspinal muscles and posterior components of the cervical spine [5, 6].

2.6 Posterior Cervical Space

The posterior cervical space is an adipose-tissue space located deep and posterior to the sternocleidomastoid muscle, and posterior to the carotid space. It surrounds the perivertebral space and contains the accessory nerve, accessory chain lymph nodes, the pre-axillary component of the brachial plexus, and the dorsal scapular nerve [5, 33].

The sternocleidomastoid muscle, scalene muscle, elevator scapulae muscle, and trapezius muscle comprise the lateral part of the neck muscles. The scalene muscles (anterior, middle, posterior) originate from the transverse processes of the cervical vertebrae (from C2 to C7) and insert into the first and second ribs. Because the cervical/brachial plexus passes between the anterior and middle scalene muscles, the scalene muscle could be an anatomical landmark for the cervical/brachial plexus. It is easily identified as a thin, cord-like, hypoechoic structure between the anterior and middle scalene muscles on US [4, 34, 35].

The phrenic nerve also passes anteriorly to the anterior scalene muscle [36]. It descends immediately behind the sternocleidomastoid muscle, lateral to the internal jugular vein, and medial to the brachial plexus roots [36].

The spinal accessory nerve passes between the posterolateral border of the sternocleidomastoid muscle and anterior border of the trapezius muscle, on the superficial aspect in the middle part of the elevator scapulae muscle, and these muscles are used as anatomical landmarks for the nerve [37, 38].

2.7 Conclusion

Knowledge of US-based anatomy may be particularly important, allowing a better identification of the target tumor or nodule and a clearer visualization of surrounding anatomical structures. In fact, due to the small volume and complex adjacent structure, it still has a certain incidence of complications for the US-guided thyroid procedures. The adjacent structures, such as RLN, anterior cervical muscles, trachea, esophagus, common carotid artery, internal jugular vein, parathyroid glands, cervical sympathetic trunk, and vagus nerve, might be damaged. Major complications were permanent voice change, caused by the involvement of the RLN or vagus nerve.

Preoperative US can estimate the risk of complication to guide the ablation process based on the location and distance from adjacent structures of the nodule. The fusion of different imaging modalities such as computed tomography and magnetic resonance imaging and the possibility of virtually navigating into a pre-acquired volume could help the operator during the ablation procedure, particularly when gas develops from the ablation, limiting the real-time US visualization [39].

References

1. Ha EJ, Baek JH, Lee JH. Ultrasonography-based thyroidal and perithyroidal anatomy and its clinical significance. Korean J Radiol. 2015;16:749–66. https://doi.org/10.3348/kjr.2015.16.4.749.
2. Papini E, Guglielmi R, Persichetti A, Pacella CM. Benign thyroid nodule laser ablation. In: Pacella CM, Jiang T, Mauri G, editors. Image-guided laser ablation. Springer. 2020. https://doi.org/10.1007/978-3-030-21748-8_7.
3. Mazzaglia PJ, Muraveika L. Normal thyroid appearance and anatomic landmarks in neck ultrasound. In: Milas M, Mandel SJ, Langer JE, editors. Advanced thyroid and parathyroid ultrasound. Springer. 2017. https://doi.org/10.1007/978-3-319-44100-9_9.
4. Gervasio A, Mujahed I, Biasio A, Alessi S. Ultrasound anatomy of the neck: the infrahyoid region. J Ultrasound. 2010;13(3):85–9. https://doi.org/10.1016/j.jus.2010.09.006.
5. Harnsberger HR, Osborn AG, Macdonald A, Ross J, Moore KR, Salzman KL, et al. Diagnostic and surgical imaging anatomy: brain, head & neck, spine. Amirsys. 2006. 126–257 p.
6. Mukherji SK, Chong V. Atlas of head and neck imaging: the extracranial head and neck. Thieme. 2004. 148–190 p.
7. Mohebati A, Shaha AR. Anatomy of thyroid and parathyroid glands and neurovascular relations. Clin Anat. 2012;25(1):19–31. https://doi.org/10.1002/ca.21220.
8. Braun EM, Windisch G, Wolf G, Hausleitner L, Anderhuber F. The pyramidal lobe: clinical anatomy and its importance in thyroid surgery. Surg Radiol Anat. 2007;29(1):21–7. https://doi.org/10.1007/s00276-006-0165-1.
9. Middleton WD, Kurtz AB, Hertzberg BS. Neck and chest. In: Ultrasound: the requisites. 2nd ed. St. Louis: Mosby; 2004. p. 244–77.
10. Bozzato A, Zenk J, Gottwald F, Koch M, Iro H. Der Einfluss der Schildknorpelossifikation bei der Larynxsonografie. Laryngo-Rhino-Otologie. 2007;86(4):276–81. https://doi.org/10.1055/s-2006-945029.
11. Mansberger AR, Wei JP. Surgical embryology and anatomy of the thyroid and parathyroid glands. Surg Clin North Am. 1993;73(4):727–46. https://doi.org/10.1016/s0039-6109(16)46082-2.
12. Fancy T, Gallagher D 3rd, Hornig JD. Surgical anatomy of the thyroid and parathyroid glands. Otolaryngol Clin North Am. 2010;43:221–7. https://doi.org/10.1016/j.otc.2010.01.001.
13. Smith SD, Benton RS. A rare origin of the superior thyroid artery. Acta Anat. 1978;101(1):91–3. https://doi.org/10.1159/000144952.
14. Umut Akyol M, Ozcan M, Ozdem C. Superior thyroid artery arising common carotid artery from the. Otolaryngol Head Neck Surg. 1997;116:701. https://doi.org/10.1016/S0194-59989770256-0.
15. Hoyes AD, Kershaw DR. Anatomy and development of the thyroid gland. Ear Nose Throat J. 1985;64(7):318–33.
16. Belli AM, Ingram CE, Heron CW, Husband JE. The appearance of the inferior thyroid veins on computed tomography. Br J Radiol. 1988;61(722):125–7. https://doi.org/10.1259/0007-1285-61-722-125.
17. Krausen AS. The inferior thyroid veins—the ultimate guardians of the trachea. Laryngoscope. 1976;86(12):1849–55. https://doi.org/10.1002/lary.5540861210.
18. Kambic V, Zargi M, Radsel Z. Topographic anatomy of the external branch of the superior laryngeal nerve. Its importance in head and neck surgery. J Laryngol Otol. 1984;98(11):1121–4. https://doi.org/10.1017/s0022215100148121.
19. Teitelbaum BJ, Wenig BL. Superior laryngeal nerve injury from thyroid surgery. Head Neck. 1995;17(1):36–40. https://doi.org/10.1002/hed.2880170108.
20. Randolph GW. Surgery of the thyroid and parathyroid glands. Philadelphia: Elsevier Science; 2003.
21. Kierner AC, Aigner M, Burian M. The external branch of the superior laryngeal nerve its topographical anatomy as related to surgery of the neck. Arch Otolaryngol Head Neck Surg. 1998;124:301–3. http://archotol.jamanetwork.com. https://doi.org/10.1001/archotol.124.3.301.
22. Cernea CR, Ferraz R, Nishio S, Dutra AJ, Hojaij FC, Medina dos Santos LR. Surgical anatomy of the external branch of the superior laryngeal nerve. Head Neck. 1992;14:380–3. https://doi.org/10.1002/hed.2880140507.
23. Sulica L. The superior laryngeal nerve: function and dysfunction. Otolaryngol Clin North Am. 2004;37(1):183–201. https://doi.org/10.1016/S0030-6665(03)00175-0.
24. Stewart GR, Mountain JC, Colcock BP. Non-recurrent laryngeal nerve. Br J Surg. 1972;59(5):379–81. https://doi.org/10.1002/bjs.1800590513.
25. Henry JF, Audiffret J, Denizot A, Plan M. The nonrecurrent inferior laryngeal nerve: review of 33 cases, including two on the left side. Surgery. 1988;104(6):977–84.

26. Hermans R, Dewandel P, Debruyne F, Delaere PR. Arteria lusoria identified on preoperative CT and nonrecurrent inferior laryngeal nerve during thyroidectomy: a retrospective study. Head Neck. 2003;25(2):113–7. https://doi.org/10.1002/hed.10180.
27. Chiou HJ, Chou YH, Chiou SY, Liu JB, Chang CY. Peripheral nerve lesions: role of high-resolution US. Radiographics. 2003;23(6):e15. https://doi.org/10.1148/rg.e15.
28. Giovagnorio F, Martinoli C. Sonography of the cervical vagus nerve: normal appearance and abnormal findings. AJR Am J Roentgenol. 2001;176(3):745–9. www.ajronline.org. https://doi.org/10.2214/ajr.176.3.1760745.
29. Knappertz VA, Tegeler CH, Hardin SJ, McKinney WM. Vagus nerve imaging with ultrasound: anatomic and in vivo validation. Otolaryngol Head Neck Surg. 1998;118(1):82–5. https://doi.org/10.1016/S0194-5998(98)70379-1.
30. Ahuia AT, Antonio GE, Griffith JF, Ho SY, Wong KT. Diagnostic and surgical imaging anatomy: ultrasound. International ed. Lippincott Williams & Wilkins. Amirsys; 2007. 178–210 p.
31. Chengazi HU, Bhatt AA. Pathology of the carotid space. Insights Imaging. 2019;10(1):21. https://doi.org/10.1186/s13244-019-0704-z.
32. Phan T, Lay J, Scali F. The alar fascia and danger space: a modern review. Cureus. 2022;14:e32871. https://doi.org/10.7759/cureus.32871.
33. Parker GD, Harnsberger HR. Radiologic evaluation of the normal and diseased posterior cervical space. AJR Am J Roentgenol. 1991;157(1):161–5. www.ajronline.org. https://doi.org/10.2214/ajr.157.1.2048512.
34. Ihnatsenka B, Boezaart AP. Applied sonoanatomy of the posterior triangle of the neck. Int J Shoulder Surg. 2010;4:63–74. https://doi.org/10.4103/0973-6042.76963.
35. Roessel T, Wiessner D, Heller AR, Zimmermann T, Koch T, Litz RJ. High-resolution ultrasound-guided high interscalene plexus block for carotid endarterectomy. Reg Anesth Pain Med. 2007;32(3):247–53. https://doi.org/10.1016/j.rapm.2006.12.007.
36. Canella C, Demondion X, Delebarre A, Moraux A, Cotten H, Cotten A. Anatomical study of phrenic nerve using ultrasound. Eur Radiol. 2010;20(3):659–65. https://doi.org/10.1007/s00330-009-1579-z.
37. Canella C, Demondion X, Abreu E, Marchiori E, Cotten H, Cotten A. Anatomical study of spinal accessory nerve using ultrasonography. Eur J Radiol. 2013;82(1):56–61. https://doi.org/10.1016/j.ejrad.2011.04.038.
38. Hong MJ, Baek JH, Kim DY, Ha EJ, Choi WJ, Choi YJ, et al. Spinal accessory nerve: ultrasound findings and correlations with neck lymph node levels. Ultraschall Med. 2016;37(5):487–91. https://doi.org/10.1055/s-0034-1385673.
39. Xiaoyin T, Ping L, Dan C, Min D, Jiachang C, Tao W, et al. Risk assessment and hydrodissection technique for radiofrequency ablation of thyroid benign nodules. J Cancer. 2018;9(17):3058–66. https://doi.org/10.7150/jca.26060.

3 Thyroid Imaging Reporting and Data Systems for Cancer Risk Determination and Artificial Intelligence (TI-RADS for Cancer Risk Determination and Artificial Intelligence)

Turtulici Giovanni and Creteanu Mihai

The rate of diagnosed thyroid nodules has increased by two to four times over the past three decades due to advances in imaging techniques [1, 2]. Ultrasonography (US) is basically a quick and available method for evaluating thyroid nodules through which the information can be obtained about the anatomical and structural properties of a nodule [3]. However, due to the operator-based result of the US leading to a different analysis of the same thyroid nodule image between several sonographers, there is a need for taking measures for the lack of precise standards in the definition and differentiation of benign nodules from malignant ones [4].

Many efforts have been made by various research groups in recent years to find a system for differentiating benign thyroid nodules from malignant ones more accurately [5].

Palpable thyroid nodules are stated in 4–7% of individuals [6]. About 5% of palpable nodules are malignant [7]. Accurate prediction of malignant and non-malignant thyroid nodules is of great importance. Pathologic findings are currently the standard for the differentiation of non-malignant from malignant lesions. As thyroid fine needle aspiration (FNA) is an invasive procedure, the determination of prognosis based on radiologic findings is currently taken into consideration [8].

Ultrasound is one of the most important imaging modalities in thyroid diagnostics. High resolution and high availability make ultrasound an efficient tool in the evaluation of thyroid diseases. In the hands of experienced users, it is the modality of choice to detect and evaluate thyroid nodules in a very short time. However, studies show that large inter- and intra-observer variabilities exist, making the assessment of thyroids highly subjective. With an incidence of up to 68% in adults, thyroid nodules are routinely found during the regular ultrasound (US) neck evaluation [9].

Since most thyroid nodules are benign, no treatment is necessary. However, benign nodules are sometimes removed for aesthetic purposes or to ease symptoms like swallowing discomfort.

Thyroid ultrasonography provides information about the characteristics of a nodule and its size, as well as to identify the presence or absence of aberrant cervical lymph nodes.

The main anatomical features of nodules including shapes, margin, structures, echogenicity, heterogeneity, echogenic dot, an extension to the capsule, vertical axis position, and nodule vascularity were evaluated for each thyroid nodule. Doppler study was mainly used to diagnose the relatively common thyroiditis and resulting white knight nodules.

The TI-RADS (Thyroid Imaging Reporting and Data System) is a proposed new classification

T. Giovanni
Ospedale Evangelico, Genoa, Italy

C. Mihai (✉)
Arcadia Hospital, Iasi, Romania

R. Valcavi et al. (eds.), *Thyroid Ablation*, https://doi.org/10.1007/978-3-031-88229-6_3

system for evaluating the malignancy risk of thyroid nodules classifying thyroid nodules into several classes according to their ultrasound shape and appearance [10]. Further research is needed to achieve the best criteria for differentiating nodules and to recognize the features that affect the increase in the incidence of malignancy, and alone or in combination with other factors, help to standardization and unifying of TI-RADS classification [11, 12].

3.1 TI-RADS Classification by Conventional Method

The thyroid nodule status of each patient was classified into different TI-RADS groups (Table 3.1). Following classification of patients according to the TI-RADS, patients in groups 3–5 with nodule sizes of greater than 1 cm were subjected to Fine Needle Aspiration Cytology (FNAC); and the rest of them were subjected to the follow-up stage [10, 13].

Table 3.2 shows the possibility of malignancy and malignancy coefficients according to the ultrasonography features of thyroid nodules.

The ultrasonography and the classification of thyroid nodules in TI-RADS system was performed by an experienced radiologist. The results of TI-RADS classifications based on conventional methods are presented in Table 3.3.

1. 1.All features with non-zero malignancy coefficients are identified in the patient.
2. All malignancy coefficients are summed together and the result is stored in S.
3. Given the S value, the TI-RADS classification is performed according to Table 3.4.

By comparing the probability of malignancy (S/Stotal) and the probability of malignancy in each of the TI-RADS classification, S-values are obtained. To simplify the use of the proposed new method, S-values for each group of TI-RADS are calculated and presented in Table 3.4.

The incidence of malignancy in each TI-RADS classification was reported based on the conventional method, and a new proposed formula was reported as a frequency table.

Four features were associated with the highest incidence of malignancy among the anatomical features of the studied thyroid nodule in TI-RADS, as the incidence of malignancy was about 85% in patients with infiltrative margin and extension to the capsule; and 74% in nodules with a vertical axis, and about 64% in marked hypo-echo.

Recent studies have also found that hypoechogenicity is associated with malignancy in more than 50–90% of cases, and hypoechogenicity increases the chance of malignancy diagnosis from 2.9 to 6 times [14, 15].

Table 3.1 TI-RADS criteria classification based on ultrasonography features of thyroid nodules

Level		Definition
TI-RADS 1	Normal thyroid	Normal thyroid
TI-RADS 2	Benign lesions	Benign lesions[a]
TI-RADS 3	Probably benign	Iso/hyperechoic nodule without suspicious feature[b]
TI-RADS 4a	Slightly suspicious	One suspicious feature
TI-RADS 4b	Suspicious	Two-three suspicious features
TI-RADS 4c	Highly suspicious	Four suspicious features
TI-RADS 5	Highly suggestive of malignancy	Five or more suspicious features
TI-RADS 6	Proven malignancy	FNA proven malignancy

[a] Simple and multinodular goiters, adenomatoid goiters (isoechoic spongiform masses), thyroiditis, white knight nodules in thyroiditis background. Cysts (simple, colloid, spongious, with or without small isoechoic mass)

[b] Suspicious features: features with malignancy coefficients equivalents 1 until 7 according to Table 3.2. (irregular shape, unclear or thick or infiltrative margin, almost solid, hypoechogenicity, micro or macrocalcification, vertical axis, extension to nodule capsule and tumoral adenopathy)

Table 3.2 Malignancy coefficients according to ultrasonography features of thyroid nodules

Thyroid nodule	Thyroid nodule features (i)	Number of patients	Patients with malignant nodules	Incidence of malignancy (Pi)	Malignancy coefficient (Wi)
Nodule shape	Regular	881	22	P1 = 2.5%	**W1 = 0**
	Irregular	**152**	71	**P2 = 46.7%**	**W2 = 3**
	Clear	699	20	P3 = 2.8%	**W3 = 0**
	Unclear	**150**	**71**	**P4 = 47.3%**	**W4 = 3**
Nodule margin	Thin halo	158	1	P5 = 0.6%	**W5 = 0**
	Thick halo	**7**	**1**	**P6 = 14.28%**	**W6 = 1**
	Infiltrative	**20**	**17**	**P7 = 85%**	**W7 = 7**
	Marginal calcification	19	0	P8 = 0%	**W8 = 0**
	Simple cyst	25	0	P9 = 0%	**W9 = 0**
	Spongy cyst	42	0	P10 = 0%	**W10 = 0**
	Colloid cyst	26	0	P11 = 0%	**W11 = 0**
Nodule structure	Cyst with small partial solidity	41	0	P12 = 0%	**W12 = 0**
	Solid with large cystic areas	143	1	P13 = 0.7%	**W13 = 0**
	Spongiform mass	224	2	P14 = 0.9%	**W14 = 0**

Table 3.3 Results of TI-RADS classifications based on conventional methods and the proposed new formula

TI-RADS classification	Number of patients		Frequency percentage		Patients with malignant nodules		Possibility of malignancy	
	C-M[a]	P-N-F[b]	C-M	P-N-F	C-M	P-N-F	C-M	P-N-F
2	224	224	21.7%	21.7%	0	0	0%	0%
3	509	577	49.3%	55.9%	2	4	0.4%	0.7%
4a	180	120	17.4%	11.6%	15	20	8.3%	16.7%
4b	52	53	5%	5%	19	23	36.5%	43.4%
4c	31	38	3%	3.7%	23	26	74.2%	68.5%
5	37	21	3.6%	2%	34	20	91.9%	95.2%

[a] Conventional Methods
[b] Proposed New Formula

Table 3.4 Relation between total malignancy coefficients (S) and TI-RADS classifications based on the proposed new formula

TI-RADS classification	Total malignancy coefficients (S)
2	0
3	1.2
4a	3–9
4b	10–16
4c	17–23
5	24–45

3.2 Fine Needle Aspiration Cytology (FNAC)

A 25 gauge needle was used for nodal aspiration. Aspirations were directly stained on 4–6 smear glass slides by May-Grunwald-Giemsa. The Bethesda system was used for the cytopathological report. All samples were examined by two skilled cytopathologists. The cytopathology results were reported based on the classification system as either benign nodules including adenomatous goiter, thyroiditis, follicular benign nodules, or malignant nodules including papillary thyroid carcinoma (PTC), suspicious for PTC, follicular thyroid carcinoma (FTC), medullary carcinoma, lymphoma, and anaplastic tumor.

In the present study, the TI-RADS classification a new proposed formula:

$$S = \sum_{i=1}^{37} X\ ixWi$$

Proposed formula for the TI-RADS classification

Was proposed for TI-RADS classification, where: S: Total malignancy coefficients per patient; i: Appearance features of thyroid nodules; X_i: Coefficient of presence or absence of thyroid in patients; (X_i = 1: a patient has appearance features of thyroid nodules; X_i = 0: the patient does not have appearance feature of thyroid nodules); Wi: Coefficient of malignancy associated with each appearance features of thyroid nodules.

The incidence of malignancy of each thyroid nodule (Pi) was first calculated based on the percentage of patients with malignant nodules in the total patients with that thyroid feature. Then, Wi value was calculated based on the Pi value. If Pi < 7%, then Wi = 0; If 7% ≤ Pi < 20%, then Wi = 1; If 20% ≤ Pi < 50%, then Wi = 3; and if 50% ≤ Pi < 90%, then Wi = 7. The Pi value > 90% was not observed in the study. Table 3.2 presents all features of thyroid nodule (i), the incidence of malignancy of each thyroid nodule (Pi) and its incidence of malignancy coefficients (Wi).

Horvat et al. have described TI-RADS classification based on an ultrasound study. They predicted the rate of malignancy in each group as follows: 0% for TI-RADS 1 and 2, less than 5% for TI-RADS 3, 5%–10% for TI-RADS 4A, 11%–65% for TI-RADS 4B, 66%–95% for TI-RADS 4C, more than 95% for TI-RADS 5, and proved malignancy in TI-RADS 6 [16].

Singaporewalla et al. compared [16] the results of TI-RADS and FNA cytology described by the Bethesda System and they reported a concordance rate of 83% cases. Sensitivity, specificity, and negative predictive values were 70.6%, 90.4%, and 93.8%. Vargas-Uricoechea et al. found that TI-RADS had an acceptable concordance with the Bethesda System [17]. As a result of the efficacy of the breast imaging reporting and data system is BIRADS for classification for breast lesions.

In BIRADS classification, a puncture will be done for nodules with BIRADS 4 and 5 and the lesions in the rest of the categories will follow up. The researchers found the risk of malignancy among TI-RADS 2, 3, 4, and 5 at 0%, 1.79%, 76.13%, and 98.85%, respectively. Using TI-RADS 4–5 to perform FNA they stated a 99.6% sensibility and 74.35% specificity [18].

The current investigation was to compare the results of TI-RADS and cytology reports in patients with thyroid nodules.

3.3 The 2D and 3D Method for Analyzing and Classifying Thyroid Nodules

Diagnostic results depend on how the operators position the probe and their ability to interpret 2D images and reconstruct 3D maps in their mind. Interpretations vary: studies for thyroid show intra- and interobserver variability for nodule volume measurements up to ±30.2% and ±44.1%, respectively. This is mainly due to the fact ultrasound is a 2D-based real-time imaging technology with relatively poor possibilities for documentation and reproducibility. Diagnosis must be made on two-dimensional cross-sectional images of a three-dimensional body while the patient is present. Subsequent evaluation and image sharing for obtaining a second opinion are very limited due to the incompleteness of image data.

However, recently, a new solution for 3D-freehand ultrasound imaging has been introduced to the market. The wireless system extends standard 2D ultrasound systems with tomographic 3D imaging capabilities. To acquire tomographic 3D images (tUS), a 2D probe is moved transversely over a thyroid while a sequence of 2D images is being recorded. A sensor attached to the probe tracks rotational information of the probe movement which is then

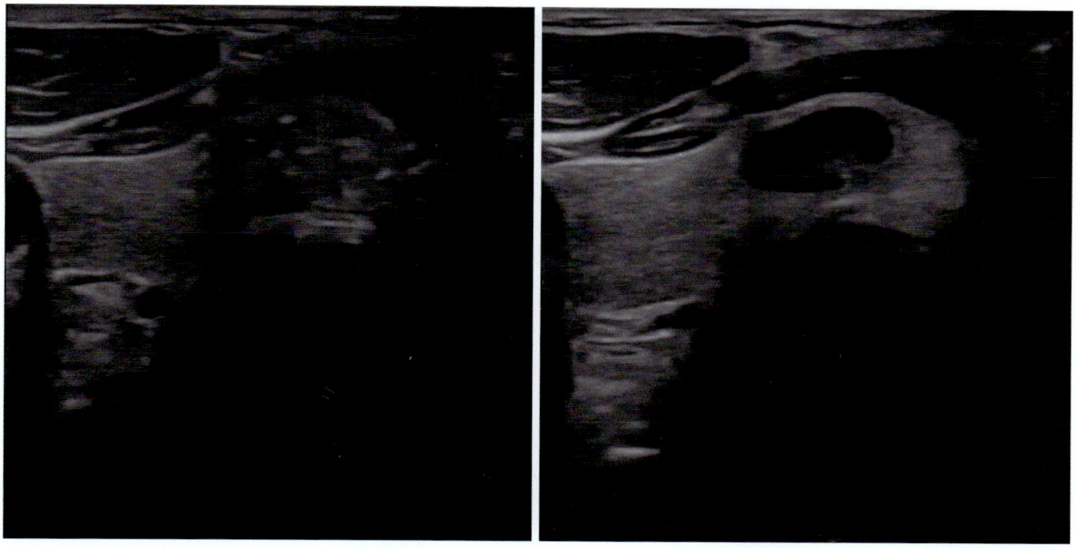

Fig. 3.1 Two different ultrasound images of the same nodule

combined with the image sequence in order to generate a volume. The trajectory of the ultrasound scan is calculated by analyzing successive images and the rotation data of the ultrasound probe (Fig. 3.1).

The image sequences are transmitted wirelessly to a computer via a video box connected to the video output of the ultrasound system. Sensor data is being transmitted via Bluetooth to the same computer. A Deep Learning-based algorithm combines the image and rotation data and calculates the associated movement of the ultrasound probe.

That way, volume images of the entire thyroid gland can be taken and reconstructed in three dimensions in just a few seconds.

Only prerequisites for a tUS image with good image quality are an ultrasound system with a digital video output. However, the system offers significant added value not only due to the fast and simple 3D acquisition, but rather due to the evaluation software specially developed for the thyroid gland. The generated ultrasound volumes can be viewed and evaluated both as 3D volume renderings and as multiplanar reconstructions (Fig. 3.2). The latest version of the software offers the possibility to evaluate and document thyroid glands and nodules quickly and efficiently with the support of artificial intelligence.

To do this, the AI fully automatically detects the thyroid gland in the ultrasound volume, performs a voxel-based measurement of the volume, and eliminates tissue that does not belong in the 3D representation. Subsequently, the user has the option to segment any thyroid nodules that may be present with AI assistance. Based on the segmentation, the volume and a classification of the nodule according to ACR TI-RADS are then calculated automatically. The user has the option to further adjust or directly accept the calculated results. These can then be summarized automatically in a report and transmitted to a PACS system. Clinical studies to confirm the clinical benefit of this 3D method for analyzing and classifying thyroid nodules are still in progress. However, Kroenke et al. recently published promising results of improved thyroid volumetry using artificial intelligence on 3D ultrasound [19].

Additional obvious benefits of tomographic 3D ultrasound that do not require clinical validation studies exist as well. Due to the imaging of the entire thyroid, documentation and follow-up comparisons of nodules can be improved. It allows temporal and spatial separation of image acquisition and image analysis, enabling clinical

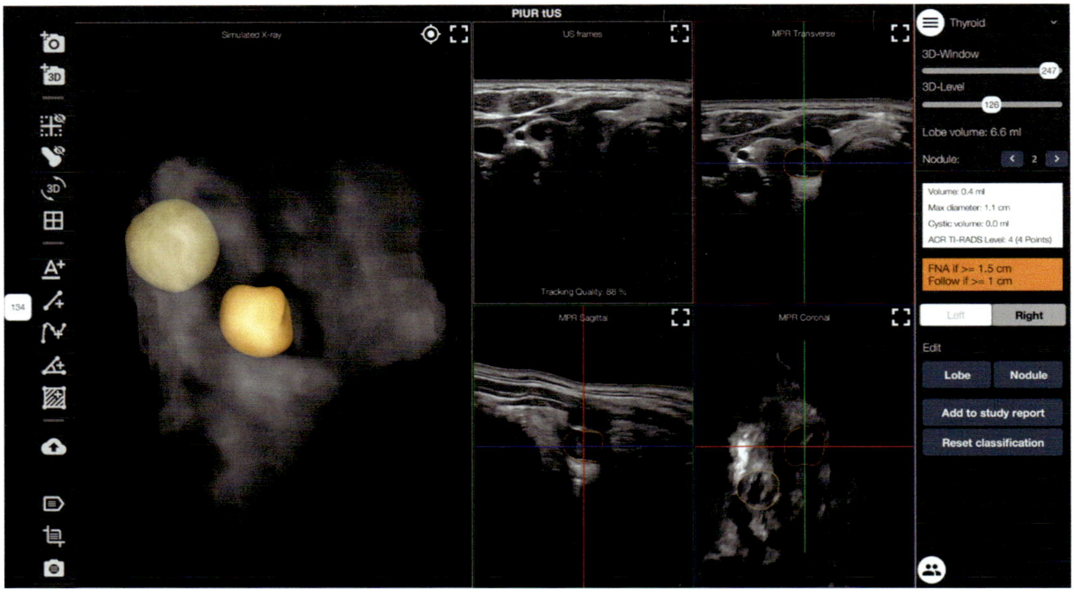

Fig. 3.2 Tomographic 3D ultrasound image of a thyroid, visualized as a volume rendering (left) and multiplanar reconstruction (right)

workflows that are mainly available in radiology these days.

Second opinions can be obtained more easily and data can be shared among referring physician and thyroid specialist in a more complete and comprehensible way. Overall, diagnoses will become more objective and also comprehensible to third parties. Once the entire procedure is fully automated and if the accuracy and robustness of the AI-algorithms can be validated by clinical studies, tomographic 3D ultrasound will lead to enormous time savings and quality improvements in clinical routine.

Thyroid diagnostics will become even more efficient—with potentially even better patient care. Previously subjective assessments will be presented objectively and transparently. It will be a major milestone in thyroid diagnostics, considering the increasing number of patients and a shrinking healthcare budget.

In recent years, several solutions have been introduced to reduce operator-dependency due to image interpretation by using artificial intelligence (AI). AI-based algorithms are applied on 2D ultrasound images of a nodule to support the physician with interpretation and classification. Applied on the same image, AI-based interpretation will always result in the same TI-RADS score, and therefore, reduce both inter- and intra-observer variability for those images. However, those algorithms still depend on the input image provided by the user.

Nodules are three-dimensional objects, and a two-dimensional image might not adequately represent the nodule's full characteristics. It is up to the user to decide on the 2D ultrasound slice that best represents the thyroid nodule in terms of size and characteristics. Figure 3.1 illustrates this challenge.

It shows two different slices of the same thyroid nodule. While the first slice suggests a mainly solid nodule with partial calcifications, and therefore, a potentially higher TI RADS score of Turtulici G, the second image clearly shows a mainly cystic nodule with a low TI-RADS score. Current AI-based TI-RADS solutions will classify this nodule differently, depending on which input image will be provided. Therefore, a strong operator-dependency remains due to image acquisition.

While the solution can be very helpful in improving efficiency and quality of image readings, they do not fully solve the issue of accurate classification of thyroid nodules. Particularly not for novice or less experienced users.

Several TI-RADS classification schemes have been introduced to improve documentation of thyroid nodules and make their evaluation more objective. However, a strong user-dependency remains also with the use of TI-RADS criteria [20]. This strong user-dependency results from two sources: (1) image acquisition and (2) image interpretation.

Some US parameters are associated with malignancy such as hypoechogenicity, irregular margins, a taller-than-wide shape, microcalcifications or increased intranodular vascularity, but none of them alone is sufficient to detect thyroid cancer accurately [21].

The first classification for thyroid nodules was in 2009, Horvath et al., Thyroid Imaging Reporting and Data System (TI-RADS), based on the Breast Imaging Reporting and Data System (BIRADS), accepted and then proposed by the American College of Radiology, followed by other scores based on various US patterns of thyroid nodules. The aim was to introduce a lexicon of sonographic features of focal thyroid lesions, to categorize finding and determine which thyroid nodule require fine needle aspiration biopsy (FNAB) or US follow-up [18].

At present, several standardized malignancy risk stratification systems are used, such as ACR TI-RADS (American College of Radiology), EU-TIRADS (European Thyroid Association), K-TIRADS (Korean Society of Thyroid Radiology), and ATA (American Thyroid Association).

3.4 ACR-TIRADS

ACR TI-RADS is a reporting system for evaluating the ultrasound characteristics of thyroid nodules proposed by the American College of Radiology (ACR).

It has been widely applied in clinical practice and has a higher specificity and reduces the number of unnecessary biopsies of benign nodules compared to other risk stratification system [22]. Compared with Color-Doppler and superb microvascular imaging (SMI), contrast-enhanced ultrasound (CEUS) is more sensitive to display the blood perfusion pattern in the region of interest [23].

In the ACR-TI-RADS, each US feature is given a specific number of points for a nodule. The nodule is then categorized as benign, not suspicious, mildly suspicious, moderately suspicious, or highly suspicious for malignancy.

The TIRADS category and cancer risk increase with higher cumulative scores. Depending on the size, the nodule's management will be established (namely FNA).

The five ultrasound features of thyroid nodules used in TI-RADS are: composition, echogenicity, shape, margin, and punctate echogenic foci. Each item is given points [24].

Composition
- **Cystic/almost completely cystic/spongiform** (**0** p)—features highly suggestive for benignity; these TN are automatically classified as TIRADS 1, with no need to further evaluate other features
- **Mixed solid-cystic** (**1**p)—the solid component will be further evaluated
- **Solid/almost completely solid** (**2**p)
- **Indeterminate** (**2**p)

Echogenicity
- **Anechoic** (**0**p)
- **Hyperechoic** or **isoechoic** (**1**p)—compared to the adjacent thyroid parenchyma
- **Indeterminate** (**1**p)
- **Hypoechoic** (**2**p)—compared to the adjacent thyroid parenchyma
- **Very hypoechoic** (**3**p)—more hypoechoic than the striated muscles in the cervical region

Shape
- **Wider-than-tall** (**0**p)
- **Taller-than-wide** (**3**p)

The evaluation is made on transversal US sections, with measurements determined parallel to the US beam for height and perpendicular to the beam for width.

Margin

- **Smooth** or **ill-defined** (**0**p)
- **Lobulated** (**2**p)—with protrusions into the adjacent parenchyma
- **Irregular** (**2**p)—spiculated
- **Extrathyroidal Extension** (**3**p)—a frank invasion of adjacent soft tissues or vascular structures

Echogenic Foci

- **None** (**0**p)
- **Large comet-tail artifacts** (**0**p)—V shape; >1 mm; present in cystic nodules; associated with the presence of colloid
- **Macrocalcifications** (**1**p)—produce an acoustic shadowing
- **Peripheral rim calcifications** (**2**p)—complete or incomplete along the edge of the nodule
- **Punctate echogenic foci** (**3**p)—without acoustic shadowing; might be the correspondent of the psammoma calcifications associated with papillary cancer.

Depending on its largest dimension, the nodule will require a biopsy or a further US. Measurements should be taken in three axes, including the halo [25].

The ACR-TIRADS system in Fig. 3.3 [25].

The risk of malignancy is:

- TR1: 0.3%
- TR2: 1.5%
- TR3: 4.8%
- TR4: 9.1%
- TR5: 35%

The ACR system does not provide a grade for "normal thyroid gland," in contrast to other thyroid reporting systems, where category 1 denotes a benign nodule.

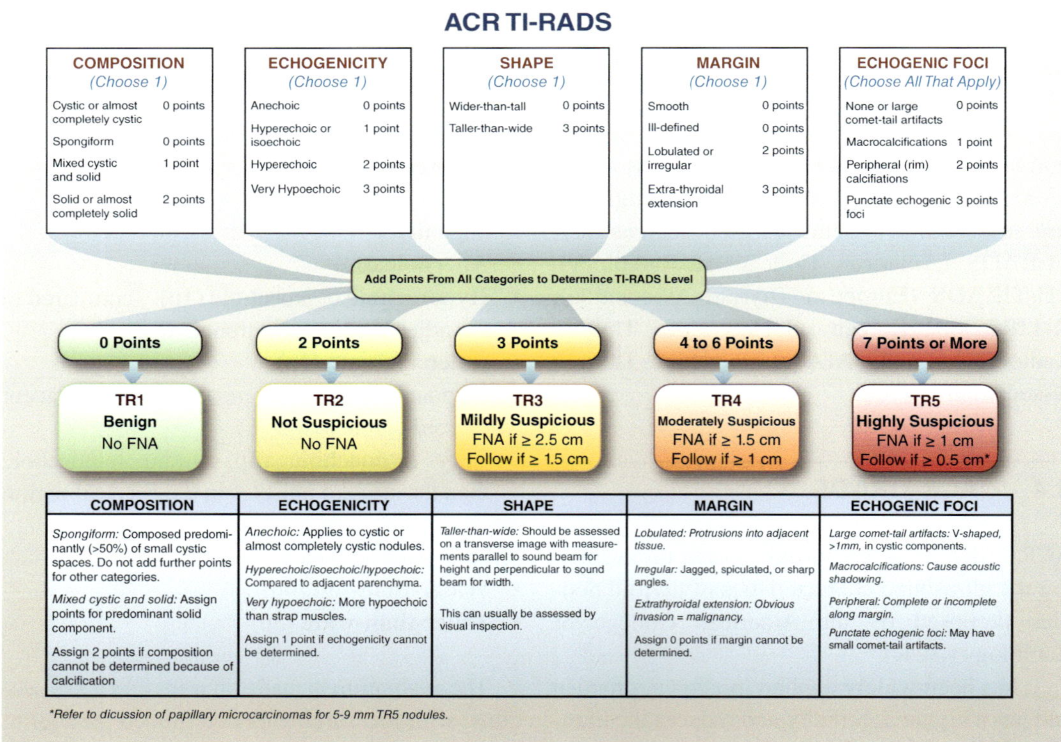

Fig. 3.3 The 2017 ACR-TIRADS system

ACR recommendations in case of multinodular thyroid nodules are as followed: report the four highest TIRADS score TN, for FNA target no more than 2 TN with the most suspicious aspect, not necessarily the largest ones [26].

3.5 EU-TIRADS

European TI-RADS is based on US pattern analysis, with a focus on echogenicity in particular (Fig. 3.4). EU-TIRADS is a pattern-based scoring system, which includes only the most important ultrasound features. As with all TI-RADS systems, the operator to be familiar with the evaluation options for the five features of composition, margin, shape, echogenity, and echogenic foci [28].

Its main objective was to create a more straightforward classification system in order to decrease interobserver variability and increase accuracy.

Classification [29]:

EU-TIRADS 1: no nodule

EU-TIRADS 2: benign (anechoic/spongiform)

EU-TIRADS 3: low risk (oval, smooth margin, iso/hyperechoic, no high-risk features)

EU-TIRADS 4: intermediate risk (oval, smooth margin, mildly hypoechoic, no high-risk features)

EU-TIRADS 5: any high-risk features (non-oval, irregular margin, microcalcifications, marked hypoechogenicity)

Recommendations

EU-TIRADS 2: no FNA required (unless for therapeutic purpose/relieve compression)

EU-TIRADS 3: >20 mm FNA

EU-TIRADS 4: >15 mm FNA

EU-TIRADS 5: >10 mm FNA, <10 mm consider FNA or active surveillance

If the nodule has at least one suspicious US feature: **marked hypoechogenicity, non-oval/round shape, irregular margin,** or **microcalcifications**, it will be classified as TI-RADS 5 (high risk); otherwise, it will be subsequently classified according to its echogenicity.

In case of multinodular thyroid nodules, at least the three most important ones (according to the risk and size criteria) should be described in detail [28].

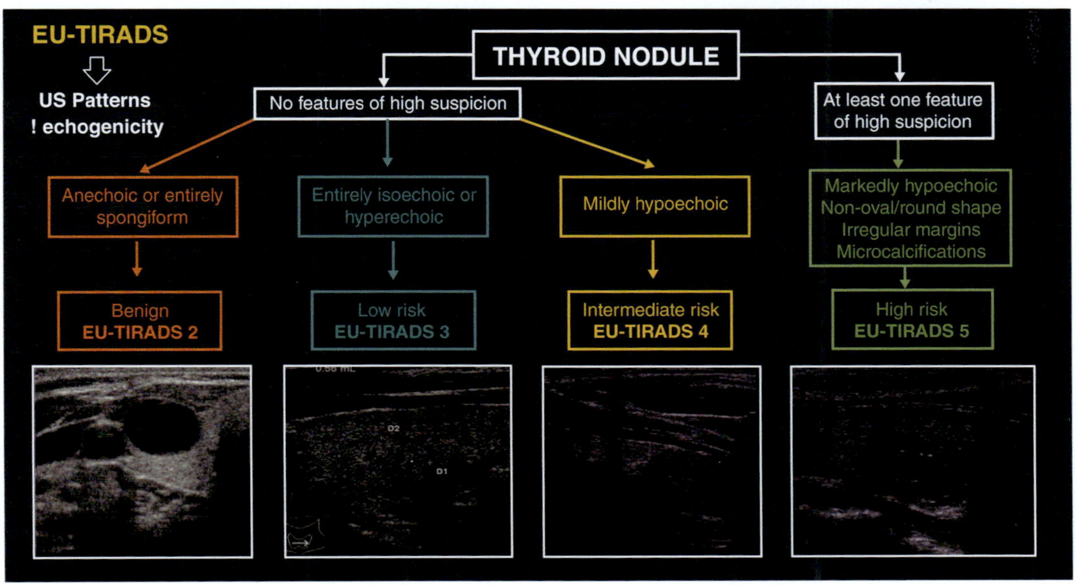

Fig. 3.4 EU-TIRADS: Algorithm Overview: Updated [27]

3.6 K-TIRADS

The Korean Thyroid Imaging Reporting and Data System (K-TIRADS) is an ultrasound (US)-based risk stratification system (RSS) for thyroid nodules that was endorsed by the Korean Society of Thyroid Radiology (KSThR) and the Korean Thyroid Association (KTA).

The Korean system was published in 2016, shortly followed by ACR TI-RADS (2017) and EU-TIRADS (2017). The K-TIRADS uses a pattern-based system instead of an individual US feature-based system or a point-based system (Fig. 3.5).

K-TIRADS is also based on US pattern analysis, with an emphasis on both composition and echogenicity [8].

K-TIRADS 1: normal thyroid gland with no nodules.

K-TIRADS 2: pure cystic nodules, partially cystic nodules with comet-tail artifacts and spongiform nodules.

K-TIRADS 3: partially cystic iso- or hyperechoic nodule without suspicious US features.

K-TIRADS 4: partially cystic iso- or hyperechoic nodule with at least one suspicious US features: non-parallel orientation, spiculated/microlobulated margin, microcalcifications, or hypoechoic solid nodule without suspicious US features.

K-TIRADS 5: hypoechoic solid nodule with at least one suspicious US features: non-parallel orientation, spiculated/microlobulated margin, microcalcifications.

Compared to the other TIRADS systems, K-TIRADS offers no recommendations for follow-up without FNA because it is disputed whether it is reliable at preventing the progression into nodal/distant metastases development [30].

3.7 ATA

To compare the diagnostic performance in determining the malignancy of thyroid nodules and the fine needle aspiration (FNA) recommendations of the guidelines set forth by the American College of Radiology in 2017 (2017 ACR-TIRADS) and the American Thyroid Association in 2015 (2015 ATA guidelines).

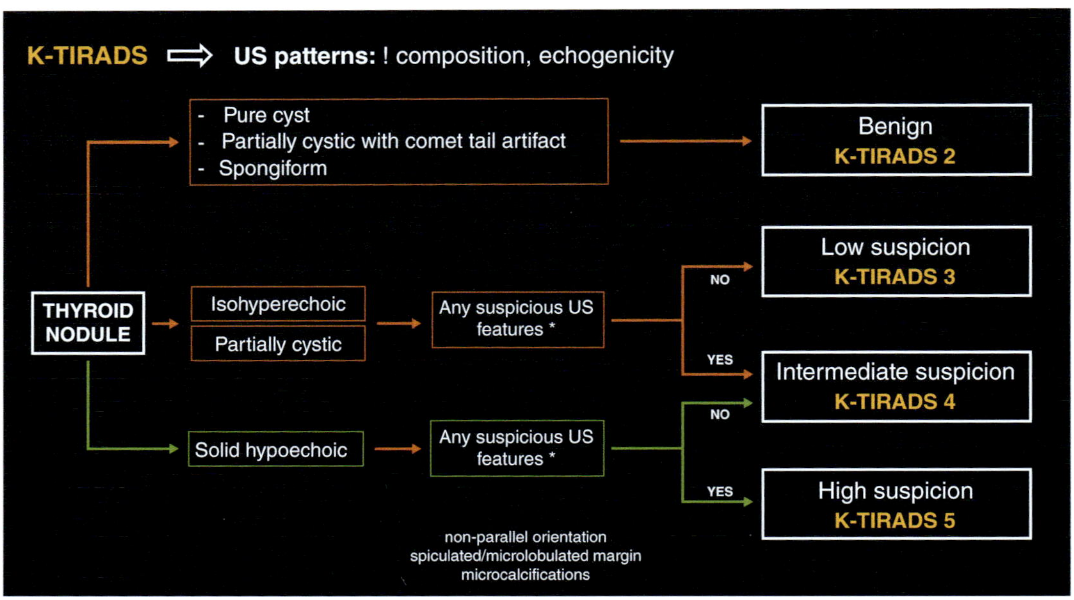

Fig. 3.5 K-TIRADS—Algorithm [30]

Based on the US features, a TN is classified into one of five categories as listed:

- benign pattern (0% risk, no biopsy): completely cystic nodules with well-defined walls, no solid nodules
- very low suspicion pattern (<3% risk, biopsy if ≥2 cm): * spongiform and partially cystic nodules, without any of the features in more suspicious patterns
- low suspicion pattern (5–10% risk, biopsy if ≥1.5 cm): isoechoic/hyperechoic nodule or partially cystic nodule with peripheral solid areas, without any of the features in more suspicious patterns
- intermediate suspicion pattern (10–20% risk, biopsy if ≥1 cm): hypoechoic solid nodule with smooth margins, without any of the features in more suspicious patterns
- high suspicion pattern (>70–90% risk, biopsy if ≥1 cm): solid hypoechoic nodule (or solid hypoechoic component of a partially cystic nodule), with at least one of these features: microcalcifications, irregular margins (infiltrative, microlobulated), extrathyroidal extension, taller than wide, rim calcifications with an extrusive soft tissue component, lymphadenopathy.

When it comes to predicting thyroid cancer in a group of surgical patients who had a relatively high incidence of malignancy, the 2015 ATA and 2017 ACR TI-RADS categorization systems seem to perform similarly overall. The study by Sara Ahmadi et al. revealed a slightly greater chance of missing malignancy in the ACR TI-RADS system than the ATA system, according to a sub-group examination of TR 3 and 4 nodules based on size. Also, in the same study 15 TN (4.4%) were unclassified based on ATA score due to the lack of criteria that suits the sonographic pattern of the nodule (solid, isoechoic with one type of calcification) [31].

A few comparative studies of the systems [31, 32] show that ACR-TIRADS has the best performance regarding unnecessary FNAB (false-positive rates) with a sensitivity ranging 75–97% and specificity ranging 53–67% [33, 34].

In a meta-analysis conducted by Kim et al., a total of 34 studies were analyzed to evaluate the diagnostic effectiveness of TIRADS, and the results indicate the highest sensitivity for the use of EU-TIRADS and the highest specificity for K-TIRADS as diagnostic tools in estimating the risk of malignancy of focal thyroid lesions [35].

The ACR scoring uses a point scale rather than a pattern recognition which makes it more time consuming compared with the other systems. However, based on a 2017 ACR white paper recommending fine needle aspiration and follow-up, a Thyroid Imaging Reporting and Data System (TI-RADS) online calculator was developed (http://tiradscalculator.com).

3.8 Artificial Intelligence

Like any other tool that humans use, AI can bring simplification and efficiency to the workflow, which in case of radiologists mean increased sensitivity and increased specificity leading to increased confidence in reported results.

ACR-TIRADS 2017 edition was considered gold standard in US and thus Gao et al. performed a retrospective study where a radiologist using TI-RADS and ATA guidelines was pitted against computer-aided diagnosis (CAD) system. While sensitivity was same for both CAD lost in terms of specificity. This finding was similar to an earlier study which compared an AI-powered CAD system to an experienced radiologist using previous ACR TI Rads classification [36].

AI gets restricted by human classification system and thus cannot compete under those parameters with an experienced radiologist. That led to the development of AI TI Rads in May 2019, which stands for the data-driven analysis and revision of the 2017 ACR TI-RADS.

Wildman-Tobriner et al. modified the ACR TI-RADS by a genetic machine learning algorithm and called it AI-TIRADS. Their proposed AI-TIRADS system revised point values based on AI interpretation, receiving 1 point for taller-than-wide shape, 2 points for hypoechogenicity, irregular and lobulated margins, peripheral echogenic foci, and 3 points for solid composition,

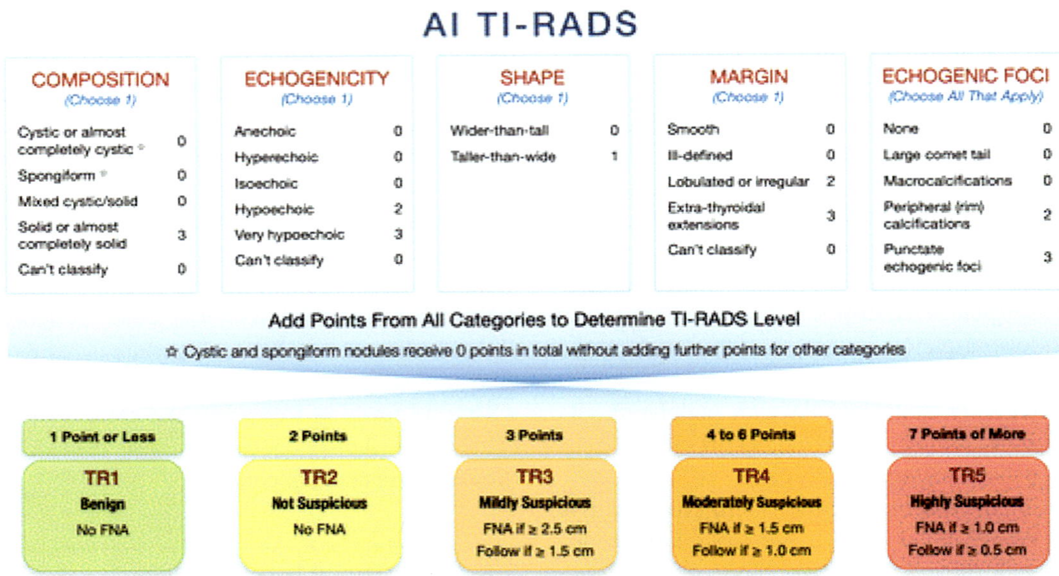

Fig. 3.6 Artificial Intelligence (AI) Thyroid Imaging Reporting and Data System (TI-RADS) classification scheme, including nodule sizes that dictate follow-up recommendations. *FNA* fine needle aspiration, *TR* TI-RADS category

very hypoechoic lesions, extrathyroidal extensions, and punctate echogenic foci. The scores for the remaining ACR-TIRADS characteristics were zero (Fig. 3.6) [37].

Sensitivity was the same (93%) between AI and ACR TI-RADS in the study by Wildman-Tobriner et al., which examined 100 TN. For AI TI-RADS, specificity increased to 65% from 47% with a single expert reader and to 55% from 47% in a group of non-expert readers. With 15 nodules not fitting the criteria for FNA, there were 43 nodules that were downcategorized (all of which were benign). Using the AI TI-RADS scoring method, no additional malignancies were missed.

Further studies for corporation of radiology AI into established classification were made, the study conducted by Sho Wang et al. used machine learning program (Google AutoML) on 249 patients with Bethesda III-IV TN for automated nodule identification and risk stratification and three blinded radiologists scored the nodules as high or low risk based on the presence of highly suspicious imaging features on TI-RADS. The AI algorithm was 100% accurate in object location, predicted the malignancy risk with a sensitivity of 73.9%, specificity of 70.8%. The radiologists performed with a sensitivity of 52.1 ± 4.4%, specificity of 65.2 ± 6.4% [38].

Both studies demonstrated the potential benefits of combining both advanced machine learning programs with experienced radiologists. It is likely essential for clinical adoption that the decision-making of an AI model be explained and validated.

The use of AI-algorithms in routine clinical practice may be able to support radiologists' decision-making processes and serve as an adjunct tool. Clinically, this strategy may make it possible to detect truly high-risk nodules more precisely on initial ultrasound and avoid invasive procedures on lower risk nodules [38].

References

1. Aslan A, Sancak S, Aslan M, Ayaz E, Inan I, Ozkanli SS, Alimoglu O, Yikilmaz A. Diagnostic value of duplex Doppler ultrasound parameters in papillary thyroid carcinoma. Acta Endocrinol (Buc). 2018;14(1):43–8.
2. Delfim RLC, de Veiga LCG, Vidal APA, Lopes FPPL, Vaisman M, de Fatima Dos Santos Teixeira

P. Likelihood of malignancy in thyroid nodules according to a proposed thyroid imaging reporting and data system (TI-RADS) classification merging suspicious and benign ultrasound features. Arch Endocrinol Metab. 2017;61(3):211–21.
3. Melany M, Chen S. Thyroid cancer: ultrasound imaging and fine-needle aspiration biopsy. Endocrinol Metab Clin. 2017;46(3):691–711.
4. Durante C, Grani G, Lamartina L, Filetti S, Mandel SJ, Cooper DS. The diagnosis and management of thyroid nodules: a review. JAMA. 2018;319(9):914–24.
5. Zhang T, Li F, Mu J, Liu J, Zhang S. Multivariate evaluation of thyroid imaging reporting and data system (TI-RADS) in diagnosis malignant thyroid nodule: application to PCA and PLS-DA analysis. Int J Clin Oncol. 2017;22(3):448–54.
6. Hawkins SP, Jamieson SG, Coomarasamy CN, Low IC. The global epidemic of thyroid cancer overdiagnosis illustrated using 18 months of consecutive nodule biopsy correlating clinical priority, ACR-TIRADS and Bethesda scoring. J Med Imaging Radiat Oncol. 2021;65:309.
7. Iwata AJ, Bhan A, Lahiri S, Williams AM, Taylor AR, Chang SS. Comparison of incidental versus palpable thyroid nodules presenting for fine-needle aspiration biopsy. Head Neck. 2018;40(7):1508–14.
8. Xie M, Gupta MK, Archibald SD, Stanley Jackson B, Young JEMT, Zhang H. The usefulness of the thyroid imaging reporting and data system in determining thyroid malignancy. Laryngoscope. 2020;10:1002.
9. Guth S, Theune U, Aberle J, Galach A, Bamberger CM. Very high prevalence of thyroid nodules detected by high frequency (13 MHz) ultrasound examination. Eur J Clin Invest. 2009;39:699–706.
10. Horvath E, Majlis S, Rossi R, Franco C, Niedmann JP, Castro A, Dominguez M. An ultrasonogram reporting system for thyroid nodules stratifying cancer risk for clinical management. J Clin Endocrinol Metabol. 2009;94(5):1748–51.
11. Zhang J, Liu BJ, Xu HX, Xu JM, Zhang YF, Liu C, Wu J, Sun LP, Guo LH, Liu LN, Xu XH, Qu S. Prospective validation of an ultrasound-based thyroid imaging reporting and data system (TI-RADS) on 3980 thyroid nodules. Int J Clin Exp Med. 2015;8(4):5911–7.
12. Hoang JK, Middleton WD, Farjat AE, Langer JE, Reading CC, Teefey SA, Abinanti N, Boschini FJ, Bronner AJ, Dahiya N, Hertzberg BS, Newman JR, Scanga D, Vogler RC, Tessler FN. Reduction in thyroid nodule biopsies and improved accuracy with American College of Radiology thyroid imaging reporting and data system. Radiology. 2018;287(1):185–93. https://doi.org/10.1148/radiol.2018172572.
13. Haugen BR, Alexander EK, Bible KC, Doherty GM, Mandel SJ, Nikiforov YE, Pacini F, Randolph GW, Sawka AM, Schlumberger M, Schuff KG, Sherman SI, Sosa JA, Steward DL, Tuttle RM, Wartofsky L. 2015 American Thyroid Association management guidelines for adult patients with thyroid nodules and differentiated thyroid cancer: the American Thyroid Association guidelines task force on thyroid nodules and differentiated thyroid cancer. Thyroid. 2016;26(1):1–133.
14. Gharib H, Papini E, Garber JR, Duick DS, Harrell RM, Hegedüs L, Paschke R, Valcavi R, Vitti P. American Association of Clinical Endocrinologists, American College of Endocrinology, and Associazione Medici Endocrinologi medical guidelines for clinical practice for the diagnosis and management of thyroid nodules—2016 update. Endocr Pract. 2016;22(5):622–39.
15. Yalcin MM, Altinova AE, Ozkan C, Toruner F, Akturk M, Akdemir O, Emiroglu T, Gokce D, Poyraz A, Taneri F, Yetkin I. Thyroid malignancy risk of incidental thyroid nodules in patients with non-thyroid cancer. Acta Endocrinol (Buc). 2016;12(2):185–90.
16. Singaporewalla RM, Hwee J, Lang TU, Desai V. Clinico-pathological correlation of thyroid nodule ultrasound and cytology using the TIRADS and Bethesda classifications. World J Surg. 2017;41(7):1807–11.
17. Vargas-Uricoechea H, Meza-Cabrera I, Herrera-Chapparo J. Concordance between the TIRADS ultrasound criteria and the Bethesda cytology criteria on the nontoxic thyroid nodule. Thyroid Res. 2017;10(1):1.
18. Horvath E, Silva CF, Majlis S, Rodriguez I, Skoknic V, et al. Prospective validation of the ultrasound based TIRADS classification: results in surgically thyroid nodules. Eur Radiol. 2017;27(6):2619–28.
19. Kroenke M, Schweiger L, Horn T, Haller B, Schwamborn K, Wurzer A, Maurer T, Wester H-J, Eiber M, Rauscher I. Validation of ^{18}F-rhPSMA-7 and ^{18}F-rhPSMA-7.3 PET imaging results with histopathology from salvage surgery in patients with biochemical recurrence of prostate cancer. J Nucl Med. 2022;63(12):1809–14. https://doi.org/10.2967/jnumed.121.2637.
20. Hoang JK, William D, Afredo M, et al. Reduction in thyroid nodule biopsies and improved accuracy with American College of Radiology Thyroid Imaging Reporting and Data System. Radiology. 2018;287(1):554–7.
21. Remonti LR, Kramer CK, Leitão CB, et al. Thyroid ultrasound features and risk of carcinoma: a systematic review and meta-analysis of observational studies. Thyroid. 2015;25:538–50.
22. Hoang JK, Middleton WD, Tessler FN. Update on ACR TI-RADS: successes, challenges, and future directions, from the AJR special series on radiology reporting and data systems. AJR Am J Roentgenol. 2021;216(3):570–8.
23. Cantisani V, Lodise P, Grazhdani H, Mancuso E, Maggini E, Di Rocco G, D'Ambrosio F, Calliada F, Redler A, Ricci P, Catalano C. Ultrasound elastography in the evaluation of thyroid pathology. Current status. Eur J Radiol. 2014;83(3):420–8. https://doi.org/10.1016/j.ejrad.2013.05.008.
24. https://radiopaedia.org/articles/acr-thyroid-imaging-reporting-and-data-system-acr-ti-rads.

25. Tessler FN, et al. ACR thyroid imaging, reporting and data system (TI-RADS): white paper of the ACR TI-RADS Committee. J Am Coll Radiol. 2017;14(5):587–95.
26. Middleton WD, Teefey SA, Reading CC, et al. Multiinstitutional analysis of thyroid nodule risk stratification using the American College of Radiology thyroid imaging reporting and data system. AJR Am J Roentgenol. 2017;208(6):1331–41.
27. Dudea SM (algorithm modified after G. Russ, et al. European Thyroid Association guidelines for ultrasound malignancy risk stratification of thyroid nodules in adults: the EU-TIRADS. Eur Thyroid J. 2017;6(5):225–237.
28. Russ G, Bonnema SJ, Erdogan MF, Durante C, Ngu R, Leenhardt L. European Thyroid Association guidelines for ultrasound malignancy risk stratification of thyroid nodules in adults: the EU-TIRADS. Eur Thyroid J. 2017;6(5):225–37.
29. https://radiopaedia.org/articles/european-thyroid-association-tirads.
30. Shin JH, Baek JH, Chung J, et al. Ultrasonography diagnosis and imaging-based management of thyroid nodules: revised Korean Society of Thyroid Radiology consensus statement and recommendations. Korean J Radiol. 2016;17(3):370–95.
31. Ahmadi S, Oyekunle T, Jiang XS, Scheri R, Perkins J, Stang M, Roman S, Sosa JA. A direct comparison of the ATA and TI-RADS ultrasound scoring systems. Endocr Pract. 2019;25(5):413–22. https://doi.org/10.4158/EP-2018-0369.
32. Xu T, Wu Y, Wu R-X, Zhang Y-Z, Gu J-Y, Ye J-H, Tang W, Xu S-H, Liu C, Wu X-H. Validation and comparison of three newly-released thyroid imaging reporting and data systems for cancer risk determination. Endocrine. 2019;64(2):299. https://doi.org/10.1007/s12020-018-1817-8.
33. Giorgio G, Livia L, Valeria A, Daniela B, Marco B, Laura G, Marianna M, Rosa F, Valeria R, Vito C, Sebastiano F, Cosimo D. Reducing the number of unnecessary thyroid biopsies while improving diagnostic accuracy: toward the "right" TIRADS. J Clin Endocrinol Metabol. 2019;104(1):95. https://doi.org/10.1210/jc.2018-01674.
34. Ha EJ, Na DG, Baek JH, Sung JY, Kim J-h, Kang SY. US fine-needle aspiration biopsy for thyroid malignancy: diagnostic performance of seven society guidelines applied to 2000 thyroid nodules. Radiology. 2018;287(3):893–900. https://doi.org/10.1148/radiol.2018171074.
35. Kim PH, Chung SR, Choi SH, Kim KW. Accuracy of thyroid imaging reporting and data system category 4 or 5 for diagnosing malignancy: a systematic review and meta-analysis. Eur Radiol. 2020;30:5611–24.
36. Gao L, Liu R, Jiang Y, Song W, Wang Y, Liu J, Wang J, Wu D, Li S, Hao A, Zhang B. Computer-aided system for diagnosing thyroid nodules on ultrasound: a comparison with radiologist-based clinical assessments. Head Neck. 2018;40(4):778–83. https://doi.org/10.1002/hed.25049. Epub 2017 Dec 29. PMID: 29286180.
37. Wildman-Tobriner B, Buda M, Hoang JK, Middleton WD, Thayer D, Short RG, et al. Using artificial intelligence to revise ACR TI-RADS risk stratification of thyroid nodules: diagnostic accuracy and utility. Radiology. 2019;292:112–9. https://doi.org/10.1148/radiol.2019182128.
38. Wang S, Xu J, Tahmasebi A, Daniels K, Liu JB, Curry J, Cottrill E, Lyshchik A, Eisenbrey JR. Incorporation of a machine learning algorithm with object detection within the thyroid imaging reporting and data system improves the diagnosis of genetic risk. Front Oncol. 2020;10:591846. https://doi.org/10.3389/fonc.2020.591846.

4 Thyroid Nodular Pathology

Kharisa N. Rachmasari and Marius N. Stan

4.1 Introduction

4.1.1 Epidemiology

Thyroid nodules are a common clinical condition. They are discrete lesions within the thyroid gland due to an abnormal focal growth of thyroid cells that are radiologically distinct from the rest of the thyroid parenchyma. The prevalence of palpable thyroid nodules is approximately 3–7% [1], and it can reach up to a third of the population if screened with thyroid ultrasound [2, 3]. In a postmortem study, thyroid nodules greater than 1 cm were found in 50% of patients who did not have any clinical history of thyroid issues [4]. Over the last few decades, the prevalence of thyroid nodules and thyroid cancer have been rising and there is an ongoing assessment of the role of increased detection of subclinical disease, possibly combined with a true increase in thyroid cancer incidence [5, 6].

The prevalence of thyroid nodule is higher in women, elderly persons, in those with iodine deficiency, and in those with a history of radiation exposure [4, 7]. A Framingham study showed that thyroid nodules in women were four times more prevalent than in men [8]. A review study found consistent findings of increasing thyroid nodule prevalence, along with multinodularity, with advancing age [9, 10]. Furthermore, in areas with iodine deficiency, besides the increased prevalence of thyroid nodules and multinodularity, it is hypothesized that prolonged thyroid hyperactivity associated with adaptation to iodine deficiency leads to thyroid growth with a tendency to mutations associated with autonomous growth and function [11].

The majority of thyroid nodules are benign, with only 4–13% representing malignant lesions [4, 12, 13]. The risk of malignancy is lower with advancing age, yet thyroid cancer in elderly tends to have a higher risk histological phenotype [9]. Increasing number of incidentally discovered thyroid nodules has partly contributed to the increased number of thyroid cancers detected [5]. The nodules detection led to a significant increase in fine-needle aspiration biopsy (FNAB) procedures. These, along with thyroidectomies performed for multinodular goiters increased the detection of thyroid cancers. These are mainly papillary thyroid microcarcinomas, which the World Health Organization has defined as papillary thyroid cancers measuring less than 1 cm in largest diameter [14].

On the other hand, the incidence of other types of thyroid cancer (follicular, medullary, and anaplastic thyroid cancers) remains relatively unchanged. Given the less aggressive character of papillary thyroid cancers, this is reassuring and argues further for an increased detection rate

K. N. Rachmasari · M. N. Stan (✉)
Division of Endocrinology, Diabetes and Nutrition, Mayo Clinic, Rochester, MN, USA
e-mail: Rachmasari.Kharisa@mayo.edu; Stan.Marius@mayo.edu

R. Valcavi et al. (eds.), *Thyroid Ablation*, https://doi.org/10.1007/978-3-031-88229-6_4

and against a general increase in thyroid carcinogenesis. Additionally, despite increased incidence in thyroid cancers, the overall mortality rate from these entities remains stable [15].

4.1.2 Clinical Presentation (Table 4.1)

In the era of increased use of cross-sectional imaging, thyroid nodules are frequently asymptomatic and often found incidentally. They are thus frequently called thyroid incidentalomas [16, 17]. These nodules may be detected during CT or MRI imaging of the chest, neck, or head, during carotid ultrasonography or during PET scans (Fig. 4.1). Although most thyroid nodules are benign, incidentally found thyroid nodules may raise concerns for malignancy as they do have the same risk for such as clinically apparent thyroid nodules. However, in the case of thyroid incidentaloma detected on PET scans with radiolabeled glucose as tracer (18F-2-fluoro-2-deoxy-d-glucose, FDG) the risk of malignancy is higher if the uptake is focal, corresponding to a specific nodule [18].

Unlike thyroid incidentalomas, visible neck masses may prompt patients themselves to seek medical evaluation. The neck mass may be apparent upon inspection or palpable on physical examination due to a large solitary thyroid nodule or a multinodular goiter. These nodules may be associated with symptoms and/or signs of local mechanical compression: dysphagia, neck tightness, positional dyspnea, or dry cough. They are related to compression on the esophagus and/or trachea (Fig. 4.2). Persistent hoarseness is rare but when it is present, it indicates compression or invasion of one of the recurrent laryngeal nerves, which may be a sign of aggressive thyroid cancer. In significantly enlarged thyroid nodules, obstruction of venous blood flow from the head can occur due to the enlarged thyroid compressing the cephalic venous return against the bony thoracic inlet. This can be noted as facial redness and engorgement within 30–90 s of the patient lifting their arms above their shoulders, a maneuver called the Pemberton sign (Fig. 4.3).

Some thyroid nodules function independent of TSH stimulation and are thus called autonomously functioning thyroid nodules (AFTN) or toxic nodules due to the increase in thyroid hormone production. They can be present as a solitary nodule or part of a toxic multinodular goiter. During history and physical exam, the clinical symptoms of thyrotoxicosis should be sought, such as palpitations, tremors, unintentional weight loss, insomnia, or increased anxiety. Lack of symptoms of thyrotoxicosis may be reassuring, but it does not rule out subclinical hyperthyroidism. With advancing age, the signs and symptoms of thyrotoxicosis may abate, resulting in the picture of apathetic thyrotoxicosis characterized just by apathy and depression associated with weight loss, weakness, and

Table 4.1 Summary of signs and symptoms of thyroid nodules

Compressive symptoms	Toxic symptoms	Aesthetic concerns
Pressure or neck tightness, dysphagia, dyspnea, dysphonia (suggestive of recurrent laryngeal nerve involvement usually associated with advanced cancer), Pemberton sign	Palpitations, tremors, weight loss, increased anxiety, insomnia, clammy skin	Neck mass and asymmetry

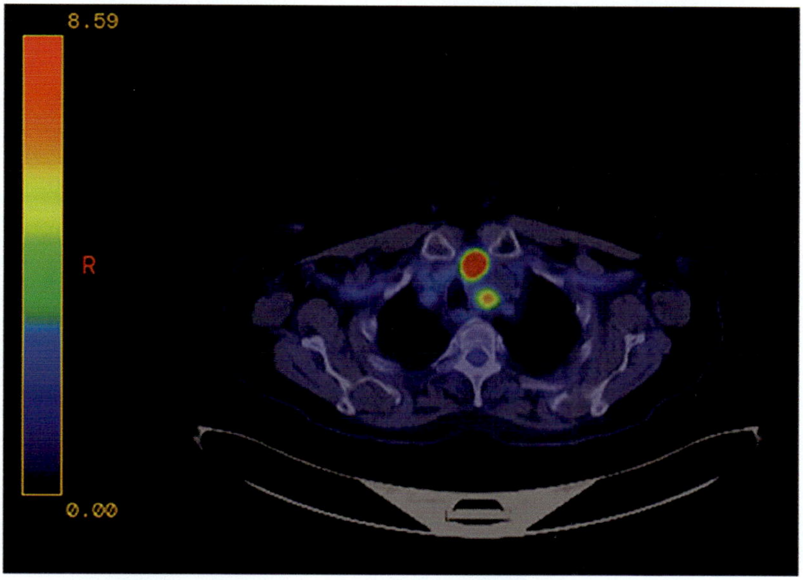

Fig. 4.1 PET scan done for a lung nodule captured two FDG avid left thyroid nodules, one slightly compressing the trachea

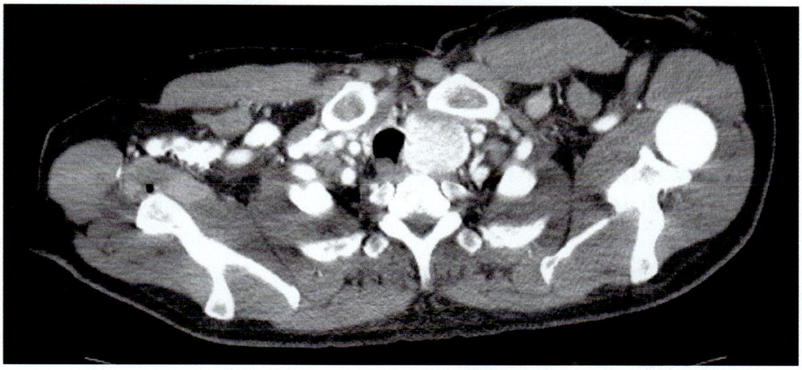

Fig. 4.2 Left-sided thyroid nodule compressing the trachea causing rightward deviation

sometimes lethargy. These patients could have delayed or missed diagnosis due to the absence of typical signs and symptoms of excitability and hyperkinesis [19].

The physical exam should seek to identify the size of the thyroid nodules, presence of tenderness, consistency, mobility regarding the surrounding structures and associated lymph nodes. It is also important to identify the presence of scars over the thyroid bed, evidence for prior radiation therapy (with decreased soft tissue elasticity) as well as the position of the nodules in relationship to the clavicles and the sternum, in order to plan appropriately for a possible biopsy. In patients with large subcutaneous/muscular structures over the neck, the definition of thyroid anatomy can be challenging. Asking the patient to swallow can be helpful, as well as evaluating the thyroid both with neck in flexion and extension.

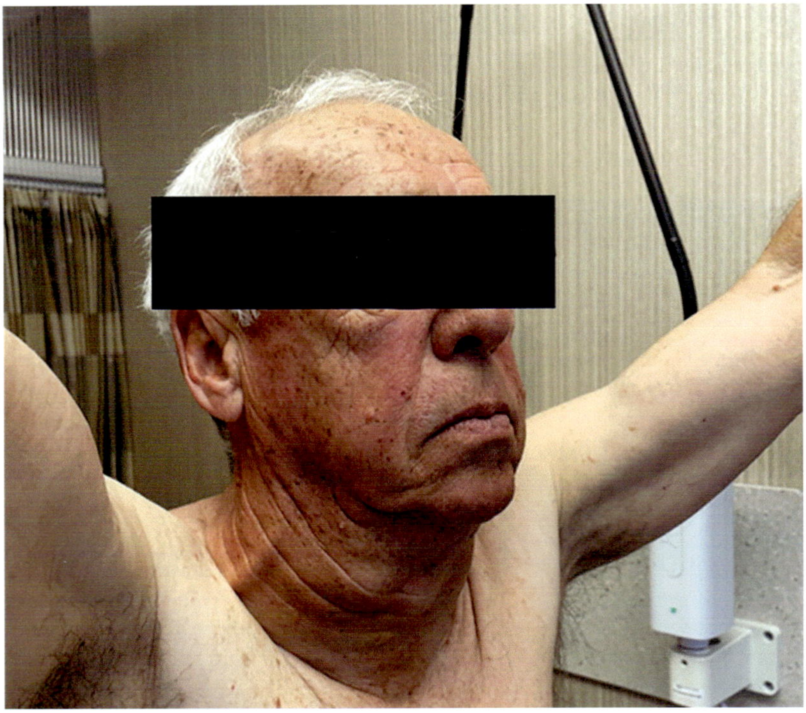

Fig. 4.3 A patient with large goiter experiencing facial redness and engorgement within 30 seconds of lifting his arms above the shoulders—Pemberton sign

4.2 Evaluation of Thyroid Nodules

The typical approach to a thyroid nodule includes obtaining the history and physical exam followed by the evaluation of thyroid function, imaging of the thyroid with ultrasound, and, when suspicion for malignancy is significant, FNAB or core biopsy. Personal history of external neck radiation, total body radiation for bone marrow transplant, smoking status, family history of thyroid cancer, syndromic disorders such as multiple endocrine neoplasia (MEN) type 2, Cowden disease, Carney complex, or familial adenomatous polyposis may put the patient at higher risk of having thyroid malignancy. Rapid growth of thyroid nodule and persistent changes in voice should also raise concern for malignancy. On physical examination, a firm nodule that is fixed or immobile and/or the presence of palpable cervical lymph nodes are highly suggestive of malignancy. Thyroid nodule size alone does not correlate with risk of malignancy [20–22]. However, data indicates that thyroid nodules greater than or equal to 4 cm in maximum diameter confer a higher incidence of malignancy and are also associated with higher risk of false-negative cytology [23]. Sometimes, patients may present with multiple nodules which can be either detected clinically or incidentally while undergoing workup for a dominant nodule. The risk of malignancy in patients with multiple thyroid nodules is the same as those with solitary nodule [24], and each nodule should be evaluated independently.

Once a thyroid nodule is identified the thyroid function should be assessed. Increasing values of serum TSH concentration, even within normal reference range, appears to be associated with an increasing risk of thyroid malignancy [25, 26]. On the other hand, the presence of overt (suppressed TSH with elevated T3 and/or T4) or subclinical thyrotoxicosis (suppressed TSH with normal T3 and T4) should lead to the investigations for possible AFTN or a toxic multinodular goiter (Fig. 4.4). This is best pursued with a combination of iodine thyroid scan and uptake and thyroid ultrasound. An AFTN should be seen as a

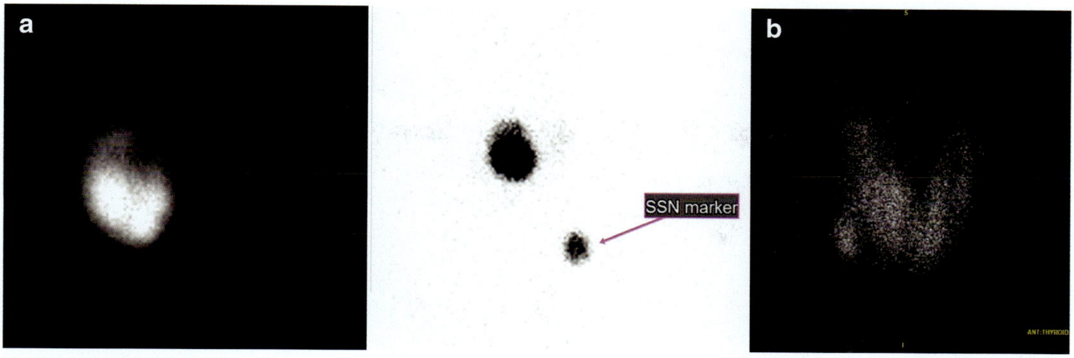

Fig. 4.4 Hot nodules. (**a**) Right thyroid nodule with increased I-123 uptake with uptake suppression in the background thyroid parenchyma. Supra-sternal notch or SSN (*Fuchsia arrow*). (**b**) Toxic multinodular goiter

focal uptake on the iodine scan, corresponding to a clearly defined thyroid nodule on the thyroid ultrasound. In the case of a toxic multinodular goiter, there are multiple areas of uptake on the iodine scan, also corresponding to nodules on thyroid ultrasound. Given that the likelihood of malignancy in these types of nodules is extremely low, most of the time the evaluation can stop here, and treatment can be discussed. However, occasionally thyroid malignancy is present in an AFTN. Therefore, nodules that are toxic yet also highly suspicious for malignancy on ultrasound should be evaluated further with FNAB.

If the patient is not thyrotoxic, then the next best step is to obtain a thyroid ultrasound. Ultrasound is the most sensitive imaging modality to assess thyroid gland, and the procedure is relatively widely available, has no ionizing radiation, and is cost effective. Cervical lymph nodes should be included in the ultrasound in order to better understand the likelihood of a thyroid malignancy. Thyroid nodules can be solid, mixed solid and cystic, or entirely cystic. Ultrasound features can be very effectively utilized to categorize nodules based on their risk of malignancy (see Chap. 2). There are a multitude of ultrasound-based criteria to help physicians decide both which nodules are very low risk for malignancy and, conversely, which nodules should then be evaluated further with FNA [27–30]. The ultrasound features that are suggestive of a benign nodule are a simple cyst structure, spongiform appearance, and iso- or hyperechoic echogenicity (Fig. 4.5). Conversely, features that are most concerning for a possible malignant nodule are hypoechoic appearance, irregular margins, presence of microcalcifications, taller than wider nodule on transverse images of the nodule, as well as the presence of pathologically appearing lymph nodes (Fig. 4.6).

Many thyroid nodules have a partial cystic component, which is the result of cystic degeneration (Fig. 4.7). Approximately 12–20% of nodules have >75% cystic components, but true cystic nodules with benign epithelial cell lining are rare [31, 32]. The risk of malignancy in pure cystic nodule is extremely low [7]; therefore, FNA is not necessary in these lesions. In complex cystic nodules, the risk of malignancy is low, and that likelihood decreases further as the cystic component increases [24]. Unfortunately, there is a higher rate of false negative [33] or non-diagnostic [31] FNAB results in cystic lesions compared to solid nodules, likely due to sampling error. Similarly, the rate of second non-diagnostic FNAB is high and directly correlated with the degree of their cystic component [31]. While cystic lesions are associated with a low rate of malignancy, thyroid nodules that are positive on FDG-PET have a rate of malignancy of 30–50% [34, 35] and FNAB is recommended for nodules ≥1 cm [28, 36].

Size is an important factor in deciding which thyroid nodules should be evaluated aggressively for the possibility of malignancy. Most guidelines [28, 36] recommend that only nodules

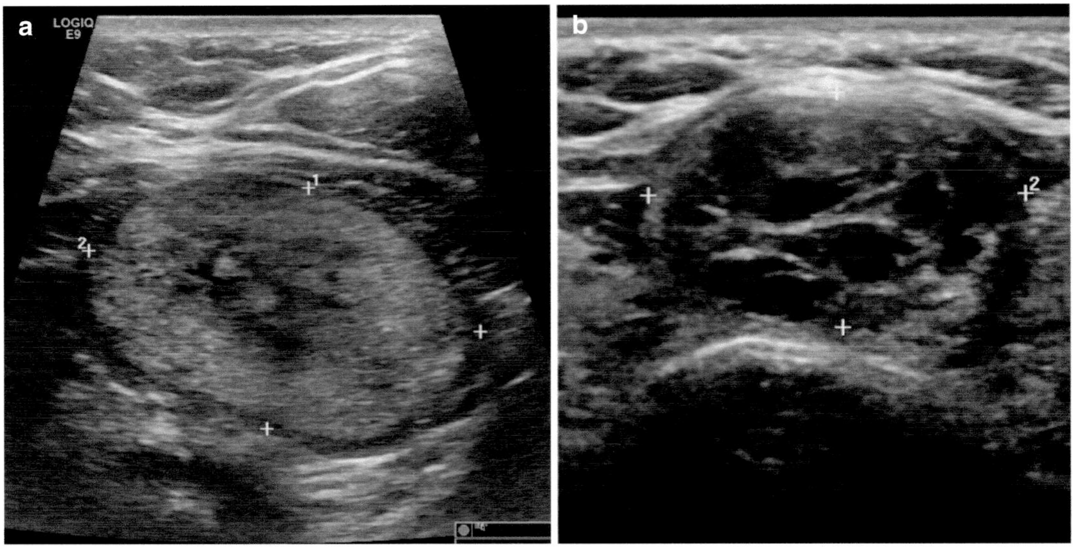

Fig. 4.5 Benign thyroid nodules. (**a**) Benign thyroid nodule appears isoechoic, well demarcated, not taller than wider. (**b**) Benign thyroid nodule with spongiform features

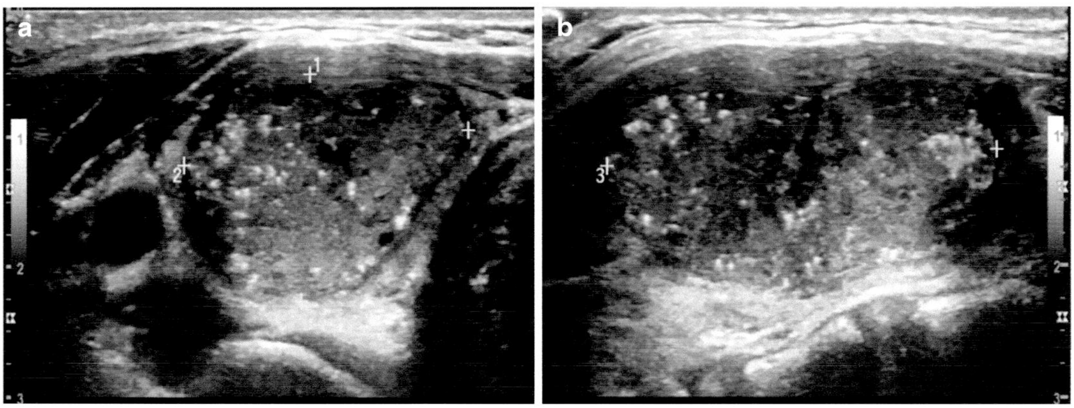

Fig. 4.6 Papillary thyroid carcinoma. Papillary thyroid carcinoma on the right thyroid lobe as seen on ultrasound, transverse view (**a**) and longitudinal view (**b**). Multiple echogenic foci are present

>1 cm should be pursued with FNAB since these nodules tend to have a greater potential to be clinically significant cancers. However, finding of a suspicious cervical lymph node mandates that even smaller thyroid nodules should be considered for an urgent and aggressive evaluation. Once a decision about biopsy has been made, almost all the time it will be FNAB. However, in rare cases where there is suspicion for lymphoma or anaplastic carcinoma, a core biopsy might be desirable to achieve a final diagnosis.

Ultimately, there is a debate whether routine screening with serum calcitonin measurement would be helpful in the initial evaluation of thyroid nodules. Proponents of the measurement argue that serum calcitonin may help detect C-cell hyperplasia and medullary thyroid cancer (MTC) at an early stage, which may improve survival [37]. However, issues with the assay's sensitivity and rarity of MTC may suggest initial evaluation with routine serum calcitonin to be less helpful and less cost-effective.

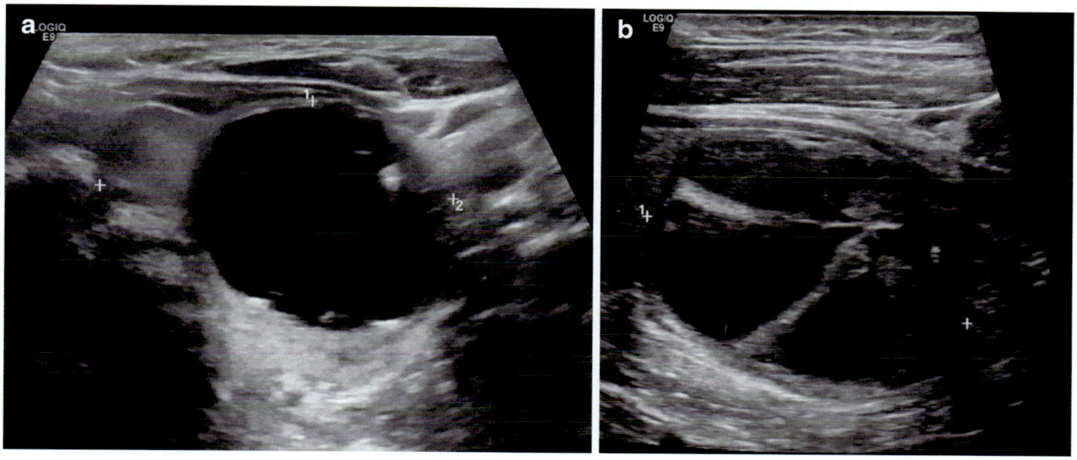

Fig. 4.7 Cystic nodules on ultrasound. (**a**) A predominantly cystic nodule on the left lower thyroid lobe. (**b**) A complex cystic nodule

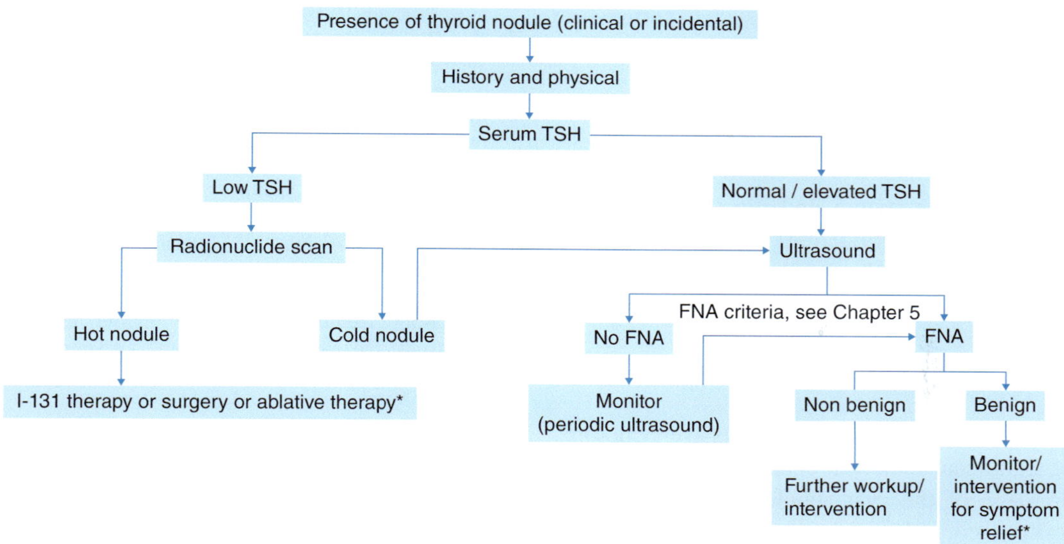

Fig. 4.8 Workup of thyroid nodule. *see Chap. 9: Nodule selection for thyroid ablation

4.3 Management Approach (Fig. 4.8)

4.3.1 Benign and Non-toxic Nodules

Benign and non-toxic nodules that are not causing compressive symptoms should be monitored over time. This should include periodic clinical examination combined with ultrasound evaluation. In a 5-year prospective study, 69% of thyroid nodules remained stable, while only 15.4% grew significantly [38] (based on the American Thyroid Association's guideline for measuring significant growth, defined as a 20% increase in more than two dimensions, with a minimum increase of 2 mm [28]). Periodic ultrasound helps clinicians assess the need for repeat FNAB evaluation. The criteria for such are increased in size or change in the appearance of thyroid nodules that raise the level of suspicion for malignancy. If the patient complains of compressive symptoms or significant esthetic concerns, then intervention for benign nodules should be discussed. This spans from surgical to ablative options, particularly considering the recent advances in thermal ablation therapies discussed elsewhere in this book (Chap. 14).

4.3.2 Benign Toxic Thyroid Nodules

These nodules should be considered for standard therapy with surgery or radioactive iodine. However, in these lesions as well, the reports of thermal ablations effectiveness suggest that this approach is rapidly becoming an equally successful alternative in centers with such expertise (see Chap. 15).

4.3.3 Malignant Thyroid Nodules

These nodules should undergo therapy as outlined in the ATA guidelines for the management of DTC [28] (see Chap. 10).

4.3.4 Fully Cystic Thyroid Lesions

At times these can cause compressive symptoms or significant esthetical concerns. In those cases, drainage of the cyst should be offered. If the lesion recurs, then the use of alcohol to induce sclerosis of the lesion should be pursued after a second drainage (see Chap. 13).

4.4 Conclusion

Thyroid nodules are a common clinical condition, and their evaluation should assess their function, risk of malignancy, and compressive symptoms and esthetic concerns. Once these aspects have been answered the management should consider the spectrum of options from observation to surgery, with the addition of ablative therapies as an exciting development in the field. The future will decide for which nodules these therapies are best suited, while excellence in their utilization should be a prerequisite for their insertion in any thyroid nodule management algorithm.

References

1. Gharib H, Papini E, Valcavi R, Baskin HJ, Crescenzi A, Dottorini ME, et al. American Association of Clinical Endocrinologists and Associazione Medici Endocrinologi medical guidelines for clinical practice for the diagnosis and management of thyroid nodules. Endocr Pract. 2006;12(1):63–102. https://doi.org/10.4158/EP.12.1.63.
2. Ezzat S, Sarti DA, Cain DR, Braunstein GD. Thyroid incidentalomas. Prevalence by palpation and ultrasonography. Arch Intern Med. 1994;154(16):1838–40. https://doi.org/10.1001/archinte.154.16.1838.
3. Tan GH, Gharib H. Thyroid incidentalomas: management approaches to nonpalpable nodules discovered incidentally on thyroid imaging. Ann Intern Med. 1997;126(3):226–31. https://doi.org/10.7326/0003-4819-126-3-199702010-00009.
4. Mortensen JD, Woolner LB, Bennett WA. Gross and microscopic findings in clinically normal thyroid glands. J Clin Endocrinol Metab. 1955;15(10):1270–80. https://doi.org/10.1210/jcem-15-10-1270.
5. Davies L, Ouellette M, Hunter M, Welch HG. The increasing incidence of small thyroid cancers: where are the cases coming from? Laryngoscope. 2010;120(12):2446–51. https://doi.org/10.1002/lary.21076.
6. Uppal A, White MG, Nagar S, Aschebrook-Kilfoy B, Chang PJ, Angelos P, et al. Benign and malignant thyroid incidentalomas are rare in routine clinical practice: a review of 97,908 imaging studies. Cancer Epidemiol Biomarkers Prev. 2015;24(9):1327–31. https://doi.org/10.1158/1055-9965.EPI-15-0292.
7. Rojeski MT, Gharib H. Nodular thyroid disease: evaluation and management. N Engl J Med. 1985;313(7):428–36. https://doi.org/10.1056/NEJM198508153130707.
8. Vander JB, Gaston EA, Dawber TR. The significance of nontoxic thyroid nodules: final report of a 15-year study of the incidence of thyroid malignancy. Ann Intern Med. 1968;69(3):537–40. https://doi.org/10.7326/0003-4819-69-3-537.
9. Kwong N, Medici M, Angell TE, Liu X, Marqusee E, Cibas ES, et al. The influence of patient age on thyroid nodule formation, multinodularity, and thyroid cancer risk. J Clin Endocrinol Metab. 2015;100(12):4434–40. https://doi.org/10.1210/jc.2015-3100.

10. Ospina NS, Papaleontiou M. Thyroid nodule evaluation and management in older adults: a review of practical considerations for clinical endocrinologists. Endocr Pract. 2021;27(3):261–8. https://doi.org/10.1016/j.eprac.2021.02.003.
11. Laurberg P, Cerqueira C, Ovesen L, Rasmussen LB, Perrild H, Andersen S, et al. Iodine intake as a determinant of thyroid disorders in populations. Best Pract Res Clin Endocrinol Metab. 2010;24(1):13–27. https://doi.org/10.1016/j.beem.2009.08.013.
12. Horlocker TT, Hay JE, James EM, Reading CC, Charboneau JW. Prevalence of incidental nodular thyroid disease detected during high-resolution parathyroid ultrasonography. Front Thyroidol. 1986;2:1309–12.
13. Komorowski RA, Hanson GA. Occult thyroid pathology in the young adult: an autopsy study of 138 patients without clinical thyroid disease. Hum Pathol. 1988;19(6):689–96.
14. Sosa JA, Hanna JW, Robinson KA, Lanman RB. Increases in thyroid nodule fine-needle aspirations, operations, and diagnoses of thyroid cancer in the United States. Surgery. 2013;154(6):1420–6; discussion 1426–7. https://doi.org/10.1016/j.surg.2013.07.006.
15. Davies L, Welch HG. Increasing incidence of thyroid cancer in the United States, 1973-2002. JAMA. 2006;295(18):2164–7. https://doi.org/10.1001/jama.295.18.2164.
16. Bahl M. Incidental thyroid nodules in the National Lung Screening Trial: estimation of prevalence, malignancy rate, and strategy for workup. Acad Radiol. 2018;25(9):1152–5. https://doi.org/10.1016/j.acra.2018.02.016.
17. Youserm DM, Huang T, Loevner LA, Langlotz CP. Clinical and economic impact of incidental thyroid lesions found with CT and MR. AJNR Am J Neuroradiol. 1997;18(8):1423–8.
18. Soelberg KK, Bonnema SJ, Brix TH, Hegedüs L. Risk of malignancy in thyroid incidentalomas detected by 18F-fluorodeoxyglucose positron emission tomography: a systematic review. Thyroid. 2012;22(9):918–25. https://doi.org/10.1089/thy.2012.0005.
19. Arnold BM, Casal G, Higgins HP. Apathetic thyrotoxicosis. Can Med Assoc J. 1974;111(9):957–8.
20. Cavallo A, Johnson DN, White MG, Siddiqui S, Antic T, Mathew M, et al. Thyroid nodule size at ultrasound as a predictor of malignancy and final pathologic size. Thyroid. 2017;27(5):641–50. https://doi.org/10.1089/thy.2016.0336.
21. Jinih M, Faisal F, Abdalla K, Majeed M, Achakzai AA, Heffron C, et al. Association between thyroid nodule size and malignancy rate. Ann R Coll Surg Engl. 2020;102(1):43–8. https://doi.org/10.1308/rcsann.2019.0156.
22. Nou E, Kwong N, Alexander LK, Cibas ES, Marqusee E, Alexander EK. Determination of the optimal time interval for repeat evaluation after a benign thyroid nodule aspiration. J Clin Endocrinol Metab. 2014;99(2):510–6. https://doi.org/10.1210/jc.2013-3160.
23. McCoy KL, Jabbour N, Ogilvie JB, Ohori NP, Carty SE, Yim JH. The incidence of cancer and rate of false-negative cytology in thyroid nodules greater than or equal to 4 cm in size. Surgery. 2007;142(6):837–844.e3. https://doi.org/10.1016/j.surg.2007.08.012.
24. Frates MC, Benson CB, Doubilet PM, Kunreuther E, Contreras M, Cibas ES, et al. Prevalence and distribution of carcinoma in patients with solitary and multiple thyroid nodules on sonography. J Clin Endocrinol Metab. 2006;91(9):3411–7. https://doi.org/10.1210/jc.2006-0690.
25. Boelaert K, Horacek J, Holder RL, Watkinson JC, Sheppard MC, Franklyn JA. Serum thyrotropin concentration as a novel predictor of malignancy in thyroid nodules investigated by fine-needle aspiration. J Clin Endocrinol Metab. 2006;91(11):4295–301. https://doi.org/10.1210/jc.2006-0527.
26. Haymart MR, Repplinger DJ, Leverson GE, Elson DF, Sippel RS, Jaume JC, et al. Higher serum thyroid stimulating hormone level in thyroid nodule patients is associated with greater risks of differentiated thyroid cancer and advanced tumor stage. J Clin Endocrinol Metab. 2008;93(3):809–14. https://doi.org/10.1210/jc.2007-2215.
27. Gharib H, Papini E, Garber JR, Duick DS, Harrell RM, Hegedüs L, et al. American Association of Clinical Endocrinologists, American College of Endocrinology, and Associazione Medici Endocrinologi medical guidelines for clinical practice for the diagnosis and management of thyroid nodules—2016 update. Endocr Pract. 2016;22(5):622–39. https://doi.org/10.4158/ep161208.Gl.
28. Haugen BR, Alexander EK, Bible KC, Doherty GM, Mandel SJ, Nikiforov YE, et al. 2015 American Thyroid Association management guidelines for adult patients with thyroid nodules and differentiated thyroid cancer: the American Thyroid Association guidelines task force on thyroid nodules and differentiated thyroid cancer. Thyroid. 2016;26(1):1–133. https://doi.org/10.1089/thy.2015.0020.
29. Russ G, Bonnema SJ, Erdogan MF, Durante C, Ngu R, Leenhardt L. European Thyroid Association guidelines for ultrasound malignancy risk stratification of thyroid nodules in adults: the EU-TIRADS. Eur Thyroid J. 2017;6(5):225–37. https://doi.org/10.1159/000478927.
30. Tessler FN, Middleton WD, Grant EG, Hoang JK, Berland LL, Teefey SA, et al. ACR thyroid imaging, reporting and data system (TI-RADS): white paper of the ACR TI-RADS Committee. J Am Coll Radiol. 2017;14(5):587–95. https://doi.org/10.1016/j.jacr.2017.01.046.
31. Alexander EK, Heering JP, Benson CB, Frates MC, Doubilet PM, Cibas ES, et al. Assessment of non-diagnostic ultrasound-guided fine needle aspirations of thyroid nodules. J Clin Endocrinol Metab. 2002;87(11):4924–7. https://doi.org/10.1210/jc.2002-020865.
32. Ma MKG, Ong GB. Cystic thyroid nodules. Br J Surg. 2005;62(3):205–6. https://doi.org/10.1002/bjs.1800620308.

33. Walfish PG, Hazani E, Strawbridge HTG, Miskin M, Rosen IB. A prospective study of combined ultrasonography and needle aspiration biopsy in the assessment of the hypofunctioning thyroid nodule. Surgery. 1977;82(4):474–82. https://doi.org/10.5555/uri:pii:0039606077901246.
34. Beech P, Lavender I, Jong I, Soo G, Ramdave S, Chong A, et al. Ultrasound stratification of the FDG-avid thyroid nodule. Clin Radiol. 2016;71(2):164–9. https://doi.org/10.1016/j.crad.2015.10.032.
35. Pattison DA, Bozin M, Gorelik A, Hofman MS, Hicks RJ, Skandarajah A. (18)F-FDG-avid thyroid incidentalomas: the importance of contextual interpretation. J Nucl Med. 2018;59(5):749–55. https://doi.org/10.2967/jnumed.117.198085.
36. Durante C, Hegedüs L, Czarniecka A, Paschke R, Russ G, Schmitt F, et al. 2023 European Thyroid Association clinical practice guidelines for thyroid nodule management. Eur Thyroid J. 2023;12(5):e230067. https://doi.org/10.1530/etj-23-0067.
37. Elisei R, Bottici V, Luchetti F, Di Coscio G, Romei C, Grasso L, et al. Impact of routine measurement of serum calcitonin on the diagnosis and outcome of medullary thyroid cancer: experience in 10,864 patients with nodular thyroid disorders. J Clin Endocrinol Metab. 2004;89(1):163–8. https://doi.org/10.1210/jc.2003-030550.
38. Durante C, Costante G, Lucisano G, Bruno R, Meringolo D, Paciaroni A, et al. The natural history of benign thyroid nodules. JAMA. 2015;313(9):926–35. https://doi.org/10.1001/jama.2015.0956.

Fine Needle Aspiration Biopsy and Core Needle Biopsy

5

Andrea Frasoldati and Simonetta Piana

5.1 Fine Needle Aspiration Biopsy

Originally introduced in the 1950s [1], thyroid fine needle aspiration biopsy (FNAB) has long been recognized as the first-line diagnostic tool for thyroid nodules. The adoption of ultrasound (US) guidance to enhance the accuracy of FNAB dates up the 1970–1980s [2] and nowadays, FNAB is routinely performed under US guidance. This is not surprising when we consider that thyroid nodule is currently defined as "a discrete lesion within the thyroid gland that is radiologically distinct from the surrounding thyroid parenchyma" [3]. In other terms, thyroid nodule is often a non-palpable lesion either visualized during US examination of the thyroid gland or incidentally spotted in the course of other imaging studies of the neck region [4, 5]. Furthermore, US plays a major role in the selection of nodules candidate to FNAB. Hence, FNAB necessarily requires to be performed under US guidance and, for practical purposes, in this chapter FNAB will be synonymous of US-guided FNAB.

5.1.1 Technique

FNAB can be performed according a variety of methods and techniques; therefore, different types of materials and devices may be used [6–9]. As well summarized by Daniel S. Duick and Susan J Mandel, literally, "there is no single best method of performing FNAB and many adaptations can be customized to individual situations" [6]. In the present section, some technical issues will be addressed with the aim of synthetizing what we know from the available evidence and what we have learned through our own experience.

5.1.2 How to Manage the Hyper-Vigilant Patients

5.1.2.1 Before Proceeding to FNAB

A successful FNAB procedure starts from the waiting room. In facts, a great proportion of our patients will experience a certain degree of anxiety, if not a major sense of fear, in undergoing FNAB. Notably, apart from texts specifically dedicate to thyroid FNAB [6–10], many well-written documents addressed to operators and patients are accessible online, which contain practical instructions and tips on how to manage

A. Frasoldati (✉)
Endocrinology Unit, Arcispedale S. Maria Nuova, Azienda USL-IRCCS di Reggio Emilia, Reggio Emilia, Italy
e-mail: Andrea.Frasoldati@ausl.re.it

S. Piana
Pathology Unit, Arcispedale S. Maria Nuova, Azienda USL-IRCCS di Reggio Emilia, Reggio Emilia, Italy
e-mail: Simonetta.Piana@ausl.re.it

R. Valcavi et al. (eds.), *Thyroid Ablation*, https://doi.org/10.1007/978-3-031-88229-6_5

the anxiety preceding biopsies and/or surgical procedures [11]. As a general premise, "life is the art of encounter," to quote the Brazilian poet and song composer Vinicius de Moraes [12]. In other words, all members of the medical and nurse staff should keep in mind that verbal as well as nonverbal communication skills are required to establish a proficient relationship with the patient [13]. Besides, a major attention should be paid by all operators to the respect of the time schedule. The patients in the waiting rooms should be timely informed of any delay and asked for collaboration. The degree of anxiety exhibited by the patient should possibly be anticipated and rated by the operators. A particular care should be reserved to the silent and apparently self-conscious patient, as an apathetic behavior may signal a major distress. The FNAB room should possibly be made an environment as much welcoming and warm as possible (soft music in the background may help) [14, 15].

5.1.2.2 The Importance of Complete Information

The clinical history of the patient with special attention to any medical conditions which may suggest a major caution in performing FNAB (e.g., increased risk of bleeding due to coagulopathy disorders and/or use of drugs which interfere with hemostasis and coagulation process) should be available to the operators and checked with the patient while having the informed consent signed [6–10]. This kind of information is usually explicated in the informed consent sheet, yet it is advisable to ask directly the patient about major health problems and/or ongoing drug therapies, as long-standing chronic disease and pharmacological treatments may often go unmentioned or be given for granted.

The FNAB procedure should be thoroughly described to the patient [6–10]. To this purpose, the patient should carefully read and subsequently sign a detailed, updated informed consent and all questions and doubts expressed by the patient need to be listened and tackled. The anxiety about the cytological result and its implications is usually as much important as the worries concerning the FNAB procedure. This issue can be effectively managed by explaining to the patient that, while performing FNA, you will evaluate the nodule and, at the end of the procedure, you will tell the patient your impressions.

Tell the patient that a mild pain/discomfort during the procedure is to be expected and gently ask not to move/mumble/swallow until the end of the maneuver. In doing this, try not to be intimidating and prescriptive: rather, the patients should feel fully involved in cooperating with the medical staff. Below, a list of practical tips:

- Show the patient that your attention is totally focused on her/him. Calling the patient by his/her first name is usually appreciated. Should you happen to be interrupted by a phone call or any other issues, tell the patient you will be back in a short while (ASAP).
- Avoid technical language: keep it simple while addressing the major concerns of the patient.
- Small talk and humor may help and do not make you less professional.
- Be empathic. Keep in mind that you deal everyday with FNAB/CNB procedure but for the patient this stuff is new and probably scary.

Last but not least, the US report by the clinician referring the patient for FNAB should be always available to the operators in charge of the procedure, in order to prevent any misunderstandings likely to compromise the clinical value of the test.

5.1.3 Materials and Procedure

5.1.3.1 Room and Patient Preparation

In the following paragraphs, some technical aspects of the FNA procedure will be briefly addressed. Before that, some general principles are to be recalled.

- FNAB room setup is a basic step. The availability of all the equipment (e.g., needles, syringes, slides, fixatives, ice packs) should be routinely checked before starting the FNAB/CNB session [6–10].

- The patient should be placed in a supine position with hyperextended neck [6–10]. Of course, due to a variety of factors, not all patients may assume the ideal position and the degree of hyperextension of the neck usually requires some negotiations: again, ask the patient to co-operate in finding a tolerable supine position.
- The adoption of anti-septic measures is mandatory: the skin should be carefully cleaned with chlorohexidine or ethanol or other products, disposable US probe cover sheaths are required and the operators should wear gloves also for protection purposes.
- Local anesthesia is not required on routine basis. As it may occasionally be helpful in some patients undergoing CNB or interventional procedures, materials for local anesthesia should be available in the operatory room [6–10].

5.1.3.2 Choice of the Needle Size/Type

FNA is usually performed using 25–27 gauge needles (Fig. 5.1). Some evidence in the literature points to the 25 gauge needles as the preferred ones although the adoption of 26–27 gauge needles may be associated with a lower rate of non-diagnostic results due to hematic contamination [6–10, 16–19]. On the other hand, larger needles may occasionally be required for drainage of viscous cystic content, or after a scarce sampling of a very firm nodule [6–10]. The use of stylet type needles (spinal needles) is profitable for FNA of posteriorly located, small lesion, because the stylet eases the straight penetration of the needle in the target tissue by making the needle stiffer. Of course, the stylet is left as far as the needle reaches the target and then is gently removed, thus avoiding uploading of cell material outside of the targeted area [6–10].

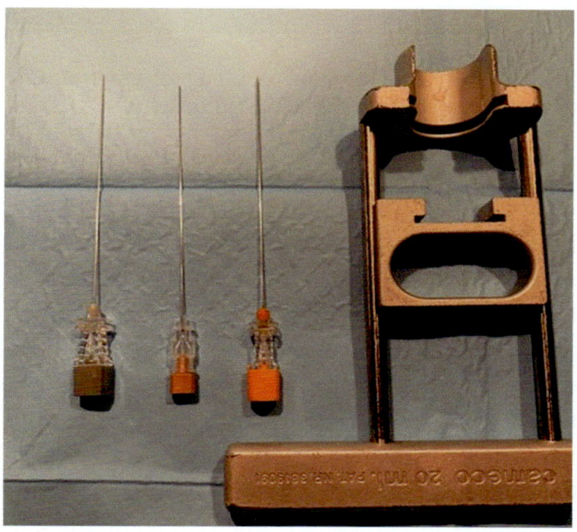

Fig. 5.1 25–27 gauge spinal needles and a Cameco pistol syringe-holder

5.1.3.3 US-Guided Approach and Visualization of the Needle

FNA can be performed either using a guiding device connected to the transducer or inserting the needle in a "free hand" manner, i.e. without any obliged trajectory of the needle [6–10]. In turn, the latter approach, more diffuse across different countries and institutions can be accomplished according two different ways: the "parallel" and the "perpendicular" approaches. In the parallel approach (Fig. 5.2), the needle is inserted at one extremity of the transducer, in parallel to the mid-plane of the long axis of the probe (sagittal plane). This approach permits to keep the needle in sight (and under full control) from its insertion throughout the entire manoeuver. In the perpendicular approach, the needle insertion into the skin and the target nodule are centered at the midpoint of the long axis of the transducer. The major problem with this approach is that the needle cannot be visualized during its penetration and descent towards the target. The needle tip will actually become visible only as it crosses the azimuthal plane of the probe. This approach may be simpler in case of superficially located nodules and may be preferred by very experienced operators because the choice of the correct angle of descent toward the nodule requires a significant skill. The routine use of US-guiding devices allows inserting the needle along a defined track, clearly visible on the US screen monitor. Although at our knowledge no systematic studies are available comparing the accuracy of FNA procedure with and without US-guiding devices, the latter approach may ensure a high precision in reaching the target

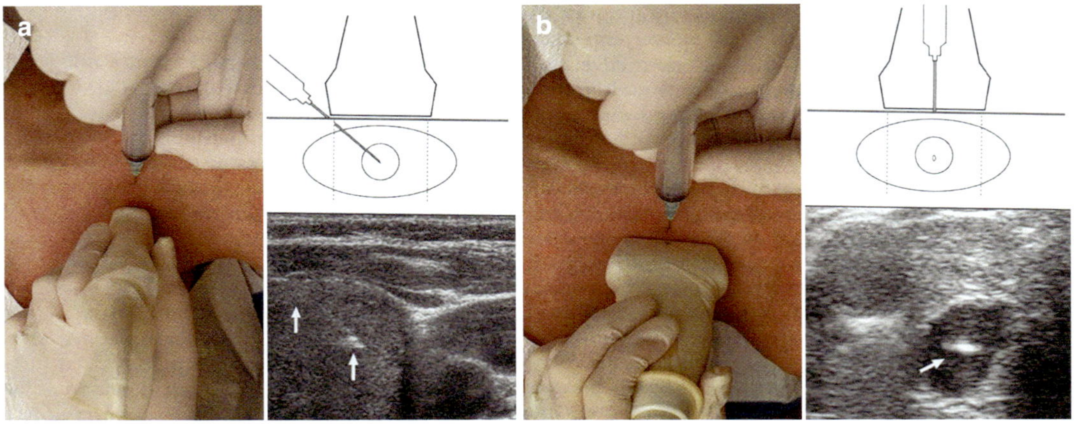

Fig. 5.2 US-guided needle insertion. (**a**) Parallel approach. The needle is inserted at one end of the transducer, in parallel to the mid-plane of the long axis of the probe (sagittal plane) and is always kept in sight along the entire procedure. (**b**) Perpendicular approach. The needle is targeted at the midpoint of the long axis of the transducer and its tip will only be visualized as it crosses the azimuthal plane of the probe. (*Modified from Duick DS, Mandel SJ (2008) Ultrasound Guided fine needle aspiration of thyroid nodules. In HJ Baskin, DS Duick, RA Levine (eds) Thyroid Ultrasound and Ultrasound guided FNA, 2nd ed. Springer New York, p 97-100* (6))

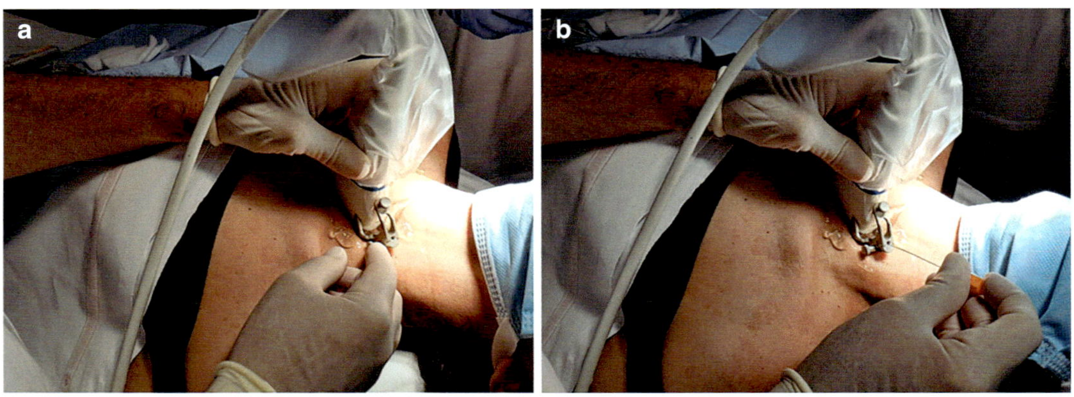

Fig. 5.3 FNAB using a needle-guiding device. (**a**) The guiding device is easily mounted over the probe protected by the sterile cover. (**b**) The needle is inserted along the device track ensuring alignment with the US imaging

lesion even when deeply located or extremely close to critical area (e.g., carotid artery). Besides, the procedure is usually more rapid and the learning curve for beginners shorter. Potential disadvantages are the higher costs (especially when disposable US-guiding devices are used) and reduced chances of adjusting the trajectory angle of the needle.

5.1.3.4 Aspiration or Capillarity?

Fundamentally, the sampling technique may be carried out either applying an active aspiration (suction) or using the capillarity principle [6–10]. While the former technique is usually accomplished with the aid of suction devices, like different types of syringe holders (which may render the maneuver a bit more complicated) (Fig. 5.1), according to the latter strategy, no suction is required and the operator simply waits for the sampling materials to spontaneously reach the needle hub (Fig. 5.3). Studies comparing the efficacy of the two techniques in terms of quality of the sampled material have obtained controversial results [16, 19–23]. In general, the routine use of suction allows the collection of a larger sample material, but this may be accompanied by a larger amount of blood that may cause a higher rate of non-diagnostic samples, especially in highly vascularized nodules. In most large spongiform nodules, aspiration is usually not necessary, whereas in small solid nodules, or in other type of target lesion, like lymph nodes or parathyroid adenomas, aspiration is generally required to avoid an insufficient sampling.

5.1.3.5 Safety

FNA is a safe procedure and major adverse events are anecdotal [6–10]. In a recently published systematic review, which included 23 studies, bleeding was reported in 0.0–6.4%, transient hoarseness in 0.03–0.9% and vase-vagal reaction in 0.02–1.3% of cases [24]. According to the available evidence, a relationship between the occurrence of bleeding and the use of antithrombotic/anticoagulant medications is questionable. The position shared by most authors is that preventive withdrawal of these classes of drugs is not always mandatory. Rather, it may be strongly advisable, if not recommended, in individual cases based on a number of factors, like the presumed degree of complexity of the procedure, mostly due to location and type of the target nodules, and the fragility of the patient [6–10].

5.2 Thyroid Cytology: Basic Notions

5.2.1 Slide Preparation

Biopsy samples obtained both by aspiration and capillarity are smeared onto glass slides for cytological examination (Fig. 5.4). As a rule, some slides are fixed in 95% ethanol for Papanicolaou staining and some are air-dried for May-Grunwald Giemsa staining, in order to emphasize nuclear and cytoplasmic characteristic of the cells, respectively. Alcohol-based fixatives are used in cytology due to their rapid action, ability to obscure blood, an overall improved morphology, and their feasibility for immunocytochemical staining. In case of cystic lesions, samples can be centrifuged at 1500 rpm for 5 min and sediment smears fixed in 95% alcohol and stained using the Papanicolaou method. Cytospin-based preparation, obtaining a consistent and reliable reduction in red cells, can represent an adjunct to standard glass slides. Cell-block material is a diagnostic tool which provides additional material for evaluation and ancillary studies and has been evaluated in many papers with good results. Cell-blocks can be obtained by using a simple sedimentation process. The specimens are therefore collected in formalin and then routinely processed into a paraffin block and stained with

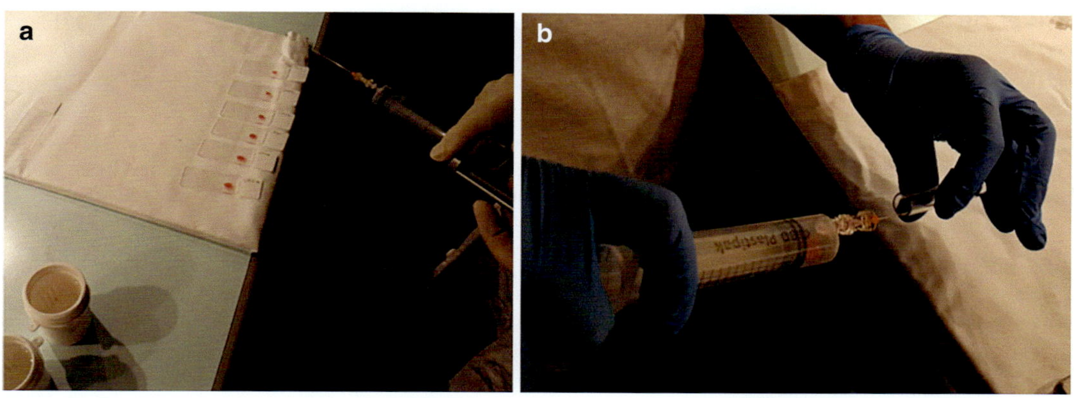

Fig. 5.4 Processing of samples obtained by FNA. (**a**) Cytological samples are gently collected onto slides before being smeared and subsequently alcohol-fixed and air-dried. (**b**) In selected cases, a small amount of the FNA sample can be collected for other purpose, as for instance hormonal (e.g., PTH, thyroglobulin, calcitonin) assay in the needle wash-outs.

hematoxylin and eosin. Cell-blocks are especially suitable when an immunocytochemical confirmation is desirable. Both stained slides and cell-blocks can be used for biomolecular prognostic and predictive analyses [25, 26].

5.2.2 Cytological Reporting Systems

The use of a standardized terminology for cytological diagnostic categories is critical for the correct interpretation of the cytological reports as well as to establish evidence-driven algorithms for the appropriate clinical management of different categories of thyroid nodules. Three major reporting systems for thyroid cytopathology, the British Thyroid Association and Royal College of Pathologists (Thy) [27], the Bethesda System for Reporting Thyroid Cytopathology [28], and the Italian Consensus (TIR) [29], are currently used in Italy. All these nomenclatures utilize a tiered system (five categories in the British and the Italian schemes and six categories in the Bethesda system) and have undergone some updating through the years [30]. The use of a standardized system is especially important in indeterminate cases, characterized by a highly variable incidence in different centres and institutions. The adoption of a unique international system with a common unique terminology would be desirable, and it would help in adjusting cytological criteria to the recent update in histological classification of thyroid neoplasms [31, 32]

5.2.3 Data Analysis and Cyto-histological Correlations

Regardless to the reporting system adopted, the systematic analysis of the distribution of cytological diagnoses within each different category (Table 5.1) as well as the constant monitoring of the correlation of cytological results with histological reports (Table 5.2) are of paramount importance in order to evaluate FNAB performance at one's own institution and to plan any possible implementation [33, 34]. More important, it should be underlined that thyroid FNAB is a team effort and a good, effective com-

Table 5.1 FNA Series at Reggio Emilia ASMN Hospital (2017–2021)

BTA class	2017 (*n*)	%	2018	%	2019	%	2020	%	2021	%	Total
THY1	320	12,9%	320	14,4%	264	12,4%	190	11,5%	302	12.5%	904
THY2	1937	77,8%	1731	77,8%	1656	78,0%	1.298	78,7%	1874	78.7%	5324
THY3a	51	2,0%	51	2,3%	51	2,4%	45	2,7%	54	2,4%	153
THY3f	91	3,7%	50	2,2%	60	2,8%	49	3,0%	57	2,4%	201
THY4	22	0,9%	16	0,7%	21	1,0%	14	0,8%	16	0,4%	59
THY5	68	2,7%	57	2,6%	71	3,3%	54	3,3%	103	4,3%	196
	2489		2225		2123		1650		2407		6837

Cytological reports are here classified according to the British Thyroid Association (BTA) reporting system [27]. Thy1 category includes also Thy1c cytological samples (= cystic nodules). Monitoring of cytological results on yearly basis permits to detect major shifts from the standard values and to implement corrective actions, when necessary

Table 5.2 Cyto-histological correlations. Reported data are referred to a 12 month-period at ASMN Reggio Emilia. Cytological smears are classified according to BTA [27]. As for cytological reports, systematic monitoring of cyto-histological correlations permits to evaluate FNA performance as well as the appropriateness of surgical referral

Histological reports	Cytological category						
	THY1	THY2	THY3a	THY3f	THY4	THY5	Total
Benign	2	14	4	8	0	0	30
Malignant	1	2	21	6	10	81	121
Not operated	198	1786	25	42	6	22	2077
Total	201	1802	50	56	16	103	2228

munication between the referring endocrinologists (physicians) and the pathologists is a fundamental prerequisite for a high-quality standard of thyroid FNAB [35].

5.3 Core Needle Biopsy

First systematic studies suggesting a potential role of CNB in the diagnosis of thyroid nodules date up to the 1990s [36–38]. Although other series of thyroid nodules diagnosed by CNB were from time to time published in the following years [39–41], a large-scale diffusion of CNB in the clinical management of thyroid nodules has not occurred, seemingly due to its higher potential harmfulness as compared to FNAB, as well as the lack of a clear diagnostic superiority. Instead, CNB has traditionally been confined to circumscribed clinical settings, likewise large thyroid masses suspicious for rare malignancies [3, 42, 43]. In the last decade, however, thyroid CNB has captured a growing interest to the point that some consensus documents have included thyroid nodules with inconclusive FNAB results among the indications for CNB [44, 45]. Besides, in some Korean and Chinese institutions, CNB has become a first-line diagnostic tool alternative to FNAB in the management of patients presenting with thyroid nodules [46–48].

5.3.1 Technique

Commercially available CNB devices usually utilize 18–21 gauge spring-activated needles. Although studies focused on possible variations in CNB performance using different needle bores have not provided definite results, the common experience is that the thinner the needles, the lower the amount of target tissue obtained in the bioptic specimen [44, 45]. Typically, CNB devices are composed of an inner needle (the "stylet") which carries a sharply profiled tip and a notch deputed to harbor the collected specimen, and of an outer needle (the "cutting cannula") which cuts and tears the tissue allowing the sampling of the tissue specimen. Fundamentally, two types of device based on a different mechanism of action and respectively defined as "automated" or "semi-automated" are available. In the automated devices, also defined as "double action," both the inner and the outer needles are spring-activated, whereas in the semi-automated devices, the inner needle is manually pushed into the tissue by the operator and only the cutting cannula is actioned by the spring (Fig. 5.5) [44, 45].

On the one hand, semi-automated devices are commonly considered to some extent safer, as the operator controls the precise positioning of the tip of the inner needle. Yet, the automated double-action devices may be more efficient should very hard, calcific, and/or fibrotic nodules be targeted [49]. As for FNAB, the needle insertion can take place using a US-guiding device or in a "free hand" manner. Of course, a much greater care is required with CNB as compared to FNAB due to the potential harmfulness of large spring-action needles (Fig. 5.6). To this purpose, US examination of the neck region must include an accurate mapping of major vessels and other critical anatomic structures located nearby the expected route of the needle. After collection, the specimen should be immediately fixed in formalin. Usually, at least two specimens are required to obtain a satisfactory bioptic sample [44, 45].

5.3.2 Clinical Use

5.3.2.1 Safety

A cumulative 4.1% complication rate was reported in the 2019 Korean Practice Guidelines for thyroid CNB, but that consensus paper also included older and small size studies [45]. A systematic review of 39 studies (14818 patients) demonstrated a 0.04% and a 1.2% rate of major and minor complications, respectively [50], observations substantially in line with another meta-analysis on over 9000 patients (13585 nodules) which reported a 0.02% and a 1.1% of major and minor complications, respectively [51]. The rate of major and minor complications reported after CNB in other recent studies are listed in Table 5.3

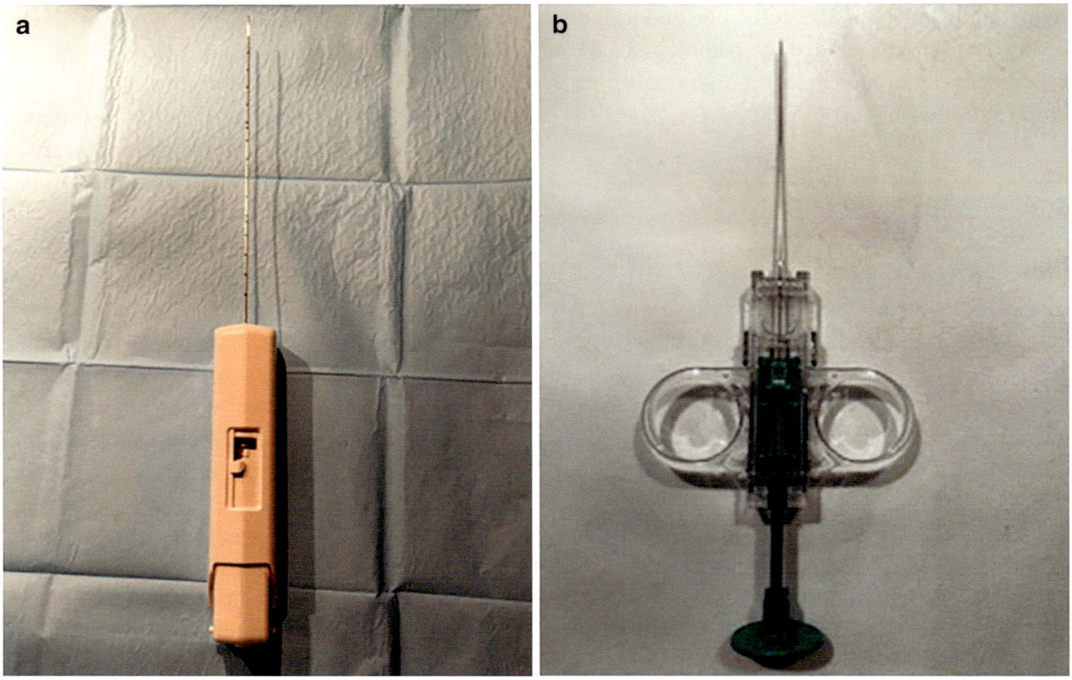

Fig. 5.5 Automated (**a**) and semi-automated (**b**) spring-activated devices for CNB

[52–55]. In all, with a rate of major complications ranging from 0.00 to 0.09% and a rate of minor complications ranging from 0.2 to 2.8%, these data confirm that CNB can be considered a safe procedure in experienced hands. Among the major complications are hematomas requiring hospital admission, permanent voice changes, and pseudoaneurysms [50–55]. In general, whereas the rate of major complication is comparably as low as that observed after FNAB, it should be underlined that the potential severity of complications reported with CNB is higher.

5.3.2.2 CNB in Thyroid Nodules with Inconclusive FNAB Results

One major point of strength of CNB as a diagnostic tool for thyroid nodules resides in the low rate (0.7–5.5%) of non-diagnostic samples [46, 47, 51, 53, 54, 56–58]. Studies in nodules with an initial non-diagnostic FNAB results, consistently show that CNB provides a higher diagnostic rate (91.7–98.8%) as compared to repeat FNAB [59–61] (Table 5.4), although a fraction of CNB results (i.e., 7.8–25.6%) in these series falls in the "indeterminate" category. Interestingly, the diagnostic value of CNB alone or as a complement to FNAB seems elevated also in calcific nodules [49, 62].

About 10–15% of thyroid nodules exhibit an indeterminate cytology, which may encompass a range of cytological pattern, from the Bethesda III (AUS/FLUS) to the Bethesda IV (follicular neoplasms) classes. CNB has been extensively evaluated in this clinical setting, with controversial results [61, 63–73]. In general, most evidence indicates that CNB provides a higher rate of conclusive results; when the analysis is limited to Bethesda III-IV (i.e., Thy 3 according to the BTA classification and Tir3 according to the Italian classification) nodules, the advantages of CNB seem less consistent.

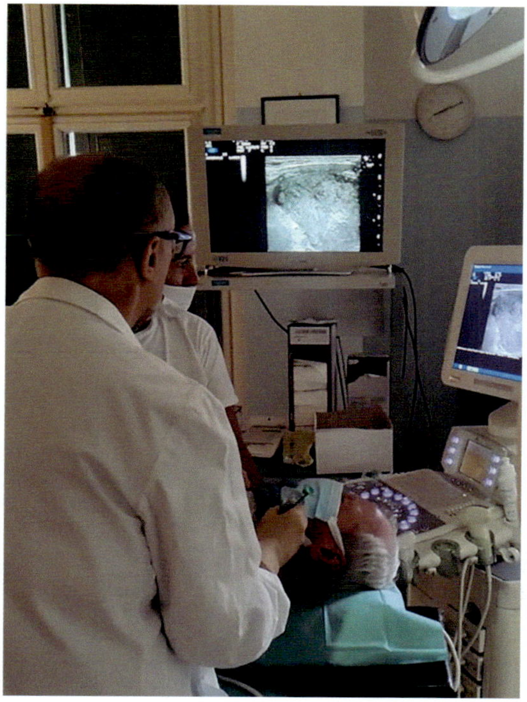

Fig. 5.6 CNB of a thyroid mass: operative setting CNB of a large inhomogeneous thyroid mass suspicious for thyroid lymphoma in an elderly patient. The procedure is performed using a semi-automated spring-activated device. The needle is manually inserted using an US-guiding device connected to the probe; its trajectory into the lesion is cautiously kept under sight on the monitor, until spring activation induces instantaneous, automated tissue sampling

5.3.2.3 CNB in Rare Thyroid Malignancies: Metastases, Thyroid Lymphoma (TL), and Anaplastic Thyroid Carcinoma (ATC)

Metastases to the thyroid gland are usually considered an uncommon finding, yet autoptic series report up to a 24% frequency of metastasis to the thyroid gland in patients deceased for non-thyroid malignancies [74–82]. In a multi-centric retrospective study, 62 cases of metastasis to the thyroid gland were found out of over 4000 patients undergoing FNAB for thyroid "nodules" which corresponded to a 0.16% frequency and a 1.9% rate of all cytologically malignant cases [83]. Kidney, lung, breast, and gastrointestinal tract are the primary tumor sites more frequently involved, with about 25% of cases originating from less common sites [78–80]. In most instances, the detection of thyroid metastasis takes place in the follow-up of patients with advanced, metastatic cancer, but in 25–30% cases it may represent an incidental finding. In some patients, the diagnosis of a thyroid metastasis may actually be the clue to the diagnosis of the primary tumor [75, 79, 81, 82].

At US examination, thyroid metastatic lesions usually present as hypoechoic, solid nodules, often with a large (>25–30 mm maximum diameter) size and an intense, predominantly peripheral, but also intranodular vascularity [82, 84–86]. The texture is often inhomogenous; a mixed pattern, which may mimic a benign colloid cystic nodule, is unusual but may occasionally be seen. Interestingly, in some series, the appearance of the majority (70–80%) of the metastatic lesions is defined as "diffuse" and not properly "nodular" [82, 84–86]. The shape of the lesion is usually oval/round, with margins described as ill-defined and/or with minor irregularities. Microcalcifications are an infrequent finding [82, 84–86]. In other terms, US features do not always identify the metastasis as a suspicious nodule/mass; a significant fraction of these lesions may be categorized on US basis as indeterminate, if not likely benign [85]. Hence, while US examination may induce at least to consider a metastatic disease in patients with a known oncological clinical history, in some cases the suspicion of metastasis may be raised only at cytological examination. Unfortunately, FNAB may not achieve a clear diagnosis in up to 24–33% of cases [74, 82, 83, 85–87]. In metastatic lesions to the thyroid, CNB show a markedly superior sensitivity as compared to FNA since CNB may provide detailed information on the architectural pattern of the lesion and on its immunohistochemical characterization [87, 88] (Fig. 5.7). Therefore, in selected cases of oncological patients presenting with a large, solid hypoechoic, thyroid nodule, CNB should be considered a complementary tool to FNAB.

In light of its high sensitivity (about 85–90%), CNB has long been recognized as a first-line diagnostic tool in patients presenting with large

Table 5.3 Major and minor complication rates of CNB

	Study design	Patients (nodules)	Major complications	Minor complications
Suh et al. (2016) [46]	Retrospective	4553 (4822)	0.03%	0.58%
Ha et al. (2017) [52]	Retrospective	6169 (6687)	0.06%	1.08%
Hong et al. (2018) [48]	Retrospective	714 (782)	0.00%	0.60%
Paja et al. (2019) [53]	Retrospective	3768 (4112)	0.09%	2.20%
Hong et al. (2020) [47]	Prospective	212 (248)	0.00%	2.80%
Aysan et al. (2022) [54]	Retrospective	3000 (3000)	0.00%	0.20%

Table 5.4 CNB in thyroid nodules with previous Thy 1 FNA results. Non-diagnostic results are confirmed only in a minority of patients (last column)

	Nodules (*n*)	Benign	Indeterminate	Suspicious/ malignant	Non-diagnostic
Choi et al. (2014) [59]	180	58.9%	7.8%	32.2%	1.1%
Yi (2015) [49]	40	77.5%	10.0%	7.5%	5.0%
Cortázar-García et al. (2020) [60]	195	62.5%	25.6%	3.6%	8.3%
Jung et al. (2021) [61]	150	69.8%	15.1%	3.2%	3.8%

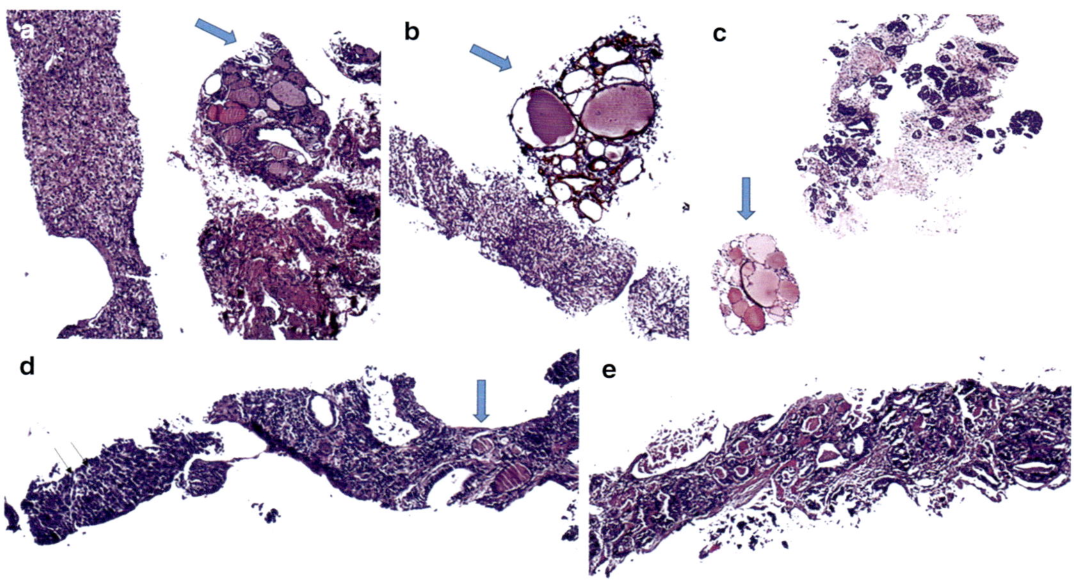

Fig. 5.7 Histological samples obtained by CNB. (**a**) Metastasis from a renal carcinoma with a solid pattern of growth. Few residual thyroid follicles are present on the right (arrow). (**b**) Metastasis from a melanoma. Again, the biopsy includes some unremarkable thyroid follicles (arrow). (**c**) Metastasis from an ovarian high-grade serous carcinoma, growing in small papillae. Few residual thyroid follicles are visible (arrow). (**d**) Metastasis from a lung squamous cell carcinoma (double arrows). In this case, rare follicles are still recognizable (arrow). (**e**) Metastasis from a colorectal adenocarcinoma. Despite the follicular appearance and the colloid-like content of the glands, all the tissue is neoplastic and no thyroid follicles are present

thyroid masses suspicious for thyroid lymphoma (TL) and anaplastic thyroid carcinoma (ATC) [89] (Fig. 5.6). In a recently published meta-analysis including 17 reports (166 patients), a 94% and 80% sensitivity were, respectively, reported for CNB in patients with TL and ATC, respectively [90]. In line with the above results, in a retrospective series of patients with large suspicious thyroid masses, diagnosis of TL was correctly achieved in 12 out of 13 cases by CNB whereas a precise diagnosis of ATC was allowed by FNAB only in a fraction (17.1%) of patients [91]. Data obtained from a series of large suspicious thyroid masses ($n = 59$) contemporarily submitted to FNA and CNB along the last two decades at our hospital are in line with the above reported evidence. In thyroid metastases, TL and ATC, CNB showed a sensitivity of 90.0%, 91.6%, and 94.7%, whereas FNAB sensitivity was confined to 70%, 50%, and 84.2%, respectively (unpublished data).

References

1. Soderstrom N. Puncture of goitres for aspiration biopsy: a preliminary report. Acta Med Scand. 1952;144:235–44. https://doi.org/10.1111/j.0954-6820.1952.tb15690.x.
2. Walfish PG, Hazani E, Strawbridge HT, Miskin M, Rosen IB. Combined ultrasound and needle aspiration cytology in the assessment and management of hypofunctioning thyroid nodule. Ann Intern Med. 1977;87:270–4. https://doi.org/10.7326/0003-4819-87-3-270_1.
3. Haugen BR, Alexander EK, Bible KC, Doherty GM, Mandel SJ, Nikiforov YE, et al. American Thyroid Association management guidelines for adult patients with thyroid nodules and differentiated thyroid cancer. Thyroid. 2016;26:1–133. https://doi.org/10.1089/thy.2015.0020.
4. Russ G, Leboulleux S, Leenhardt L, Hegedüs L. Thyroid incidentalomas: epidemiology, risk stratification with ultrasound and workup. Eur Thyroid J. 2014;3:154–63. https://doi.org/10.1159/000365289.
5. Fisher SB, Perrier ND. The incidental thyroid nodule. CA Cancer J Clin. 2018;68:97–105. https://doi.org/10.3322/caac.21447.
6. Duick DS, Mandel SJ. Ultrasound guided fine needle aspiration of thyroid nodules. In: Baskin HJ, Duick DS, Levine RA, editors. Thyroid ultrasound and ultrasound guided FNA. 2nd ed. Boston: Springer; 2008. p. 97–100. https://doi.org/10.1007/978-0-387-77634-7_7.
7. Levine RA, Interlandi J. The procedure of ultrasound guided percutaneous biopsy of thyroid and cervical lymph nodes: technical steps, pitfalls and pearls. In: Milas M, Mandel SJ, Langer JF, editors. Advanced thyroid and parathyroid ultrasound. Cham: Springer; 2017. p. 309–32. https://doi.org/10.1007/978-3-319-44100-9_28.
8. Sacks B. Thyroid fine needle aspiration and biopsy technique for lesions in the neck. In: Eldeiry LS, Laver NMV, Randolph GW, Sacks B, Garber JR, editors. Handbook of thyroid and neck ultrasonography. Cham: Springer Nature; 2023. p. 53–68. https://doi.org/10.1007/978-3-031-18448-2_3.
9. Jasim S, Dean DS, Gharib H. Fine-needle aspiration of the thyroid gland. [Updated 2023 Mar 23]. In: Feingold KR, Anawalt B, Blackman MR, et al., editors. Endotext [internet]. South Dartmouth: MDText.com, Inc.; 2000. https://www.ncbi.nlm.nih.gov/books/NBK285544/.
10. Smith T, Kaufman CS. Ultrasound guided thyroid biopsy. Tech Vasc Interv Radiol. 2021;24(3):100768. https://doi.org/10.1016/j.tvir.2021.100768.
11. What can help relieve anxiety before surgery? 2006 [Updated 2018 Feb 8]. InformedHealth.org [internet]. Cologne: Institute for Quality and Efficiency in Health Care (IQWiG); 2006. https://www.ncbi.nlm.nih.gov/books/NBK279557/.
12. de Moraes V, Powell B. "Samba da Bênção" (from the Album "Vinicius", 1967).
13. Miller LS, Shelby RA, Balmadrid MH, Yoon S, Baker JA, Wildermann L, Soo MS. Patient anxiety before and immediately after imaging-guided breast biopsy procedures: impact of radiologist-patient communication. J Am Coll Radiol. 2013;10:423–31. https://doi.org/10.1016/j.jacr.2012.11.005.
14. Bradt J, Dileo C, Shim M. Music interventions for preoperative anxiety. Cochrane Database Syst Rev. 2013;2013(6):CD006908. https://doi.org/10.1002/14651858.cd006908.pub2.
15. Ashour ASA, Abd-ElGawad M, Yohanna M, El-Nagar M, Fadl AN, et al. Is music intervention effective in reducing anxiety and pain during breast biopsy procedure? A systematic review and meta-analysis of randomized controlled trials. Support Care Cancer. 2022;30:10379–89. https://doi.org/10.1007/s00520-022-07414-7.
16. Cerit M, Yücel C, Göçün PU, Poyraz A, Cerit ET, Taneri F. Ultrasound-guided thyroid nodule fine-needle biopsies—comparison of sample adequacy with different sampling techniques, different needle sizes, and with/without onsite cytological analysis. Endokrynol Pol. 2015;66:295–300. https://doi.org/10.5603/ep.2015.0037.
17. Dong Y, Gao L, Sui Y, Mao M, Zhan W, Zhou J. Comparison of ultrasound-guided fine-needle cytology quality in thyroid nodules with 22-, 23-, and 25-gauge needles. Anal Cell

Pathol (Amst). 2021;2021:5544921. https://doi.org/10.1155/2021/5544921.
18. Saraph S, Cohen H, Ronen O. Effect of needle gauge on thyroid FNA diagnostic rate. Endocrine. 2021;74:625–31. https://doi.org/10.1007/s12020-021-02797-9.
19. Wang CY, Zhou Y, Ren YY, Luan YS, Jiang ZC, Wang ZX. Analysis of the influencing factors on fine-needle aspiration biopsy results of the thyroid. Front Surg. 2022;9:907086. https://doi.org/10.3389/fsurg.2022.907086.
20. Tublin ME, Martin JA, Rollin LJ, Pealer K, Kurs-Lasky M, Ohori NP. Ultrasound-guided fine-needle aspiration versus fine-needle capillary sampling biopsy of thyroid nodules: does technique matter? J Ultrasound Med. 2007;26:1697–701. https://doi.org/10.7863/jum.2007.26.12.1697.
21. Song H, Wei C, Li D, Hua K, Song J, Maskey N, Fang L. Comparison of fine needle aspiration and fine needle nonaspiration cytology of thyroid nodules: a meta-analysis. Biomed Res Int. 2015;2015:796120. https://doi.org/10.1155/2015/796120.
22. Zhou JQ, Zhang JW, Zhan WW, Zhou W, Ye TJ, Zhu Y, et al. Comparison of fine-needle aspiration and fine-needle capillary sampling of thyroid nodules: a prospective study with emphasis on the influence of nodule size. Cancer Cytopathol. 2014;122:266–73. https://doi.org/10.1002/cncy.21382.
23. Archana E, Vijayakumar C, Raj Kumar N, Balasubramanian G, Srinivasan K, Sreenath GS, et al. Comparative study of fine-needle aspiration and non-aspiration cytology diagnosis in thyroid lesions. Niger J Surg. 2020;26:147–52. https://doi.org/10.4103/njs.NJS_29_20.
24. Park JI, Choi W, Hong AR, Yoon LH, Kim HK, Kang H-C. Comprehensive assessment of the harms of fine-needle aspiration biopsy for thyroid nodules: a systematic review. Endocrinol Metab. 2023;38:104–16. https://doi.org/10.3803/EnM.2023.1669.
25. Baloch ZW, Cibas ES, Clark DP, Layfield LJ, Ljung BM, Pitman MB, et al. The National Cancer Institute thyroid fine needle aspiration state of the science conference: a summation. Cytojournal. 2008;5:6. https://doi.org/10.1186/1742-6413-5-6.
26. Vance J, Dubin K, Manglik N, Gilani SM. Diagnostic utility of cell block in fine needle aspiration cytology of thyroid gland. Diagn Cytopathol. 2019;47:1245–50. https://doi.org/10.1002/dc.24304.
27. Cross P, Chandra A, Giles T, Johnson S, Kocjan G, Poller D, Stephenson T. Guidance on the reporting of thyroid cytology specimens. Royal College of Pathologists; 2019. https://www.rcpath.org/static/d40af26c-0e49-4d40-8fce4a38f2a5c44b/G089-Guidance-on-the-reporting-of-thyroid-cytology-specimensFor-Publication.pdf.
28. Cibas ES, Ali SZ. The Bethesda system for reporting thyroid cytopathology. Thyroid. 2019;19:1159–65. https://doi.org/10.1089/thy.2017.0500.
29. Nardi F, Basolo F, Crescenzi A, Fadda G, Frasoldati A, Orlandi F, et al. Italian consensus for the classification and reporting of thyroid cytology. J Endocrinol Invest. 2014;37:593–9. https://doi.org/10.1007/s40618-014-0062-0.
30. Collins J, Rossi ED, Chandra A, Ali SZ. Terminology and nomenclature schemes for reporting thyroid cytopathology: an overview. Semin Diagn Pathol. 2015;32:258–63. https://doi.org/10.1053/j.semdp.2014.12.007.
31. Poller DN, Cochand-Priollet B, Trimboli P. Thyroid FNA terminology: the case for a single unified international system for thyroid FNA reporting. Cytopathology. 2021;32:714–7. https://doi.org/10.1111/cyt.13017.
32. Rossi ED, Baloch Z. The impact of the 2022 WHO classification of thyroid neoplasms on everyday practice of cytopathology. Endocr Pathol. 2023;34:23–33. https://doi.org/10.1007/s12022-023-09756-2.
33. Piana S, Frasoldati A, Ferrari M, Valcavi R, Froio E, Barbieri V, et al. Is a five-category reporting scheme for thyroid fine needle aspiration cytology accurate? Experience of over 18,000 FNAs reported at the same institution during 1998-2007. Cytopathology. 2011;22:164–73. https://doi.org/10.1111/j.1365-2303.2010.00777.x.
34. Torregrossa L, Poma AM, Macerola E, Rago T, Vignali P, Romani R, et al. The Italian consensus for the classification and reporting of thyroid cytology: cytohistologic and molecular correlations on 37,371 nodules from a single institution. Cancer Cytopathol. 2022;130:899–912. https://doi.org/10.1002/cncy.22618.
35. Oertel YC. Fine needle aspiration of the thyroid: a pathologist's perspective. J Clin Pathol. 2008;61:785–6. https://doi.org/10.1136/jcp.2008.057216.
36. Quinn SF, Nelson HA, Demlow TA. Thyroid biopsies: fine-needle aspiration biopsy versus spring-activated core biopsy needle in 102 patients. J Vasc Interv Radiol. 1994;5:619–23. https://doi.org/10.1016/s1051-0443(94)71565-7.
37. Liu Q, Castelli M, Gattuso P, Prinz RA. Simultaneous fine-needle aspiration and core-needle biopsy of thyroid nodules. Am Surg. 1995;61:628–32.
38. Taki S, Kakuda K, Kakuma K, Annen Y, Katada S, Yamashita R, et al. Thyroid nodules: evaluation with US-guided core biopsy with an automated biopsy gun. Radiology. 1997;202:874–7. https://doi.org/10.1148/radiology.202.3.9051050.
39. Screaton NJ, Berman LH, Grant JW. US-guided core-needle biopsy of the thyroid gland. Radiology. 2003;226:827–32. https://doi.org/10.1148/radiol.2263012073.
40. Novoa E, Gurtler N, Arnoux A, Kraft M. Role of ultrasound-guided core-needle biopsy in the assessment of head and neck lesions: a meta-analysis and systematic review of the literature. Head Neck. 2012;34:1497–503. https://doi.org/10.1002/hed.21821.
41. Trimboli P, Nasrollah N, Guidobaldi L, Taccogna S, Cicciarella Modica DD, et al. The use of core

needle biopsy as first-line in diagnosis of thyroid nodules reduces false negative and inconclusive data reported by fine-needle aspiration. World J Surg Oncol. 2014;12:61–6. https://doi.org/10.1186/1477-7819-12-61.
42. Perros P, Boelaert K, Colley S, Evans C, Evans RM, Gerrard Ba G, et al. Guidelines for the management of thyroid cancer. Clin Endocrinol. 2014;81(Suppl 1):1–122. https://doi.org/10.1111/cen.12515.
43. Gharib H, Papini E, Garber JR, Duick DS, Harrel RM, Hegedus L, et al. American Association of Clinical Endocrinologists, American College of Endocrinology, and Associazione Medici Endocrinologi medical guidelines for clinical practice for the diagnosis and management of thyroid nodules: 2016 update. Endocr Pract. 2016;22:622–39. https://doi.org/10.4158/ep161208.gl.
44. Na DG, Baek JH, Jung SL, Kim J-H, Sung JY, Kim KS, et al. Core needle biopsy of the thyroid: 2016 consensus statement and recommendations from Korean Society of Thyroid Radiology. Korean J Radiol. 2017;18:217–37. https://doi.org/10.3348/kjr.2017.18.1.217.
45. Jung CK, Baek JH, Na DG, Oh YL, Yi KH, Kang H-C. 2019 practice guidelines for thyroid core needle biopsy: a report of the Clinical Practice Guidelines Development Committee of the Korean Thyroid Association. J Pathol Transl Med. 2020;54:64–86. https://doi.org/10.4132/jptm.2019.12.04.
46. Suh CH, Baek JH, Lee JH, ,Choi HJ, Kim JK, Sung T-Y et al. The role of core-needle biopsy as a first-line diagnostic tool for initially detected thyroid nodules. Thyroid 2016;26: 395–403. https://doi.org/10.1089/thy.2015.0404.
47. Hong MJ, Na DG, Kim SJ, Kim DS. Role of core needle biopsy as a first-line diagnostic tool for thyroid nodules: a retrospective cohort study. Ultrasonography. 2018;37:244–53. https://doi.org/10.14366/usg.17041.
48. Hong MJ, Na DG, Lee H. Diagnostic efficacy and safety of core needle biopsy as a first-line diagnostic method for thyroid nodules: a prospective cohort study. Thyroid. 2020;115:1141–9. https://doi.org/10.1089/thy.2019.0444.
49. Yi KS, Kim JH, Na DG, Seo H, Min HS, Won JK, et al. Usefulness of core needle biopsy for thyroid nodules with macrocalcifications: comparison with fine-needle aspiration. Thyroid. 2015;25:657–64. https://doi.org/10.1089/thy.2014.0596.
50. Ha EJ, Suh CH, Baek JH. Complications following ultrasound guided core needle biopsy of thyroid nodules: a systematic review and meta-analysis. Eur Radiol. 2018;28:3848–60. https://doi.org/10.1007/s00330-018-5367-5.
51. Chung SR, Suh CH, Baek JH, Choi YJ, Lee JH. The role of core needle biopsy in the diagnosis of initially detected thyroid nodules: a systematic review and meta-analysis. Eur Radiol. 2018;28:4909–18. https://doi.org/10.1007/s00330-018-5494-z.
52. Ha EJ, Baek JH, Lee JH, Kim JK, Choi YJ, Sung TY, et al. Complications following US-guided core-needle biopsy for thyroid lesions: a retrospective study of 6,169 consecutive patients with 6,687 thyroid nodules. Eur Radiol. 2017;27:1186–94. https://doi.org/10.1007/s00330-018-5367-5.
53. Paja M, Del Cura JL, Zabala R, Korta I, Ugalde A, Lopez JI. Core needle biopsy in thyroid nodules: performance, accuracy, and complications. Eur Radiol. 2019;29:4889–96. https://doi.org/10.1007/s00330-019-06038-6.
54. Aysan E, Guler B, Kiran T, Idiz UO. Core needle biopsy in the diagnosis of thyroid nodules. Am Surg. 2023;89:5170–4. https://doi.org/10.1177/00031348221142570.
55. Choe J, Baek JH, Park HS, Choi YJ, Lee JH. Core needle biopsy of thyroid nodules: outcomes and safety from a large single-center single-operator study. Acta Radiol. 2018;59:924–31. https://doi.org/10.1177/0284185117741916.
56. Liu N, Meng Z, Jia Q, He X, Tian W, Tan J, et al. Ultrasound-guided core needle biopsy for differential diagnosis of thyroid nodules: a systematic review and meta-analysis. Mol Clin Oncol. 2017;6:825–32. https://doi.org/10.3892/mco.2017.1246.
57. Wolinski K, Stangierski A, Ruchala M. Comparison of diagnostic yield of core-needle and fine-needle aspiration biopsies of thyroid lesions: Systematic review and meta-analysis. Eur Radiol. 2017;27:431–6. https://doi.org/10.1007/s00330-016-4356-9.
58. Lan L, Luo Y, Zhou M, Huo L, Chen H, Zuo Q, et al. Comparison of diagnostic accuracy of thyroid cancer with ultrasound-guided fine-needle aspiration and core-needle biopsy: a systematic review and meta-analysis. Front Endocrinol. 2020;13(11):44. https://doi.org/10.3389/fendo.2020.00044.
59. Choi SH, Baek JH, Lee JH, Choi YJ, Hong MJ, Song DE, et al. Thyroid nodules with initially nondiagnostic, fine-needle aspiration results: comparison of core-needle biopsy and repeated fine-needle aspiration. Eur Radiol. 2014;24:2819–26. https://doi.org/10.1007/s00330-014-3325-4.
60. Cortázar-García R, Martín-Escalante MD, Robles-Cabeza L, Martínez-Santos C. Usefulness of ultrasound-guided core biopsy in thyroid nodules with inconclusive fine-needle aspiration biopsy findings. Radiologia (Engl Ed). 2022;64:195–205. https://doi.org/10.1016/j.rxeng.2020.06.005.
61. Jung SM, Koo HR, Jang KS, Chung MS, Song CM, Ji YB, Park JS, et al. Comparison of core-needle biopsy and repeat fine-needle aspiration for thyroid nodules with inconclusive initial cytology. Eur Arch Otorhinolaryngol. 2021;278:3019–25. https://doi.org/10.1007/s00405-020-06473-y.
62. Na DG, Kim DS, Kim SJ, Ryoo JW, Jung SL. Thyroid nodules with isolated macrocalcification: malignancy risk and diagnostic efficacy of fine-needle aspiration and core needle biopsy. Ultrasonography. 2016;35:212–9. https://doi.org/10.14366/usg.15074.
63. Na DG, Kim JH, Sung JY, Baek JH, Jung KC, Lee H, et al. Core-needle biopsy is more useful than repeat fine-needle aspiration in thyroid nodules read

as nondiagnostic or atypia of undetermined significance by the Bethesda system for reporting thyroid cytopathology. Thyroid. 2012;22:468–75. https://doi.org/10.1089/thy.2011.0185.
64. Min HS, Kim JH, Ryoo I, Jung SL, Jung CK. The role of core needle biopsy in the preoperative diagnosis of follicular neoplasm of the thyroid. APMIS. 2012;122:993–1000. https://doi.org/10.1111/apm.12244.
65. Na DG, Min HS, Lee H, Won JK, Seo HB, Kim JH. Role of core needle biopsy in the management of atypia/follicular lesion of undetermined significance thyroid nodules: comparison with repeat fine-needle aspiration in subcategory nodules. Eur Thyroid J. 2015;4:189–96. https://doi.org/10.1159/000437051.
66. Choi YJ, Baek JH, Suh CH, Shim WH, Jeong B, Kim JK, et al. Core-needle biopsy versus repeat fine-needle aspiration for thyroid nodules initially read as atypia/follicular lesion of undetermined significance. Head Neck. 2017;39:361–9. https://doi.org/10.1002/hed.24597.
67. Yim Y, Baek JH. Core needle biopsy in the management of thyroid nodules with an indeterminate fine-needle aspiration report. Gland Surg. 2019;8(Suppl 2):S77–85. https://doi.org/10.21037/gs.2018.09.07.
68. Joo L, Na DG, Kim JH, Seo H. Comparison of core needle biopsy and repeat fine-needle aspiration in avoiding diagnostic surgery for thyroid nodules initially diagnosed as atypia/follicular lesion of undetermined significance. Korean J Radiol. 2022;23:280–8. https://doi.org/10.3348/kjr.2021.0619.
69. Kim JY, Chang S, Kwon AY, Park EY, Kim TH, Choi S, et al. Core needle biopsy and ultrasonography are superior to fine needle aspiration in the management of follicular variant papillary thyroid carcinomas. Endocrine. 2022;75:437–46. https://doi.org/10.1007/s12020-021-02864-1.
70. Pyo JS, Sohn JH, Kang G. Core needle biopsy is a more conclusive follow-up method than repeat fine needle aspiration for thyroid nodules with initially inconclusive results: a systematic review and meta-analysis. J Pathol Transl Med. 2016;50:217–24. https://doi.org/10.4132/jptm.2016.02.15.
71. Suh CH, Baek JH, Park C, Choi YJ, Lee JH. The role of core needle biopsy for thyroid nodules with initially indeterminate results on previous fine-needle aspiration: a systematic review and meta-analysis. Am J Neuroradiol. 2017;38:1421–6. https://doi.org/10.3174/ajnr.a5182.
72. Trimboli P, Giovanella L. Reliability of core needle biopsy as a second-line procedure in thyroid nodules with an indeterminate fine-needle aspiration report: a systematic review and meta-analysis. Ultrasonography. 2018;37:121–8. https://doi.org/10.14366/usg.17066.
73. Ahn SH. Usage and diagnostic yield of fine-needle aspiration cytology and core needle biopsy in thyroid nodules: a systematic review and meta-analysis of literature published by Korean authors. Clin Exp Otorhinolaryngol. 2021;14:116–30. https://doi.org/10.21053/ceo.2020.00199.
74. Kim TY, Kim WB, Gong G, Hong SJ, Shong YK. Metastasis to the thyroid diagnosed by fine-needle aspiration biopsy. Clin Endocrinol. 2005;62:236–41. https://doi.org/10.1111/j.1365-2265.2005.02206.x.
75. Moghaddan PA, Cornejo KM, Khan A. Metastatic carcinoma to the thyroid gland: a single institution 20-year experience and review of the literature. Endocr Pathol. 2013;24:116–24. https://doi.org/10.1007/s12022-013-9257-8.
76. Papi G, Fadda G, Corsello SM, Corrado S, Rossi ED, Radighieri E, et al. Metastases to the thyroid gland: prevalence, clinicopathological aspects and prognosis: a 10-year experience. Clin Endocrinol. 2007;66:565–71. https://doi.org/10.1111/j.1365-2265.2007.02773.x.
77. Chung AY, Tran TB, Brumund KT, Weisman RA, Bouvet M. Metastases to the thyroid: a review of the literature from the last decade. Thyroid. 2012;22:258–68. https://doi.org/10.1089/thy.2010.0154.
78. Hegerova L, Griebeler ML, Reynolds JP, Henry MR, Gharib H. Metastasis to the thyroid gland: report of a large series from the Mayo Clinic. Am J Clin Oncol. 2015;38:338–42. https://doi.org/10.1097/COC.0b013e31829d1d09.
79. Nixon IJ, Coca-Pelaz A, Kaleva AI, Triantafyllou A, Angelos P, Owen RP, et al. Metastasis to the thyroid gland: a critical review. Ann Surg Oncol. 2017;24:1533–9. https://doi.org/10.1245/s10434-016-5683-4.
80. Ghossein CA, Khimraj A, Dogan S, Xu B. Metastasis to the thyroid gland: a single-institution 16-year experience. Histopathology. 2021;78:508–19. https://doi.org/10.1111/his.14246.
81. Nguyen M, He G, Lam AK. Clinicopathological and molecular features of secondary cancer (metastasis) to the thyroid and advances in management. Int J Mol Sci. 2022;23:3242. https://doi.org/10.3390/ijms23063242.
82. Battistella E, Pomba L, Mattara G, Franzato B, Toniato A. Metastases to the thyroid gland: review of incidence, clinical presentation, diagnostic problems and surgery, our experience. J Endocrinol Invest. 2020;43:1555–60. https://doi.org/10.1007/s40618-020-01282-w.
83. Pusztaszeri M, Wang H, Cibas ES, Powers CN, Bongiovanni M, Ali S, et al. Fine-needle aspiration biopsy of secondary neoplasms of the thyroid gland: a multi-institutional study of 62 cases. Cancer Cytopathol. 2015;123:19–29. https://doi.org/10.1002/cncy.21494.
84. Saito Y, Sugitani I, Toda K, Yamada K, Fujimoto Y. Metastatic thyroid tumors: ultrasonographic features, prognostic factors and outcomes in 29 cases. Surg Today. 2014;44:55–61. https://doi.org/10.1007/s00595-013-0492-x.
85. Yoon JH, Kim EK, Kwak JY, Moon HJ, Kim GR. Sonographic features and ultrasonography-

guided fine-needle aspiration of metastases to the thyroid gland. Ultrasonography. 2014;33:40–8. https://doi.org/10.14366/usg.13014.
86. Tang Z, Gao L, Wang X, Zhang J, Zhan W, Zhou W. Metastases to the thyroid gland: ultrasonographic findings and diagnostic value of fine-needle aspiration cytology. Front Oncol. 2022;12:939965. https://doi.org/10.3389/fonc.2022.939965.
87. Choi SH, Baek JH, Ha EJ, Choi YJ, Song DE, Kim JK, et al. Diagnosis of metastasis to the thyroid gland: comparison of core-needle biopsy and fine-needle aspiration. Otolaryngol Head Neck Surg. 2016;154:618–25. https://doi.org/10.1177/0194599816629632.
88. Rahman M, Okada AR, Guan K, Tauchi-Nishi P. Metastatic neoplasms to the thyroid diagnosed by fine-needle aspiration/core needle biopsy: clinicopathologic and cytomorphologic correlation. Cytojournal. 2017;14:16. https://doi.org/10.4103/cytojournal.cytojournal_50_16.
89. Ha EJ, Baek JH, Lee JH, Kim JK, Song DE, Kim WB, Hong SJ. Core needle biopsy could reduce diagnostic surgery in patients with anaplastic thyroid cancer or thyroid lymphoma. Eur Radiol. 2016;26:1031–6. https://doi.org/10.1007/s00330-015-3921-y.
90. Vander Poorten V, Goedseels N, Triantafyllou A, Sanabria A, Clement PM, Cohen O, et al. Effectiveness of core needle biopsy in the diagnosis of thyroid lymphoma and anaplastic thyroid carcinoma: a systematic review and meta-analysis. Front Endocrinol (Lausanne). 2022;13:971249. https://doi.org/10.3389/fendo.2022.971249.
91. Matrone A, De Napoli L, Torregrossa L, Aghababyan A, Papini P, Ambrosini CE, et al. Core needle biopsy can early and precisely identify large thyroid masses. Front Oncol. 2022;12:854755. https://doi.org/10.3389/fonc.2022.854755.
92. Cao C, Jasim S, Cherian A, Nassar A, Chindris AM, Rivas AM, et al. Patient discomfort in relation to thyroid nodule fine-needle aspiration (FNA) performed with or without parenteral and/or topical anesthetic. Endocr Pract. 2020;26:1497–504. https://doi.org/10.4158/ep-2020-0403.

6 Molecular Testing of Thyroid Nodules

Marialuisa Sponziello, Leslie Eldeiry, and Cosimo Durante

6.1 Introduction

The molecular pathogenesis of thyroid tumors has been extensively investigated. Advances in high-throughput technologies have enabled comprehensive genomic profiling of thyroid tumors and identification of novel biomarkers, which are essential not only to inform tumor diagnosis and prognosis, but also to tailor therapeutic decisions. Most thyroid neoplasms have a "quiet" genome, with a low tumor mutational burden compared to other cancers [1]. The molecular alterations involved in the pathogenesis of thyroid tumors are mainly represented by somatic mutations that likely occur in the early steps of tumorigenesis and cause dysregulation of the mitogen-activated protein kinase (MAPK) and phosphatidylinositol-3 kinase (PI3K)-AKT pathways. The main drivers of these pathways are *BRAF* and *RAS* point mutations and *RET* rearrangement, which drive thyroid cell transformation in a mutually exclusive manner. Most encapsulated tumors exhibit a *RAS*-like molecular profile. Tumors with papillary and/or infiltrative growth have a *BRAF*^{V600E}-like profile. Two scoring methods were introduced by the TCGA study to evaluate differentiation of thyroid cells and activation of the MAPK signaling pathway: the thyroid differentiation score (TDS) and the ERK score. *BRAF*^{V600E}-like tumors have a low TDS, while *RAS*-like tumors have a high TDS score. TDS negatively correlates with ERK score in both molecular subtypes [2]. Thyroid cancer progression and dedifferentiation involves additional mutations, such as those in *TP53*, *TERT* promoter (*pTERT*), SWI/SNF complexes, and WNT/β--catenin pathway [3].

RET point mutations are driver events in multiple endocrine neoplasia, type 2 (MEN2) syndrome and in 40-65% of sporadic medullary thyroid cancers [4]. Mutations in *RAS* genes (mainly *H*- and *KRAS*) are found in 13–28% of sporadic MTC [3, 5].

Molecular alterations other than gene mutations and fusions include copy number alterations (CNA) and dysregulation of microRNA expression. CNAs, defined as somatically acquired gains or losses of a DNA segment, can be driver events in thyroid tumorigenesis [2, 6]. MicroRNAs (miRNA) are small noncoding RNAs that play an important role in the post-transcriptional regulation of gene expression. Several miRNAs have been characterized in thyroid cancer, and some of them have also been associated with thyroid cancer progression. Due to their tissue specificity, the development of miRNA-based molecular assays is an attractive

M. Sponziello (✉) · C. Durante
Department of Translational and Precision Medicine, SAPIENZA University of Rome, Rome, Italy
e-mail: marialuisa.sponziello@uniroma1.it; cosimo.durante@uniroma1.it

L. Eldeiry
Department of Endocrinology, Harvard Vanguard Medical Associates/Atrius Health, Boston, MA, USA
e-mail: Leslie_Eldeiry@atriushealth.org

R. Valcavi et al. (eds.), *Thyroid Ablation*, https://doi.org/10.1007/978-3-031-88229-6_6

strategy for thyroid cancer diagnosis and prognostication [7].

Molecular markers are increasingly being used in precision medicine to provide diagnostic, prognostic, and therapeutic information and to support clinical decision-making. Molecular testing of fine needle aspirates (FNA) improves the diagnostic accuracy of detecting cancer in cytologically indeterminate thyroid nodules and may also provide prognostic information. Moreover, molecular markers enable targeted therapeutic options in advanced thyroid cancers. In this chapter, we will summarize the genomic landscape of thyroid tumors classified according to the latest edition of WHO, the available molecular tests for thyroid cancer, and their clinical utility.

6.2 Genetics and Genomics of Thyroid Tumors

The fifth edition of the WHO Classification of Endocrine and Neuroendocrine Tumors of the thyroid gland subclassifies thyroid tumors into several new categories based on the cell of origin, pathologic features, molecular classification, and biological behavior. Follicular cell-derived tumors are divided into benign, low-risk, and malignant neoplasms (Fig. 6.1a). The only

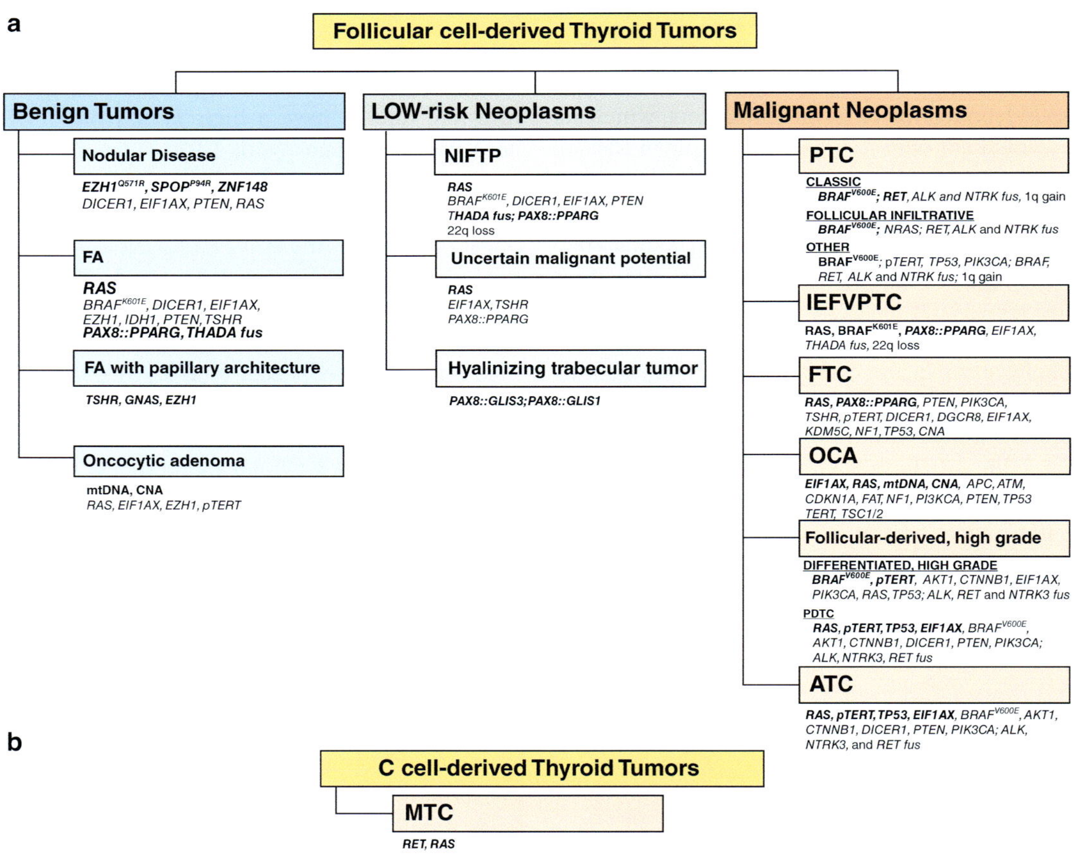

Fig. 6.1 Molecular markers of thyroid tumors classified according to the fifth edition of WHO. (**a**) Follicular cell-derived Thyroid Tumors; (**b**) C cell-derived Thyroid Tumors. Abbreviations: *ATC* anaplastic thyroid cancer; *CNA* copy number alterations; *FA* follicular adenoma; *FTC* follicular thyroid cancer; *Fus* gene fusions; *IEFVPTC* invasive encapsulated follicular variant papillary carcinoma; *MTC* medullary thyroid cancer; *mtDNA* mitochondrial DNA mutations; *NIFTP* noninvasive follicular neoplasm with papillary-like nuclear features; *OCA* oncocytic carcinoma; *PTC* papillary thyroid cancer

C-cell-derived neoplasm is medullary thyroid carcinoma [8] (Fig. 6.1b).

6.2.1 Follicular Cell-Derived Neoplasms

6.2.1.1 Benign Tumors

Benign lesions include nodular disease, follicular adenoma (FA), follicular adenoma with papillary architecture, and oncocytic adenoma [8].

Thyroid follicular nodular disease is an umbrella term proposed in the latest WHO classification that refers to nodules within a multinodular goiter, previously classified as colloid nodules, adenomatous nodules or incorrectly named as hyperplastic nodules [8]. At the molecular level, hyperplasia is a polyclonal proliferation of untransformed cells, unlike adenomas, which are defined as clonal proliferation of follicular cells [9]. Extensive genomic profiling of adenomatous nodules has revealed a unique molecular signature characterized by mutually exclusive $SPOP^{P94R}$, $EZH1^{Q571R}$, and *ZNF148* mutations and distinctive gene expression patterns. Sequencing of these genes in indeterminate thyroid nodules may provide "rule out" information, thus increasing the diagnostic accuracy of the current molecular diagnostic assays for thyroid cancer [10].

The molecular profile of FA is very similar to that of minimally invasive follicular thyroid carcinoma (miFTC), providing evidence for a continuum of evolution [11]. These tumors are characterized by *RAS* mutations, along with mutations in *DICER1*, *EIF1AX*, *IDH1*, *PTEN*, and *PAX8::PPARG*. No significant transcriptional difference has been described between FA and miFTC [11, 12].

FA with papillary architecture is characterized by encapsulation and papillary architecture that lacks nuclear features of papillary thyroid carcinoma (PTC). Nearly 70% of these tumors harbor activating *TSHR* mutations that constitutively activate the cAMP cascade and induce growth and hyperfunction of thyroid follicular cells and, ultimately, thyroid autonomy. A small minority have *GNAS* and/or *EZH1* mutations. Molecular analysis of FNA samples can detect these mutations, thus avoiding unnecessary or aggressive treatments [8].

Oncocytic adenomas have distinctive genetic alterations in the mitochondrial genome [13], and 38% of them display CNAs. Mutations in *RAS*, *EIF1AX*, *EZH1*, and p*TERT* have also been associated with oncocytic adenoma. Unlike in oncocytic carcinoma, these mutations never co-occur with CNAs [14]. Gene expression profiles of oncocytic adenomas are comparable to that of minimally invasive oncocytic carcinoma [15].

6.2.1.2 Low-Risk Neoplasms

Low-risk neoplasms include noninvasive follicular thyroid neoplasm with papillary-like nuclear features (NIFTP), thyroid tumors of uncertain malignant potential (UMP), and hyalinizing trabecular tumors (HTT) [8].

According to the latest WHO classification, NIFTPs are follicular encapsulated tumors characterized by <1% papillae, <30% of solid/trabecular/insular growth patterns and absence of psammoma bodies, high-grade morphology, vascular or capsular invasion. At the molecular level, 40–70% of NIFTPs are driven by *RAS* mutations. Further oncogenic alterations include BRAF p.K601E, *DICER1*, *EIF1AX*, and *PTEN* mutations, 22q loss, *THADA::IGF2BP3* and *PAX8::PPARG* [16, 17]. BRAF p.V600E, *RET*, *NTRK*, or *ALK* fusions never occur in NIFTP [8]. NIFTPs display different gene expression profiles, which can be similar to FA (FA-like) or to the infiltrative follicular subtype of PTC (IFVPTC-like) [18]. Downregulation of miR-7-5p distinguishes NIFTP from hyperplasia [19]. miR-152-3p, miR-185-5p, and miR-574-3p are significantly downregulated in NIFTPs compared with FA, whereas miR-10a-5p and miR-320e can distinguish between NIFTPs and IFVPTCs [20].

Thyroid tumors of UMP present equivocal capsular or vascular invasion [8]. They are characterized by a high prevalence of *RAS*-like mutations, including those in *H/K/N-RAS*, *EIF1AX*, *TSHR*, and *PAX8::PPARG* [21].

HTTs are well-demarcated thyroid nodules with PTC-like nuclear changes, trabecular architecture, and abundant intratrabecular hyalinization [8]. *GLIS* gene rearrangements are genomic hallmarks of HTT, with *PAX8::GLIS3* being the most prevalent fusion, followed by *PAX8::GLIS1* [22].

6.2.1.3 Malignant Neoplasms

Malignant neoplasms encompass papillary thyroid cancer (PTC), invasive encapsulated follicular variant papillary carcinoma (IEFVPTC), follicular thyroid cancer (FTC), oncocytic carcinoma (OCA, previously called Hürthle cell carcinoma), high-grade carcinoma, and anaplastic thyroid cancers (ATC) [8].

PTC is the most common thyroid malignancy, characterized by either peculiar nuclear features or a papillary growth pattern. PTCs include multiple subtypes, with classical and follicular being the most common. IEFVPTC is classified in a separate section of the WHO based on clinical features and molecular alterations, which are closer to FTC than PTC. Conversely, IFVPTCs typically behave like classic PTCs, with a propensity to spread to lymph nodes [16]. Aggressive subtypes include tall cell, columnar cell, and hobnail PTCs, which are associated with advanced disease and lymph node metastases at diagnosis. From a molecular perspective, there are two main classes of mutations in PTC: *BRAF*^{V600E}-like mutations result in cancers with clear nuclear atypia (mainly IFVPTC, classic and tall cell cancers), while *RAS*-like mutations result in cancers with less clear nuclear atypia and a follicular growth pattern [8]. BRAF p.V600E is the most common alteration in PTC [8], with a prevalence ranging from 29 to 83% [3]. Rare *BRAF* mutations include *BRAF* p.K601E and small in-frame insertions/deletions, which are mainly associated with indolent follicular-patterned tumors, unless additional genetic events are present [23]. *RAS* mutations are found in 12.9% of PTCs, mainly in encapsulated follicular-patterned tumors with a high degree of differentiation [2]. Gene fusions also contribute to PTC pathogenesis, with *RET* fusions being the most frequent (6.8%) [2], especially in radiation-induced cancers (17%) [24], followed by *BRAF* (2.7%), *NTRK* (1.2%), *THADA* (1.2%), *ALK* (0.8%) fusions, and *PAX8::PPARG* (0.8%) [2]. The TCGA study of PTC extended the set of known drivers to include *EIF1AX*, *PPM1D*, and *CHEK2* [2]. Somatic CNAs are identified in 27% of PTCs. The most common are 22q loss, which are found mainly in follicular subtype of PTCs, and 1q gain, which occurs frequently in tall cell and classic subtypes [2]. Late secondary hits in p*TERT*, *TP53*, or *PIK3CA* frequently occur in cancers with distant metastases [25]. Thus, their identification in an indeterminate thyroid nodule increases the odds that a thyroid lesion represents an aggressive cancer. A subset of miRNAs has been consistently found to be deregulated in PTCs, including miR-146b, miR-221, miR-222, miR-21, and miR-204. Some miRNAs discriminate specific PTC subtypes [7, 26]. MicroRNAs can potentially be used as diagnostic, prognostic, and predictive biomarkers in liquid biopsy samples [7, 27].

FTC is a predominantly *RAS*-like neoplasm with a follicular pattern, which lacks nuclear features of PTC. FTCs, like PTCs, display a low mutational burden (0.38 mutations/Mb), with no marked difference in the mutational signatures between minimally invasive and widely invasive subtypes [28]. Most FTCs are characterized by mutually exclusive mutations in *RAS* genes (17–57%) and *PAX8::PPARG* (12–53%) [3]. *TSHR*, *DICER1*, *DGCR8*, *EIF1AX*, *KDM5C*, *NF1*, *PTEN*, *PIK3CA*, *pTERT*, and *TP53* mutations have also been reported in FTC [28, 29], as well as recurrent 22q losses, 5q and 7q gains [28]. Since *RAS* mutations are common drivers in benign and malignant follicular thyroid lesions, attempts to identify additional preoperative biomarkers have been made. Several miRNAs display histotype-specific deregulations, some of which (miR-146b-5p, miR-144-3p, and miR-451a) can discriminate between *RAS*-mutant benign (FA) and *RAS*-mutant neoplasms (NIFTP, PTC, FTC), thus serving as potential diagnostic biomarkers. miR-145-5p is the only miRNA that has been found to be specifically deregulated in FTC versus FA [30].

OCA is characterized by more than 75% oncocytic cells, with a unique biological behavior and mutational signature [8]. OCA displays a higher mutational burden (2.6 mutations/Mb) than other differentiated thyroid cancers (DTC). Somatic mutations affect canonical signal-transduction (MAPK, PI3K/AKT/mTOR, Wnt/beta-catenin pathways) and tumor-suppressor pathways (DNA damage and DNA repair pathways) [15, 31]. Epigenetic-modifying gene mutations are also common in these carcinomas, along with near-homoplasmic mutations of mitochondrial DNA and genome-wide loss of heterozygosity. *TERT* mutations are present in 22% of OCA, with a higher frequency in widely invasive (32%) than in minimally invasive (5%) cancers, which are also characterized by marked differences in gene expression profiles [32].

High-grade carcinoma defines a group of malignant lesions with an intermediate prognosis between the favorable outcome of DTCs and the poor outcome of ATC. It includes differentiated high-grade thyroid carcinoma (DHGTC) and poorly differentiated thyroid carcinoma (PDTC) [8]. PDTCs are typically *RAS*-driven tumors, whereas DHGTCs frequently harbor BRAF p. V600E mutation, or more rarely *RET* or *NTRK3* fusions. Secondary mutations in *pTERT*, *PIK3CA*, and *TP53* frequently occur in both PDTC and DHGTC [8, 33].

ATC is characterized by early and late genetic events, which suggests a multi-step model of progression from DTC, DHGTC, and PDTC. Early events include *BRAF* or *RAS* mutations, whereas late events are mainly mutations of p*TERT* and *TP53*. Mutations of *CDKN2A/B* and genes involved in DNA mismatch repair, chromatin remodeling, and histone modification are frequently reported [8, 33, 34].

6.2.2 Thyroid C-Cell-Derived Carcinoma

MTC is the only C-cell-derived neoplasm, which can be either sporadic (75%) or familial (25%). Activating point mutations of *RET* are the main drivers, occurring in 40–65% and 98% of sporadic and familial cases, respectively. Rare small insertions/deletions of *RET* can also occur [4, 35], as well as *RAS* mutations in 13–28% of sporadic cases [3, 5]. Somatic CNAs occur in 65% of sporadic MTCs, with a higher prevalence in *RET*-mutant cancers [36]. *RET/RAS*-negative MTCs can harbor *NF1* gene inactivation [37] or *ETV6::NTRK2* [38]. Among the rare *RET*-negative familial MTCs, *MET* [39], and *ESR2* [40] germline mutations have been documented. Circulating expression levels of miR-26b-5p and miR-451a are reported to be promising noninvasive diagnostic biomarkers for MTC [41].

6.3 Molecular Tests

Comprehensive molecular profiling of thyroid tumors has enhanced the development of ancillary molecular tests that can reduce the need for diagnostic surgery in cytologically indeterminate thyroid nodules [42].

Molecular tests can be categorized into two subtypes, depending on their ability to confirm ("rule-in tests") or exclude ("rule-out tests") malignancy. Rule-in tests have high specificity and positive predictive values (PPV). Rule-out tests have high sensitivity and negative predictive values (NPV). An ideal test should be both highly sensitive and specific, in order to accurately distinguish benign from malignant thyroid lesions. However, increasing sensitivity often leads to decreased specificity, and vice versa. Notably, predictive values are not static properties of a diagnostic test but vary with the pretest probability of disease. Therefore, the prevalence of thyroid cancer should be evaluated at each institution to accurately assess the malignancy risk of a cytologically indeterminate thyroid nodule associated with molecular test findings.

The tests developed so far are based on three molecular approaches for the identification of a molecular signature associated with thyroid cancer: testing for somatic mutations, evaluation of expression profiles at the transcriptional (mRNA) or post-transcriptional (microRNA) level, or combination of multiple biomarkers (mutations, mRNA and/or miRNAs).

6.3.1 Methodologies

6.3.1.1 Identification of Somatic Mutations

Molecular testing for somatic mutations is currently the most employed molecular diagnostic approach in FNA specimens. Conventional Sanger sequencing, which involves sequencing of one or a few DNA fragments that were initially amplified by PCR, was the gold standard for the identification of mutations until the late 2000s and it is still used as an orthogonal method to confirm previously detected mutations. However, it requires long analysis times and is associated with high costs if multiple DNA regions need to be analyzed. Moreover, the method is suboptimal for identifying somatic mutations due to its low sensitivity of approximately 20% (meaning that 20% of the sequenced DNA molecules need to contain the mutation to be reliably detected) [43].

Other conventional assays include immunohistochemistry (IHC), fluorescence in situ hybridization (FISH), and reverse transcription polymerase chain reaction (RT-PCR). IHC can detect protein change that results from DNA rearrangement (e.g., pan-TRK assay to detect all NTRK fusions [44] and ALK assays [45]) and point mutations (BRAF p.V600E, clone VE1, or pan-RAS Q61R [45]). FISH has been the gold-standard method for identifying DNA rearrangements, and it is frequently employed to validate gene-level amplifications when IHC results are inconclusive. Using break-apart probes which are each directed to the 5′ and 3′ ends of a target gene, FISH analysis can identify the presence of a fusion event without knowing the fusion partner [46]. RT-PCR can identify gene fusions with high specificity and sensitivity; however, it does not detect new fusion partners since it uses preselected primers.

Advantages of these conventional methods include the wide availability in clinical laboratories, low cost, and fast turnaround. However, each biomarker needs to be specifically defined to be found.

Conversely, next-generation sequencing (NGS) is a high-throughput method that allows for simultaneous sequencing of multiple genes. Compared with Sanger sequencing, NGS has greater sensitivity for detecting low-level mutations (2–5% of variant allele frequency) and allows for quantitative evaluation of the mutant allele. A wide range of genomic changes, including point mutations, small insertion/deletion, copy number alterations, and gene fusions, can be analyzed simultaneously using NGS. In comparison to serial single-biomarker analyses, it offers a more effective, economical, and tissue-saving tumor analysis [46].

6.3.1.2 Evaluation of mRNA and MicroRNA Expression Levels

High-throughput RNA-sequencing technologies can currently be used to analyze gene expression on a large scale. It is the technique that enables the most informative, simultaneous analysis of the expression patterns of a huge number of targets. Targeted sequencing, microarray, real-time PCR, or digital PCR assays can be used to identify relative differences in gene or miRNA expression on selected targets [47].

6.3.2 Single Gene/Small Panels

Testing for single-gene mutations in thyroid nodules is one strategy used in cytopathology. Most studies have focused on BRAF p.V600E detection. Although the assay is highly specific (rule-in test), low cost, and simple to perform in most diagnostic laboratories, it is not sensitive enough to diagnose thyroid cancer when used alone [48]. The seven-gene panel is a more comprehensive approach, which covers the genetic alterations found in nearly 70% of thyroid cancers, namely BRAF p.V600E, *HRAS*, *NRAS*, *KRAS*, *RET-PTC1*, *RET-PTC3*, and *PAX8::PPARG*. This assay has certainly improved sensitivity over the single molecular test; however, the overall sensitivity as a rule-out test remains low. Discrepancies in test performance have been revealed among different series with sensitivity ranging from 18 to 100% and specificity from 82 to 100%. Inconsistent results are mainly attributed to local variations in cancer prevalence rates and inter-observer variability in the cytological and histological diagnosis of thyroid lesions [48, 49].

6.3.3 Thyroid-Specific Panels

Commonly used commercially available molecular tests in North America are ThyroSeq v.3 [50], Afirma Genomic Sequencing Classifier/ Xpression Atlas (GSC/XA) [51], and ThyGeNEXT/ThyraMIR [52]. These tests combine identification of somatic mutations with evaluation of mRNA or miRNA expression profiles to refine the preoperative risk stratification of cytologically indeterminate thyroid nodules (Table 6.1).

Table 6.1 Commercially available molecular panels in the United States and South America: comparison of test characteristics and performance in cytologically indeterminate thyroid nodules

Parameter	ThyroSeq v3 [50]	Afirma GSC/XA [51, 54]	ThyGenNEXT/ ThyraMIR [52]	ThyroidPrint [55]	miR-THYpe [57]
Molecular sample	One fresh pass in preservative solution or direct smears	Two fresh passes in preservative solution	One fresh pass or direct smears or ThinPrep slides	Two fresh passes in preservative solution	Direct smears
Methodology	Targeted NGS on DNA and RNA	Whole transcriptome RNA-sequencing	Targeted NGS for mutational analysis. Real-time PCR for miRNA expression analysis	Real-time PCR	Real-time PCR
SNV and/or small ins/del	112 genes	905 variants[a]	10 genes	None	None
Gene fusions	>150	235[a]	28	None	None
CNA	10	LoH	37	None	None
GEA	19 genes	>10,000 genes (1115 for classifier)	4 genes	10 genes	None
microRNA	–	–	11 miRNAs	–	12 miRNAs
Molecular results	Negative	GSC benign	Negative (low risk)	Benign	Negative
	Currently negative	GSC suspicious	Moderate risk	Suspicious	Positive
	Positive		Positive (high risk)		
Validation study; sample size	Multicentered, blinded prospective; $N = 257$	Multicentered, blinded prospective; $N = 191$	Multicentered, blinded retrospective; $N = 178$	Multicentered, blinded prospective; $N = 270$	Real-world, multicentered prospective; $N = 440$
Cancer prevalence	27%	24%	30%	32%	29%
Sensitivity	94	91	Neg 100%; Mod 98%; Pos 81%	91%	89%
Specificity	82	68	Neg 0%; Mod 86%; Pos 98%	88%	82%
NPV	97	96	Neg 99%; Mod 93%; Pos 70%	95%	95%
PPV	66	47	Neg 30%; Mod 75%; Pos 96%	78%	66%

Abbreviations: *CNA* copy number alteration; *GEA* gene expression alteration; *GSC/XA* Genomic Sequencing Classifier/ Xpression Atlas; *LoH* Loss of Heterozygosity; *Mod* moderate threshold; *Neg* negative threshold; *NGS* next-generation sequencing; *Pos* positive threshold; *SNV* single nucleotide variants

[a] Afirma XA panel includes 593 genes informing on 905 variants and 235 fusions

ThyroSeq Genomic Classifier, currently in its third version, uses targeted NGS to analyze 112 thyroid cancer-related genes for point mutations, small insertions/deletions, gene fusions, copy number alterations, and gene expression alterations. Findings are classified as positive (high cancer probability) or negative (very low probability of cancer) by a unique Genomic Classifier. Negative samples can further be subcategorized as "negative for all tested genetic alterations" (risk of malignancy, ROM, 3%), and "currently negative due the presence of a low-risk mutation" (ROM, 10–15%). Validation on 257 indeterminate nodules with surgical pathology reports revealed high sensitivity (94%) and specificity (82%), with 97% NPV and 66% PPV. In this study, up to 61% of individuals with indeterminate nodules did not require diagnostic surgery [50].

The Afirma GSC is the latest version of the Afirma gene expression classifier (GEC), the first test designed to rule out thyroid cancer in indeterminate thyroid nodules. Afirma GSC combines RNA-sequencing with advanced machine learning algorithms to provide a *benign* or a *suspicious* result, based on the expression levels of more than 10,000 genes and 7 further components (i.e., parathyroid, MTC, BRAF p.V600E cassettes, RET/PTC1 and RET/PTC3 fusion modules to detect specific and rare patient subgroups; follicular content, oncocytic cell, and oncocytic neoplasm indexes to further improve the benign vs. suspicious classification performance). Clinical validation on 191 indeterminate thyroid nodules through a prospective, blinded, multicenter study showed 91% sensitivity, 68% specificity, 96% NPV, and 47% PPV [51]. Meta-analysis of 13 independent studies in multiple clinical settings outperformed the validation study with 97% sensitivity, 88% specificity, 99% NPV, and 65% PPV [53]. By using the same RNA-sequencing methodology, indeterminate thyroid nodules with an Afirma GSC suspicious result or cytologically suspicious/malignant nodules may also take advantage of the Afirma Xpression Atlas (XA) to detect expressed variants and gene fusions in 593 genes, thus optimizing personalized treatment decisions [54].

ThyGeNEXT/ThyraMIR v.2 is a multiplatform assay that combines a mutation panel test with a microRNA risk classifier. Samples first undergo mutational testing. If a strong driver ($BRAF^{V600E}$-like mutations) is found, miRNA classifier is not performed. Samples with a weak-driver (*RAS*-like mutations) or no mutations at all undergo miRNA testing through pairwise analysis of individual growth-promoting and growth-suppressing miRNAs. Results are classified in three categories as *negative* (low risk), *moderate-risk*, or *positive* (high risk) with respect to cancer probability. Test performance was separately evaluated for the three categories on 178 indeterminate thyroid nodules collected in a multicentered, blinded retrospective trial, showing NPV ranging from 70 to 99% and PPV from 30 to 96%, with improvement of the negative threshold to 99% and positive threshold to 96% afforded by the pairwise analysis [52].

Two further commercial tests developed in South America are ThyroidPrint [55] and miR-THYPE [56] assays that are uniquely based on an mRNA expression classifier and miRNA expression classifier, respectively (Table 6.1).

ThyroidPrint was designed in a multiplex real-time PCR diagnostic kit to analyze expression levels of 10 genes. Test performance was evaluated in two independent, ethnically diverse, prospective multicenter trials revealing 91% sensitivity, 88% specificity, 95% NPV, and 78% PPV. This indicates that a benign result reduces the risk of malignancy to less than 5%, allowing avoidance of many unnecessary diagnostic surgery [55].

miR-THYpe can be performed on an FNA cytology smear slide with no additional sampling required. Data from a real-world, prospective, multicenter study on 440 indeterminate thyroid nodules showed 89.3% sensitivity, 81.65% specificity, 95% NPV, and 66.2% PPV, with a rate of avoided surgeries of 52.5% [57].

Other molecular tests, mainly developed in research settings, have been designed in Europe [58, 59] and East Asia [60] with promising results.

6.4 Clinical Utility of Molecular Tests

In clinical practice, molecular marker testing has become an important adjunctive tool to clinical, radiologic, and cytology data. The 2011 National Comprehensive Cancer Network (NCCN) Task Force Report evaluating the clinical utility of tumor markers in oncology defined four types of molecular markers: diagnostic, predictive, prognostic, and companion diagnostic. Both analytic validity and clinical utility, ideally demonstrated by prospective clinical trials, are needed for these tests to become part of the routine management of thyroid nodules and malignancy [61].

Despite rapid progress in this field, several limitations and challenges to the clinical application of these tools exist, including the correlation of genetic alterations with both benign and malignant pathology, identifying the molecular profile associated with the relatively new pathologic entity, NIFTP, and the lack of long-term follow-up or histology data for nodules without molecular alterations. Moreover, the criteria for selecting nodules for molecular testing vary widely and the optimal use of these tools in clinical practice, including selecting appropriate candidates for testing and cost-effective use, are areas of ongoing research. Current guidelines recommend consideration of molecular testing in patients who have indeterminate thyroid nodules, which includes three categories: atypia of undetermined significance (AUS), follicular neoplasm (FN), and suspicious for malignancy. Surgery is generally performed for nodules that are cytologically suspicious (Bethesda V) because of the high malignancy probability in this category (~74%), thereby simplifying treatment decisions [62] (Table 6.2).

Table 6.2 The Bethesda System for Reporting Thyroid Cytopathology: implied risk of malignancy (ROM) with expected ranges based on follow-up of surgically resected nodules with recommended clinical management [62]

Diagnostic category	ROM[a] Mean% (range)	Usual management[b]
Nondiagnostic	13 (5–20)[c]	Repeat FNA[d] with ultrasound guidance
Benign	4 (2–7)[e]	Clinical and sonographic follow-up
Atypia of undetermined significance[f]	22 (13–30)	Repeat FNA[d], molecular testing, diagnostic lobectomy, or surveillance
Follicular neoplasm[g]	30 (23–34)	Molecular testing[h], diagnostic lobectomy
Suspicious for malignancy	74 (67–83)	Molecular testing[h], lobectomy, or near-total thyroidectomy[i]
Malignant	97 (97–100)	Lobectomy or near-total thyroidectomy[i]

Adapted, with permission, from Ali and VanderLaan [62]

[a] These ROM estimates are skewed by selection bias, as many thyroid nodules (especially those diagnosed as Benign or AUS) may not undergo surgical excision

[b] Actual management may depend on other factors (e.g., clinical, sonographic) besides the FNA interpretation

[c] The risk of malignancy varies with the type/structure of the nodule, i.e., solid vs. complex vs. ≥50% cystic. Nondiagnostic aspirates from solid nodules are associated with a higher risk of malignancy as compared to those showing ≥50% cystic change and low-risk ultrasonographic features

[d] Studies have shown diagnostic resolution with repeat FNA

[e] This ROM estimate is based on follow-up of surgically resected nodules, which is skewed by selection bias since the vast majority of thyroid nodules classified as benign do not undergo surgical excision. Based on long-term follow-up studies, the best overall ROM estimate for a benign FNA is approximately 1–2%

[f] This category can be further subclassified into specimens with nuclear vs. non-nuclear atypia; the ROM appears to be higher for cases with nuclear atypia

[g] Includes cases of follicular neoplasm with oncocytic features (Hürthle cell neoplasm)

[h] Molecular analysis can be performed to assess the type of surgical procedure (lobectomy vs. total thyroidectomy)

[i] In the case of "Suspicious for metastatic tumor" or a "Malignant" interpretation indicating metastatic tumor rather than a primary thyroid malignancy, surgery may not be indicated

6.4.1 Bethesda II

In general, there is no role for molecular marker testing of Bethesda II nodules in the clinical setting. In some cases, testing is performed at the discretion of the clinician, for example, in the setting of suspicious ultrasound findings, large or growing nodules or in validation studies of new molecular tests.

A minority of patients with Bethesda II nodules undergo surgery, usually on the basis of large size, nodule growth or clinical symptoms, and a smaller minority of those patients have a malignancy on final histopathology. One study of nearly 550 FNAs identified single mutations (*BRAF*, *KRAS*, *HRAS*, or *NRAS*) or fusion transcripts (*PAX8::PPARG* or *RET/PTC*) in all Bethesda categories, including a positivity rate ranging from 3.5% for benign nodules to 80% for malignant nodules [63].

A prospective cohort study examining the performance of ACR-TIRADS, FNA cytology, and molecular marker testing in which molecular testing was performed only in Bethesda II nodules that were classified as ACR-TIRADS suspicious or based on the examiner's recommendation, showed a mutation detection rate of 10.1% and a surprisingly high cancer prevalence (including NIFTP and tumor of UMP) of 37.5% [64]. Another study of greater than 4 cm Bethesda II nodules that went to surgery reported a 10.4% false-negative benign cytology rate. Although molecular testing aided risk stratification of nodules with genetic alterations, it remains uncertain whether this tool can or should be applied to all Bethesda II nodules to rule out malignancy [65].

6.4.2 Bethesda III, IV, and V

In clinical practice, molecular testing has been used primarily for the evaluation of thyroid nodules with indeterminate cytology, for both diagnosis and potentially for guiding the decision regarding extent of surgery.

The management of AUS and FN nodules, which are associated with a more moderate risk of malignancy (10–30%) compared to the suspicious for malignancy category, poses a challenging dilemma. In a recent meta-analysis comparing various molecular tests, it was estimated that up to 85% of surgeries for indeterminate nodules could be avoided with negative molecular testing results [66]. A small pilot cohort study of patients with Bethesda III/IV nodules that underwent surgery found that diagnostic molecular marker testing may be unnecessary in the setting of high-risk ultrasound (US) features but may enhance clinical decision-making when US features are low-to-intermediate risk [67].

In the case of Bethesda III and IV cytology, studies have shown that repeat FNA of indeterminate nodules may help avoid diagnostic surgery by re-classification to benign cytology [68]. Moreover, a restrictive model of performing molecular testing only on nodules with two separate biopsies showing Bethesda III/IV cytology may significantly reduce the rate of diagnostic surgery for histologically benign nodules while missing only rare low-risk tumors or NIFTP, an approach by which the benefit of more selective testing and surgery appears to outweigh the potential harm of missed cancer diagnoses [69].

The PPV of several molecular tests has been demonstrated to decrease when NIFTP is classified as a nonmalignant lesion, though a "positive" test in this context should not exclude the appropriate conservative management, which is usually surgical lobectomy [70].

6.4.3 Bethesda VI

Molecular testing of nodules with Bethesda VI cytology is generally not performed prior to surgery, as surgery is the recommended treatment for these lesions. Use of molecular markers for guiding extent of surgery has been debated, and currently there is no evidence for improved long-term outcomes in this context. In addition to clinicopathologic data, genomic alterations are being increasingly used for prognostication of thyroid cancer. Use of novel techniques for ongoing disease monitoring, including microRNA, circulating long noncoding RNA, circulating tumor

DNA, and circulating tumor cells, are still in the early stages of investigation.

A systematic literature review published in 2021 examined the potential use of preoperative molecular testing in Bethesda VI nodules for risk stratification utilizing different molecular testing methods. Most nodules with malignant cytology that were sampled harbored a genetic alteration, with BRAF p.V600E mutation being the most common (70–75%), followed by p*TERT* mutations [71].

While the identification of BRAF p.V600E mutation has been associated with more aggressive clinicopathologic features, including higher mortality rates in older patients and more advanced staging, the significance of the isolated mutation, independent of other risk factors, is uncertain. Comprehensive oncogene panel testing that includes prognostic and actionable gene alterations, for example p*TERT* mutations or *RET* and *NTRK* gene rearrangements, can aid both surgical decision-making and individualized treatment decisions through selection of targeted therapies and the identification of radioiodine-refractory tumors.

Combination testing with a miRNA expression classifier to investigate for altered genetic material in mutation-negative cells or in nodules positive for *RAS* mutations may further raise the risk profile and the diagnostic yield.

Additional study is needed to fully assess the role of molecular testing for the preoperative risk stratification of malignant nodules and apply the findings to clinical decision-making.

6.4.4 Advanced Thyroid Cancers

Molecular testing may provide valuable information that can help determine targeted therapeutic options for advanced thyroid cancer.

Current first-line or salvage therapy for radioiodine-refractory DTC is centered around multikinase inhibitors (MKIs), including sorafenib, lenvatinib, cabozantinib, and pazopanib, which each target multiple kinases to varying degrees including VEGFR1-3, PDGFR, RET, FLT, FGFR1–4, and KIT.

Due to a significant risk of high-grade adverse events with these drugs, therapeutic options with more favorable side effect profiles are needed. The agents selpercatinib and pralsetinib have more recently been introduced into clinical care for the treatment of *RET* fusion-positive DTC. *ALK*- and *NTRK* fusions are other genomic lesions which are present in DTC, albeit rarely, and the NTRK inhibitors larotrectinib and entrectinib have U.S. Food and Drug Administration (FDA) approvals for NTRK fusion-positive malignancies agnostic of tissue-of-origin.

The combination of dabrafenib (BRAF inhibitor) plus trametinib (MEK inhibitor) has also been FDA-approved for use in the United States in locally advanced or metastatic ATC with BRAF p.V600E mutation that is ineligible for treatment with surgery or radiotherapy, due to a phase II non-randomized trial demonstrating an impressive 80% 12-month overall survival rate. Rapid identification of targetable mutations and gene rearrangements through sequencing platforms is an important challenge in the management of ATC, a highly aggressive cancer. In MTC, several MKIs that inhibit RET among other kinases, including vandetanib and cabozantinib, have demonstrated improved overall response rates and progression-free survival. Selpercatinib and pralsetinib were also approved by the U.S. FDA in 2020 for the treatment of *RET*-mutant MTC [72].

6.4.5 Neoadjuvant Therapy

Use of targeted therapy for tumor bulk reduction of unresectable tumors or borderline resectable disease that would be associated with significant surgical morbidity is an emerging area of investigation. Selection of optimal candidates for this approach, i.e., those who would benefit from targeted therapy pre-surgery to avoid incomplete resection while also avoiding drug-resistant disease progression requires further elucidation through ongoing clinical trials [73].

Neoadjuvant BRAF-directed therapy has been used to reduce the extent of surgery and surgical morbidity for BRAF-mutated ATC. Early promising data should be confirmed in prospective clinical trials [74].

A small case series of patients with RET-mutated locoregionally advanced MTC treated with neoadjuvant selpercatinib followed by surgical resection showed both significant radiographic responses and surgical preservation of major neurovascular structures, raising the prospect of achieving locoregional disease control with reduced morbidity by this novel approach [75].

6.4.6 Cost-Effective Use of Molecular Testing

Studies examining the cost-effectiveness of molecular testing have generally supported the use of this tool for Bethesda III and IV nodules, on the basis that the information gleaned from testing leads to fewer diagnostic surgeries and completion surgeries, as compared to surgery performed without molecular testing. One study utilizing hypothetical modeling showed that molecular testing is only cost-effective for indeterminate nodules that have low- or intermediate-risk sonographic features [76]. It should be noted, however, that the costs of surgery vs. clinical follow-up are variable, are impacted by many patient- and hospital-related factors, and studies in this area have generally not taken into account the long-term costs of surveillance of patients who do not have surgery [77].

6.5 Conclusions

The PPV for cancer prediction by a specific genomic alteration depends on the individual variant or fusion identified, keeping in mind that the finding of high-risk mutations predicting more aggressive tumor behavior that is not already clinically evident is a relatively rare occurrence. Clinical decision-making regarding use of molecular testing should be individualized and patients should be informed about both the benefits and limitations of such testing. Selective, rather than routine, use of molecular testing when the results of testing would alter management, and when the clinical, cytology, and imaging data do not provide adequate guidance, is favored [78]. Directed therapy toward known cancers is an evolving and promising area of clinical application.

References

1. Lawrence MS, Stojanov P, Polak P, Kryukov GV, Cibulskis K, Sivachenko A, et al. Mutational heterogeneity in cancer and the search for new cancer-associated genes. Nature. 2013;499:214–8. https://doi.org/10.1038/nature12213.
2. Agrawal N, Akbani R, Aksoy BA, Ally A, Arachchi H, Asa SL, et al. Integrated genomic characterization of papillary thyroid carcinoma. Cell. 2015;159:676–90. https://doi.org/10.1016/j.cell.2014.09.050.
3. Prete A, Borges de Souza P, Censi S, Muzza M, Nucci N, Sponziello M. Update on fundamental mechanisms of thyroid cancer. Front Endocrinol (Lausanne). 2020;11:102. https://doi.org/10.3389/FENDO.2020.00102.
4. Verrienti A, Grani G, Sponziello M, Pecce V, Damante G, Durante C, et al. Precision oncology for RET-related tumors. Front Oncol. 2022;12:992636. https://doi.org/10.3389/FONC.2022.992636.
5. Ciampi R, Romei C, Ramone T, Prete A, Tacito A, Cappagli V, et al. Genetic landscape of somatic mutations in a large cohort of sporadic medullary thyroid carcinomas studied by next-generation targeted sequencing. IScience. 2019;20:324–36. https://doi.org/10.1016/j.isci.2019.09.030.
6. Araujo AN, Camacho CP, Mendes TB, Lindsey SC, Moraes L, Miyazawa M, et al. Comprehensive assessment of copy number alterations uncovers recurrent AIFM3 and DLK1 copy gain in medullary thyroid carcinoma. Cancers (Basel). 2021;13:1–17. https://doi.org/10.3390/CANCERS13020218.
7. Celano M, Rosignolo F, Maggisano V, Pecce V, Iannone M, Russo D, et al. MicroRNAs as biomarkers in thyroid carcinoma. Int J Genomics. 2017;2017:6496570. https://doi.org/10.1155/2017/6496570.
8. Baloch ZW, Asa SL, Barletta JA, Ghossein RA, Juhlin CC, Jung CK, et al. Overview of the 2022 WHO classification of thyroid neoplasms. Endocr Pathol. 2022;33:27–63. https://doi.org/10.1007/S12022-022-09707-3.
9. Mete O, Asa SL. Pitfalls in the diagnosis of follicular epithelial proliferations of the thyroid. Adv Anat Pathol. 2012;19:363–73. https://doi.org/10.1097/PAP.0B013E318271A5AC.
10. Ye L, Zhou X, Huang F, Wang W, Qi Y, Xu H, et al. The genetic landscape of benign thyroid nodules revealed by whole exome and transcriptome sequencing. Nat Commun. 2017;8:15533. https://doi.org/10.1038/NCOMMS15533.

11. Yoo SK, Lee S, Kim SJ, Jee HG, Kim BA, Cho H, et al. Comprehensive analysis of the transcriptional and mutational landscape of follicular and papillary thyroid cancers. PLoS Genet. 2016;12:e1006239. https://doi.org/10.1371/JOURNAL.PGEN.1006239.
12. Dom G, Frank S, Floor S, Kehagias P, Libert F, Hoang C, et al. Thyroid follicular adenomas and carcinomas: molecular profiling provides evidence for a continuous evolution. Oncotarget. 2017;9:10343–59. https://doi.org/10.18632/ONCOTARGET.23130.
13. Gasparre G, Porcelli AM, Bonora E, Pennisi LF, Toller M, Iommarini L, et al. Disruptive mitochondrial DNA mutations in complex I subunits are markers of oncocytic phenotype in thyroid tumors. Proc Natl Acad Sci USA. 2007;104:9001–6. https://doi.org/10.1073/PNAS.0703056104.
14. Doerfler WR, Nikitski AV, Morariu EM, Paul Ohori N, Chiosea SI, Landau MS, et al. Molecular alterations in Hürthle cell nodules and preoperative cancer risk. Endocr Relat Cancer. 2021;28:301–9. https://doi.org/10.1530/ERC-20-0435.
15. Ganly I, Filho JR, Eng S, Ghossein R, Morris LGT, Liang Y, et al. Genomic dissection of Hurthle cell carcinoma reveals a unique class of thyroid malignancy. J Clin Endocrinol Metab. 2013;98:E962–72. https://doi.org/10.1210/JC.2012-3539.
16. Brandler TC, Zhou F, Liu CZ, Serrano A, Sun W, Nikiforov YE, et al. Molecular profiles of noninvasive, minimally invasive, and invasive follicular patterned thyroid neoplasms with papillary nuclear features. Thyroid. 2023;33:715–23. https://doi.org/10.1089/THY.2023.0047.
17. Chu YH, Sadow PM. Noninvasive follicular thyroid neoplasm with papillary-like nuclear features (NIFTP): diagnostic updates and molecular advances. Semin Diagn Pathol. 2020;37:213–8. https://doi.org/10.1053/J.SEMDP.2020.06.001.
18. Giannini R, Ugolini C, Poma AM, Urpì M, Niccoli C, Elisei R, et al. Identification of two distinct molecular subtypes of non-invasive follicular neoplasm with papillary-like nuclear features by digital RNA counting. Thyroid. 2017;27:1267–76. https://doi.org/10.1089/THY.2016.0605.
19. Jahanbani I, Al-Abdallah A, Ali RH, Al-Brahim N, Mojiminiyi O. Discriminatory miRNAs for the management of papillary thyroid carcinoma and noninvasive follicular thyroid neoplasms with papillary-like nuclear features. Thyroid. 2018;28:319–27. https://doi.org/10.1089/THY.2017.0127.
20. Borrelli N, Denaro M, Ugolini C, Poma AM, Miccoli M, Vitti P, et al. miRNA expression profiling of "noninvasive follicular thyroid neoplasms with papillary-like nuclear features" compared with adenomas and infiltrative follicular variants of papillary thyroid carcinomas. Mod Pathol. 2017;30:39–51. https://doi.org/10.1038/MODPATHOL.2016.157.
21. Duan H, Liu X, Ren X, Zhang H, Wu H, Liang Z. Mutation profiles of follicular thyroid tumors by targeted sequencing. Diagn Pathol. 2019:14. https://doi.org/10.1186/S13000-019-0817-1.
22. Nikiforova MN, Nikitski AV, Panebianco F, Kaya C, Yip L, Williams M, et al. GLIS rearrangement is a genomic hallmark of hyalinizing trabecular tumor of the thyroid gland. Thyroid. 2019;29:161–73. https://doi.org/10.1089/THY.2018.0791.
23. De Leo A, Serban D, Maloberti T, Sanza V, Coluccelli S, Altimari A, et al. Expanding the spectrum of BRAF non-V600E mutations in thyroid nodules: evidence-based data from a tertiary referral centre. Int J Mol Sci. 2023;24:4057. https://doi.org/10.3390/IJMS24044057.
24. Morton LM, Karyadi DM, Stewart C, Bogdanova TI, Dawson ET, Steinberg MK, et al. Radiation-related genomic profile of papillary thyroid carcinoma after the Chernobyl accident. Science. 2021;372:eabg2538. https://doi.org/10.1126/SCIENCE.ABG2538.
25. Yip L, Gooding WE, Nikitski A, Wald AI, Carty SE, Karslioglu-French E, et al. Risk assessment for distant metastasis in differentiated thyroid cancer using molecular profiling: a matched case-control study. Cancer. 2021;127:1779–87. https://doi.org/10.1002/CNCR.33421.
26. Rosignolo F, Memeo L, Monzani F, Colarossi C, Pecce V, Verrienti A, et al. MicroRNA-based molecular classification of papillary thyroid carcinoma. Int J Oncol. 2017;50:1767–77. https://doi.org/10.3892/ijo.2017.3960.
27. Rosignolo F, Sponziello M, Giacomelli L, Russo D, Pecce V, Biffoni M, et al. Identification of thyroid-associated serum microRNA profiles and their potential use in thyroid cancer follow-up. J Endocr Soc. 2017;1:3–13. https://doi.org/10.1210/js.2016-1032.
28. Nicolson NG, Murtha TD, Dong W, Paulsson JO, Choi J, Barbieri AL, et al. Comprehensive genetic analysis of follicular thyroid carcinoma predicts prognosis independent of histology. J Clin Endocrinol Metab. 2018;103:2640–50. https://doi.org/10.1210/JC.2018-00277.
29. Paulsson JO, Rafati N, Dilorenzo S, Chen Y, Haglund F, Zedenius J, et al. Whole-genome sequencing of follicular thyroid carcinomas reveal recurrent mutations in MicroRNA processing subunit DGCR8. J Clin Endocrinol Metab. 2021;106:3265–82. https://doi.org/10.1210/CLINEM/DGAB471.
30. Macerola E, Poma AM, Vignali P, Proietti A, Torregrossa L, Ugolini C, et al. MicroRNA expression profiling of RAS-mutant thyroid tumors with follicular architecture: microRNA signatures to discriminate benign from malignant lesions. J Endocrinol Investig. 2023;46:1651–62. https://doi.org/10.1007/s40618-023-02023-5.
31. Santana NO, Lerario AM, Schmerling CK, Marui S, Alves VAF, Hoff AO, et al. Molecular profile of Hürthle cell carcinomas: recurrent mutations in the Wnt/β-catenin pathway. Eur J Endocrinol. 2020;183:647–56. https://doi.org/10.1530/EJE-20-0597.
32. Ganly I, Makarov V, Deraje S, Dong YY, Reznik E, Seshan V, et al. Integrated genomic analysis of Hürthle cell cancer reveals oncogenic drivers, recur-

rent mitochondrial mutations, and unique chromosomal landscapes. Cancer Cell. 2018;34:256–270.e5. https://doi.org/10.1016/J.CCELL.2018.07.002.
33. Landa I, Ibrahimpasic T, Boucai L, Sinha R, Knauf JA, Shah RH, et al. Genomic and transcriptomic hallmarks of poorly differentiated and anaplastic thyroid cancers. J Clin Invest. 2016;126:1052–66. https://doi.org/10.1172/JCI85271.
34. Volante M, Lam AK, Papotti M, Tallini G. Molecular pathology of poorly differentiated and anaplastic thyroid cancer: what do pathologists need to know? Endocr Pathol. 2021;32:63–76. https://doi.org/10.1007/S12022-021-09665-2.
35. Elisei R, Ciampi R, Matrone A, Prete A, Gambale C, Ramone T, et al. Somatic RET Indels in sporadic medullary thyroid cancer: prevalence and response to Selpercatinib. J Clin Endocrinol Metab. 2022;107:2195–202. https://doi.org/10.1210/CLINEM/DGAC325.
36. Ramone T, Romei C, Ciampi R, Casalini R, Valetto A, Bertini V, et al. Chromosomal alterations in sporadic medullary thyroid carcinoma and correlation with outcome. Endocr Relat Cancer. 2023;30:e220251. https://doi.org/10.1530/ERC-22-0251.
37. Ciampi R, Ramone T, Romei C, Casalini R, Matrone A, Prete A, et al. NF1 gene inactivation acts as tumor driver in RET/RAS negative medullary thyroid carcinomas. Eur J Endocrinol. 2023;188:430–7. https://doi.org/10.1093/EJENDO/LVAD051.
38. Alsharif O, Panella T, Nodit L, Hu MI. Letter to the editor: ETV6-NTRK2 fusion identified in a patient with medullary thyroid carcinoma. Thyroid. 2023;33:774–6. https://doi.org/10.1089/THY.2022.0630.
39. Sponziello M, Benvenuti S, Gentile A, Pecce V, Rosignolo F, Virzì AR, et al. Whole exome sequencing identifies a germline MET mutation in two siblings with hereditary wild-type RET medullary thyroid cancer. Hum Mutat. 2018;39:371–7. https://doi.org/10.1002/humu.23378.
40. Smith J, Read ML, Hoffman J, Brown R, Bradshaw B, Campbell C, et al. Germline ESR2 mutation predisposes to medullary thyroid carcinoma and causes up-regulation of RET expression. Hum Mol Genet. 2016;25:1836–45. https://doi.org/10.1093/hmg/ddw057.
41. Besharat ZM, Trocchianesi S, Verrienti A, Ciampi R, Cantara S, Romei C, et al. Circulating miR-26b-5p and miR-451a as diagnostic biomarkers in medullary thyroid carcinoma patients. J Endocrinol Investig. 2023;46:2583–99. https://doi.org/10.1007/S40618-023-02115-2.
42. Grani G, Sponziello M, Pecce V, Ramundo V, Durante C. Contemporary thyroid nodule evaluation and management. J Clin Endocrinol Metab. 2020;105:2869–83. https://doi.org/10.1210/CLINEM/DGAA322.
43. Kamps R, Brandão RD, van den Bosch BJ, Paulussen ADC, Xanthoulea S, Blok MJ, et al. Next-generation sequencing in oncology: genetic diagnosis, risk prediction and cancer classification. Int J Mol Sci. 2017;18:308. https://doi.org/10.3390/IJMS18020308.
44. Haddad R, Elisei R, Hoff AO, Liu Z, Pitoia F, Pruneri G, et al. Diagnosis and management of tropomyosin receptor kinase fusion-positive thyroid carcinomas: a review. JAMA Oncol. 2023;9:1132–41. https://doi.org/10.1001/JAMAONCOL.2023.1379.
45. Agarwal S, Bychkov A, Jung CK. Emerging biomarkers in thyroid practice and research. Cancers (Basel). 2021;14:204. https://doi.org/10.3390/CANCERS14010204.
46. Malone ER, Oliva M, Sabatini PJB, Stockley TL, Siu LL. Molecular profiling for precision cancer therapies. Genome Med. 2020;12:8. https://doi.org/10.1186/S13073-019-0703-1.
47. Narrandes S, Xu W. Gene expression detection assay for cancer clinical use. J Cancer. 2018;9:2249–65. https://doi.org/10.7150/JCA.24744.
48. Bellevicine C, Sgariglia R, Nacchio M, De Luca C, Pisapia P, Pepe F, et al. Molecular testing of thyroid fine-needle aspiration: local issues and solutions. An interventional cytopathologist perspective. J Mol Pathol. 2021;2:233–40. https://doi.org/10.3390/jmp2030020.
49. Nishino M. Molecular cytopathology for thyroid nodules: a review of methodology and test performance. Cancer Cytopathol. 2016;124:14–27. https://doi.org/10.1002/CNCY.21612.
50. Nikiforov YE, Steward DL, Carty SE, Sippel RS, Yang SP, Sosa JA, et al. Performance of a multigene genomic classifier in thyroid nodules with indeterminate cytology: a prospective blinded multicenter study. JAMA Oncol. 2019;5:204–12. https://doi.org/10.1001/JAMAONCOL.2018.4616.
51. Patel KN, Angell TE, Babiarz J, Barth NM, Blevins T, Duh QY, et al. Performance of a genomic sequencing classifier for the preoperative diagnosis of cytologically indeterminate thyroid nodules. JAMA Surg. 2018;153:817–24. https://doi.org/10.1001/JAMASURG.2018.1153.
52. Finkelstein SD, Sistrunk JW, Malchoff C, Thompson DV, Kumar G, Timmaraju VA, et al. A retrospective evaluation of the diagnostic performance of an interdependent pairwise microRNA expression analysis with a mutation panel in indeterminate thyroid nodules. Thyroid. 2022;32:1362–71. https://doi.org/10.1089/THY.2022.0124.
53. Nasr CE, Andrioli M, Endo M, Harrell RM, Livhits MJ, Osakwe I, et al. Real-world performance of the Afirma genomic sequencing classifier (GSC)—a meta-analysis. J Clin Endocrinol Metab. 2023;108:1526–32. https://doi.org/10.1210/CLINEM/DGAC688.

54. Krane JF, Cibas ES, Endo M, Marqusee E, Hu MI, Nasr CE, et al. The Afirma Xpression atlas for thyroid nodules and thyroid cancer metastases: insights to inform clinical decision-making from a fine-needle aspiration sample. Cancer Cytopathol. 2020;128:452–9. https://doi.org/10.1002/CNCY.22300.
55. Zafereo M, McIver B, Vargas-Salas S, Domínguez JM, Steward DL, Holsinger FC, et al. A thyroid genetic classifier correctly predicts benign nodules with indeterminate cytology: two independent, multicenter, prospective validation trials. Thyroid. 2020;30:704–12. https://doi.org/10.1089/THY.2019.0490.
56. Dos Santos MT, Buzolin AL, Gama RR, Da Silva ECA, Dufloth RM, Figueiredo DLA, et al. Molecular classification of thyroid nodules with indeterminate cytology: development and validation of a highly sensitive and specific new miRNA-based classifier test using fine-needle aspiration smear slides. Thyroid. 2018;28:1618–26. https://doi.org/10.1089/THY.2018.0254.
57. Santos MT, Rodrigues BM, Shizukuda S, Oliveira AF, Oliveira M, Figueiredo DLA, et al. Clinical decision support analysis of a microRNA-based thyroid molecular classifier: a real-world, prospective and multicentre validation study. EBioMedicine. 2022;82:104137. https://doi.org/10.1016/J.EBIOM.2022.104137.
58. Sponziello M, Brunelli C, Verrienti A, Grani G, Pecce V, Abballe L, et al. Performance of a dual-component molecular assay in cytologically indeterminate thyroid nodules. Endocrine. 2020;68:458–65. https://doi.org/10.1007/S12020-020-02271-Y.
59. Sgariglia R, Nacchio M, Migliatico I, Vigliar E, Malapelle U, Pisapia P, et al. Moving towards a local testing solution for undetermined thyroid fine-needle aspirates: validation of a novel custom DNA-based NGS panel. J Clin Pathol. 2021;0:1–7. https://doi.org/10.1136/JCLINPATH-2021-207429.
60. Song Y, Xu G, Ma T, Zhu Y, Yu H, Yu W, et al. Utility of a multigene testing for preoperative evaluation of indeterminate thyroid nodules: a prospective blinded single center study in China. Cancer Med. 2020;9:8397–405. https://doi.org/10.1002/CAM4.3450.
61. NCCN Biomarkers compendium. www.nccn.org/professionals/biomarkers/default.aspx.
62. Ali SZ, Vanderlaan PA, editors. The Bethesda system for reporting thyroid cytopathology. 3rd ed. Springer; 2023. https://doi.org/10.1007/978-3-031-28046-7.
63. Beaudenon-Huibregtse S, Alexander EK, Guttler RB, Hershman JM, Babu V, Blevins TC, et al. Centralized molecular testing for oncogenic gene mutations complements the local cytopathologic diagnosis of thyroid nodules. Thyroid. 2014;24:1479–87. https://doi.org/10.1089/THY.2013.0640.
64. Grimmichova T, Pacesova P, Hill M, Pekova B, Vankova M, Moravcova J, et al. Thyroid cancer detection in a routine clinical setting: performance of ACR TI-RADS, FNAC, and molecular testing in prospective cohort study. Biomedicines. 2022;10:954. https://doi.org/10.3390/BIOMEDICINES10050954.
65. Wharry LI, McCoy KL, Stang MT, Armstrong MJ, Lebeau SO, Tublin ME, et al. Thyroid nodules (≥4 cm): can ultrasound and cytology reliably exclude cancer? World J Surg. 2014;38:614–21. https://doi.org/10.1007/S00268-013-2261-9.
66. Vargas-Salas S, Martínez JR, Urra S, Domínguez JM, Mena N, Uslar T, et al. Genetic testing for indeterminate thyroid cytology: review and meta-analysis. Endocr Relat Cancer. 2018;25:R163–77. https://doi.org/10.1530/ERC-17-0405.
67. Gomes-Lima CJ, Auh S, Thakur S, Zemskova M, Cochran C, Merkel R, et al. A novel risk stratification system for thyroid nodules with indeterminate cytology-a pilot cohort study. Front Endocrinol (Lausanne). 2020;11:53. https://doi.org/10.3389/FENDO.2020.00053.
68. Papazian MR, Dublin JC, Patel KN, Oweity T, Jacobson AS, Brandler TC, et al. Repeat fine-needle aspiration with molecular analysis in management of indeterminate thyroid nodules. Otolaryngol Head Neck Surg. 2023;168:738–44. https://doi.org/10.1177/01945998221093527.
69. Nishino M, Mateo R, Kilim H, Feldman A, Elliott A, Shen C, et al. Repeat fine needle aspiration cytology refines the selection of thyroid nodules for Afirma gene expression classifier testing. Thyroid. 2021;31:1253–63. https://doi.org/10.1089/THY.2020.0969.
70. Jug RC, Datto MB, Jiang XS. Molecular testing for indeterminate thyroid nodules: performance of the Afirma gene expression classifier and ThyroSeq panel. Cancer Cytopathol. 2018;126:471–80. https://doi.org/10.1002/CNCY.21993.
71. Labourier E, Fahey TJ. Preoperative molecular testing in thyroid nodules with Bethesda VI cytology: clinical experience and review of the literature. Diagn Cytopathol. 2021;49:E175–80. https://doi.org/10.1002/DC.24637.
72. Miller KC, Chintakuntlawar AV. Molecular-driven therapy in advanced thyroid cancer. Curr Treat Options in Oncol. 2021;22:24. https://doi.org/10.1007/S11864-021-00822-7.
73. Cavalheiro BG, Shah JP, Randolph GW, Medina JE, Tufano RP, Zafereo M, et al. Management of recurrent well-differentiated thyroid carcinoma in the neck: a comprehensive review. Cancers (Basel). 2023;15:923. https://doi.org/10.3390/CANCERS15030923.
74. Zhao X, Wang JR, Dadu R, Busaidy N, Xu L, Learned K, et al. Surgery after BRAF-directed therapy is associated with improved survival in BRAFV600E mutant anaplastic thyroid cancer: a single-center retrospec-

tive cohort study. Thyroid. 2023;33:484–91. https://doi.org/10.1089/THY.2022.0504.
75. Contrera KJ, Gule-Monroe MK, Hu MI, Cabanillas ME, Busaidy NL, Dadu R, et al. Neoadjuvant selective RET inhibitor for medullary thyroid cancer: a case series. Thyroid. 2023;33:129–32. https://doi.org/10.1089/THY.2022.0506.
76. Zanocco KA, Wang MM, Yeh MW, Livhits MJ. Selective use of molecular testing based on sonographic features of cytologically indeterminate thyroid nodules: a decision analysis. World J Surg. 2020;44:393–401. https://doi.org/10.1007/S00268-019-05177-7.
77. Wu SY, Terrell J, Park A, Perrier N. Understanding thyroidectomy cost variations among National Cancer Institute-designated cancer centers. World J Surg. 2020;44:385–92. https://doi.org/10.1007/S00268-019-05176-8.
78. Khan TM, Zeiger MA. Thyroid nodule molecular testing: is it ready for prime time? Front Endocrinol (Lausanne). 2020;11:590128. https://doi.org/10.3389/FENDO.2020.590128.

7 Selection of Minimally Invasive Treatment Modality by Indication for Thyroid Disease

Salem I. Noureldine, Tatiana Ferraro, and Chelsey K. Baldwin

7.1 Introduction

The selection and appropriateness of minimally invasive treatments (MIT) for the management of thyroid disease is dependent upon the physical characteristics of the target lesion, including solid composition, size, and location relative to high-risk structures within the neck. Additionally, the target lesion classification as a neoplasm vs. hyperplastic etiology also has implications for efficacy. In this chapter, we aim to highlight the most commonly used MIT modalities and their relative efficacy by indication.

S. I. Noureldine · T. Ferraro
Department of Surgery, School of Medicine and Health Sciences, The George Washington University, Washington, DC, USA
e-mail: snoureldine@mfa.gwu.edu; tferraro@mfa.gwu.edu

C. K. Baldwin (✉)
Department of Endocrinology, School of Medicine and Health Sciences, The George Washington University, Washington, DC, USA
e-mail: cbaldwin@mfa.gwu.edu

7.2 MIT Modalities for Management of Thyroid Disease

7.2.1 Ethanol Ablation

Ethanol Ablation (EA) refers to the use of high concentration (95–99%) ethanol injection into a target lesion. Ethanol in high concentration induces caustic injury leading to coagulative and ischemic necrosis as well as endothelial damage resulting in thrombosis of small vessels. Safety concerns for use of ethanol within the thyroid and adjacent tissue include heterogenous diffusion within solid tissue and unintended leak of ethanol into adjacent structures due to absence or injury of target lesion capsule. This results in severe pain requiring immediate cessation of injection and discontinuation of procedure, limiting the ablative effect.

7.2.2 Laser Ablation (LA)

Laser Ablation (LA) is the use of variable length light electromagnetic (EM) energy wavelengths to deliver collimated, monochromatic light energy, usually generated by a diode or a Nd:YAG source, to target tissue via one or more optical fibers resulting in a small area of direct cell injury (active ablation) and subsequent heat production leading to injury of

R. Valcavi et al. (eds.), *Thyroid Ablation*, https://doi.org/10.1007/978-3-031-88229-6_7

adjacent tissue through thermal conductance (passive ablation). Laser ablation's reliance on passive ablation can be associated with longer procedure times [1] for large nodules which require multiple wires and serial wire pull back to treat entire volume [2]. Cost of procedure is directly related to number of optical fibers required [3]. Suggested strengths of laser ablation include reliable small spherical treatment zones [4] improving safety for structures adjacent to nodule border or for management of small rounded lesions like metastatic lymph nodes.

7.2.3 Radiofrequency Ablation (RFA)

Radiofrequency Ablation (RFA) is the application of EM waves with frequencies ranging from 450 to 1200 kHz resulting the rapid alternation of ions within the target tissue which generates frictional heat. Similar to LA, RFA results in a small area of active ablation due to frictional heat generation and a larger volume of tissue undergoes thermal injury from thermal conductance (passive ablation) [5]. The moving shot technique allows free hand variable allocation of energy deposition throughout a nodule, tailoring lower energy deposition at borders and increased energy within the center of the nodule resulting in safe and complete treatment. Mauri et al. proposed a higher degree of technical expertise is required due to the free hand nature of the RF probe manipulation, compared to LA [1]. Additionally, due to reliance on thermal conductance for the majority of treatment zone, RFA is associated with longer procedure times and consideration must be given to target characteristics that effect thermal conductance such as vaporization, carbonization, tissue heterogeneity, and acknowledgment of susceptibility to vascular flow heat sink effect [2]. The delay in attaining lethal temperatures may be protective, allowing for detection and discontinuation when patient symptomatology is consistent with unintentional heat delivery to adjacent nerves or aerodigestive structures.

7.2.4 Microwave Ablation (MWA)

Microwave Ablation (MWA) utilizes EM wave frequencies ranging from 915 MHz to 2.45 GHz inducing dielectric hysteresis or rapid realignment of polar molecules, predominantly water, with an alternating electrical field creating frictional heat. The technique is identical to RFA. The probe is introduced into the lesion under ultrasound guidance, followed by multiple overlapping burns. Microwave ablation results in high energy deposition within the target tissue and allows for the attainment of higher temperatures and larger areas of active ablation compared to LA and RFA. MWA relies less on thermal conductance therefore less susceptible to factors that impair heat spread compared to other thermal ablation modalities [5]. Potential concerns regarding the use of MWA within the thyroid include the risk of inadvertent near immediate delivery of lethal thermal energy to adjacent critical structures [6, 7].

7.3 Additional Modalities

7.3.1 High-Intensity Focused Ultrasound (HIFU)

This is the only currently available completely noninvasive ablation modality [8]. HIFU uses low-intensity sound waves to target a specific lesion. High-intensity ultrasound then transfers sufficient energy to induce coagulative necrosis via molecular vibration, frictional heating, and cavitation. A key challenge in using this modality is the safe delivery of energy to the target lesion without causing damage to intervening and surrounding tissues. This can be accomplished by focusing the high-intensity waves from numerous sources outside the body onto the same target, avoiding significant energy accumulation in the propagation path. This can be easily achieved in wide surface areas like the abdomen, with limited applicability within the neck's confined spaces. Real-time magnetic resonance thermometry during sonification has been described to limit damage to surrounding tissues; this however can limit this modalities application in an outpatient clinic setting [9]. This also led to the development of interstitial high-intensity therapeutic ultrasound percutaneous applicators like RFA, voiding the noninvasive advantage of this modality [10].

7.3.2 Cryoablation

This modality produces localized tissue necrosis by inducing cycles of tissue freezing down to temperatures of −40 to −160 °C and then thawing. Cryoablation is a well-established treatment option for kidney and prostate cancers, with recent successful applications for lung, breast, and pancreatic tumors. Pressured argon gas is released from the applicators tip into the tissue causing expansion and rapid cooling via the Joule-Thomson effect. An expanding "ice ball" is then formed in the targeted tissue causing osmotic insult, cell wall crystal injury, and microvascular thrombosis. Unlike hyperthermia-induced necrosis, there is less disruption of the tissue architecture, partly reducing the risk of vascular and nerve injury [11]. This technique is generally less painful than heat-based technologies. One of the major limitations of this modality is that the ice ball is only visible on computerized tomography and magnetic resonance imaging and, less distinctly, with ultrasound examination. Therefore, this procedure cannot be done reliably in an outpatient clinic setting with real-time monitoring using ultrasound.

7.4 MIT Efficacy by Indication

7.4.1 Pure Cysts and Predominantly Cystic Lesions

Ethanol ablation (EA) is supported by all current guidelines for MIT as first-line intervention for symptomatic pure or predominantly cystic lesions [12–17]. Ethanol ablation is efficacious for volume reduction of pure and predominantly cystic lesions with a reported volume reduction ratio (VRR) of 85–98.5% [18]. When compared to thermal ablation, Sung et al. found EA to be non-inferior to radiofrequency ablation (RFA) regarding VRR, therapeutic success (defined as >50% VRR), improvement in cosmetic scoring. However, the number of treatments needed to achieve outcomes was significantly fewer in the EA treated group vs. RFA, 1.2 vs. 1.7 ($p < 0.03$) [19]. The authors concluded that the cost and technical simplicity of EA procedure made it the ideal first-line indication for pure and predominantly cystic nodules. However, a novel concern particularly within the United States is the rising cost of ethanol [20] that will impact that cost-benefit ratio in decision to treat with EA vs. RFA.

The efficacy of ethanol ablation for management of symptomatic mixed solid cystic nodules is indirectly related to the percentage of the solid component of the nodule [21, 22]. Patient satisfaction with outcomes has been reported to decrease once the target nodule exceeds 20% solid content [23]. In such nodules, a stepwise approach of EA followed by RFA has been proposed for nodules that fail to meet therapeutic success goals after EA. Jang et al. reported that RFA after single session of EA was able to significantly reduce compressive and cosmetic symptoms scores and mean nodule volume from 11.3 to 0.9 mL ($p < 0.001$) [23]. Yoon et al. proposed that EA be used as an initial step in the treatment of mixed solid cystic nodules to prevent post-cystic evacuation hemorrhage prior to RFA [24].

7.4.2 Predominantly Solid Benign Symptomatic Nodules

Efficacy of EA for volume reduction of nodules in which the solid component exceeds 50% is 38–47% [18]. Improved VRR, 70–71%, have been reported when the average number of treatment sessions increase to 5–7.4 [25, 26], compared to 1–1.9 treatments reported in studies with lower VRR. Reduced efficacy of EA in solid nodules may be related to heterogenous distribution of ethanol within the target tissue. Additional safety concerns include injury to adjacent structures due to unintended seepage of ethanol [26, 27].

Thermal ablative MIT have been shown to have a higher VRR compared to EA for the treatment of predominantly solid nodules [18]. Several single and multicenter studies have attempted to directly compare thermal ablation modalities for the management of benign thyroid nodules and are summarized in Table 7.1.

7.4.2.1 RFA vs. LA

Early comparisons of thermal ablation techniques in benign thyroid nodules included systematic review of LA and RFA by Ha et al. in 2015 in which the outcomes of single modality studies were pooled and reported to demonstrated superiority of RFA vs. LA regarding VRR (76.1% vs. 49.9%, respectively) [28]. However, Mauri et al. argued that LA and RFA were equally efficacious in VRR (70 vs. 74%, $p > 0.05$) and safe when compared directly and performed by the same highly trained operators [1]. Additional studies that attempted to directly compare RFA and LA are conflicting as to which modality provides superior VRR [3, 29, 30]. Papini et al. suggested that the variability in laser VRR outcomes within

Table 7.1 Primary studies comparing outcomes of MIT modalities for Benign Symptomatic Thyroid Nodules

Study	MIT modality (n = treated nodules)	Study design	VRR (%) at last follow-up	Key points
	RFA vs. LA			
Mauri et al. (2017)	RFA ($n = 59$) vs. LA ($n = 31$)	BTN	70 (LA) vs. 74 (RFA) $p > 0.05$	RFA is faster but requires higher energy. Equally safe and effective. Baseline critique of study: volumes for RF treated nodules significantly larger than those treated with LA (32.7 mL vs. 20.3 mL; $p = 0.003$)
Pacella et al. (2017)	RFA ($n = 138$) vs. LA ($n = 138$)	Solid or predominantly solid (>70%) BTN Multi center	62 (RFA) vs. 70 (LA) $p = 0.001$ Subset analysis of nodules >30 mL: 54 (RFA) vs. 73 (LA) $p = 0.001$	Both modalities are effect, LA achieved significantly larger VRR particular in large nodules >30 mL
Cesareo et al. (2021)	RFA ($n = 29$) vs. LA ($n = 29$)	Single center randomized control trial of solid and predominantly solid BTN	70.9 (RF) vs. 60 (LA) $p = 0.024$)	No significant differences in cosmetic and compressive symptom reduction between groups
Bernardi et al. (2020)	Single session of RFA ($n = 216$) or LA ($n = 190$)	Retrospective multi center of BTN w 5-year follow-up	77 (RFA) vs. 57 (LA) $p < 0.001$ Propensity matched subset ($n = 76$ in both treatment groups) 75 (RFA) vs. 56%)	Risk of regrowth (20% vs. 38%, $p < 0.001$) and retreatment (12% vs. 24%, $p < 0.001$) lower in RFA group than in LA. 35 36 randomized control trial
	RFA vs. MWA			

(continued)

Table 7.1 (continued)

Study	MIT modality (n = treated nodules)	Study design	VRR (%) at last follow-up	Key points
Yue et al. (2017)	RFA ($n = 102$); MWA ($n = 102$)	Multicenter retrospective propensity score matched study of solid BTN > 2 cm	83.6 vs. 81.6 ($p = 0.144$)	No significant differences in outcomes
Cheng et al. (2017)	RFA ($n = 687$); MWA ($n = 664$)	Multicenter prospective study of BTN	91.3 vs. 81.1 ($p = 0.045$)	VRR greater with RFA vs. MWA at and after 6 months follow-up No significant differences in major side effects
Korkusuz et al. (2017)	RFA ($n = 40$) MWA ($n = 40$)	Prospective single center study of BTN	50 (RFA) vs. 44 (MWA) $p > 0.05$	No significant differences in VRR at end follow-up which was limited to 3 months
Vorländer et al. (2018)	RFA ($n = 36$); MWA ($n = 24$)	Single center retrospective study of thyroid nodules	51.21 (RFA) vs. 53.54 (MWA) ($p > 0.65$)[a]	No significant difference in VRR. No significant difference in energy deposition ($p > 0.97$)
Hu et al. (2019)	RFA ($n = 72$) MWA ($n = 100$)	Retrospective single center of BTN	85.4 (RFA) vs. 75.8 (MWA)	No significant difference in VRR until 6 months at which time significantly higher VRR seen in RFA vs. MWA
Jin et al. (2021)	RFA ($n = 289$); MWA ($n = 289$)	Single center retrospective propensity matched study of BTN	89.2 (RFA) vs. 91.7 (MWA) $p = 0.58$	No significant differences between energy delivery ($p = 0.89$) VRR ($p = 0.058$), quality-of-life scores ($p = 0.67$), nor complication rates ($p = 0.73$)

BTN Benign thyroid nodule
[a] Last follow-up at 3 months

the literature is linked to operator experience [31] and is the probable cause for inconsistent benefit of one modality over the other. Overall, both RFA and LA were successful in obtainment therapeutic success of VRR >50% and are supported as first-line indications for the management of symptomatic BTN [16].

7.4.2.2 RFA vs. MWA

More recently, MWA has been introduced as an effective MIT for benign thyroid nodules [32–34]. MWA is associated with rapid ablation times [32] and in theory is capable of higher temperature and energy deposition compared with RFA [5]. Several retrospective analyses of RFA vs. MWA showed no difference in VRR between the modalities [6, 7, 35]. A single prospective study demonstrated a small benefit to VRR for RFA vs. MWA (91.3 vs. 81.1; $p = 0.045$) [36]. In a meta-analysis published by Guo et al. in 2021, reported no significant differences in VRR at 3 and 6 months however by 12 months follow-up VRR was significantly increased in RF treated group compared to MWA (86.2% vs. 82.0% $p = 0.036$) suggestive of better long-term outcomes with RFA. The authors proposed higher temperatures achieved with MWA increased frequency of tissue carbonization in MWA treated nodules, the presence of which impairs nodule absorption and therefore VRR apparent at time points greater than 6 months. No differences in cosmetic and compressive symptoms were reported between the treatment groups, which significantly improved in both [37]. Additionally, two studies report no significant increase in energy deposition for nodules treated with MWA vs. RFA despite this theoretic advantage of MWA [7, 35]; Energy delivery is limited by patient tolerability and safety concerns. Safety of both procedures has been reported to be similar [35, 37]. However, in the context of a single patient with reported sympathetic nerve injury after MWA, Vorlander et al. proposed the lack of susceptibility of MWA to heat sink effect of the carotid may increase risk of injury to vagal nerve or sympathetic ganglion compared to RFA [7].

Special considerations for modality selection may be warranted in very large thyroid nodules. Given the increased risk of false-negative preprocedural fine needle aspiration (FNA) for underlying malignancy in nodules >4 cm [38], thermal ablation of large thyroid nodules should be limited those with two benign FNAs and benign ultrasound features. Additionally, Huh et al. demonstrated thyroid nodules >20 mL were more likely to have an inadequate therapeutic response after a single session of RFA [39]. Yao and colleagues proposed that effective single session RFA for large thyroid nodules, average volume 27.49 ± 7.90 mL, was feasible with the addition of hydrodissection, to allow for the safe and complete treatment of nodule portions adjacent to high-risk structures (e.g., danger triangle). Additionally, intraprocedural contrast-enhanced ultrasound (CEUS) was used to assure immediate treatment of persistent viable thyroid nodule tissue. In this study, CEUS lead to additional ablation in nearly half of the treated nodules, resulting in VRR of 83.41% at 6 months follow-up [40]. Similarly, Dong et al. was able to demonstrate 90% VRR at 12 months follow-up of nodules >4 cm treated with MWA; this group also reported routine use of pre- and intraprocedural CEUS [41].

7.4.3 Autonomous Functioning Thyroid Nodules

In contrast to the robust data supporting the use of MIT for management of BTN, there is limited and variable evidence for the use of MIT for the definitive management autonomously functioning thyroid nodules (AFTN) in patients refusing or with contraindication to standards of care, surgery or radioactive iodine ablation (RAIA) [42–44]. When compared to single RAIA, a single session of LA achieved similar VRR ($p = 0.73$); however, LA was significantly less likely to normalize TSH (100 vs. 50%, $p < 0.001$) [43]. Similar study designs comparing single RAIA to RFA and MWA showed no significant differences regarding VRR and resolution of nodular overproduction of thyroid hormone (baseline average volumes of 14.3 mL and 8.08 mL, for nodules treated with RFA and MWA, respectively). However, in both studies RAIA demonstrated 20% risk of post-treatment hypothyroidism (low triiodothyronine or thyroxine) compared to no cases in thermal ablation groups [42, 44]. Potential avoidance of life-long thyroid hormone replacement has been of particular interest to clinicians and patients in considering MIT use for AFTN in which successful outcomes are predicted [15]. Current literature has suggested several factors for predicting therapeutic success of thermal ablation for AFTN to include baseline nodule volume, number of treatment sessions, VRR, and pre-toxic scintigraphy classification.

7.4.3.1 Baseline Nodule Volume

Cesaero and colleagues published a prospective study that demonstrated baseline nodule volume predicted successful treatments of AFTN with RF: nodules <12 mL had significantly higher cure rates (86 vs. 45% $p < 0.001$) [45]. Similarly, therapeutic success was achieved in all very small AFTN, baseline volume 3.15 ± 1.26 mL, treated with LA [46]; which was consistent with subsequent studies that showed the rate of methimazole discontinuation was inversely related with the baseline volume of autonomous nodules treated with LA, 90.2% (5–15 mL), 61.1% (15–25 mL), and 28.5% (>25 mL) [47]. EA success in treatment of AFTN also correlated to nodule volume, nodules >15 mL was associated with treatment failure [48].

7.4.3.2 Number of Treatment Sessions

Sung et al., in a multicenter retrospective study of 44 AFTN, demonstrated normalization of TSH in 79.5% of patients with larger nodule volumes (18.5 ± 30.1 mL) after repeat RF sessions, an average of 1.8 sessions with a max of 6 treatment sessions assuring treatment of the marginal zones of the nodule [49]. LA too achieved 100% clinical success in single AFTN and 50% of functional multinodular goiter, baseline volume 4.7–39.2 mL, when treated with 1–5 (average 3) LA sessions [50].

7.4.3.3 Volume Reduction Ratio (VRR)

The influence of VRR on TSH normalization has been inconsistent within the available literature. Bernardi et al. suggested a threshold of adequate treatment after single session of RFA that resulted in an average VRR of 81% was predictive of complete responses compared to those with a partial response with an average VRR of 68% [51]. Higher success rates of TSH normalization after LA by Amabile et al. compared to a prior study by Dossing et al. (88.5 vs. 50%) [43, 52] was thought by some authors to be related to the differences in VRR, 77.3 vs. 44%, respectively [53]. However, a subsequent large retrospective analysis of 361 patients with AFTN treated with a single session of RFA or LA found that only at 2 month, 6 month, and 12-month follow-up did VRR >80% correlate with significant improvement in TSH, which lost significance at follow-ups 24 and 36 months ($p > 0.05$). In this same study, there was a significantly larger VRR in those treated with RFA vs. LA at final follow-up (83.8 vs. 67.3%, $P < 0.001$); however, this finding did not correlate with significant differences in TSH values ($p = 0.828$) [54].

7.4.3.4 Pre-toxic AFTN

Spiezia and colleagues also reported pre-toxic nodules, defined as nodules not suppressing the surrounding thyroid parenchyma on scintigraphy, as a positive predictive factor for therapeutic success. In their prospective study that included 28 patients with autonomously functioning thyroid nodules treated with RFA, 100% of pre-toxic nodules were able to discontinue anti-thyroidal treatment compared to only 53% of toxic nodules [55]. Similarly, scintigraphy consistent with pre-toxic AFTN correlated to significantly better outcomes in nodules treated with EA. [56]

7.4.4 Thyroid Neoplasms

7.4.4.1 Papillary Thyroid Microcarcinoma (PTMC), T1bN0 Papillary Thyroid Cancer

Conservative management of PTMC has been proposed given the low rates of clinical progression [57]. Clinician and patient shared decision-making plays a significant role in individualizing care for PTMC ranging from surveillance to total thyroidectomy. MIT strategies may appeal to patients and clinicians desiring an intermediary intervention between the therapeutic option extremes. Ethanol ablation has been described as an effective MIT for the management of PTMC by Brito and colleagues. They reported a cohort of 14 PTMC treated with EA with mean VRR 82%, no evidence of nodal metastasis development during follow-up (15–95 months) [58]. A meta-analysis of 11 studies examining thermal ablation techniques for the management of PTMC found all TA techniques to be effective with RFA demonstrating the greatest VRR compared to MWA and LA (99.3, 95.3, and 88.6%, respectively, $p < 0.001$) [59]. In a subsequent multicenter retrospective study of 725 patient with PTMC treated with RFA and MWA found no significant differences in rates of tumor disappearance ($p = 0.15$), disease progression ($p = 0.96$), or complication rates ($p = 0.96$) between treatment modalities [60]. Disease progression, local recurrence, or development of lymph node metastasis, in single center retrospective study was reported to occur a frequency of 6.8% after thermal ablation of PTMC [61]. When compared to routine surgery to thermal ablation for the management of PTMC, a meta-analysis demonstrated lower rates of pooled complications (OR 0.24), hospital stay length (SMD −3.14), and cost in perioperative period for those treated with thermal ablation compared to routine surgery. There were no differences between rates of recurrence and recurrence-free survival ($p = 0.88$) [62].

The use of thermal ablation has been expanded by some groups to treat papillary thyroid cancer <2 cm without evidence of metastatic lymph nodes (T1bN0) although the literature is limited. A multicenter retrospective analysis of 172 patients with T1bN0 tumors treated with thermal ablation (MWA = 123; RFA = 49) of tumor and safety margin resulted in significant volume reduction from tumor baseline after 6 months (VRR at 6 months 45% and 48 months 99% $p > 0.005$), with 61.6% of tumors completely resolving. Low rates of lymph node metastasis (0.6%), new tumor development (1.2%) were reported over mean follow-up of 24.9 + 14 months. Over all complications occurred at a frequency of 5.2%, of which 4.6% (8/172) were major, all 8 patients experienced hoarseness, and 0.6% minor complication, one patient with post-procedural fever [63]. Differences between the thermal ablation treatment modalities were not reported; however, suggesting overall thermal ablation is a safe and effective management for papillary thyroid cancers <2 cm without lymph node involvement, particularly in patients who are ineligible or refusing surgery.

7.4.4.2 Locally Metastatic/Recurrent Papillary Thyroid Cancer: Chelsey Start Here with Sources

In patients with PTC that undergo surgical resection/thyroidectomy, 20–30% of patients develop nodal metastases in the cervical region [64]. While surgical re-excision remains the established treatment approach for regional thyroid cancer recurrence to achieve biochemical and structural remission, re-operating may not be the best option for some patients or, the patient may not be a surgical candidate. Therefore, MIT modalities can be considered as an option for carefully selected patients with recurrent/persistent disease to treat low volume metastatic disease in the neck.

Ethanol ablation has been utilized for over 30 years and reported in multiple single center case series to be a safe, inexpensive, and effective modality in achieving local disease control in select patients with low volume metastatic disease in the neck [65, 66]. Multiple ethanol ablation sessions are usually required for complete ablation, with VRR ranging from 30 to 100% [67]. This wide range of volume reduction is the main limitation of ethanol ablation which is due to the uneven and unpredictable area of ablation when this modality is used. Ethanol leakage into the cervical tissue is also frequently reported requiring cessation of the ablation session. This can result in suboptimal ablation and complications to include recurrent laryngeal nerve injury that can be temporary or permanent when the target lesion is within the central compartment of the neck. Despite this, Heilo et al. have been able to demonstrate complete ablation in 84% of cases of recurrent/persistent disease over a 3-year median follow-up period with no major complications [65]. The durability of lesion reduction has also been proven in long-term follow-up data exceeding 5 years [68, 69]. With the widespread use of thermal ablative techniques, studies have recently compared the use of ethanol ablation to RFA and found ethanol ablation to have inferior results with regards to VRR, local progression, and recurrence of disease [70, 71]. Ethanol ablations remains frequently used today due to it being inexpensive and easily available.

Thermal ablation of nodal metastasis is an area of increasing interest; however, there are no specific guidelines on nodal characteristics that correspond to improved outcomes with ablative techniques. In the meta-analysis of 498 treated lymph nodes by Zhang et al., the characteristics of metastatic nodes meeting criteria for ablation were vastly underreported [72]. With use of a minimally invasive technique (LA, RFA, MWA) all have comparable outcomes with respect to reduction of nodal volume and maximum diameter [73]. Overall, the volume reduction rate of cervical lymph node metastases was between 50 and 80% [72]. In up to 80% of cases following ablation, patients experience a complete disappearance of the initial metastatic node [73]. Thyroglobulin was trended before and after ablation, with a significant reduction across all modalities following treatment [72–75]. Cao et al. boasts the advantages of MWA in that it achieves high temperatures quickly, making it possible to ablate a larger surface area while minimizing procedure duration. Nevertheless, there is no reported superiority in effectiveness or improved outcomes between LA, RFA, and MWA for reducing nodal size or recurrence.

7.4.4.3 Follicular Neoplasm

The surgical management of follicular neoplasm is first-line management and inherently necessary to render a diagnosis which is dependent on post-surgical histology. General consensus suggests that treating follicular neoplasms with thermal ablation is contraindicated due to the risk of unintentional treatment of follicular thyroid cancer and the likely higher risk of recurrent benign disease due to the underlying neoplastic origin. However, most thyroid follicular neoplasms are benign [76] and some authors have ventured to use thermal ablation for their management. Dobrinja and colleagues reported thermal ablation of six ultrasonographically bland follicular neoplasms (baseline volume range: 2–40 mL) in patients refusing or ineligible for surgery [61]. Two of six nodules, both greater than 20 mL at baseline, regrew >50% from nadir volume and surgery was recommended. On final pathology, one case was diagnosed as minimally invasive follicular carcinoma and the other follicular neoplasm of indeterminate malignant behavior. Dobrinja et al. in conclusion warned against the use of RFA for follicular neoplasms suggesting it delayed the diagnosis of follicular carcinoma [77]. However, Ha and colleagues subsequently reported the successful treatment of 1–2 cm cytologic follicular neoplasms in ten patients refusing surgery with a VRR of 99.5%, 80% completely disappearing, and no recurrence at 5-year follow-up [78]. Yang et al. also described the safe and effective use of MWA for 46 Bethesda IV (cytology consistent with follicular neoplasm or suspicious for follicular neoplasm) nodules (baseline volume 7.47 + 6.68 mL) with 85% VRR at 12 months and lower incidence of complications, treatment time, and cost compared to surgery ($p < 0.001$) [79]. Experts have suggested that baseline volume of follicular neoplasm may be predictive of successful outcomes after thermal ablation [80] given the increased rate of malignancy in nodules greater than 4 cm [81] and the near-zero rate of metastatic disease associated with follicular neoplasms <2 cm [82].

7.5 Conclusions

The selection of MIT modality is dependent on the target lesions characteristics. While there is little debate that EA is the best first-line option for purely cystic nodules, superiority of a given MIT modality in mixed solid cystic and solid nodules of both hyperplastic and neoplastic origin has been variable in the literature. EA, LA, MWA, and RFA have all been shown to be effective for the management of thyroid structural disease and the variability between modalities is likely a product of operator expertise.

References

1. Mauri G, Cova L, Monaco CG, Sconfienza LM, Corbetta S, Benedini S, et al. Benign thyroid nodules treatment using percutaneous laser ablation (PLA) and radiofrequency ablation (RFA). Int J Hyperth. 2017;33(3):295–9. https://doi.org/10.1080/02656736.2016.1244707.
2. Baek JH, Lee JH, Valcavi R, Pacella CM, Rhim H, Na DG. Thermal ablation for benign thyroid nodules: radiofrequency and laser. Korean J Radiol. 2011;12(5):525–40. https://doi.org/10.3348/kjr.2011.12.5.525.
3. Bernardi S, Giudici F, Cesareo R, Antonelli G, Cavallaro M, Deandrea M, et al. Five-year results of radiofrequency and laser ablation of benign thyroid nodules: a multicenter study from the Italian minimally invasive treatments of the thyroid group. Thyroid. 2020;30(12):1759–70. https://doi.org/10.1089/thy.2020.0202.

4. Cheng Z, Liang P. Advances in ultrasound-guided thermal ablation for symptomatic benign thyroid nodules. Adv Clin Exp Med. 2020;29(9):1123–9. https://doi.org/10.17219/acem/125433.
5. Kim C. Understanding the nuances of microwave ablation for more accurate post-treatment assessment. Future Oncol. 2018;14(17):1755–64. https://doi.org/10.2217/fon-2017-0736.
6. Yue WW, Wang SR, Lu F, Sun LP, Guo LH, Zhang YL, et al. Radiofrequency ablation vs. microwave ablation for patients with benign thyroid nodules: a propensity score matching study. Endocrine. 2017;55(2):485–95. https://doi.org/10.1007/s12020-016-1173-5.
7. Vorländer C, David Kohlhase K, Korkusuz Y, Erbelding C, Luboldt W, Baser I, et al. Comparison between microwave ablation and bipolar radiofrequency ablation in benign thyroid nodules: differences in energy transmission, duration of application and applied shots. Int J Hyperth. 2018;35(1):216–25. https://doi.org/10.1080/02656736.2018.1489984.
8. Orgera G, Monfardini L, Della Vigna P, Zhang L, Bonomo G, Arnone P, et al. Highintensity focused ultrasound (HIFU) in patients with solid malignancies: evaluation of feasibility, local tumour response and clinical results. Radiol Med. 2011;116(5):734–48.
9. Partanen A, Ellens N, Noureldine S, Burdette E, Tufano R, Farahani K. We-EF-Bra-12: magnetic resonance-guided high-intensity focused ultrasound for localized ablation of head and neck tissue structures: a feasibility study in an animal model. Med Phys. 2015;42(6):3677.
10. Ellens N, Partanen A, Ghoshal G, Burdette E, Farahani K. SU-E-J-04: integration of interstitial high intensity therapeutic ultrasound applicators on a clinical MRI-guided high intensity focused ultrasound treatment planning software platform. Med Phys. 2015;42(6Part7):3264.
11. Cazzato RL, Garnon J, Ramamurthy N, Koch G, Tsoumakidou G, Caudrelier J, et al. Percutaneous image-guided cryoablation: current applications and results in the oncologic field. Med Oncol. 2016;33(12):140. https://doi.org/10.1007/s12032-016-0848-3.
12. Kim JH, Baek JH, Lim HK, Ahn HS, Baek SM, Choi YJ, et al. 2017 thyroid radiofrequency ablation guideline: Korean Society of Thyroid Radiology. Korean J Radiol. 2018;19(4):632–55. https://doi.org/10.3348/kjr.2018.19.4.632.
13. Gharib H, Papini E, Garber JR, Duick DS, Harrell RM, Hegedüs L, et al. American Association of Clinical Endocrinologists, American College of Endocrinology, and Associazione Medici Endocrinologi Medical Guidelines for clinical practice for the diagnosis and Management of Thyroid Nodules—2016 update. Endocr Pract. 2016;22(5):622–39. https://doi.org/10.4158/EP161208.GL.
14. National Institute for Health and Care Excellence. Ultrasound-guided percutaneous radiofrequency ablation for benign thyroid nodules. Interventional procedure guidance [IPT562]. London: National Institute for Health and Care Excellence; 2016. https://www.nice.org.uk/guidance/ipg562.
15. Papini E, Pacella CM, Solbiati LA, Achille G, Barbaro D, Bernardi S, et al. Minimally-invasive treatments for benign thyroid nodules: a Delphi-based consensus statement from the Italian minimally-invasive treatments of the thyroid (MITT) group. Int J Hyperth. 2019;36(1):376–82. https://doi.org/10.1080/02656736.2019.1575482.
16. Papini E, Monpeyssen H, Frasoldati A, Hegedüs L. 2020 European thyroid association clinical practice guideline for the use of image-guided ablation in benign thyroid nodules. Eur Thyroid J. 2020;9(4):172–85. https://doi.org/10.1159/000508484.
17. Orloff LA, Noel JE, Stack BC Jr, Russell MD, Angelos P, Baek JH, et al. Radiofrequency ablation and related ultrasound-guided ablation technologies for treatment of benign and malignant thyroid disease: an international multidisciplinary consensus statement of the American Head and Neck Society Endocrine Surgery Section with the Asia Pacific Society of Thyroid Surgery, Associazione Medici Endocrinologi, British Association of Endocrine and Thyroid Surgeons, European Thyroid Association, Italian Society of Endocrine Surgery Units, Korean Society of Thyroid Radiology, Latin American Thyroid Society, and Thyroid Nodules Therapies Association. Head Neck. 2022;44(3):633–60. https://doi.org/10.1002/hed.26960.
18. Ha EJ, Baek JH. Advances in nonsurgical treatment of benign thyroid nodules. Future Oncol. 2014;10(8):1399–405. https://doi.org/10.2217/fon.14.59.
19. Sung JY, Kim YS, Choi H, Lee JH, Baek JH. Optimum first-line treatment technique for benign cystic thyroid nodules: ethanol ablation or radiofrequency ablation? AJR Am J Roentgenol. 2011;196(2):W210–4. https://doi.org/10.2214/AJR.10.5172.
20. Meyer H. FDA seeks a new way to review old drugs without causing prices to soar. KFF Health News. 2021. https://kffhealthnews.org/news/article/the-fda-seeks-a-new-way-to-review-old-drugs-without-causing-prices-to-soar/. Accessed 4 July 2023.
21. Basu N, Dutta D, Maisnam I, Basu S, Ghosh S, Chowdhury S, et al. Percutaneous ethanol ablation in managing predominantly cystic thyroid nodules: an eastern India perspective. Indian J Endocrinol Metab. 2014;18(5):662–8. https://doi.org/10.4103/2230-8210.139229.
22. Alcântara-Jones DM, Araújo LM, Almeida Ade M, Jones Dde A, Cardoso LJ, Passos MC. Efeito da injeção percutânea de etanol na redução de nódulos tireoideanos [Percutaneous ethanol injection for the treatment of thyroid nodules]. Arq Bras Endocrinol Metabol. 2006;50(1):97–104. Portuguese. https://doi.org/10.1590/s0004-27302006000100014.
23. Jang SW, Baek JH, Kim JK, Sung JY, Choi H, Lim HK, et al. How to manage the patients with unsatisfactory results after ethanol ablation for thyroid

nodules: role of radiofrequency ablation. Eur J Radiol. 2012;81(5):905–10. https://doi.org/10.1016/j.ejrad.2011.02.039.
24. Yoon HM, Baek JH, Lee JH, Ha EJ, Kim JK, Yoon JH, et al. Combination therapy consisting of ethanol and radiofrequency ablation for predominantly cystic thyroid nodules. AJNR Am J Neuroradiol. 2014;35(3):582–6. https://doi.org/10.3174/ajnr.A3701.
25. Caraccio N, Goletti O, Lippolis PV, Casolaro A, Cavina E, Miccoli P, et al. Is percutaneous ethanol injection a useful alternative for the treatment of the cold benign thyroid nodule? Five years' experience. Thyroid. 1997;7(5):699–704. https://doi.org/10.1089/thy.1997.7.699.
26. Zingrillo M, Collura D, Ghiggi MR, Nirchio V, Trischitta V. Treatment of large cold benign thyroid nodules not eligible for surgery with percutaneous ethanol injection. J Clin Endocrinol Metab. 1998;83(11):3905–7. https://doi.org/10.1210/jcem.83.11.5257.
27. Gharib H, Hegedüs L, Pacella CM, Baek JH, Papini E. Clinical review: nonsurgical, image-guided, minimally invasive therapy for thyroid nodules. J Clin Endocrinol Metab. 2013;98(10):3949–57. https://doi.org/10.1210/jc.2013-1806. Epub 2013 Aug 16
28. Ha EJ, Baek JH, Kim KW, Pyo J, Lee JH, Baek SH, et al. Comparative efficacy of radiofrequency and laser ablation for the treatment of benign thyroid nodules: systematic review including traditional pooling and bayesian network meta-analysis. J Clin Endocrinol Metab. 2015;100(5):1903–11. https://doi.org/10.1210/jc.2014-4077.
29. Cesareo R, Manfrini S, Pasqualini V, Ambrogi C, Sanson G, Gallo A, et al. Laser ablation versus radiofrequency ablation for thyroid nodules: 12-month results of a randomized trial (LARA II study). J Clin Endocrinol Metab. 2021;106(6):1692–701. https://doi.org/10.1210/clinem/dgab102.
30. Pacella CM, Mauri G, Cesareo R, Paqualini V, Cianni R, De Feo P, et al. A comparison of laser with radiofrequency ablation for the treatment of benign thyroid nodules: a propensity score matching analysis. Int J Hyperth. 2017;33(8):911–9. https://doi.org/10.1080/02656736.2017.1332395.
31. Papini E, Rago T, Gambelunghe G, Valcavi R, Bizzarri G, Vitti P, et al. Long-term efficacy of ultrasound-guided laser ablation for benign solid thyroid nodules. Results of a three-year multicenter prospective randomized trial. J Clin Endocrinol Metab. 2014;99(10):3653–9. https://doi.org/10.1210/jc.2014-1826.
32. Honglei G, Shahbaz M, Farhaj Z, Ijaz M, Kai SY, Davrieux CF, et al. Ultrasound guided microwave ablation of thyroid nodular goiter and cystadenoma: a single center, large cohort study. Medicine (Baltimore). 2021;100(34):e26943. https://doi.org/10.1097/MD.0000000000026943.
33. Feng B, Liang P, Cheng Z, Yu X, Yu J, Han Z, et al. Ultrasound-guided percutaneous microwave ablation of benign thyroid nodules: experimental and clinical studies. Eur J Endocrinol. 2012;166(6):1031–7. https://doi.org/10.1530/EJE-11-0966.
34. Yue W, Wang S, Wang B, Xu Q, Yu S, Yonglin Z, et al. Ultrasound guided percutaneous microwave ablation of benign thyroid nodules: safety and imaging follow-up in 222 patients. Eur J Radiol. 2013;82(1):e11–6. https://doi.org/10.1016/j.ejrad.2012.07.020.
35. Jin H, Fan J, Lu L, Cui M. A propensity score matching study between microwave ablation and radiofrequency ablation in terms of safety and efficacy for benign thyroid nodules treatment. Front Endocrinol (Lausanne). 2021;12:584972. https://doi.org/10.3389/fendo.2021.584972.
36. Cheng Z, Che Y, Yu S, Wang S, Teng D, Xu H, et al. US-guided percutaneous radiofrequency versus microwave ablation for benign thyroid nodules: a prospective multicenter study. Sci Rep. 2017;7(1):9554. https://doi.org/10.1038/s41598-017-09930-7.
37. Guo DM, Chen Z, Zhai YX, Su HH. Comparison of radiofrequency ablation and microwave ablation for benign thyroid nodules: a systematic review and meta-analysis. Clin Endocrinol. 2021;95(1):187–96. https://doi.org/10.1111/cen.14438.
38. McCoy KL, Jabbour N, Ogilvie JB, Ohori NP, Carty SE, Yim JH. The incidence of cancer and rate of false-negative cytology in thyroid nodules greater than or equal to 4 cm in size. Surgery. 2007;142(6):837–44; discussion 844.e1–3. https://doi.org/10.1016/j.surg.2007.08.012.
39. Huh JY, Baek JH, Choi H, Kim JK, Lee JH. Symptomatic benign thyroid nodules: efficacy of additional radiofrequency ablation treatment session–prospective randomized study. Radiology. 2012;263:909–16. https://doi.org/10.1148/radiol.12111300.
40. Yao Z, Wu T, Zheng B, Tan L, Lian Y, Liu B, et al. A novel strategy for single-session ultrasound-guided radiofrequency ablation of large benign thyroid nodules: a pilot cohort study. Front Endocrinol (Lausanne). 2020;7(11):560508. https://doi.org/10.3389/fendo.2020.560508.
41. Dong P, Wu XL, Sui GQ, Luo Q, Du JR, Wang H, et al. The efficacy and safety of microwave ablation versus lobectomy for the treatment of benign thyroid nodules greater than 4 cm. Endocrine. 2021;71(1):113–21. https://doi.org/10.1007/s12020-020-02338-w.
42. Ertürk MS, Cekic B, Celik M, Demiray UI. Microwave ablation of autonomously functioning thyroid nodules: a comparative study with radioactive iodine therapy on the functional treatment success. Endokrynol Pol. 2021;72(2):120–5. https://doi.org/10.5603/EP.a2020.0088.
43. Døssing H, Bennedbaek FN, Bonnema SJ, Grupe P, Hegedüs L. Randomized prospective study comparing a single radioiodine dose and a single laser therapy session in autonomously functioning thyroid nodules. Eur J Endocrinol. 2007;157(1):95–100. https://doi.org/10.1530/EJE-07-0094.

44. Cervelli R, Mazzeo S, Boni G, Boccuzzi A, Bianchi F, Brozzi F, et al. Comparison between radioiodine therapy and single-session radiofrequency ablation of autonomously functioning thyroid nodules: a retrospective study. Clin Endocrinol. 2019;90(4):608–16. https://doi.org/10.1111/cen.13938.
45. Cesareo R, Naciu AM, Iozzino M, Pasqualini V, Simeoni C, Casini A, et al. Nodule size as predictive factor of efficacy of radiofrequency ablation in treating autonomously functioning thyroid nodules. Int J Hyperth. 2018;34(5):617–23. https://doi.org/10.1080/02656736.2018.1430868.
46. Spiezia S, Vitale G, Di Somma C, Pio Assanti A, Ciccarelli A, Lombardi G, et al. Ultrasound-guided laser thermal ablation in the treatment of autonomous hyperfunctioning thyroid nodules and compressive nontoxic nodular goiter. Thyroid. 2003;13(10):941–7. https://doi.org/10.1089/105072503322511346.
47. Gambelunghe G, Stefanetti E, Colella R, Monacelli M, Avenia N, De Feo P. A single session of laser ablation for toxic thyroid nodules: three-year follow-up results. Int J Hyperth. 2018;34(5):631–5. https://doi.org/10.1080/02656736.2018.1437931.
48. Lippi F, Ferrari C, Manetti L, Rago T, Santini F, Monzani F, et al. Treatment of solitary autonomous thyroid nodules by percutaneous ethanol injection: results of an Italian multicenter study. The Multicenter Study Group. J Clin Endocrinol Metab. 1996;81(9):3261–4. https://doi.org/10.1210/jcem.81.9.8784080.
49. Sung JY, Baek JH, Jung SL, Kim JH, Kim KS, Lee D, et al. Radiofrequency ablation for autonomously functioning thyroid nodules: a multicenter study. Thyroid. 2015;25(1):112–7. https://doi.org/10.1089/thy.2014.0100.
50. Barbaro D, Orsini P, Lapi P, Pasquini C, Tuco A, Righini A, et al. Percutaneous laser ablation in the treatment of toxic and pretoxic nodular goiter. Endocr Pract. 2007;13(1):30–6. https://doi.org/10.4158/EP.13.1.30.
51. Bernardi S, Stacul F, Michelli A, Giudici F, Zuolo G, de Manzini N, et al. 12-month efficacy of a single radiofrequency ablation on autonomously functioning thyroid nodules. Endocrine. 2017;57(3):402–8. https://doi.org/10.1007/s12020-016-1174-4.
52. Amabile G, Rotondi M, Pirali B, Dionisio R, Agozzino L, Lanza M, Buonanno L, Di Filippo B, Fonte R, Chiovato L. Interstitial laser photocoagulation for benign thyroid nodules: time to treat large nodules. Lasers Surg Med. 2011;43(8):797–803. https://doi.org/10.1002/lsm.21114.
53. Pacella CM, Mauri G. Is there a role for minimally invasive thermal ablations in the treatment of autonomously functioning thyroid nodules? Int J Hyperth. 2018;34(5):636–8. https://doi.org/10.1080/02656736.2018.1462537.
54. Mauri G, Papini E, Bernardi S, Barbaro D, Cesareo R, De Feo P, et al. Image-guided thermal ablation in autonomously functioning thyroid nodules. A retrospective multicenter three-year follow-up study from the Italian Minimally Invasive Treatment of the Thyroid (MITT) Group. Eur Radiol. 2022;32(3):1738–46. https://doi.org/10.1007/s00330-021-08289-8.
55. Spiezia S, Garberoglio R, Milone F, Ramundo V, Caiazzo C, Assanti AP, et al. Thyroid nodules and related symptoms are stably controlled two years after radiofrequency thermal ablation. Thyroid. 2009;19(3):219–25. https://doi.org/10.1089/thy.2008.0202.
56. Monzani F, Caraccio N, Goletti O, Casolaro A, Lippolis PV, Cavina E, et al. Treatment of hyperfunctioning thyroid nodules with percutaneous ethanol injection: eight years' experience. Exp Clin Endocrinol Diabetes. 1998;106(Suppl 4):S54–8. https://doi.org/10.1055/s-0029-1212058.
57. Ito Y, Miyauchi A, Kihara M, Higashiyama T, Kobayashi K, Miya A. Patient age is significantly related to the progression of papillary microcarcinoma of the thyroid under observation. Thyroid. 2014;24(1):27–34. https://doi.org/10.1089/thy.2013.0367.
58. Brito JP, Hay ID. Management of papillary thyroid microcarcinoma. Endocrinol Metab Clin N Am. 2019;48(1):199–213. https://doi.org/10.1016/j.ecl.2018.10.006.
59. Choi Y, Jung SL. Efficacy and safety of thermal ablation techniques for the treatment of primary papillary thyroid microcarcinoma: a systematic review and meta-analysis. Thyroid. 2020;30(5):720–31. https://doi.org/10.1089/thy.2019.0707.
60. Cao XJ, Yu MA, Zhu YL, Qi L, Cong ZB, Yan GZ, et al. Ultrasound-guided thermal ablation for papillary thyroid microcarcinoma: a multicenter retrospective study. Int J Hyperth. 2021;38(1):916–22. https://doi.org/10.1080/02656736.2021.1936218.
61. Lu C, Li X, Chu X, Li R, Li J, Wang J, et al. Clinical effects of microwave ablation in the treatment of low-risk papillary thyroid microcarcinomas and related histopathological changes. Front Endocrinol (Lausanne). 2020;12:751213. https://doi.org/10.3389/fendo.2021.751213.
62. Shen K, Xue S, Xie Y, Wang H, Li J, Sun Y, et al. Comparison of thermal ablation and routine surgery for the treatment of papillary thyroid microcarcinoma: a systematic review and meta-analysis. Int J Hyperth. 2020;37(1):913–24. https://doi.org/10.1080/02656736.2020.1777331.
63. Cao XJ, Liu J, Zhu YL, Qi L, Liu G, Wang HL, et al. Efficacy and safety of thermal ablation for solitary T1bN0M0 papillary thyroid carcinoma: a multicenter study. J Clin Endocrinol Metab. 2021;106(2):e573–81. https://doi.org/10.1210/clinem/dgaa776. Erratum in: J Clin Endocrinol Metab. 2021;106(6):e2466.
64. Hay ID, Hutchinson ME, Gonzalez-Losada T, McIver B, Reinalda ME, Grant CS, et al. Papillary thyroid microcarcinoma: a study of 900 cases observed in a 60-year period. Surgery. 2008;144(6):980–7;

discussion 987–8. https://doi.org/10.1016/j.surg.2008.08.035.

65. Heilo A, Sigstad E, Fagerlid KH, Hskjold OI, Grholt KK, Berner A, et al. Efficacy of ultrasound-guided percutaneous ethanol injection treatment in patients with a limited number of metastatic cervical lymph nodes from papillary thyroid carcinoma. J Clin Endocrinol Metab. 2011;96(9):2750–5. https://doi.org/10.1210/jc.2010-2952.
66. Lewis BD, Hay ID, Charboneau JW, McIver B, Reading CC, Goellner JR. Percutaneous ethanol injection for treatment of cervical lymph node metastases in patients with papillary thyroid carcinoma. Am J Roentgenol. 2002;178:699–704. https://doi.org/10.2214/ajr.178.3.1780699.
67. Kim BM, Kim MJ, Kim EK, Il PS, Park CS, Chung WY. Controlling recurrent papillary thyroid carcinoma in the neck by ultrasonography-guided percutaneous ethanol injection. Eur Radiol. 2008;18:835–42. https://doi.org/10.1007/s00330-007-0809-5.
68. Kim SY, Kim SM, Chang H, Kim BW, Lim CY, Lee YS, et al. Long-term outcomes of ethanol injection therapy for locally recurrent papillary thyroid cancer. Eur Arch Otorrinolaringol. 2017;274(9):3497–501. https://doi.org/10.1007/s00405-017-4660-2.
69. Hay ID, Lee RA, Davidge-Pitts C, Reading CC, Charboneau JW. Long-term outcome of ultrasound-guided percutaneous ethanol ablation of selected "recurrent" neck nodal metastases in 25 patients with TNM stages III or IVA papillary thyroid carcinoma previously treated by surgery and 131I therapy. Surg (United States). 2013;154:1448–54. https://doi.org/10.1016/j.surg.2013.07.007.
70. Guenette JP, Monchik JM, Dupuy DE. Image guided ablation of postsurgical locoregional recurrence of biopsy-proven well-differentiated thyroid carcinoma. J Vasc Interv Radiol. 2013;24(5):672–9.
71. Suh CH, Baek JH, Choi YJ, Lee JH. Efficacy and safety of radiofrequency and ethanol ablation for treating locally recurrent thyroid cancer: a systematic review and meta-analysis. Thyroid. 2016;26(3):420–8. https://doi.org/10.1089/thy.2015.0545.
72. Zhang X, Ni T, Zhang W. Ultrasonography-guided thermal ablation for cervical lymph node metastasis of recurrent papillary thyroid carcinoma: is it superior to surgical resection? Front Endocrinol (Lausanne). 2022;13:907195. https://doi.org/10.3389/fendo.2022.907195.
73. Zhu Y, Wang Y, Liu F, Liao Y, Wang Q, Xiao X. Thermal ablation for cervical lymph node metastasis from papillary thyroid carcinoma: a meta-analysis. Medicine (Baltimore). 2022;101(51):e32193. https://doi.org/10.1097/MD.0000000000032193.
74. Cao XJ, Wei Y, Zhao ZL, Peng LL, Li Y, Yu MA. Efficacy and safety of microwave ablation for cervical metastatic lymph nodes arising post resection of papillary thyroid carcinoma: a retrospective study. Int J Hyperth. 2020;37(1):450–5. https://doi.org/10.1080/02656736.2020.1759829.
75. Korkusuz Y, Gröner D, Raczynski N, Relin O, Kingeter Y, Grünwald F, et al. Thermal ablation of thyroid nodules: are radiofrequency ablation, microwave ablation and high intensity focused ultrasound equally safe and effective methods? Eur Radiol. 2018;28(3):929–35. https://doi.org/10.1007/s00330-017-5039-x.
76. Gulcelik NE, Gulcelik MA, Kuru B. Risk of malignancy in patients with follicular neoplasm: predictive value of clinical and ultrasonographic features. Arch Otolaryngol Head Neck Surg. 2008;134(12):1312–5. https://doi.org/10.1001/archotol.134.12.1312.
77. Dobrinja C, Bernardi S, Fabris B, Eramo R, Makovac P, Bazzocchi G, et al. Surgical and pathological changes after radiofrequency ablation of thyroid nodules. Int J Endocrinol. 2015;2015:576576. https://doi.org/10.1155/2015/576576.
78. Ha SM, Sung JY, Baek JH, Na DG, Kim JH, Yoo H, et al. Radiofrequency ablation of small follicular neoplasms: initial clinical outcomes. Int J Hyperth. 2017;33(8):931–7. https://doi.org/10.1080/02656736.2017.1331268.
79. Yang J, Zhang Y, Li X, Zhao Y, Han X, Chen G, Chu X, Li R, Wang J, Huang F, Liu C, Xu S. Efficacy and safety of ultrasound-guided microwave ablation versus surgical resection for Bethesda category IV thyroid nodules: a retrospective comparative study. Front Endocrinol (Lausanne). 2022;13:924993. https://doi.org/10.3389/fendo.2022.924993.
80. Baldwin CK, Natter MB, Patel KN, Hodak SP. Minimally invasive techniques for the management of thyroid nodules. Endocrinol Metab Clin N Am. 2022;51(2):323–49. https://doi.org/10.1016/j.ecl.2022.01.001.
81. Paramo JC, Mesko T. Age, tumor size, and in-office ultrasonography are predictive parameters of malignancy in follicular neoplasms of the thyroid. Endocr Pract. 2008;14(4):447–51. https://doi.org/10.4158/EP.14.4.447.
82. Machens A, Holzhausen HJ, Dralle H. The prognostic value of primary tumor size in papillary and follicular thyroid carcinoma. Cancer. 2005;103(11):2269–73. https://doi.org/10.1002/cncr.21055.

Nodule Selection for Thyroid Ablation

8

Amanda Silver Karcioglu
and Hervé Monpeyssen

8.1 Introduction

Ablative techniques for thyroid nodules offer an alternative to surgery in patients with benign symptomatic nodules and may be considered in select cases of autonomous functioning nodules or thyroid malignancy. Surgery to remove half of the thyroid (thyroid lobectomy with or without isthmusectomy) or the entire thyroid gland (total thyroidectomy) has been the standard of care; however, nonsurgical ablative techniques to treat benign symptomatic nodules have been gaining acceptance. With over two decades of clinical use, there is a growing body of literature to support efficacy and safety of ablative techniques applied to thyroid nodules. Of the available technologies, radiofrequency ablation (RFA) at present haves the widest acceptance and utilization [1–4]. Optimal nodule and patient selection are critical, and this chapter will focus on the selection of thyroid nodules and metastatic lymph nodes for ablative techniques. The treatment of parathyroid glands will not be addressed.

In the selection of a thyroid nodule for treatment with ablation, patient factors as well as nodule characteristics and resource availability should be considered. Ablative techniques are not equally suited for all nodules and therefore the merits and limitations of different ablative techniques, such as radiofrequency ablation (RFA; Chaps. 14, 15, 17, and 18), Ethanol ablation (EA, Chap. 13), Laser Ablation (LA; Chap. 19), Microwave ablation (MA; Chaps. 21 and 22) and High Intensity Focused Ultrasound (HIFU; Chap. 20), are to be thought of in light of patient and nodule factors as well as clinician experience and skill, blended with institutional resource availability and implications for longer term surveillance. Importantly, for each patient on an individual basis, ablative techniques should be compared to appropriate and applicable alternatives of observation and/or surgery. Prior to ablative procedures, treatment expectations and careful discussion of post-procedure surveillance of thyroid nodule ablation performed in lieu of observation or surgery are to be discussed with patients. This is crucial because ablative techniques often do not resolve thyroid nodules completely and result in sonographic changes of the nodules [5] that must be accounted for during sonographic surveillance post-treatment, although importantly RFA does not appear to result in malignant transformation of benign nodules [6].

Comprehensive ultrasonography skills are a prerequisite for successful ultrasound-guided

A. S. Karcioglu (✉)
Division of Otolaryngology-Head and Neck Surgery, Department of Surgery, Endeavor Health - Teaching Affiliate of the University of Chicago, Chicago, IL, USA

Pritzker School of Medicine, University of Chicago, Chicago, IL, USA

H. Monpeyssen
Thyroid Unit, American Hospital of Paris, Neuilly-sur-Seine, France
e-mail: hm@thyroide.org

R. Valcavi et al. (eds.), *Thyroid Ablation*, https://doi.org/10.1007/978-3-031-88229-6_8

thermal ablative techniques [1]. Due to the inherent operator variability in thyroid ultrasonography, reliance on ultrasonography performed by another individual may result in less favorable outcomes [7].

8.2 Patient Factors

Patients with symptomatic nodules who are unwilling or unfit (due to other medical factors) to undergo surgery may be considered for appropriate forms of thyroid ablation, depending on nodule characteristics and availability of treatment modalities. A list of common indications for thermal ablation of thyroid nodules is shown in Table 8.1.

The procedure is generally performed with the patient in supine position with head extension and after the administration of local anesthetic. Patients therefore should be willing and able to tolerate an awake procedure and accept generally mild associated symptoms that may occur during the procedure [1], such as some degree of local and/or referred discomfort to the ear, teeth, jaw or head, chest and/or back and possibly the appreciation of sound from the heat effect on the thyroid tissue.

Prior to performing radiofrequency ablation, several international guidelines endorse the use of pre-procedure checklists to ensure thorough work-up and discussion of treatment expectations and informed consent [1–3]. Informed consent (written and/or oral) for ablative procedures to treat thyroid nodules should include a detailed discussed of the following [1, 2]:

- The risks and benefits of the various available treatment options including observation, thermal ablation, or surgery.
- Modalities of thermal ablative techniques, including a description of the offered procedure to prepare and set patient expectations.
- Risks and potential complications of each treatment option.
- For thermal ablative techniques, a discussion about the expected decrease in nodule size, including the (often low) probability of complete nodule disappearance.
- Importance of long-term continued clinical and ultrasonographic surveillance.
- Possible nodule regrowth over time and implications surveillance and for additional treatments including repeat thermal ablative procedures and/or surgery.

Patients at risk for bleeding, including those taking anticoagulation medications, require careful pre-procedure evaluation and consideration. A summary of recommendations for international guidelines for the discontinuation of anticoagulation medications prior to RFA is outlined in Table 8.2.

Thyroid nodules treated with thermal ablation require post-treatment surveillance for treatment efficacy and assessment of potential regrowth, which may occur many years after treatment. Universal post-procedure protocols delineating the timing and elements of follow-up visits however are lacking. Nevertheless, patients consenting to ablative treatment should be willing and

Table 8.1 Common indications for treatment with thermal ablation

- Symptoms referable to large thyroid nodule including but not limited to:
  - Compressive symptoms
  - Dysphagia
  - Respiratory symptoms
  - Cough
- Cosmetic concerns related to the nodule
- Benign nodule with evidence of growth

Table 8.2 Recommendations for discontinuation of anticoagulation medications prior to TA

Medication	Hold prior to procedure	Resume after procedure
Aspirin	7–10 days	1 day
Clopidogrel	7–10 days	1 day
Warfarin	3–5 days	Evening following
Direct oral anticoagulants (dabigatran, rivaroxaban, apixaban, edoxaban)	24–36 h	1 day
Heparin	4–6 h	2–6 h

Note: Management of antiplatelet therapy with platelet aggregation inhibitors (i.e., clopidogrel, ticlopidine, and prasugrel) recommended to be done in consultation with treating cardiologist based on patient individual clinical history and risk factors

Source: Adopted from Kim JH et al. 2017 and Orloff et al. 2021 [1, 3]

able to adhere to the post-procedure follow-up as recommended by the treating physician, typically involving clinical examination, serial ultrasounds and serologic assessment of thyroid function (with at least TSH) [2]. Should physicians performing ablative thyroid procedures not anticipate providing longitudinal follow-up, they are recommended to ensure adequate transition of care to providers experiences in the management of nodular thyroid conditions, including the nuances of sonographic evaluation of nodules post-treatment, given the sonographic changes that occur [1].

8.3 Nodule Factors

8.3.1 Benign Nodules and General Considerations

Thyroid nodules are common and present in up to two thirds of adults [8, 9]. Although most thyroid nodules are benign and typically asymptomatic, symptomatic benign nodules are treated generally [10]. Symptoms due to large or poorly positioned nodules may include compressive symptoms of pressure, dysphagia, foreign body sensation, cough, discomfort, or pain. Depending on nodule location, cosmetic concerns may be present and may be an indication for treatment.

Several guidelines recommend confirmation that a nodule is benign with two ultrasound-guided fine needle aspirations (FNAs) or core need biopsy (CNB) prior to ablation [1, 3]. Although the risk of malignancy in a nodule with benign cytopathology is low (<4%) [11, 12], a second biopsy is recommended in nodules with suspicious features on ultrasound to reduce the false-negative rate [13–15]. In cases of benign features on ultrasound (i.e., isoechoic spongiform nodule or benign-appearing cystic nodules with intracystic comet tail artifact), a single confirmatory FNA may be considered [3]. The use of FNA in the context of thermal ablation is discussed in further detail in Chap. 5.

Solid nodules generally respond more favorably to thermal ablation compared to mixed solid/cystic nodules. Completely cystic nodules are best treated by non-thermal ablation such as ethanol ablation if observation or surgery is not desired. Furthermore nodules with significant calcifications are not as amenable to treatment with thermal ablation such as RFA [3] (Fig. 8.1). Table 8.3 summarizes the nodule characteristics to be evaluated prior to ablative therapy.

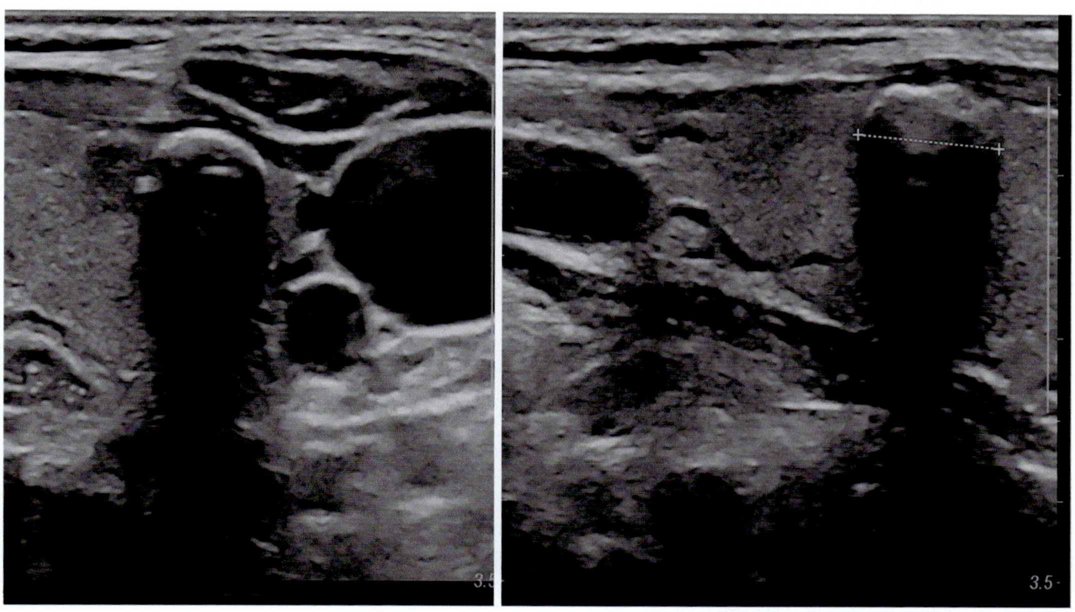

Fig. 8.1 Nodule with eggshell calcification

There are no definite criteria for size or volume qualifications for thyroid ablation [3] and strict universally accepted size criteria is challenging to establish. The 2017 Korean Society of Thyroid Radiology Guidelines recommends 2 cm as the minimum size blended with presence of symptoms [3], while the 2020 ETA guidelines suggest a minimum size of 3 cm [2]. It should be kept in mind that nodules of similar size may result in different symptoms based on body habitus. Nodule size therefore is best considered in the context of location within the thyroid gland and also overall patient stature as a patient's overall size may influence the impact of the nodule on referable symptoms [1, 3]. An isthmic or anteriorly positioned nodule may be of cosmetic concern for instance, while a similarly sized nodule that is more posterior situated may be asymptomatic. In general, posterior nodules are more likely to lead to compressive symptoms, and not cosmetic symptoms, when sufficiently large (Fig. 8.5). A visual analog scale (grade 0–10 with 0 = no symptoms and 10 = maximal symptoms) provides patient self-reported symptom score and a cosmetic score can be calculated by a physician using a four point scale (1 = no palpable mass, 2 = palpable mass without cosmetic problem, 3 = cosmetic problem on swallowing only, and 4 = readily detected cosmetic problem) [16–19] (Fig. 8.5).

Treatment of smaller nodules generally results in greater volume reduction as calculated by the

Table 8.3 Consideration of nodule characteristics for treatment with Thermal Ablation (TA)

Nodule features	Notes
Nodule composition (Fig. 8.2)	
• Solid nodule	• Generally well treated with TA
• Mixed solid/cystic nodules	• Consider EA for cystic component
• Cystic nodule	• EA preferred technique
Nodule location	
• Surrounded by rim of normal thyroid tissue (Fig. 8.3)	• "Danger Zone", trachea and great vessels during ablation (Fig. 8.4)
Other	
• Single large nodule	• In case of multinodular goiter, symptomatic dominant nodule
Nodule cytology	
• Benign	• Consider 2 FNA (or if necessary CNB) with benign cytology or 1 FNA (or if necessary CNB) if ultrasound demonstrates benign morphology
• Autonomous functioning	• Traditionally considered second line to RAI or surgery • Single benign FNA (Bethesda Class 2) sufficient
• Malignant	• Low-risk molecular pattern

Note: Role of molecular testing remains to be defined (see Chap. 7)

Abbreviations: *TA* thermal ablation; *EA* ethanol ablation; *FNA* fine needle aspiration; *CNB* core needle biopsy

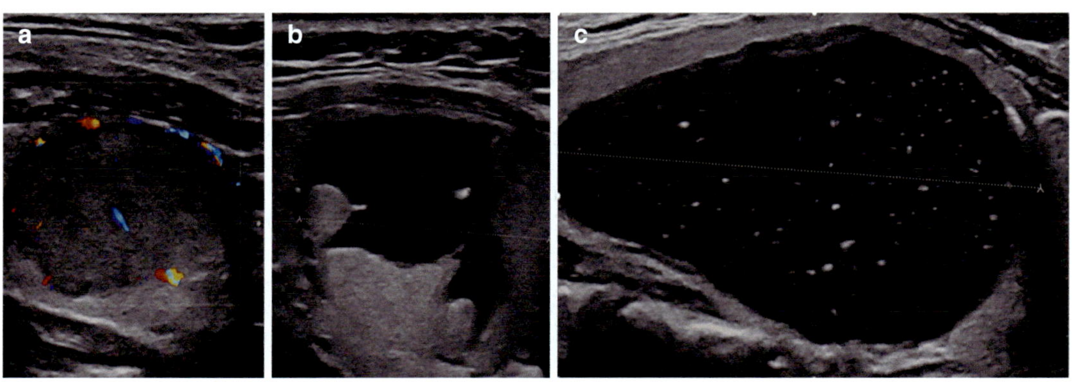

Fig. 8.2 Nodule echostructure: (**a**) solid; (**b**) mixed; (**c**) fluid

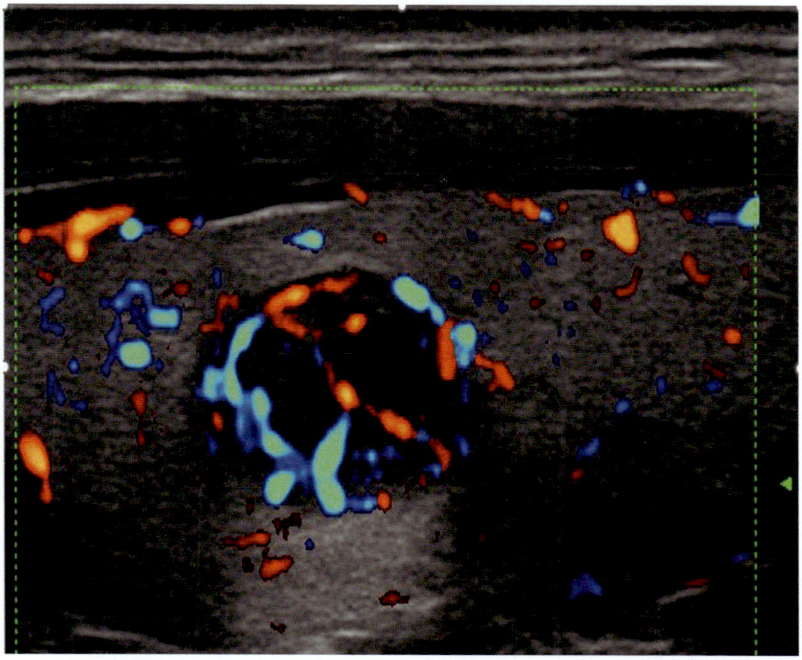

Fig. 8.3 Autonomous thyroid nodule with normal surrounding tissue is a candidate for treatment with thermoablation

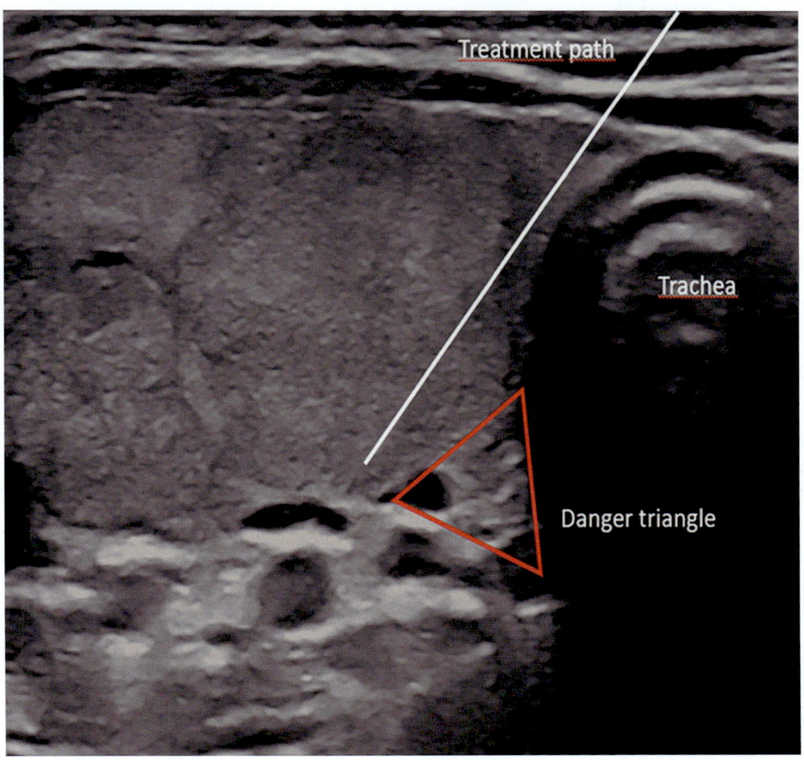

Fig. 8.4 Dominant nodule in multinodular goiter with deeper aspect abutting the "Danger triangle"

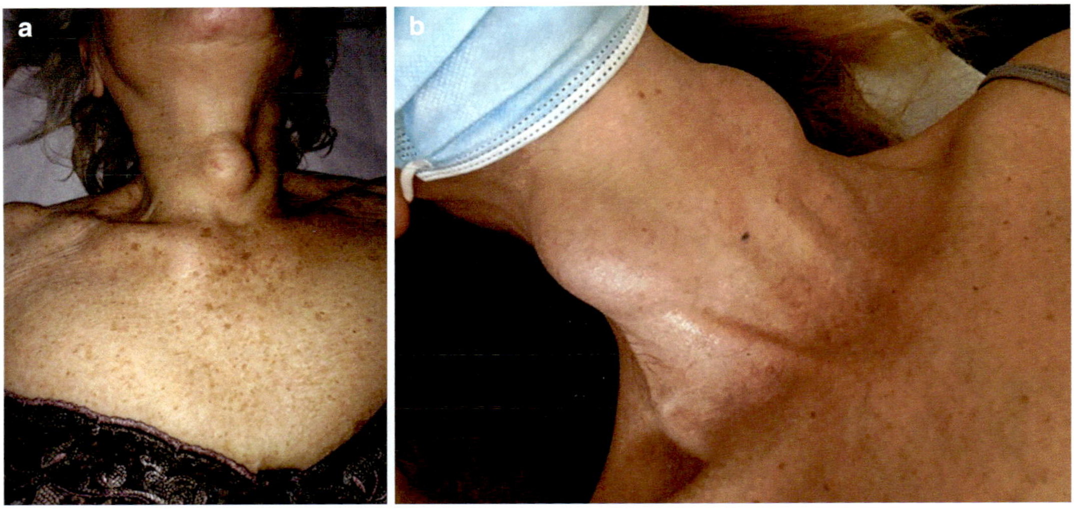

Fig. 8.5 Thyroid nodules causing cosmetic concerns: Isthmus nodule (**a**) and bilateral enlarged superior thyroid poles (**b**)

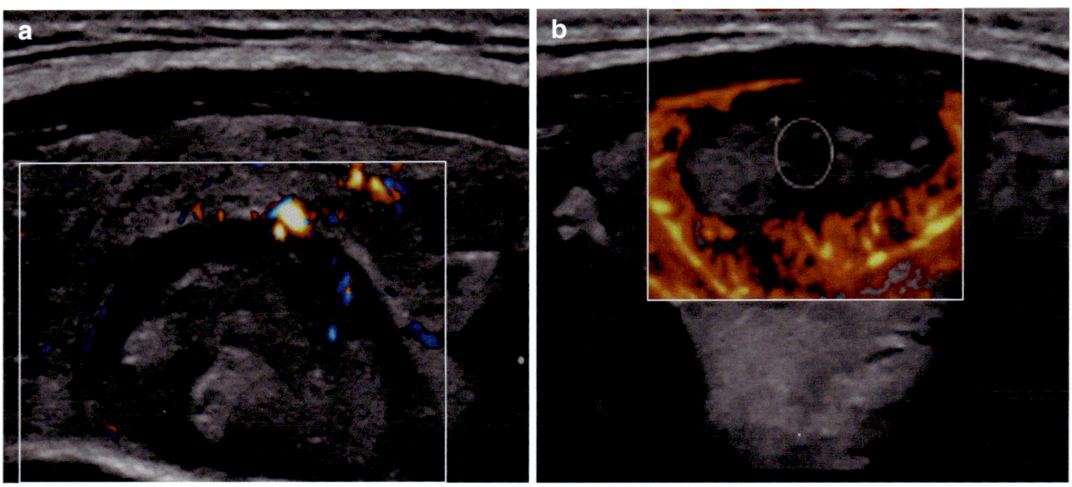

Fig. 8.6 Images of thyroid nodules two months after treatment with microwave thermoablation: Nodule completely treated (**a**) and nodule with deeper component still active (not yet treated) (**b**)

volume reduction ratio (VRR (%) = [100 × (initial volume − final volume)]/initial volume) [20, 21]. Larger nodules and nodules exhibiting rapid growth prior to initial treatment may be more likely to regrow compared to nodules with a slower growth trajectory [22]. Residual untreated peripheral tissue may lead to marginal regrowth over time, requiring additional treatment [22–24] (Fig. 8.6).

Although thermal ablation is minimally invasive, patients and clinicians should consider the risks of thyroid nodule thermal ablation to be similar to those of open surgery [1, 25]. Reported rates of complications range from 0 to 17% with major complications occurring in up to 3.8% of cases [26–29] (Fig. 8.7). A summary of potential complications is shown in Table 8.4. The most frequent complication involves injury of the recurrent laryngeal nerve, which may result in changes in voice and swallowing function, and less commonly the external branch of the supe-

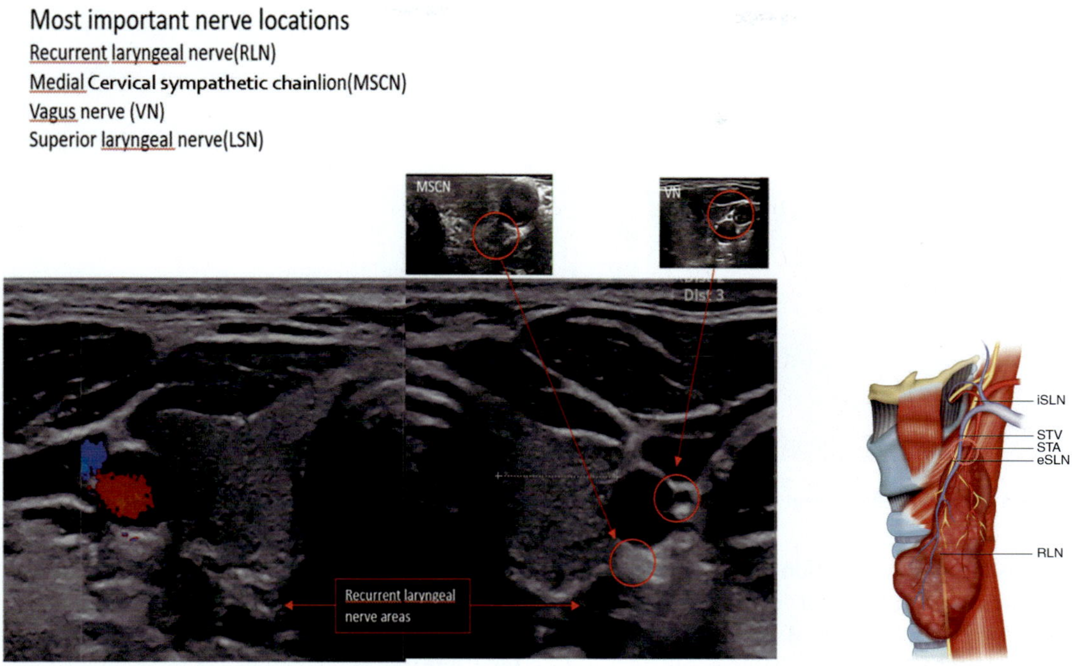

Fig. 8.7 Critical cervical nerves at risk during ablative procedures

Table 8.4 Summary of potential complications for thermal ablation with reported incidence [25, 27, 28, 30, 32–34]

Major complications		Minor complications	
Nerve injury	1.0–2.0%	Pain	0.0–100.0%
Nodule rupture	0.2–0.5%	Bleeding (hematoma/hemorrhage)	0.0–17.0%
Tracheal injury	Rare (2 reported cases)	Skin burn	0.3–3.7%
Horner's syndrome	Rare		

rior laryngeal nerve resulting in voice change [28, 30]. Depending on the location of the nodule or lymph node to be treated, the vagus nerve, the sympathetic chain posterior to the carotid artery, the brachial plexus in the supraclavicular fossa, and the phrenic nerve are potentially at risk. Thermal ablation also carries a risk of thyroid nodule rupture (Fig. 8.8), the second most frequently reported major complication, which may present in a delayed fashion several weeks following the procedure [30]. Thermal injury to the overlying cervical skin can result in cutaneous scar which may be temporary or permanent, or when occurring more deeply thermal injury may damage adjacent structures such as the trachea [31]. In general, the presence of normal thyroid tissue circumferentially around the nodule to be treated—especially deep, medial, and lateral to the nodule—affords a margin of greater safety during ablation. Treatment of anteriorly located nodules carries less risk (other than to skin) compared to nodules located laterally and closer to the carotid sheath or deeper and closer to the danger triangle (Fig. 8.4).

8.3.2 Follicular Thyroid Nodules

The role of thermal ablation for follicular neoplasms is unclear. Distinguishing thyroid follicular adenomas from follicular thyroid carcinoma, which account for 10–20% of all thyroid carcino-

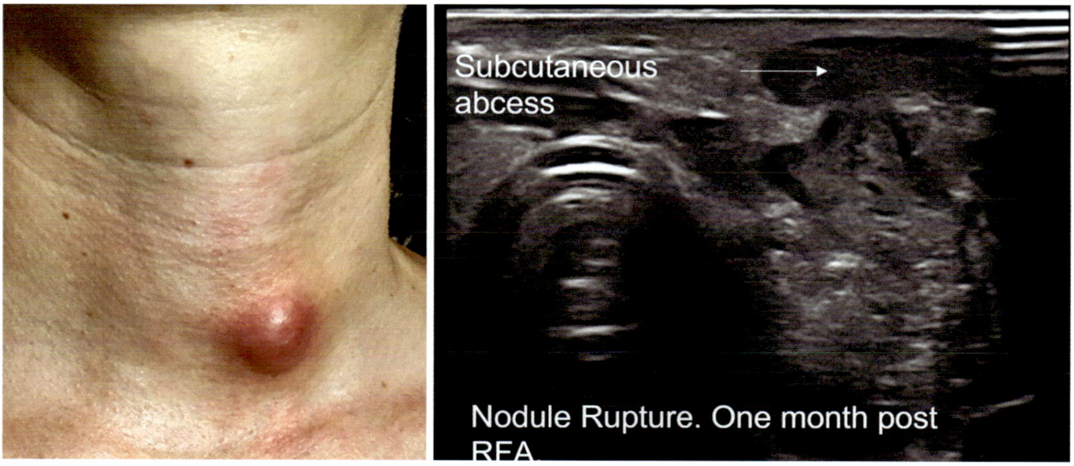

Fig. 8.8 Thyroid nodule upture with subcutaneous abscess one month following radiofrequency ablation

mas, is based on evaluation of the thyroid nodule capsule, vascular and/or extrathyroidal extension, and the presence of metastasis to lymph nodes or distant sites [9, 35]. For follicular neoplasms, although a CNB may reduce the rate of false-negative cytopathologic results [12, 36, 37], it should be kept in mind that surgery (without for preoperative CNB) remains the standard of care [9, 11, 35]. The role of molecular testing in the diagnosis of these lesions continues to evolve [9, 11].

Size of follicular neoplasms may predict clinical behavior with follicular carcinomas <2 cm less likely to metastasize [38]. One study that evaluated RFA to treat follicular lesions <2 cm demonstrated no recurrences or metastatic lesions during the 5-year follow-up period [39]. Another study of 30 patients with Bethesda Class IV nodules treated with thermal ablation extending 3 mm beyond the margin of the nodule similarly found no recurrences or evidence of local or distal metastases in a follow-up of up to 24 months [40]. Nodules >2 cm treated with RFA, followed by surgery because of continued growth, however have been found to be malignant [41]. Treatment with thermal ablation does not aid in the diagnosis or guarantee complete resolution of the nodule in question and therefore currently the use of thermal ablation for follicular neoplasms is not endorsed by guidelines [1–3].

8.3.3 Autonomous Functioning Thyroid Nodules (AFTNs)

First-line treatment options for autonomous functioning thyroid nodules (AFTNs) includes antithyroid medications, radioactive iodine (RAI) therapy and surgery [42]. Patient seeking to avoid post-treatment hypothyroidism or who cannot undergo the standard treatment of surgery or RAI, however may be considered for ablative treatment [43–46].

In general, AFTNs may be considered similarly to benign symptomatic nodules. Smaller nodules (< 3 cm) are treated more effectively due in part to the greater nodule volume reduction seen with smaller thyroid nodules [1, 2]. Thermal ablation is less effective for Grave's disease or toxic multinodular goiter and therefore scintigraphy is recommended to confirm a single AFTN [2, 47]. In addition, the 2020 European Thyroid Association guidelines do not endorse the use of RFA for Grave's disease or for toxic multinodular goiter [2].

A single benign FNA (or CNB) is sufficient to proceed with thermal ablation [2, 3]. Most AFTNs are benign; however, there have been reports of AFTNs ultimately proven to be malignant [48, 49]. Pre-toxic nodules, which carry a 4% annual risk of conversion to overtly toxic nodules [50] may also be considered for treatment [3].

The treatment of smaller nodules with RFA appears more likely to reestablish a euthyroid state [51], although larger AFTNs causing compressive symptoms, or compression of adjacent structures, cosmetic concerns, and/or symptoms of hyperthyroidism may be candidates for thermal ablation when first-line therapy is not possible [2]. Results from thermal ablation may be less predictable, possibly due to increased vascularity of AFTN; [52] however, a meta-analysis of over 200 AFTNs followed for up to 2 years after treatment with RFA found a pooled rate of TSH normalization in 57% of patients (with smaller baseline nodule volume associated with TSH normalization) and an optimal response on scintigraphy in 60% with a pooled VRR at 1 year of 79% [46].

8.4 Malignant Nodules

Differentiated thyroid cancer typically is indolent, with an overall 5-year survival rate of 98%, however recurrence may be seen in up to 30% of patients and when present (locally or distally) may dramatically lower survival [10, 53]. Standard treatment of thyroid cancer involves surgery and in some cases post-operative radioactive iodine (RAI) therapy [9]. Malignancy (primary or recurrent) should be established with cytology (FNA or CNB) serum thyroglobulin levels and FNA thyroglobulin wash out as needed [54]. Due to the risk of medullary thyroid cancers having indeterminate cytology and absence of high-risk features on ultrasound, the 2020 ETA guidelines include consideration of a single serum calcitonin measurement [2].

In cases where surgery cannot be performed or is refused, there is a growing international experience of radiofrequency ablation to treat certain low-risk primary papillary thyroid carcinoma [55–58] as well as recurrent papillary thyroid carcinoma [59–64]. Treatment intent—cure vs. palliation—should be clearly established [1]. Similar to the care of benign thyroid disease, a multidisciplinary comprehensive discussion with the patient of the risks, benefits, and alternatives of treatment options is recommended. A full discussion of the application of ablative technology for malignant thyroid disease can be found in Chap. 25.

8.4.1 Primary Thyroid Carcinoma

In certain patients unwilling or unable to undergo surgery for primary thyroid carcinoma, ablative therapy may be considered, with the largest body of evidence describing use of RFA for papillary thyroid carcinomas [3, 54, 65, 66]. Ideally, primary tumors should have the following characteristics [54, 56, 67] (Fig. 8.9):

- Unifocal microcarcinoma confined to the thyroid gland and without capsular contact
- Papillary thyroid carcinoma without evidence of aggressive subtype on cytology
- No evidence of metastatic lymphadenopathy
- Patient at high risk or unable to undergo surgery or who decline surgery

Low-risk papillary thyroid microcarcinoma (PTMC) that otherwise may be considered for active surveillance with excellent outcomes have been treated with RFA [56, 66–71], LA [72, 73], and MA [74, 75]. In a study of 182 patients treated for solitary T1bNoMo PTC with RFA or surgery ($n = 91$/group), Xiao J et al. found no significant difference in local tumor progression between the two groups [76]. A multicenter retrospective study of 847 patients who refused or were unable to undergo surgery and were treated with either RFA or MA found complete disappearance of tumors in 68% (577 of 847) of patients (69% of T1a (466 of 673) and 64% of T1b PTC (111 of 174) $p < 0.001$) [77]. The disease progression rate after ablation was 1.1% (9 of 847 with 6/673 T1a patients and 3/174 of T1b patients; $P = 0.54$). He et al. evaluated 204 patients with pT1bNoMo PTC treated with RFA ($n = 94$) or surgery ($n = 110$) and followed over 12 months and found no significant difference in disease progression or complications between the two groups, while the RFA group incurred less cost [78]. A retrospective study of 358 patients with solitary T1N0M0 PTC treated with RFA and followed for over 5 years, reported a 5% overall

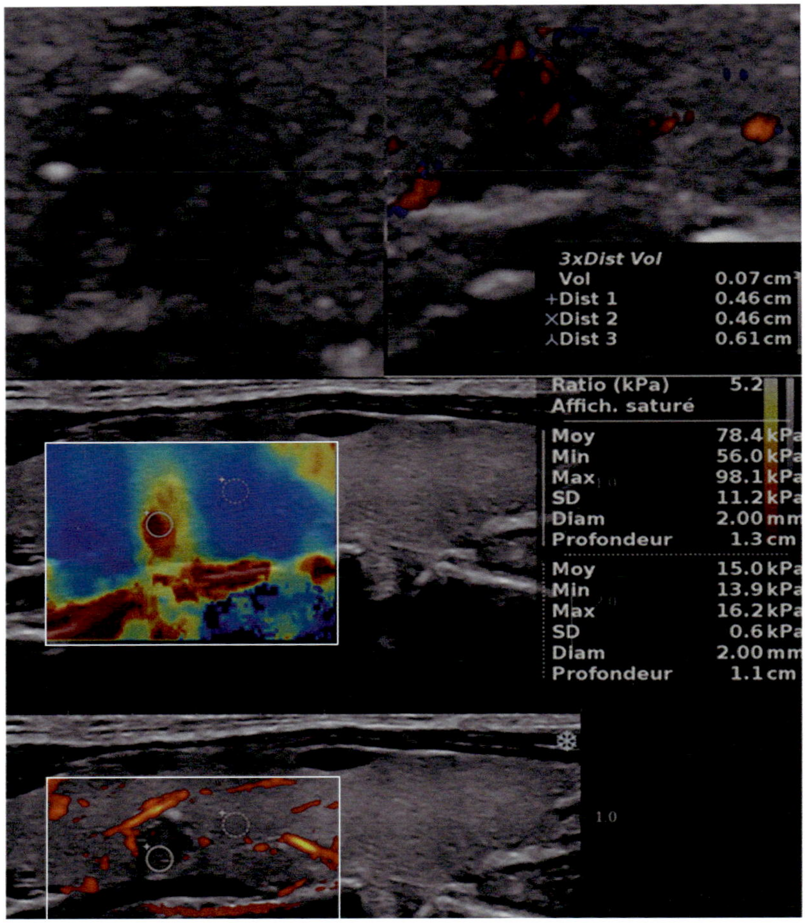

Fig. 8.9 Ultrasound of papillary microcarcinoma

disease progression rate with T1a and T1b groups having similar incidence of disease progression (5.0% vs. 5.5%, $p = 1.000$), lymph node metastasis (1.3% vs. 1.8%, $p = 0.568$), recurrent tumor (3.3% vs. 1.8%, $p = 0.872$), persistent tumors (0.3% vs. 1.8%, $p = 0.284$), and 5-year recurrence-free survival (95.4% vs. 96.4%, $p = 0.785$) [79].

Roughly 80% of follicular thyroid neoplasms are benign; however, cytology alone remains insufficient to differentiation benign from malignant lesions [80] and therefore as discussed above, the role of thermal ablation in the management of these lesions remains in question. The role of thermal ablation in the treatment of medullary thyroid carcinoma similarly remains limited at present to patients ineligible for surgery (the treatment of choice) or for inoperable regional recurrence after prior surgical resection [81, 82]. In general due to lack of sufficient evidence of efficacy, the role of ablation in the setting of anaplastic thyroid carcinoma remains questionable beyond palliation. Jeong SY et al. described the use of RFA to treat nine thyroid cancers with more promising results for thyroid papillary micro- and macrocarcinomas than the one anaplastic thyroid carcinoma treated [83].

8.4.2 Recurrent or Metastatic Thyroid Cancer

Revision surgery to treat cancer recurrences involves increased risk, particularly to the recurrent laryngeal nerve and the parathyroid glands due to scarring in the field. Treatment of recurrent papillary and follicular carcinomas by RFA was first reported in 2001 [84]. For patients deemed to be at high surgical risk or who refuse revision surgery, thermal ablation may offer local control. Universal guidelines for the application of thermal ablation in this setting are lacking and a multidisciplinary approach is recommended so that patients may be informed of the relative risks and benefits of all treatment options available and treatment goals (cure vs. palliation) can be established [9, 54]. At present, RFA has been shown to be most effective for indolent metastases <10 mm and/or <3–4 foci of localized cervical recurrent thyroid cancer without metastases beyond the neck [54, 59, 62, 85]. Fig. 8.10 illustrates a lymph node metastasis suitable for treatment with thermal ablation.

A meta-analysis of 321 patients with 498 cervical lymph node metastases (CLNM) treated with thermal ablation (RFA or LA or MWA) and followed for longer than 6 months (up to 127 months) found a significant reduction in volume of the CLNM ($P < 0.0001$) with an 88% VRR and 283 of the 498 CLMN (57%) disappearing completely on imaging [64]. Another meta-analysis of 312 patients with 559 CLMN reported a pooled VRR 91% [95% confidence interval (CI): 86.60–95.97%] and complete disappearance rate of 67.9% [95% CI: 53.1–81.1%] and recurrence of CMLNs rate of 7.8% [95% CI: 3.0–14.1%] [86]. In this study, the respective pooled rate of overall and major complications were 2.9% [95% CI: 0.3–7.1%] and 0.3% [95% CI: 0–1.9%] respectively.

8.4.3 Palliative Treatment

Palliative treatment with thermal ablation may be considered in cases where surgical or other treatment is not feasible or acceptable [3, 87]. There are no established guidelines for the application of palliative thermal ablation for thyroid cancer and treatment with RFA may be considered when reduction in the size of the disease is judged to reduce symptoms and improve quality of life [1, 54].

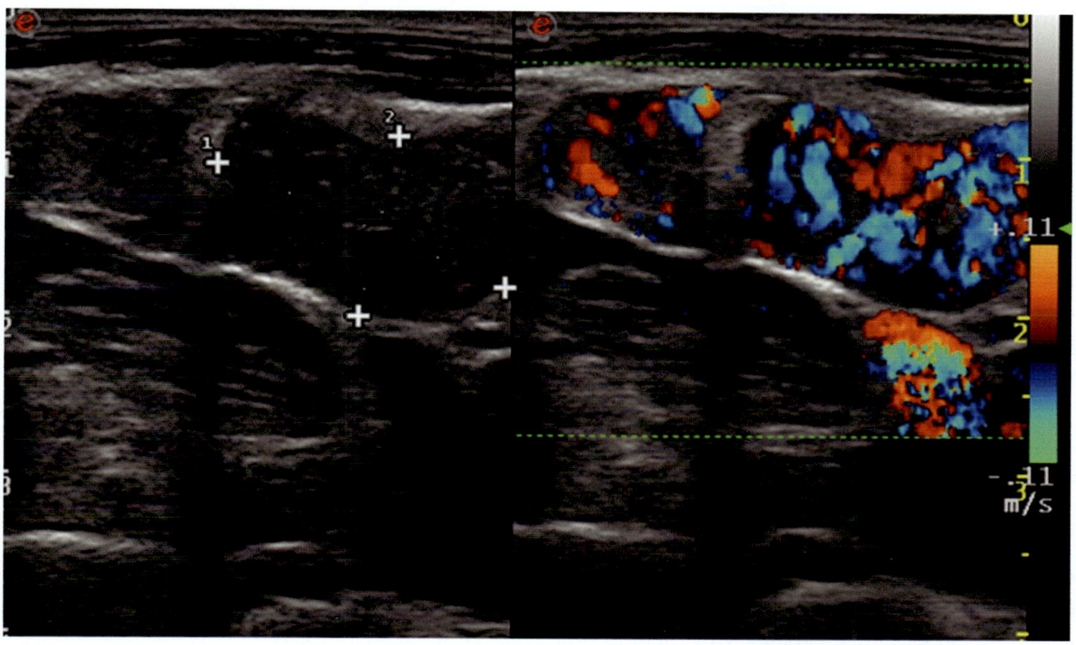

Fig. 8.10 Ultrasound of cervical lymph node with metastatic papillary thyroid carcinoma (grayscale image (left) and doppler imaging (right)

8.5 Molecular Testing

The role of molecular testing in the evaluation and management of thyroid nodules continues to evolve. Testing is not universally available, and indications or application vary by country. In general, however where available molecular testing is not recommended for nodules with benign cytology [88] (Bethesda class II) as the risk of malignancy is low (0–4%) [11]. The risk of malignancy is higher and ranges from 13 to 3-% however for cytologically indeterminant nodules (Bethesda class III or atypia of undetermined significance (AUS) and 23 - 34% for follicular neoplasms (Bethesda class IV) [11]. Molecular testing of these nodules may assist in risk stratification and given the high negative predictive value of commercially available molecular tests, nodules with negative molecular profiles may be managed as benign nodules [89]. Nodules suspicious for malignancy (Bethesda class V) have a risk of malignancy of 67 to 83% [11] and therefore molecular testing is generally not indicated and surgery is recommended [89].

When available molecular profiling may improve risk stratification however the prognostic value of molecular profiling remains an area of active investigation [90, 91]. Similarly, the application of molecular testing in the work-up of a thyroid nodule for consideration of ablative therapy remains in question. The presence of high-risk molecular patterns favor surgery over ablative therapy, while in the appropriate clinical context, negative molecular testing may support the use of ablative therapy in patients unable to undergo or refusing surgery [54]. A full discussion of the role of molecular testing in the context of thermal ablation can be found in Chap. 7.

8.6 Summary

Thermal ablation of carefully selected nodules in the appropriate clinical context with consideration of goals of care and availability of resources and clinician expertise expands treatment option for patients with nodular thyroid disease. As experience with the various ablative technologies expands and the duration of follow-up increases, the application of these technologies is expected to expand. A multidisciplinary approach is advocated for optimal care.

References

1. Orloff LA, Noel JE, Stack BC, Russell MD, Angelos P, Baek JH, et al. Radiofrequency ablation and related ultrasound-guided ablation technologies for treatment of benign and malignant thyroid disease: an international multidisciplinary consensus statement of the American Head and Neck Society Endocrine Surgery Section with the Asia Pacific Society of Thyroid Surgery, Associazione Medici Endocrinologi, British Association of Endocrine and Thyroid Surgeons, European Thyroid Association, Italian Society of Endocrine Surgery Units, Korean Society of Thyroid Radiology, Latin American Thyroid Society, and Thyroid Nodules Therapies Association. Head Neck. 2022;44(3):633–60. https://doi.org/10.1002/hed.26960.
2. Papini E, Monpeyssen H, Frasoldati A, Hegedüs L. 2020 European thyroid association clinical practice guideline for the use of image-guided ablation in benign thyroid nodules. Eur Thyroid J. 2020;9(4):172–85. https://doi.org/10.1159/000508484.
3. Kim JH, Baek JH, Lim HK, Ahn HS, Baek SM, Choi YJ, et al. 2017 thyroid radiofrequency ablation guideline: Korean Society of Thyroid Radiology. Korean J Radiol. 2018;19(4):632–55. https://doi.org/10.3348/kjr.2018.19.4.632.
4. Papini E, Crescenzi A, D'Amore A, Deandrea M, De Benedictis A, Frasoldati A, et al. Italian guidelines for the management of non-functioning benign and locally symptomatic thyroid nodules. Endocr Metab Immune Disord Drug Targets. 2023;23(6):876–85. https://doi.org/10.2174/187153032366623020110411 2.
5. Wu MH, Chen KY, Chen A, Chen CN. Differences in the ultrasonographic appearance of thyroid nodules after radiofrequency ablation. Clin Endocrinol. 2021;95(3):489–97. https://doi.org/10.1111/cen.14480.
6. Ha SM, Shin JY, Baek JH, Song DE, Chung SR, Choi YJ, et al. Does radiofrequency ablation induce neoplastic changes in benign thyroid nodules: a preliminary study. Endocrinol Metab Seoul Korea. 2019;34(2):169–78. https://doi.org/10.3803/EnM.2019.34.2.169.
7. Ben Hamou A, Ghanassia E, Muller A, Cao CD, Drui D, Leboulleux S, et al. SFE-AFCE-SFMN 2022 consensus on the management of thyroid nodules: thermal ablation. Ann Endocrinol. 2022;83(6):423–30. https://doi.org/10.1016/j.ando.2022.10.011.

8. Tan GH, Gharib H. Thyroid incidentalomas: management approaches to nonpalpable nodules discovered incidentally on thyroid imaging. Ann Intern Med. 1997;126(3):226–31. https://doi.org/10.7326/0003-4819-126-3-199702010-00009.
9. Haugen BR, Alexander EK, Bible KC, Doherty GM, Mandel SJ, Nikiforov YE, et al. 2015 American Thyroid Association management guidelines for adult patients with thyroid nodules and differentiated thyroid cancer: the American Thyroid Association guidelines task force on thyroid nodules and differentiated thyroid cancer. Thyroid. 2016;26(1):1–133. https://doi.org/10.1089/thy.2015.0020.
10. Suresh NV, De Ravin E, Barrette LX, Rasad A, Romeo D, Ng J, et al. Quality appraisal of clinical practice guidelines for the use of radiofrequency ablation in the treatment of thyroid nodules and cancer. Am J Otolaryngol. 2022;43(4):103508. https://doi.org/10.1016/j.amjoto.2022.103508.
11. Ali SZ, Baloch ZW, Cochand-Priollet B, Schmitt FC, Vielh P, VanderLaan PA. The 2023 Bethesda System for Reporting Thyroid Cytopathology. Thyroid. 2023;33(9):1039–44. https://doi.org/10.1089/thy.2023.0141.
12. Na DG, Baek JH, Jung SL, Kim JH, Sung JY, Kim KS, et al. Core needle biopsy of the thyroid: 2016 consensus statement and recommendations from Korean Society of Thyroid Radiology. Korean J Radiol. 2017;18(1):217–37. https://doi.org/10.3348/kjr.2017.18.1.217.
13. Erdoğan MF, Kamel N, Aras D, Akdoğan A, Başkal N, Erdoğan G. Value of re-aspirations in benign nodular thyroid disease. Thyroid Off J Am Thyroid Assoc. 1998;8(12):1087–90. https://doi.org/10.1089/thy.1998.8.1087.
14. Orlandi A, Puscar A, Capriata E, Fideleff H. Repeated fine-needle aspiration of the thyroid in benign nodular thyroid disease: critical evaluation of long-term follow-up. Thyroid Off J Am Thyroid Assoc. 2005;15(3):274–8. https://doi.org/10.1089/thy.2005.15.274.
15. Oertel YC, Miyahara-Felipe L, Mendoza MG, Yu K. Value of repeated fine needle aspirations of the thyroid: an analysis of over ten thousand FNAs. Thyroid Off J Am Thyroid Assoc. 2007;17(11):1061–6. https://doi.org/10.1089/thy.2007.0159.
16. Baek JH, Kim YS, Lee D, Huh JY, Lee JH. Benign predominantly solid thyroid nodules: prospective study of efficacy of sonographically guided radiofrequency ablation versus control condition. AJR Am J Roentgenol. 2010;194(4):1137–42. https://doi.org/10.2214/AJR.09.3372.
17. Lee JH, Kim YS, Lee D, Choi H, Yoo H, Baek JH. Radiofrequency ablation (RFA) of benign thyroid nodules in patients with incompletely resolved clinical problems after ethanol ablation (EA). World J Surg. 2010;34(7):1488–93. https://doi.org/10.1007/s00268-010-0565-6.
18. Jang SW, Baek JH, Kim JK, Sung JY, Choi H, Lim HK, et al. How to manage the patients with unsatisfactory results after ethanol ablation for thyroid nodules: role of radiofrequency ablation. Eur J Radiol. 2012;81(5):905–10. https://doi.org/10.1016/j.ejrad.2011.02.039.
19. Deandrea M, Limone P, Basso E, Mormile A, Ragazzoni F, Gamarra E, et al. US-guided percutaneous radiofrequency thermal ablation for the treatment of solid benign hyperfunctioning or compressive thyroid nodules. Ultrasound Med Biol. 2008;34(5):784–91. https://doi.org/10.1016/j.ultrasmedbio.2007.10.018.
20. Cesareo R, Pasqualini V, Simeoni C, Sacchi M, Saralli E, Campagna G, et al. Prospective study of effectiveness of ultrasound-guided radiofrequency ablation versus control group in patients affected by benign thyroid nodules. J Clin Endocrinol Metab. 2015;100(2):460–6. https://doi.org/10.1210/jc.2014-2186.
21. Deandrea M, Sung JY, Limone P, Mormile A, Garino F, Ragazzoni F, et al. Efficacy and safety of radiofrequency ablation versus observation for nonfunctioning benign thyroid nodules: a randomized controlled international collaborative trial. Thyroid. 2015;25(8):890–6. https://doi.org/10.1089/thy.2015.0133.
22. Sim JS, Baek JH. Unresolved clinical issues in thermal ablation of benign thyroid nodules: regrowth at long-term follow-up. Korean J Radiol. 2021;22(8):1436–40. https://doi.org/10.3348/kjr.2021.0093.
23. Huh JY, Baek JH, Choi H, Kim JK, Lee JH. Symptomatic benign thyroid nodules: efficacy of additional radiofrequency ablation treatment session—prospective randomized study. Radiology. 2012;263(3):909–16. https://doi.org/10.1148/radiol.12111300.
24. Monpeyssen H, Alamri A, Ben Hamou A. Long-term results of ultrasound-guided radiofrequency ablation of benign thyroid nodules: state of the art and future perspectives-a systematic review. Front Endocrinol. 2021;12:622996. https://doi.org/10.3389/fendo.2021.622996.
25. Lim JY, Kuo JH. Thyroid nodule radiofrequency ablation: complications and clinical follow up. Tech Vasc Interv Radiol. 2022;25(2):100824. https://doi.org/10.1016/j.tvir.2022.100824.
26. Muhammad H, Santhanam P, Russell JO. Radiofrequency ablation and thyroid nodules: updated systematic review. Endocrine. 2021;72(3):619–32. https://doi.org/10.1007/s12020-020-02598-6.
27. Jeong WK, Baek JH, Rhim H, Kim YS, Kwak MS, Jeong HJ, et al. Radiofrequency ablation of benign thyroid nodules: safety and imaging follow-up in 236 patients. Eur Radiol. 2008;18(6):1244–50. https://doi.org/10.1007/s00330-008-0880-6.
28. Baek JH, Lee JH, Sung JY, Bae JI, Kim KT, Sim J, et al. Complications encountered in the treatment of benign thyroid nodules with US-guided radiofrequency ablation: a multicenter study. Radiology. 2012;262(1):335–42. https://doi.org/10.1148/radiol.11110416.

29. Cho SJ, Baek JH, Chung SR, Choi YJ, Lee JH. Long-term results of thermal ablation of benign thyroid nodules: a systematic review and meta-analysis. Endocrinol Metab Seoul Korea. 2020;35(2):339–50. https://doi.org/10.3803/EnM.2020.35.2.339.
30. Chung SR, Baek JH, Sung JY, Ryu JH, Jung SL. Revisiting rupture of benign thyroid nodules after radiofrequency ablation: various types and imaging features. Endocrinol Metab Seoul Korea. 2019;34(4):415–21. https://doi.org/10.3803/EnM.2019.34.4.415.
31. van Baardewijk LJ, Plaisier ML, van den Broek FJC, van Poppel PCMW, Kurban S, Kruimer JWH. Tracheal necrosis following radiofrequency ablation of a benign thyroid nodule. Cardiovasc Intervent Radiol. 2021;44(1):170–1. https://doi.org/10.1007/s00270-020-02632-0.
32. Wang JF, Wu T, Hu KP, Xu W, Zheng BW, Tong G, et al. Complications following radiofrequency ablation of benign thyroid nodules: a systematic review. Chin Med J. 2017;130(11):1361–70. https://doi.org/10.4103/0366-6999.206347.
33. Feldkamp J, Grünwald F, Luster M, Lorenz K, Vorländer C, Führer D. Non-surgical and non-radioiodine techniques for ablation of benign thyroid nodules: consensus statement and recommendation. Exp Clin Endocrinol Diabetes. 2020;128(10):687–92. https://doi.org/10.1055/a-1075-2025.
34. Ben Hamou A, Monpeyssen H. Horner's syndrome during high-intensity focused ultrasound ablation for a benign thyroid nodule. AACE Clin Case Rep. 2021;7(3):164–8. https://doi.org/10.1016/j.aace.2020.11.035.
35. Wu MH, Chen KY, Hsieh MS, Chen A, Chen CN. Risk stratification in patients with follicular neoplasm on cytology: use of quantitative characteristics and sonographic patterns. Front Endocrinol. 2021;12:614630. https://doi.org/10.3389/fendo.2021.614630.
36. Joo L, Na DG, Kim JH, Seo H. Comparison of core needle biopsy and repeat fine-needle aspiration in avoiding diagnostic surgery for thyroid nodules initially diagnosed as atypia/follicular lesion of undetermined significance. Korean J Radiol. 2022;23(2):280–8. https://doi.org/10.3348/kjr.2021.0619.
37. Yoon RG, Baek JH, Lee JH, Choi YJ, Hong MJ, Song DE, Kim JK, Yoon JH, Kim WB. Diagnosis of thyroid follicular neoplasm: fine-needle aspiration versus core-needle biopsy. Thyroid. 2014;24(11):1612–7. https://doi.org/10.1089/thy.2014.0140.
38. Machens A, Holzhausen HJ, Dralle H. The prognostic value of primary tumor size in papillary and follicular thyroid carcinoma. Cancer. 2005;103(11):2269–73. https://doi.org/10.1002/cncr.21055.
39. Ha SM, Sung JY, Baek JH, Na DG, Kim JH, Yoo H, et al. Radiofrequency ablation of small follicular neoplasms: initial clinical outcomes. Int J Hyperth. 2017;33(8):931–7. https://doi.org/10.1080/02656736.2017.1331268.
40. Li X, Lan Y, Li N, Yan L, Xiao J, Zhang M, et al. Ultrasound-guided thermal ablation of Bethesda IV thyroid nodules: a pilot study. Front Endocrinol. 2021;12:674970. https://doi.org/10.3389/fendo.2021.674970.
41. Dobrinja C, Bernardi S, Fabris B, Eramo R, Makovac P, Bazzocchi G, et al. Surgical and pathological changes after radiofrequency ablation of thyroid nodules. Int J Endocrinol. 2015;2015:576576. https://doi.org/10.1155/2015/576576.
42. Ross DS, Burch HB, Cooper DS, Greenlee MC, Laurberg P, Maia AL, Rivkees SA, Samuels M, Sosa JA, Stan MN, Walter MA. 2016 American Thyroid Association guidelines for diagnosis and management of hyperthyroidism and other causes of thyrotoxicosis. Thyroid. 2016;26(10):1343–421. https://doi.org/10.1089/thy.2016.0229. Erratum in: Thyroid. 2017;27(11):1462.
43. Ha EJ, Baek JH, Lee JH, Sung JY, Lee D, Kim JK, Shong YK. Radiofrequency ablation of benign thyroid nodules does not affect thyroid function in patients with previous lobectomy. Thyroid. 2013;23(3):289–93. https://doi.org/10.1089/thy.2012.0171.
44. Ji Hong M, Baek JH, Choi YJ, Lee JH, Lim HK, Shong YK, et al. Radiofrequency ablation is a thyroid function-preserving treatment for patients with bilateral benign thyroid nodules. J Vasc Interv Radiol. 2015;26(1):55–61. https://doi.org/10.1016/j.jvir.2014.09.015.
45. Garberoglio R, Aliberti C, Appetecchia M, Attard M, Boccuzzi G, Boraso F, et al. Radiofrequency ablation for thyroid nodules: which indications? The first Italian opinion statement. J Ultrasound. 2015;18(4):423–30. https://doi.org/10.1007/s40477-015-0169-y.
46. Cesareo R, Palermo A, Benvenuto D, Cella E, Pasqualini V, Bernardi S, et al. Efficacy of radiofrequency ablation in autonomous functioning thyroid nodules. A systematic review and meta-analysis. Rev Endocr Metab Disord. 2019;20(1):37–44. https://doi.org/10.1007/s11154-019-09487-y.
47. Cesareo R, Palermo A, Pasqualini V, Manfrini S, Trimboli P, Stacul F, et al. Radiofrequency ablation on autonomously functioning thyroid nodules: a critical appraisal and review of the literature. Front Endocrinol. 2020;11:317. https://doi.org/10.3389/fendo.2020.00317.
48. Lee ES, Kim JH, Na DG, Paeng JC, Min HS, Choi SH, et al. Hyperfunction thyroid nodules: their risk for becoming or being associated with thyroid cancers. Korean J Radiol. 2013;14(4):643–52. https://doi.org/10.3348/kjr.2013.14.4.643.
49. Lau LW, Ghaznavi S, Frolkis AD, Stephenson A, Robertson HL, Rabi DM, et al. Malignancy risk of hyperfunctioning thyroid nodules compared with non-toxic nodules: systematic review and a meta-analysis. Thyroid Res. 2021;14(1):3. https://doi.org/10.1186/s13044-021-00094-1.
50. Sandrock D, Olbricht T, Emrich D, Benker G, Reinwein D. Long-term follow-up in patients with

autonomous thyroid adenoma. Acta Endocrinol. 1993;128(1):51–5. https://doi.org/10.1530/acta.0.1280051.
51. Cesareo R, Naciu AM, Iozzino M, Pasqualini V, Simeoni C, Casini A, et al. Nodule size as predictive factor of efficacy of radiofrequency ablation in treating autonomously functioning thyroid nodules. Int J Hyperth. 2018;34(5):617–23. https://doi.org/10.1080/02656736.2018.1430868.
52. Tufano RP, Pace-Asciak P, Russell JO, Suárez C, Randolph GW, López F, et al. Update of radiofrequency ablation for treating benign and malignant thyroid nodules. The future is now. Front Endocrinol. 2021;12:698689. https://doi.org/10.3389/fendo.2021.698689.
53. Grønlund MP, Jensen JS, Hahn CH, Grønhøj C, von Buchwald C. Risk factors for recurrence of follicular thyroid cancer: a systematic review. Thyroid. 2021;31(10):1523–30. https://doi.org/10.1089/thy.2020.0921.
54. Mauri G, Hegedüs L, Bandula S, Suárez C, Randolph GW, López F, et al. European thyroid association and cardiovascular and interventional radiological Society of Europe 2021 clinical practice guideline for the use of minimally invasive treatments in malignant thyroid lesions. Eur Thyroid J. 2021;10(3):185–97. https://doi.org/10.1159/000516469.
55. Lim HK, Cho SJ, Baek JH, Lee KD, Son CW, Son JM, et al. US-guided radiofrequency ablation for low-risk papillary thyroid microcarcinoma: efficacy and safety in a large population. Korean J Radiol. 2019;20(12):1653–61. https://doi.org/10.3348/kjr.2019.0192.
56. Yan L, Lan Y, Xiao J, Lin L, Jiang B, Luo Y. Long-term outcomes of radiofrequency ablation for unifocal low-risk papillary thyroid microcarcinoma: a large cohort study of 414 patients. Eur Radiol. 2021;31(2):685–94. https://doi.org/10.1007/s00330-020-07128-6.
57. Yan L, Zhang M, Song Q, Luo Y. Ultrasound-guided radiofrequency ablation versus thyroid lobectomy for low-risk papillary thyroid microcarcinoma: a propensity-matched cohort study of 884 patients. Thyroid. 2021;31(11):1662–72. https://doi.org/10.1089/thy.2021.0100.
58. Cho SJ, Baek SM, Lim HK, Lee KD, Son JM, Baek JH. Long-term follow-up results of ultrasound-guided radiofrequency ablation for low-risk papillary thyroid microcarcinoma: more than 5-year follow-up for 84 tumors. Thyroid Off J Am Thyroid Assoc. 2020;30(12):1745–51. https://doi.org/10.1089/thy.2020.0106.
59. Baek JH, Kim YS, Sung JY, Choi H, Lee JH. Locoregional control of metastatic well-differentiated thyroid cancer by ultrasound-guided radiofrequency ablation. AJR Am J Roentgenol. 2011;197(2):W331–6. https://doi.org/10.2214/AJR.10.5345.
60. Guenette JP, Monchik JM, Dupuy DE. Image-guided ablation of postsurgical locoregional recurrence of biopsy-proven well-differentiated thyroid carcinoma. J Vasc Interv Radiol JVIR. 2013;24(5):672–9. https://doi.org/10.1016/j.jvir.2013.02.001.
61. Kim JH, Yoo WS, Park YJ, Park DJ, Yun TJ, Choi SH, et al. Efficacy and safety of radiofrequency ablation for treatment of locally recurrent thyroid cancers smaller than 2 cm. Radiology. 2015;276(3):909–18. https://doi.org/10.1148/radiol.15140079.
62. Lee SJ, Jung SL, Kim BS, Ahn KJ, Choi HS, Lim DJ, et al. Radiofrequency ablation to treat loco-regional recurrence of well-differentiated thyroid carcinoma. Korean J Radiol. 2014;15(6):817–26. https://doi.org/10.3348/kjr.2014.15.6.817.
63. Chen WC, Chou CK, Chang YH, Chiang PL, Lim LS, Chi SY, et al. Efficacy of radiofrequency ablation for metastatic papillary thyroid cancer with and without initial biochemical complete status. Front Endocrinol. 2022;13:933931. https://doi.org/10.3389/fendo.2022.933931.
64. Zhang X, Ni T, Zhang W. Ultrasonography-guided thermal ablation for cervical lymph node metastasis of recurrent papillary thyroid carcinoma: is it superior to surgical resection? Front Endocrinol. 2022;13:907195. https://doi.org/10.3389/fendo.2022.907195.
65. Choi Y, Jung SL. Efficacy and safety of thermal ablation techniques for the treatment of primary papillary thyroid microcarcinoma: a systematic review and meta-analysis. Thyroid. 2020;30(5):720–31. https://doi.org/10.1089/thy.2019.0707.
66. Cho SJ, Baek SM, Na DG, Lee KD, Shong YK, Baek JH. Five-year follow-up results of thermal ablation for low-risk papillary thyroid microcarcinomas: systematic review and meta-analysis. Eur Radiol. 2021;31(9):6446–56. https://doi.org/10.1007/s00330-021-07808-x.
67. Zhang M, Tufano RP, Russell JO, Zhang Y, Zhang Y, Qiao Z, et al. Ultrasound-guided radiofrequency ablation versus surgery for low-risk papillary thyroid microcarcinoma: results of over 5 years' follow-up. Thyroid. 2020;30(3):408–17. https://doi.org/10.1089/thy.2019.0147.
68. Ding M, Tang X, Cui D, Chi J, Shi Y, Wang T, et al. Clinical outcomes of ultrasound-guided radiofrequency ablation for the treatment of primary papillary thyroid microcarcinoma. Clin Radiol. 2019;74(9):712–7. https://doi.org/10.1016/j.crad.2019.05.012.
69. Zhang M, Luo Y, Zhang Y, Tang J. Efficacy and safety of ultrasound-guided radiofrequency ablation for treating low-risk papillary thyroid microcarcinoma: a prospective study. Thyroid. 2016;26(11):1581–7. https://doi.org/10.1089/thy.2015.0471.
70. Chung SR, Baek JH, Choi YJ, Lee JH. Thermal ablation for the Management of Papillary Thyroid Microcarcinoma in the era of active surveillance and Hemithyroidectomy. Curr Oncol Rep. 2022;24(8):1045–52. https://doi.org/10.1007/s11912-022-01268-2.

71. Kim JH, Baek JH, Sung JY, Min HS, Kim KW, Hah JH, et al. Radiofrequency ablation of low-risk small papillary thyroidcarcinoma: preliminary results for patients ineligible for surgery. Int J Hyperth. 2017;33(2):212–9. https://doi.org/10.1080/02656736.2016.1230893.
72. Papini E, Guglielmi R, Gharib H, Misischi I, Graziano F, Chianelli M, et al. Ultrasound-guided laser ablation of incidental papillary thyroid microcarcinoma: a potential therapeutic approach in patients at surgical risk. Thyroid. 2011;21(8):917–20. https://doi.org/10.1089/thy.2010.0447.
73. Zhang L, Zhou W, Zhan W, Peng Y, Jiang S, Xu S. Percutaneous laser ablation of Unifocal papillary thyroid microcarcinoma: utility of conventional ultrasound and contrast-enhanced ultrasound in assessing local therapeutic response. World J Surg. 2018;42(8):2476–84. https://doi.org/10.1007/s00268-018-4500-6.
74. Yue W, Wang S, Yu S, Wang B. Ultrasound-guided percutaneous microwave ablation of solitary T1N0M0 papillary thyroid microcarcinoma: initial experience. Int J Hyperth. 2014;30(2):150–7. https://doi.org/10.3109/02656736.2014.885590.
75. Teng DK, Li WH, Du JR, Wang H, Yang DY, Wu XL. Effects of microwave ablation on papillary thyroid microcarcinoma: a five-year follow-up report. Thyroid. 2020;30(12):1752–8. https://doi.org/10.1089/thy.2020.0049.
76. Xiao J, Zhang Y, Zhang M, Lan Y, Yan L, Luo Y, et al. Ultrasonography-guided radiofrequency ablation vs. surgery for the treatment of solitary T1bN0M0 papillary thyroid carcinoma: a comparative study. Clin Endocrinol. 2021;94(4):684–91. https://doi.org/10.1111/cen.14361.
77. Cao XJ, Wang SR, Che Y, Liu J, Cong ZB, He JF, et al. Efficacy and safety of thermal ablation for treatment of solitary T1N0M0 papillary thyroid carcinoma: a multicenter retrospective study. Radiology. 2021;300(1):209–16. https://doi.org/10.1148/radiol.2021202735.
78. He H, Wu R, Zhao J, Song Q, Zhang Y, Luo Y. Ultrasound-guided radiofrequency ablation versus surgical resection for the treatment of T1bN0M0 papillary thyroid carcinoma in different age groups. Front Endocrinol. 2021;12:734432. https://doi.org/10.3389/fendo.2021.734432.
79. Yan L, Li Y, Li XY, Xiao J, Tang J, Luo Y. Clinical outcomes of ultrasound-guided radiofrequency ablation for solitary T1N0M0 papillary thyroid carcinoma: a retrospective study with more than 5 years of follow-up. Cancer. 2023;129(16):2469–78. https://doi.org/10.1002/cncr.34802.
80. Baloch ZW, Fleisher S, LiVolsi VA, Gupta PK. Diagnosis of "follicular neoplasm": a gray zone in thyroid fine-needle aspiration cytology. Diagn Cytopathol. 2002;26(1):41–4. https://doi.org/10.1002/dc.10043.
81. Tong MY, Li HS, Che Y. Recurrent medullary thyroid carcinoma treated with percutaneous ultrasound-guided radiofrequency ablation: a case report. World J Clin Cases. 2021;9(4):864–70. https://doi.org/10.12998/wjcc.v9.i4.864.
82. Biamonte E, Solbiati L, Ierace T, Colombo P, Lavezzi E, Mazziotti G, et al. Medullary thyroid carcinoma treated with percutaneous ultrasound-guided radiofrequency ablation. Endocrine. 2019;65(3):515–9. https://doi.org/10.1007/s12020-019-01995-w.
83. Jeong SY, Baek JH, Choi YJ, Chung SR, Sung TY, Kim WG, et al. Radiofrequency ablation of primary thyroid carcinoma: efficacy according to the types of thyroid carcinoma. Int J Hyperth. 2018;34(5):611–6. https://doi.org/10.1080/02656736.2018.1427288.
84. Dupuy DE, Monchik JM, Decrea C, Pisharodi L. Radiofrequency ablation of regional recurrence from well-differentiated thyroid malignancy. Surgery. 2001;130(6):971–7. https://doi.org/10.1067/msy.2001.118708.
85. Lim HK, Baek JH, Lee JH, Kim WB, Kim TY, Shong YK, et al. Efficacy and safety of radiofrequency ablation for treating locoregional recurrence from papillary thyroid cancer. Eur Radiol. 2015;25(1):163–70. https://doi.org/10.1007/s00330-014-3405-5.
86. Tang W, Tang X, Jiang D, Zhang X, Wang R, Niu X, et al. Safety and efficacy of thermal ablation for cervical metastatic lymph nodes in papillary thyroid carcinoma: a systematic review and meta-analysis. Front Endocrinol. 2022;13:967044. https://doi.org/10.3389/fendo.2022.967044.
87. Park KW, Shin JH, Han BK, Ko EY, Chung JH. Inoperable symptomatic recurrent thyroid cancers: preliminary result of radiofrequency ablation. Ann Surg Oncol. 2011;18(9):2564–8. https://doi.org/10.1245/s10434-011-1619-1.
88. Alexander EK, Doherty GM, Barletta JA. Management of thyroid nodules. Lancet Diabetes Endocrinol. 2022;10(7):540–8. https://doi.org/10.1016/S2213-8587(22)00139-5.
89. Kobaly K, Kim CS, Mandel SJ. Contemporary Management of Thyroid Nodules. Annu Rev Med. 2022;73:517–28. https://doi.org/10.1146/annurev-med-042220-015032.
90. Bernet VJ, Chindris AM. Update on the evaluation of thyroid nodules. J Nucl Med Off Publ Soc Nucl Med. 2021;62(Suppl 2):13S–9S. https://doi.org/10.2967/jnumed.120.246025.
91. Russell MD, Shonka DC, Noel J, Karcioglu AS, Ahmed AH, Angelos P, et al. Preoperative evaluation of thyroid cancer—a review of current best practices. Endocr Pract. 2023;29(10):811–21. https://doi.org/10.1016/j.eprac.2023.05.009.

9 Vital Structures Protection

Catherine F. Sinclair and Jose Higino Steck

9.1 General Safety Principles for Vital Structures Protection

9.1.1 Pre-procedural Counseling and Consent

The thyroid gland sits in a crowded and complex area of the neck, surrounded by multiple critical structures including the trachea, esophagus, laryngeal nerves, and carotid sheath (Fig. 9.1).

As such, although ablative procedures are widely touted as "safer" than comparative surgical procedures, in actuality the inability to directly visualize some (particularly neural) structures during these procedures pose unique challenges. Extensive counseling of procedural risks prior to a patient electing to proceed with ablation is critical for facilitating a strong patient-proceduralist relationship, ensuring the patient is able to comply with peri-procedural safety protocols, and addressing and correcting unrealistic outcome expectations [1–4]. Pre-procedural ultrasound assessment of nodule structure and location weighs heavily into this counseling process by identifying disease factors that may increase a given risk of visceral or neurovascular injury. Some examples of situations where adequate and specific counseling regarding vital structures may be particularly important include:

- Nodules abutting the posterior or lateral thyroid capsule. These nodules are almost invariably adjacent to one or more vital structure, including the recurrent laryngeal nerves, a medially placed vagus nerve and/or the esophagus. Although use of lower power and careful applicator positioning adjacent to these structures is essential to minimize injury, such safety strategies can lead to potential undertreatment of the area and increased likelihood of regrowth.
- Isthmic nodules due to their proximity to tracheal cartilages.
- Large retrosternal goiters where the possibility of requiring repeat procedures is high and the associated risks to retrosternal vital structures (subclavian vessels, trachea, esophagus) may be elevated.
- Patients who have had prior neck surgery, where scar tissue may distort normal anatomy and cause vital structures to lie in unexpected locations.

Patients who have had prior neck surgery and/or who have pre-existing dysphonia should undergo laryngeal assessment prior to ablation

C. F. Sinclair (✉)
Department of Surgery, Monash University, Melbourne, VIC, Australia

Icahn School of Medicine at Mount Sinai, New York, NY, USA
e-mail: catherine@melbournethyroidsurgery.com.au

J. H. Steck
Campinas State University, Sao Paulo, Brazil

R. Valcavi et al. (eds.), *Thyroid Ablation*, https://doi.org/10.1007/978-3-031-88229-6_9

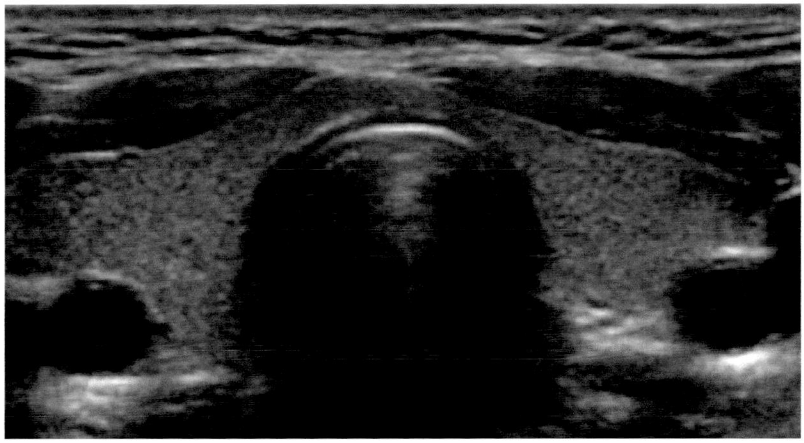

Fig. 9.1 Axial neck ultrasound image showing proximity of the thyroid gland to surrounding vital structures. *CCA* common carotid artery; *ESO* esophagus; *SM* strap musculature; *SCM* sternomastoid muscle

[1–8]. Similarly, patients planned for bilateral ablations need to have their larynx assessed prior to commencing ablation on the second side. Laryngeal assessment can determine whether:

- A patient has a pre-existing vocal fold paralysis on the ipsi- or contralateral side which may indicate the need for further etiologic work-up and/or procedure cancellation.
- A patient has a pre-existing vocal fold hypomobility that may make that nerve more susceptible to peri-procedural injury.
- A patient has sustained a nerve injury causing vocal fold immobility during ablation of the first side in a bilateral ablation—in this case the second side ablation should not be commenced.
- A patient has pre-procedural dysphonia that is unrelated to vocal fold mobility issues. This type of dysphonia should not be significantly altered by ablation but is similarly unlikely to be improved by ablation.

A thorough pre-procedural work-up with appropriate and targeted counseling for patients with identified risk factors for vital structures injury will enhance the patient-proceduralist relationship and ensure patients are fully informed and accepting of the risks discussed.

9.1.2 Peri-procedural Considerations for Vital Structures Protection

Hydrodissecton refers to the use of fluid to lift critical structures off the surface of the ablation target [1–4]. Anteriorly, local anesthetic agents can be used for hydrodissection, where they serve dual roles of analgesia and subcutaneous tissue protection. More laterally near the carotid sheath and posteriorly near the recurrent laryngeal nerves, a non-anesthetic agent is preferred as anesthesia in these areas can cause transient neuropraxia and hoarseness, thus interfering with the ability of the proceduralist to monitor the patient's voice during the ablative procedure. In these areas, a non-conducting fluid such as 5% dextrose is appropriate. Cold fluid is preferable as it also acts to dissipate heat in perithyroidal tissues and thereby lessen peri-procedural patient discomfort.

The trans-isthmic approach and moving-shot technique are two widely described and utilized techniques for optimizing vital structure safety during thyroid ablative procedures. The trans-isthmic approach allows for "buffer zone" anteriorly between the active tip of the applicator and the skin/subcutaneous tissues. This buffer zone enables heat dissipation in the case of inadvertent withdrawal of the proximal active tip outside of the desired ablation zone, thereby preventing injury to superficial neck tissues. The moving-shot technique provides another mechanism for heat dissipation as withdrawal of the applicator in a posterior to anterior or lateral to medial direction prevents an excessive build-up of heat in any one area of the thyroid. This is of particular importance when ablating along the capsule adjacent to nerves, viscera, and vasculature. Choice of electrode active tip size and ablation power are other important parameters to consider when trying to minimize heat transfer out of a given nodule. Generally, the smaller the active tip size and lower the power, the narrower the field of heat transfer. Power can be adjusted during a case such that lower power is utilized in the periphery of a nodule when ablating close to vital structures.

9.1.3 Prerequisite Training

The experience and skill of the operator performing the thyroid RFA plays a significant role in preventing complications to critical structures. Operators should be well-trained in neck ultrasound and familiar with the anatomy of the neck to ensure accurate needle placement and safe energy delivery. Studies have shown that there is a learning curve for RFA. Physicians who preexisting expertise in US and FNA can pass the initial learning phase after performing at least 20–30 cases of thyroid ablation however consolidation and proficiency in these skills, with achievement of consistent results requires upwards of 60 procedures [1, 10, 11].

9.2 Unique Considerations for Individual Vital Structures

9.2.1 Nerves

Anatomic Principles The recurrent laryngeal nerve (RLN) is a branch of the vagus nerve (cranial nerve X) that supplies motor and sensory innervation to the larynx. It takes a recurrent course, giving it its name. The right RLN loops around the right subclavian artery and ascends to the larynx, while the left RLN loops around the aortic arch and ascends in a similar manner, along the tracheoesophageal groove towards the larynx, passing under the inferior constrictor muscle and entering the larynx to innervate the vocal cord muscles.

The sympathetic trunk runs parallel to the cervical spine and is situated posterior to the carotid sheath. It plays a role in controlling functions such as blood pressure and pupil dilation. A sympathetic trunk lesion in the neck causes Horner's syndrome, characterized by:

- Ptosis (drooping of the upper eyelid)
- Miosis (constricted pupil)
- Anhidrosis (lack of sweating) on the affected side of the face

The vagus nerve courses through the neck alongside the carotid sheath. The carotid sheath contains the common carotid artery (CCA) and internal jugular vein (IJV) and the position of the vagus nerve in relation to the vessels is variable. Most commonly, the nerve is located between the CCA and IJV, but it can be located anterior, medial, or posterior to these vessels. The vagus nerve gives rise to multiple branches as it courses through the neck. These branches contribute to a wide range of functions:

- Pharyngeal Branches: Innervate the muscles of the pharynx and contribute to swallowing and speech.
- Superior Laryngeal Nerve: Provides sensory innervation to the larynx and contributes to reflexes like the cough reflex.
- Recurrent Laryngeal Nerve**:** Loops around the aorta on the left side and the subclavian artery on the right side. It innervates the intrinsic muscles of the larynx, controlling vocal cord movement.

Specific Strategies for Preventing Periprocedural Injury Hydrodissection creates a protective barrier around neural structures, thereby mitigating the risk of thermal injury. Cold 5% dextrose is the optimal injection fluid.

Peri-procedurally, the patient can be asked to vocalize intermittently between ablation runs to monitor for voice changes caused by inadvertent heat delivery to the vocal nerves [1–7]. A continuous auditory voice assessment (CAVA) protocol, where the patient is asked to count in a monotonal voice whenever ablation is occurring in nerve danger zones, can also be adopted. *Monotonal* counting prevents significant vertical motion of the axial ultrasound image during vocalization and thus prevents unexpected electrode motion [9]. This protocol can identify voice changes in real time, thereby allowing prompt cessation of ablation if voice change occurs to facilitate rapid nerve recovery.

When ablating nodules in bilateral thyroid lobes, vocal fold mobility on the contralateral side should be assessed via real-time larynx ultrasound or by laryngoscopy if laryngeal ultrasound is not possible. Ablation of the second side must be staged if immobility of the vocal fold on the first side is identified to prevent bilateral vocal cord paralysis and airway compromise [1, 2].

9.2.2 Aerodigestive Structures

Anatomic Principles The thyroid gland is situated in close proximity to the trachea. It wraps around the anterior and lateral aspects of the trachea, with its lobes on either side of the midline. The isthmus of the thyroid gland rests anteriorly over the trachea, just below the cricoid cartilage. The trachea is susceptible to injury during ablation procedures of nodules, especially isthmus nodules. Damage to the trachea can lead to airway compromise, perforation, and other serious complications.

The esophagus is posterior to the thyroid gland and needs to be carefully avoided during ablation procedures. Injury to the esophagus can lead to severe complications including perforation and mediastinitis.

Strategies for Preventing Peri-procedural Injury Precise identification of anatomic landmarks, such as the midline and lateral borders of the thyroid gland, helps in maintaining a safe distance from the trachea and esophagus during ablation. Real-time ultrasound guidance enables visualization of these landmarks to ensure accurate electrode placement. During the procedure, continuous monitoring of the patient's responses, including any changes in voice quality or breathing, can provide early indications of potential damage to nearby structures. Coughing or worsening discomfort can be warning signs of proximity to the trachea.

9.2.3 Vasculature

Anatomic Principles Major vascular structures in the thyroid region include the common carotid artery (CCA), internal jugular vein (IJV), subclavian vessels, and the anterior jugular veins. The CCA sits immediately adjacent to the lateral capsule of the thyroid lobe and can oppose it closely with laterally located nodules. The IJV generally sits lateral and slightly anterior to the CCA and is more at risk during ablation of metastatic nodal disease than during thyroid nodule ablation. Subclavian vessels assume particular importance during ablation of retrosternal goiters, where both the artery and vein can immediately oppose the goiter on its anterior, inferior, or posterior aspect depending on the direction of goiter extension (Fig. 9.2).

Assessment of the subclavian artery is always important even without retrosternal disease as its absence on the right may indicate the presence of a non-recurrent laryngeal nerve. The anterior jugular veins can easily be punctured by the ablation applicator upon insertion through the skin. Bleeding from these veins can be profuse and may not manifest until applicator withdrawal at completion of the procedure, leading to large anterior neck hematomas. Luckily, prolonged direct pressure to the area is usually sufficient to control bleeding if recognized early.

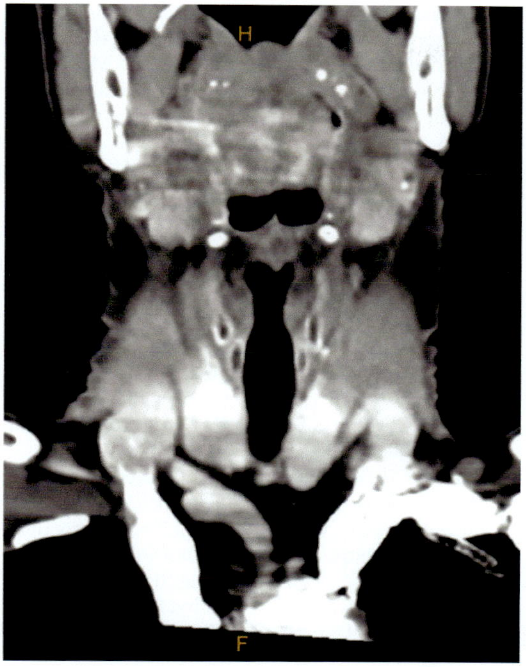

Fig. 9.2 Contrast enhanced coronal CT scan of the neck at mid thyroid level demonstrating the proximity of the subclavian artery and carotid sheath to the thyroid. *CCA* common carotid artery; *IJV* internal jugular vein; *SA* subclavian artery

Specific Strategies for Preventing Peri-procedural Injury Hydrodissection is an important technique for CCA and IJV protection. For the CCA, any transmitted heat is dissipated quickly due to the high blood flow within the vessel. However, lifting the CCA off the lateral thyroid capsule is important not only to protect the artery from injury but also to mitigate patient pain. Pain often radiates to the ipsilateral ear, jaw, or tooth and can be difficult to control unless the artery is moved off the thyroid capsule. Identification and avoidance of the subclavian vessels is the best method to prevent injury—cross-sectional imaging can be helpful in assessing extent and direction of retrosternal goiter extension and the presence of aberrant vascular patterns. Assessment of the location of the right subclavian artery is of particular importance pre-ablation as its absence indicates the presence of a non-recurrent laryngeal nerve on the right side, allowing appropriate procedural precautions to be taken.

9.2.4 Skin and Superficial Tissues

Anatomic Principles The thyroid gland is enveloped by muscles, connective tissues, and skin. The strap musculature (sternohyoid and sternothyroid muscles) covers the lobes directly and, in the case of a large goiter, the sternomastoid muscles can also overly the anterolateral lobe.

Specific Strategies for Preventing Peri-procedural Injury Internally cooled applicators help prevent superficial tissue injury during ablation by preventing heat transfer outside of the active tip region. A trans-isthmic approach also provides a buffer zone to superficial tissue injury. Nodules within the isthmus frequently have a very thin layer of connective tissue separating them from the skin. Hydrodissection anteriorly for these nodules is of particular importance to lift the skin and connective tissues off the anterior surface of the nodule, facilitating a more thorough ablation with lower risk. Use of cold hydrodissection fluid for this purpose acts as a further dissipation measure against thermal injury.

9.3 Conclusion

There are many strategies that can, and should, be utilized to protect the vital structures that are proximate to the thyroid lobes. These strategies range from careful patient selection and pre-procedural work-up, through to peri-procedural techniques. Proceduralists performing ablative procedures must have a sound understanding of these principles and be prepared to alter their technique depending on individual case considerations.

References

1. Sinclair CF, Baek JH, Hands KE, Hodak SP, Huber TC, et al. General principles for the safe performance, training, and adoption of ablation techniques for benign thyroid nodules: an American Thyroid Association statement. Thyroid. 2023;33(10):1150–70. https://doi.org/10.1089/thy.2023.0281.

2. Orloff LA, Noel JE, Stack BC Jr, Russell MD, Angelos P, et al. Radiofrequency ablation and related ultrasound-guided ablation technologies for treatment of benign and malignant thyroid disease: an international multidisciplinary consensus statement of the American Head and Neck Society Endocrine Surgery Section with the Asia Pacific Society of Thyroid Surgery, Associazione Medici Endocrinologi, British Association of Endocrine and Thyroid Surgeons, European Thyroid Association, Italian Society of Endocrine Surgery Units, Korean Society of Thyroid Radiology, Latin American Thyroid Society, and Thyroid Nodules Therapies Association. Head Neck. 2022;44(3):633–60. https://doi.org/10.1002/hed.26960.
3. Cheng KL, Lin WC. Thyroid radiofrequency ablation guideline: the Korean Society of Thyroid Radiology. Korean J Radiol. 2018;19(6):1196–7. https://doi.org/10.3348/kjr.2018.19.6.1196.
4. Baek JH, Lee JH, Valcavi R, Pacella CM, Rhim H, Na DG. Thermal ablation for benign thyroid nodules: radiofrequency and laser. Korean J Radiol. 2011;12(5):525–40. https://doi.org/10.3348/kjr.2011.12.5.525.
5. Shin JH, Baek JH, Ha EJ, Lee JH. Radiofrequency ablation of thyroid nodules: basic principles and clinical application. Int J Endocrinol. 2012;2012:1. https://doi.org/10.1155/2012/919650.
6. Dobnig H, Zechmann W, Hermann M, Lehner M, Heute D, Mirzaei S, et al. Radiofrequency ablation of thyroid nodules: "good clinical practice recommendations" for Austria: an interdisciplinary statement from the following professional associations: Austrian Thyroid Association (ÖSDG), Austrian Society for Nuclear Medicine and Molecular Imaging (OGNMB), Austrian Society for Endocrinology and Metabolism (ÖGES), Surgical Endocrinology Working Group (ACE) of the Austrian Surgical Society (OEGCH). Wien Med Wochenschr. 2020;170:6. https://doi.org/10.1007/s10354-019-0682-2.
7. Baek JH, Lee JH, Sung JY, Bae JI, Kim KT, Sim J, et al. Korean Society of Thyroid Radiology. Complications encountered in the treatment of benign thyroid nodules with US-guided radiofrequency ablation: a multicenter study. Radiology. 2012;262(1):335–42. https://doi.org/10.1148/radiol.11110416.
8. Chung SR, Suh CH, Baek JH, et al. Safety of radiofrequency ablation of benign thyroid nodules and recurrent thyroid cancers: a systematic review and meta-analysis. Int J Hyperth. 2017;33:920. https://doi.org/10.1080/02656736.2017.1337936.
9. Sinclair CF. Early recognition and prevention of voice change during thyroid radiofrequency ablation: continuous auditory voice assessment. VideoEndocrinol. 2024;11:11. https://doi.org/10.1089/ve.2024.0002.
10. Kuo CY, Liu CL, Tsai CH, Cheng SP. Learning curve analysis of radiofrequency ablation for benign thyroid nodules. Int J Hyperth. 2021;38(1):1536–40. https://doi.org/10.1080/02656736.2021.1993358.
11. Bom WJ, Joosten FBM, van Borren MMGJ, Bom EP, van Eekeren RRJP, de Boer H. Radiofrequency ablation for symptomatic, non-functioning, thyroid nodules: a single-center learning curve. Endocr Connect. 2022;11(1):e210304. https://doi.org/10.1530/EC-21-0304.

10 Learning Curve of Thyroid Ablative Procedures

Gilles Russ

10.1 Introduction

Thyroid ablative procedures have encountered growing acceptance in the medical community and by patients. The more numerous practitioners will be to perform these procedures, the more important it will to ensure a homogeneous quality of practice in terms of efficacy and security. This necessarily implies mastering a learning curve. The demonstration of its existence and the way to optimize it are discussed in this chapter. The underlying technical tips and skills are described in other parts of the book.

Supplementary Information The online version contains supplementary material available at https://doi.org/10.1007/978-3-031-88229-6_10.

G. Russ (✉)
Endocrinology Unit, Ospedale Regionale di Lugano, Ente Ospedaliero Cantonale (EOC), Lugano, Switzerland

10.2 The Learning Curve of Thyroid Ablation

10.2.1 Learning Curve of RFA in Other Than Thyroid Organs and of Non-RFA Thyroidal Procedures

A learning curve is a general process of all neuronal activities. They take a particular importance in thyroid RFA as the anatomy of the region is complex and involve numerous vital organs.

The existence of a learning curve has been demonstrated in non-RFA thyroidal procedures.

- In a report on 1067 US-guided fine-needle aspirates (UG-FNA), Fernandes et al. showed that the adequacy rate from adoption into practice improved from 71 to 85% over 300 cases [1]. Moreover, when UG-FNA was subsequently taught to trainees, non-diagnostic rates were higher earlier in training. Interestingly, adequacy was not related to size or palpability, but cystic lesions yielded more inadequate specimens.
- The learning curve of robotic thyroidectomy has been studied by Kim et al. [2]. A total of 172 robotic total thyroidectomies were performed by a single surgeon. Cumulative summation analysis revealed that it took 50 cases for the surgeon to significantly improve the operation time. Mean operation time was significantly shorter after the first 50 cases. On

R. Valcavi et al. (eds.), *Thyroid Ablation*, https://doi.org/10.1007/978-3-031-88229-6_10

the other hand, the surgeon was competent after the 75th case when postoperative transient hypoparathyroidism was used as the outcome measure. The incidence of hypoparathyroidism gradually decreased from 52.0%, for the first 75 cases, to 40.2% after the 76th case. These results indicated that the criteria used to assess proficiency greatly influenced the interpretation of the learning curve. Incorporation of the operation time, complications, and oncologic outcomes should be considered in learning curve assessment.

The learning curve of RFA for organs other than the thyroid gland has also been studied.

- RFA can be used to treat Barrett's esophagus (BE). Pasricha et al. analyzed the effects of the number of patients treated by individual endoscopists and individual centers on safety and efficacy outcomes of RFA [3]. They found that as case experience of endoscopists and centers increased, the numbers of treatment sessions required to achieve complete eradication of Barrett's esophagus (CEIM) decreased. Interestingly, they also showed that center experience was not significantly associated with overall rates of CEIM. It was concluded that the number of sessions needed to achieve CEIM increased with case volume, indicating a learning curve effect. This trend began to disappear after treatment of approximately 30 patients by the center or individual endoscopist. On the other hand, no learning curve was observed with regard to risks of stricture, gastrointestinal bleeding, perforation, or hospitalization.
- A prospective study of the learning curve of RFA for treating pulmonary metastases from colorectal carcinoma was performed in 70 consecutive cases [4]. A comparison between the initial 35 cases (group 1) and the subsequent 35 cases (group 2) was performed. There was a significant decline in the incidence of overall morbidity, pneumothorax, and chest drain requirement in group 2 as compared with group 1. The authors concluded that there was a learning curve for percutaneous lung RFA. With accumulated experience in this procedure, a low morbidity rate could be achieved.
- The learning curve for RFA of liver tumors has been studied in a prospective analysis of initial 100 patients in a tertiary institution [5]. Poon et al. compared the data of the first 50 patients (group I) and the second 50 patients (group II). Group II had significantly shorter hospital stay, lower morbidity rate, and higher complete ablation rate (100% versus 85.7%) than group I. By multivariate analysis, treatment period (group I versus group II) was an independent significant factor affecting the morbidity rate and complete ablation rate. Thus, the authors concluded that there was a significant learning curve in RFA for liver tumors.

Consequently, the study of the literature of RFA of non-thyroidal procedures, thyroid US-FNA, and robotic surgery constantly indicates that there is a learning curve. The figures converge between 30 and 75 cases to acquire proficiency, both in terms of efficiency and security.

10.3 Criteria to Assess the Learning Curve of Thyroid Ablative Procedures

It is an obligation for all practitioners to self-evaluate their efficacy and to assess and understand the complications encountered. This in turn allows to improve one's practice. Knowledge of the criteria used to assess this is useful. More precisely, especially for beginners, practical knowledge on how to correctly obtain these data can be meaningful.

10.3.1 Regarding Efficacy, All Usual Criteria Should Be Taken into Account

- Symptoms, both compressive and esthetic. They should be very precisely described in the report before the procedure, so as to be able to interrogate the patient with the same words that he/she has used to describe them. They can be evaluated by a visual or oral analog scale from 1 to 5 or 1 to 10. They can also be very simply evaluated after the procedure as unchanged, improved, or cured as described by Mauri et al. [6]. They should be compared before and after the treatment and assessed at each follow-up consultation.

- Technical efficacy. Defined as a nodular volume reduction ratio (VRR) >50%. The interest of this criterion is that a volume reduction of 50% is usually sufficient to induce a complete disappearance of pressure symptoms. It can also be of interest to quantify the % of procedures where the VRR is superior to 50%. Once the learning curve is over, the vast majority of the results should be over this value.
- Volume reduction Ratio (VRR). The values obtained should be calculated at each visit. This supposes that a precise calculation is obtained and the intra-observer reproducibility of it assessed by taking two or three consecutive measures. Particular attention should be paid to the measurement of thickness as it can vary between the longitudinal and transverse planes if the nodule is not parallel to the skin. The halo of the nodule should be included in the measurements.
- Ablation Ratio (AR). Identification of the destroyed remaining tissue is a multiparametric evaluation. Using B Mode, this area is usually hypoechoic, more rarely isoechoic. Doppler is mandatory to assert the absence of vascularity, but technical parameters have a great influence. If only color Doppler is available, the gain should be set to the highest level before the signal to noise ratio drops, showing lots of tiny colored dots on the screen. The velocities should be set to 6 cm/s. The most precise evaluation can be acquired through the use of contrast-enhanced US, but unfortunately is not allowed for thyroid assessment in all countries by local authorities (e.g., France). Thus, if available, microvascular (also called super-resolution) Doppler should be used because its sensitivity for the detection of slow blood flows is an undeniable advantage in that situation. Last, the destroyed area shows high stiffness. Strain elastography is of simpler use to delineate the rigid area but shear-wave allows for a quantitative measuring of stiffness in kPa or m/s. Once the volume of the destroyed zone has been calculated as precisely as possible (knowing that its shape and borders are quite frequently irregulars), the ablation ratio can easily be obtained by the following formula:
- AR = 100 × (initial volume − total remaining volume + destroyed volume)/initial volume.
- The literature shows [7] that a satisfactory ablation ratio is longer to acquire than symptoms alleviation or volume reduction ratio are. Aiming at more than 75–85% is recommended.
- Regrowth: The occurrence of it is rare during the first year after ablation and should trigger the possibility of malignancy, which can be the case in 2–3% of treated nodules [8]. Thus, in most cases regrowth is only detected after 3–5 years and will not be a relevant indicator in the early phase of the learning curve, but a late one. Taking note of the smallest volume reached after ablation for a specific nodule (the nadir) is important, so as to compare it with the results during the next follow-up consultations. An increase of more than 50% in volume is considered to be relevant.

10.3.2 Criteria Used to Assess Safety

Exhaustive reporting of all side-effects and minor or major complications is advised for self-evaluation and improvement.

- Minor complications: These can be defined as not life threatening, with no necessity for rehospitalization or permanent sequelae. Thus, should be included in that category:
  - transient voice alterations, sometimes only perceived by the patient: loss of power, raspy voice, change in tone
  - transient drooping eyelid or red conjunctiva

  - minor skin burns (simple erythema)
  - nodular rupture with a favorable outcome
- Pain and procedure completion (pauses, complete interruption): Pain should be evaluated by the patient both by expressing it with his/her usual vocabulary and with an oral or visual analog scale. Moreover, it can be very useful to take note of the number of interruptions of the procedure caused by pain, all the more if it leads to a premature complete interruption of it.
- Major complications: Defined as life threatening, necessitating a rehospitalization or causing permanent sequelae. Severe skin burn, tracheal burn, brachial plexus injury, permanent inferior, and superior laryngeal nerve damages are included in this category.

10.4 Literature Analysis of RFA Thyroid Learning Curve

Russ et al. studied the learning curve of thyroid RFA in the first 90 patients treated by a single operator, in a referral thyroid center [7]. Patients were divided into three groups according to their chronological treatment rank: patients 1–30 (G1), 31–60 (G2), and 61–90 (G3). The operator was a radiologist with more than 20 years of experience in thyroid imaging, fine-needle aspirations, core-needle biopsies, percutaneous ethanol therapy, and had performed 40 laser thyroid ablation procedures before starting RFA. There was no significant difference in nodular median initial volume between the three groups. Median treated volume was 21 mL [3–72 mL].

Regarding efficacy, no significant differences were observed between the three treated groups for pressure symptoms and esthetic complaints reduction. A significant improvement in technical efficacy (TE), VRR, and AR was found between groups 1 and 2, but not between groups 2 and 3. However, in the subgroup of small and medium nodules (< 30 mL), AR did continue to improve between groups 2 and 3. In large nodules, TE only improved between groups 1 and 2, whereas it also improved between groups 1 and 3 in VRR and AR.

Possible explanations were searched. Two factors were independently associated with VRR and AR. Nodular baseline volume was negatively associated with these two criteria and energy delivered per mL positively associated. Time trend correlation showed a significant increase in delivered energy per volume and ablation duration with experience.

All in all, the main result of the study was that no learning curve was demonstrated for clinical efficacy. The satisfactory clinical efficacy observed during the initial phase of the learning curve could be attributed to the fact that a 50% volume reduction is most often sufficient to improve patients' symptoms. TE, VRR, and AR were clearly identified as subjected to a learning curve. However, after 60 patients, improvement only persisted in the latter and for small to medium nodules. Regarding large (>30 mL) nodules, an improvement was observed between groups 3 and 1 in AR and the authors speculated that these nodules could require even a larger experience than 90 cases to learn how to ablate them more completely.

Regarding safety, three minor complications were observed. A transient vocal cord palsy was recorded in patient n°79 (group 3), due to recurrent laryngeal nerve injury. A nodular rupture (patient n°41, group 2) was detected 1 month after RFA. A vaso-vagal reaction forcing to interrupt the procedure was observed in patient no. 73 (group 3).

Kuo et al. studied the learning curve of thyroid RFA of a single operator, an endocrine surgeon, with 5 years of experience in thyroid ultrasound and ultrasound-guided FNA [9]. 102 nodules in 93 patients (82 women and 11 men) were analyzed. The mean baseline nodule volume was 24.7 mL (range, 0.9–98.9). In all, 58 were solid; 18 predominantly solid; 20 predominantly cystic; and six cystic. At 6 months post-RFA, the mean VRR of 102 nodules was 55.9% (range: 23.5–98.8%). Interestingly, sequential case number was not associated with the VRR. The only predictor of the VRR after RFA was nodule composition. As expected, cystic nodules were associated with a higher VRR. However, when calculating the composition-adjusted VRR for each nodule, gradual increase was shown along with the chronological treatment order. In the subgroup of solid nodules, a similar trend of slowly increasing VRR was noted. Two inflection points of the learning curve were identified at the 20th and 65th cases, respectively. Based on the results of the learning curve analysis, all patients were divided into three phases: initial learning phase (case 1–20), technical consolidation phase (case 21–65), and proficiency phase (case 66–102), accompanied by increased volume reduction.

It is interesting to note that the learning curve was associated with the acquisition of technical tips. Longer (10 mm) active tips of RF electrodes and higher power output were used by the operator during the later phase. A significantly longer treatment time in the later phase of the learning curve was spent ablating thyroid nodules.

Regarding complications and regrowth, one patient had a minor complication in the consolidation phase, a transient vocal cord palsy that recovered spontaneously. At 6 months post-RFA, two patients (one in the consolidation phase and the other in the proficiency phase) underwent a second-session RFA for regrowth of thyroid nodules.

Bom et al. performed a retrospective cohort study of the first 103 consecutive patients with symptomatic, benign, predominantly solid nodules receiving RFA treatment in a teaching hospital [10]. RFA was performed by a team consisting of two dedicated radiologists, always acting together during each procedure. The median nodule volume at baseline was 12.0 mL (range 2.0–58.0 mL). Cystic degeneration was present in 18 nodules. The median amount of deposited energy was 6.6 kCal (range 1.5–10.2 kCal) or 0.5 kCal/mL nodule (equivalent to 2093 J/mL). Over time, the applied energy gradually increased from 0.32 to 0.84 kCal/mL.

At baseline, all patients had symptoms, mainly local pressure sensations or difficulty in swallowing. After 12 months, 84 (89%) patients had become asymptomatic. At 6-months follow-up, initially, the results of RFA were poor. Only 9 (45%) of the first 20 patients had a 6-month VRR >50%, and this increased to 15 (75%) of the next 20 patients and then to 50 (79%) of the following 63 subjects. The median 6-month VRR was 56.1% in the first 40 patients, and this rose to 62.7% in the following 63 patients. The degree of volume reduction was related to the applied energy.

Regarding safety, a transient loss of voice occurred in one patient during the RFA procedure. The ablation was stopped immediately, and an ice pack was put on the area of treatment. About 30 min later, the voice was back to normal.

The authors concluded that it takes about 40 RFA procedures before a 6-month VRR of 50% has become a realistic goal in most patients. They also hypothesized that in a teaching setting with experienced instructors to guide novices, the numbers needed to treat to achieve a consistent VRR >50% may be lower.

Dobnig et al. described the 1-year results of RFA in 277 consecutive patients and reported a gradual improvement in VRR with increasing experience [11]. In the first 15 patients, the mean VRRs at 3 and 12 months were 58% and 70%, respectively, and this gradually increased to a plateau value of 70 and 80% when the number of procedures was greater than 45.

In the study by Sung et al. [12], it was shown that RFA of autonomous functioning nodules performed by six radiologists who were trained in thyroid RFA during a program organized by the Korean Society of Thyroid Radiology (KSThR) lead to a final volume reduction of 81.7%. As a multicenter study including five institutions, it validated the concept that RFA performed by well-trained radiologists could provide reproducible results.

Deandrea et al. also published a randomized controlled trial reporting the efficacy of RFA in non-autonomous nodules and comparing the results of two centers [13]. The Korean center (the "more experienced group" in this field) had an experience of about 3000 cases of thyroid RFA; the Italian center (the "less experienced group" in this field) had a significant experience in interventional US-guided therapies (both PEI and thermal ablation by other devices) and had previously treated 50 cases of benign nodules

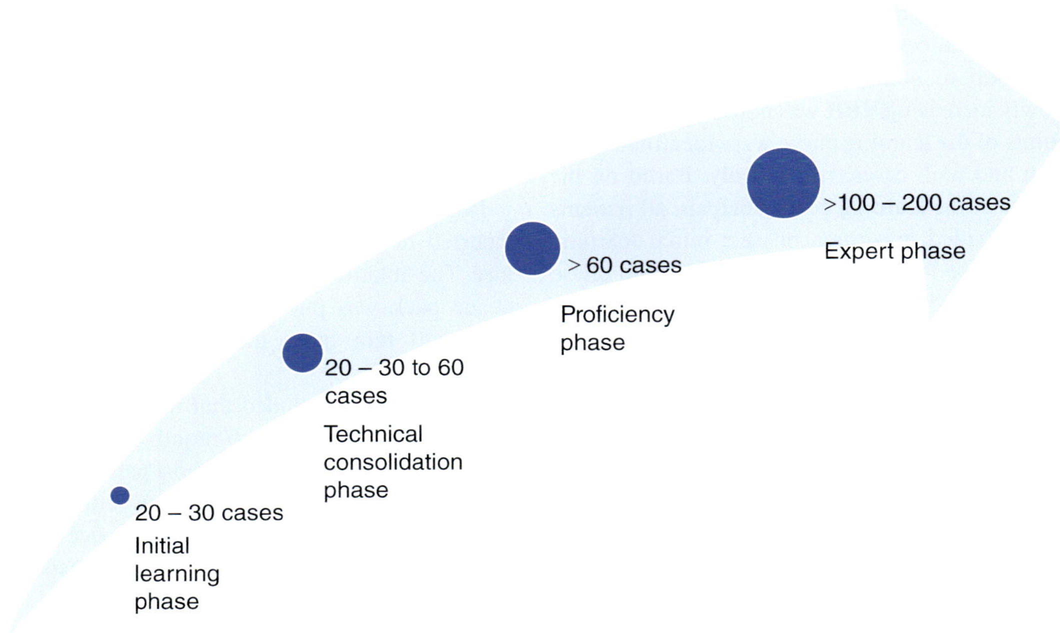

Fig. 10.1 The learning curve of thyroid RFA can be grossly divided into four phases, according to the number of procedures the operator has performed. However, initial training and benefiting from a mentor's experience, as well as individual skills are factors that can very probably reduce this period

with the moving-shot technique, after an initial instruction given by a Korean radiologist. No significant difference in volume reduction was seen at 6-months evaluation between the two groups (Korean group: 77% vs. Italian group: 66%).

Therefore, the analysis of the published literature shows that a learning curve exists for thyroid RFA. Improvement in VRR is acquired during the 40–60 first cases (initial and technical consolidation phases) (Fig. 10.1). Improvement in AR persists during the next 30 cases (proficiency phase), especially for small and medium nodules. However, AR is still imperfect for larger (>30 mL) nodules at this phase and may be even longer to master. All these references show that technical knowledge was developed during these three phases. This included using higher power output, longer active tips, higher energy delivered in J/mL, and distributing the energy to the marginal zone of the nodules with growing operator skills in electrode maneuvering. Thus, it could be speculated that proctoring by a highly trained physician could permit to shorten considerably the learning curve of thyroid RFA.

10.5 How to Begin: Environment and Nodules (Table 10.1)

The first step is to establish a care course. More or less depending on the specialty of the practitioner who performs the ablation, a multidisciplinary approach is always helpful. On the one hand, the aim is to set the care course which will provide with referring selected patients to the operator. On the other hand, the goal is to discuss the best treatment modality, active surveillance, surgery or RFA, between endocrinologists, sur-

Table 10.1 Tips to begin one's activity in thyroid RFA

Establish a care course and work in a multidisciplinary team
Avoid difficult morphotypes
Choose nodules with a likely good response: – small to intermediate sized nodules, less than 20 mL – of mixed composition – with a central vascularity of low to medium intensity
Avoid nodules extending towards the deep part of the neck or the thoracic inlet

geons, and radiologists. Multidisciplinary team meetings, similar to the ones organized in oncology, can be an excellent approach.

The second step is to carefully select the nodules and patients that will be treated during the initial phase of the learning curve of the operator. Regarding patients, it is advised to avoid difficult morphotypes, such as a short, stocky neck, or a morbid obesity. Regarding nodules, a selection of potential good responders is helpful. These would be small to intermediate sized nodules (inferior to 20–30 mL for non-secreting nodules and 10 mL for autonomous ones), of mixed composition (Fig. 10.2a and b), with a central vascularity of low to medium intensity (Fig. 10.3a and b). Avoiding nodules extending towards the deep part of the neck or the thoracic inlet is also advised.

10.6 Prior Knowledge, Training, and Qualifications (Table 10.2)

10.6.1 Local Health Authorities Required Qualifications

Physicians who perform US-guided thyroid RFA should be licensed medical practitioners who have a thorough understanding of the indications

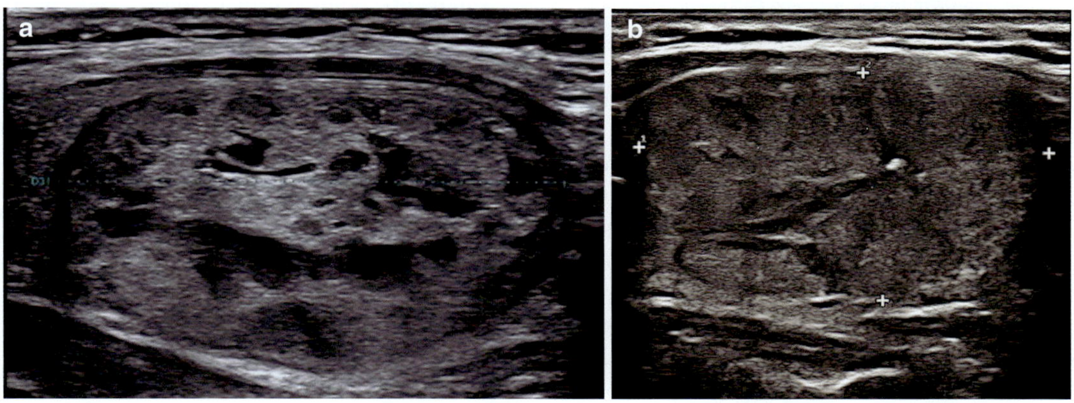

Fig. 10.2 (**a** and **b**) The composition of the nodule should be taken into account when planning the first procedures. Nodules with a mixed composition as the one shown on (**a**) are better responders, easier to ablate, than exclusively solid nodules like the one shown in (**b**)

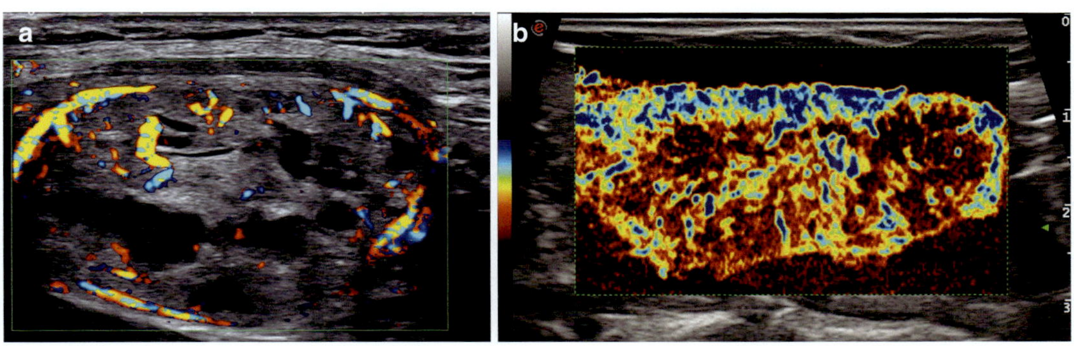

Fig. 10.3 (**a** and **b**) The vascularity of the nodule should be taken into account when planning the first procedures. Nodules with a moderate central vascularity as the one shown in (**a**) are better responders, easier to ablate, than nodules with an intense central vascularity like the one shown in (**b**)

Table 10.2 Advised prerequisites before beginning thyroid RFA

Proficiency in neck and thyroid ultrasound imaging – Identification of thyroid nodules and ability to assess their risk of malignancy using a risk stratification system – Three dimensions and volume nodule measurements with correct intra- and inter-observer reproducibility – Knowledge on thyroid US reporting – Anatomic knowledge of nerves and vessels of the thyroid region – Laryngeal ultrasonography to assess the function of vocal cords in real time. This may help prevent permanent injury to the laryngeal inferior nerve
Proficiency in fine-needle and/or core-needle biopsy of thyroid nodules
Learn how to perform perithyroidal local anesthesia
Practice on phantoms
Attend teaching courses
Attend treatment procedures and participate in patient management

and guidelines for this technique as well as familiarity with its basic physical principles and limitations. They should be familiar with alternative treatments and thyroid diseases and have some knowledge of clinical and biological aspects.

In certain countries, performing RFA could be submitted to legal rules. These rules can apply to the type of medical specialty likely to be allowed to practice RFA, but also to sub-specialty training or diploma such as interventional radiology. Moreover, the setting where RFA takes place and the paramedical staff can also be imposed by law, as could be a minimal number of annual procedures.

10.6.2 Thyroid US

Physicians responsible for thyroid RFA should be able to demonstrate familiarity with the anatomy, physiology, and pathophysiology of the cervical region. Proficiency in imaging anatomy of the neck and in thyroid ultrasound imaging is mandatory. It is difficult to set a valid numeral cut-off on how many thyroid US should have been performed prior to beginning performing thyroid RFA because there is no evidence on the subject. However, the American Institute of Ultrasound in Medicine (AIUM) considers in its training guidelines that an acceptable clinical experience can be documented by demonstrating evidence of being involved with the performance, evaluation, interpretation, and reporting of at least 100 diagnostic thyroid, parathyroid, and neck ultrasound examinations within the previous 36 months [14]. The maintenance of competence is also considered to need performing at least 100 examinations per year.

More specifically, it could be advised to be proficient on the following points:

- Identification of thyroid nodules
- Ability to assess their risk of malignancy using a risk stratification system
- Three dimensions and volume nodule measurements with correct intra- and inter-observer reproducibility (Fig. 10.4a and b)
- Knowledge on thyroid US reporting
- Anatomic knowledge of nerves and vessels of the thyroid region
- Laryngeal ultrasonography to assess the function of vocal cords in real time. This may help prevent permanent injury to the laryngeal inferior nerve [15].

10.6.3 Thyroid FNA and CNB

Learning and mastering thyroid FNA seems legitimate prior to starting thyroid RFA. Indeed, learning to visualize and displace the needle to the desired location by will under US guidance is a very good preliminary to the moving-shot approach currently used for thyroid RFA. This is particularly true as the appearance of bubbles and acoustic shadows, induced by the heating effect of RFA, creates a challenging environment for US guidance. The tip of the electrode can become difficult to identify. Thus, having learned to visualize the tip of the needle used for FNA in several and complex situations will facilitate the identification of the tip of the RF electrode. There again, there is no such evidence-based number of FNA to perform prior to beginning RFA, but the AIUM states that a minimum of 10 ultrasound-guided fine-needle aspirations per year are recommended

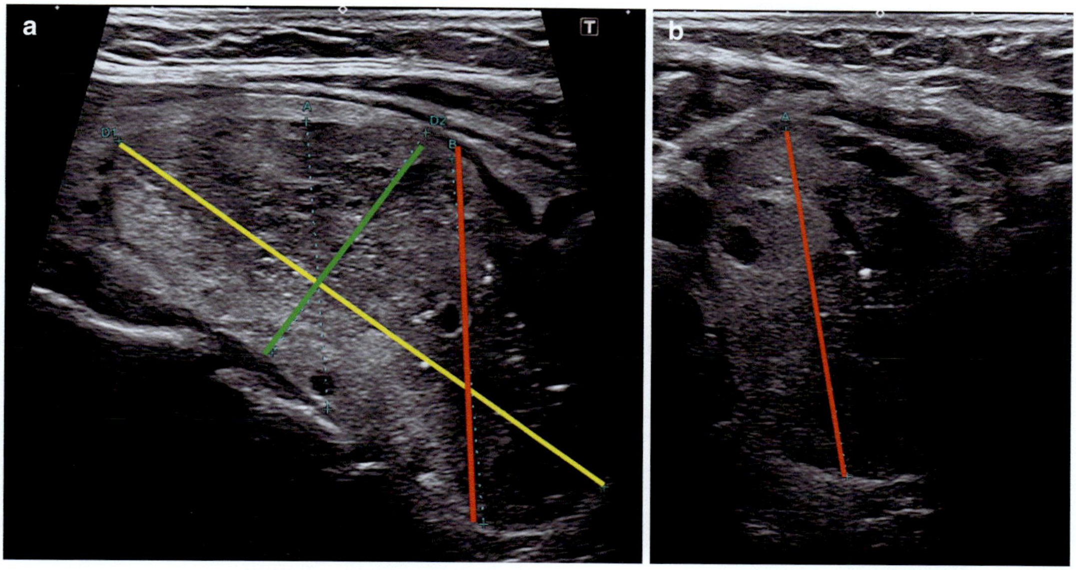

Fig. 10.4 (**a** and **b**) Measures in longitudinal plane (**a**). If the nodule is not parallel to the skin, as the one shown here, care should be taken to measure its thickness in the longitudinal plane. The length is shown in yellow. The proper way to measure the thickness is shown in green. If the thickness is measured on the transverse plane (**b**, in red), it is considerably overestimated, as explained by the projection of this measure on the longitudinal plane (in red also). The volume calculation leads in one case to 69 × 29 × 29 = 30 mL (using the thickness in green) and to 69 × 29 × 39 = 41 mL (using the thickness in red): gross overestimation

to maintain the physician's skills [14]. Using the parallel approach, rather than the perpendicular one during US guidance seems here more logical as it will be the case during RFA.

Thyroid CNB practice can also be very useful. In fact, it is a way to learn how to puncture the thyroid gland through the trans-isthmic approach and to perform a peri-capsular local anesthesia.

10.6.4 Phantoms (Video 10.1)

Li et al. have used a food training model of thyroid RFA [16]. Chicken hearts were simulated into thyroid nodules, three-layer pork meats into peri-thyroid structure, and gel bottles into trachea, respectively. Successful training ablations were defined as chicken hearts that were fully cooked. After repeating training ablations of chicken hearts at least 100 times with a nearly 100% success rate for three young endocrinologists trainees, they served as the first assistant for the real procedures of thyroid RFA and then were qualified to perform thyroid RFA on real patients under the supervision of one experienced interventional radiologist. Twenty-three real patients were then treated with RFA by the three trainees. The median VRR at 12 months was 82%. Two major complications were transient hoarseness, and three minor complications were wound pain. All complications were completely recovered within 3 days. The authors concluded that for young and RFA-naive physicians without any basic skills of ultrasound-guided intervention, this food model of thyroid RFA was useful for medical training and education. A control group with three trainees not having benefited from this food-training model would have been ideal to judge its efficacy.

Other sorts of phantoms have been developed, such as three-dimensional printing ones [17] or less costly ones [18, 19] and could also be used for that purpose.

Thus, the use of practice phantoms could be recommended to treat nodule-like targets that can be excised from the phantom after the session and then examined to assess completeness of ablation with particular attention to the marginal zones. When the operator is able to consistently and thoroughly ablate such targets in phantoms, they then could be considered ready to attempt treatment in patients.

10.7 RFA Teaching Courses

Dedicated thyroid-RFA courses organized at a national or international level by scientific associations or societies are another way to engage in this practice, both for beginners and skilled operators and an occasion to share experience.

10.7.1 Proctoring

Although not evidence-based in thyroid RFA, mentoring obviously is of great value. Humanistic teaching practices are always well received by beginners and help address a gap by building skills in their training. A mentorship program should ideally be implemented in high-volume centers and visiting these encouraged.

10.8 Participating in Patient Management

The selection of patients to be treated with RFA is often medically complex and therefore requires both comprehensive pre-treatment evaluation and post-treatment follow-up. It can be advised:

- to attend pre-procedural consultations, to understand how to select patients for RFA, but also how to deliver the best information on the benefit and risks compared with surveillance and surgery
- to attend multiple procedures performed by skilled operators
- to participate in the follow-up of treated patients.

10.9 Self-Assessment

This takes a very important place in the learning curve, as it is a tool to improve more rapidly. It is very useful when beginning thyroid RFA to follow the patients early after the treatment, in terms of volume reduction ratio and ablation ratio. More precisely, evaluating these parameters a few weeks after each initial treatment will lead to a shortened understanding on how to improve. Numerous pictures of the pre- and immediate post-procedural aspects of the treated nodules should be taken and then be compared with what is seen during follow-up. This in turn allows to integrate the subtle differences of echogenicity that should be looked for at the end of the procedure, especially at the margins of the nodules, to achieve complete ablation.

10.10 Conclusion

A learning curve clearly exists for thyroid RFA. Its duration is of course dependent on the previous expertise of the operator in thyroid US and thyroid FNA. However, it can probably be shortened if proper steps are systematically taken. These include knowledge of the criteria used to assess efficacy and safety, learning thyroid US and guided procedures, practicing on phantoms whenever possible, attending specialized courses and being mentored. If all these conditions are gathered, safe and quick procedural mastering can be expected.

References

1. Fernandes VT, Magarey MJ, Kamdar DP, Freeman JL. Surgeon performed ultrasound-guided fine-needle aspirates of the thyroid: 1067 biopsies and learning curve in a teaching center. Head Neck. 2016;38(Suppl 1):E1281–4. https://doi.org/10.1002/hed.24212.
2. Kim H, Kwon H, Lim W, Moon BI, Paik NS. Quantitative assessment of the learning curve for robotic thyroid surgery. J Clin Med. 2019;8(3):402. https://doi.org/10.3390/jcm8030402.

3. Pasricha S, Cotton C, Hathorn KE, Li N, Bulsiewicz WJ, Wolf WA, et al. Effects of the learning curve on efficacy of radiofrequency ablation for Barrett's esophagus. Gastroenterology. 2015;149(4):890–6.e2. https://doi.org/10.1053/j.gastro.2015.06.012.
4. Yan TD, King J, Sjarif A, Glenn D, Steinke K, Morris DL. Learning curve for percutaneous radiofrequency ablation of pulmonary metastases from colorectal carcinoma: a prospective study of 70 consecutive cases. Ann Surg Oncol. 2006;13(12):1588–95. https://doi.org/10.1245/s10434-006-9010-3.
5. Poon RT, Ng KK, Lam CM, Ai V, Yuen J, Fan ST, et al. Learning curve for radiofrequency ablation of liver tumors: prospective analysis of initial 100 patients in a tertiary institution. Ann Surg. 2004;239(4):441–9. https://doi.org/10.1097/01.sla.0000118565.21298.0a.
6. Mauri G, Pacella CM, Papini E, Solbiati L, Goldberg SN, Ahmed M, et al. Image-guided thyroid ablation: proposal for standardization of terminology and reporting criteria. Thyroid. 2019;29(5):611–8. https://doi.org/10.1089/thy.2018.0604.
7. Russ G, Ben Hamou A, Poirée S, Ghander C, Ménégaux F, Leenhardt L, et al. Learning curve for radiofrequency ablation of benign thyroid nodules. Int J Hyperth. 2021;38(1):55–64. https://doi.org/10.1080/02656736.2021.1871974.
8. Bernardi S, Giudici F, Cesareo R, Antonelli G, Cavallaro M, Deandrea M, et al. Five-year results of radiofrequency and laser ablation of benign thyroid nodules: a multicenter study from the Italian minimally invasive treatments of the thyroid group. Thyroid. 2020;30(12):1759–70. https://doi.org/10.1089/thy.2020.0202.
9. Kuo CY, Liu CL, Tsai CH, Cheng SP. Learning curve analysis of radiofrequency ablation for benign thyroid nodules. Int J Hyperth. 2021;38(1):1536–40. https://doi.org/10.1080/02656736.2021.1993358.
10. Bom WJ, Joosten FBM, van Borren MMGJ, Bom EP, van Eekeren RRJP, et al. Radiofrequency ablation for symptomatic, non-functioning, thyroid nodules: a single-center learning curve. Endocr Connect. 2022;11(1):e210304. https://doi.org/10.1530/EC-21-0304.
11. Dobnig H, Amrein K. Monopolar radiofrequency ablation of thyroid nodules: a prospective Austrian single-center study. Thyroid. 2018;28(4):472–80. https://doi.org/10.1089/thy.2017.0547.
12. Sung JY, Baek JH, Jung SL, Kim JH, Kim KS, Lee D, et al. Radiofrequency ablation for autonomously functioning thyroid nodules: a multicenter study. Thyroid. 2015;25(1):112–7. https://doi.org/10.1089/thy.2014.0100.
13. Deandrea M, Sung JY, Limone P, Mormile A, Garino F, Ragazzoni F, et al. Efficacy and safety of radiofrequency ablation versus observation for nonfunctioning benign thyroid nodules: a randomized controlled international collaborative trial. Thyroid. 2015;25(8):890–6. https://doi.org/10.1089/thy.2015.0133. Epub 2015 Jul 13
14. AIUM Training Guidelines for Physicians Who Evaluate and Interpret Diagnostic Thyroid, Parathyroid, and Neck Ultrasound Examinations. https://www.aium.org/resources/ptGuidelines.aspx
15. Fung MMH, Lang BHH. Using intra-operative laryngeal ultrasonography as a real-time tool in assessing vocal cord function during radiofrequency ablation of the thyroid gland. World J Surg. 2022;46(9):2206–11. https://doi.org/10.1007/s00268-022-06596-9.
16. Li YR, Chou WY, Chan WK, Cheng KL, Sun JH, Liu FH, et al. Successful applications of food-assisted and -simulated training model of thyroid radiofrequency ablation. Front Endocrinol (Lausanne). 2022;13:809835. https://doi.org/10.3389/fendo.2022.809835.
17. Baba M, Matsumoto K, Shindo H, Matsumoto M, Otsubo R, Tanaka A, et al. Development and evaluation of an original phantom model of ultrasonography-guided thyroid gland biopsy for the training of surgical residents and students. Surg Today. 2023;53(4):443–50. https://doi.org/10.1007/s00595-022-02582-9.
18. Schwartz CM, Ivancic RJ, McDermott SM, Bahner DP. Designing a low-cost thyroid ultrasound phantom for medical student education. Ultrasound Med Biol. 2020;46(6):1545–50. https://doi.org/10.1016/j.ultrasmedbio.2020.01.033.
19. Hakimi AA, Armstrong WB. Improving on the do-it-yourself ultrasound-guided fine-needle aspiration simulation phantom. J Ultrasound Med. 2021;40(4):815–9. https://doi.org/10.1002/jum.15461.

11 Percutaneous Ethanol Injection (PEI) and Radiofrequency Ablation of Thyroid Cysts and Cystic Thyroid Nodules

Devaprabu Abraham and Nikita R. Abraham

11.1 Introduction

Thyroid nodules and cysts are common conditions seen in 30–70% of the general population [1]. Cranial, neck and chest imaging fortuitously identify these subclinical tumors, evoking further evaluations. Although several nodule risk-assessment systems (RSS) have shaped biopsy, management, and follow-up recommendations for nodules with suspicious features, there is no clear consensus for the optimal management of benign nodules or cysts [2]. Larger size, cosmetic concerns, and the development of compression symptoms are the commonly used indications for intervention. About 10–20% are large enough to cause compression symptoms. Many of the cystic thyroid nodules result from spontaneous degeneration of solid nodules, which constitutes about 10% of the nodules. Larger cysts (>4 cm) are less common in the general population [3]. Percutaneous interventions such as percutaneous ethanol injection (PEI) and radiofrequency ablation (RFA) have gained popularity, which are reviewed in this chapter.

Supplementary Information The online version contains supplementary material available at https://doi.org/10.1007/978-3-031-88229-6_11.

D. Abraham (✉)
Division of Endocrinology, Department of Internal Medicine, University of Utah Health, Salt Lake City, UT, USA
e-mail: dev.Abraham@hsc.utah.edu

N. R. Abraham
Molecular Medicine Program (U2M2), Office of Research Integrity and Compliance, University of Utah, Salt Lake City, UT, USA
e-mail: nikita.abraham@hsc.utah.edu

11.2 Practice Patterns and Worldwide Differences in the Management of Thyroid Nodules and Cysts

Surgical removal is the primary therapeutic modality utilized for the treatment of thyroid nodules and cysts in the USA. Although surgery is definitive with no risk of recurrence, it is associated with anesthetic, intra- and postoperative risks [4]. The complication rates vary significantly with the procedure volume of the surgeon and the centers performing these procedures [2]. Some patients are averse to surgery because of the ensuing scar or loss of thyroid function. Non-surgical interventions such as PEI and RFA have gained popularity over the past 30 years in Europe and Asia. The growing worldwide popularity of PEI and RFA is due to the avoidance of a visible scar, conservation of thyroid function, outpatient procedure, cost containment, and short recuperation times [5]. The ATA guidelines recommend surgical removal or PEI for recurrent benign cystic nodules as weak recommendation and low-quality evidence (recommendation 28) [2]. The Korean and European guidelines endorse PEI and

R. Valcavi et al. (eds.), *Thyroid Ablation*, https://doi.org/10.1007/978-3-031-88229-6_11

RFA for the treatment of cystic thyroid nodules [6, 7]. Despite the proven efficacy of PEI, a recent European survey of 860 physicians in 40 countries revealed that PEI was conducted only by 22.1% of the respondents [8]. Although the effectiveness is established, the procedural training, individual learning curve, certification standards, national guidelines, and provider acceptance are quite variable across the health care systems in different countries.

11.3 Sonographic Anatomy of the Neck Relevant to PEI and RFA Procedures

A thorough understanding of the anatomic orientation of critical neck structures in relation to the target for ablation is the cornerstone to the successful percutaneous intervention and eliminating complications [9]. The at-risk areas are the following (Fig. 11.1):

1. The external jugular veins are located within the subcutaneous planes lateral to the thyroid gland. These veins are variable in size and location. There are branches of the external jugular veins that course medially. The most prominent is the anterior jugular vein, a branch of the external jugular vein. These veins are susceptible to injury during intervention.
2. The posteromedial aspect of the thyroid gland contains the esophagus, larynx, and trachea. The recurrent laryngeal nerves (RLN) course along the length of the thyroid gland medially within the trachea-esophageal grooves.
3. The vagus nerve, the common carotid artery, the internal jugular vein, and the sympathetic trunk are the laterally located structures, which are susceptible to injury. The cervical portion of the vagus nerve is commonly located posterolateral (80% of the subjects) to the common carotid artery within the carotid sheath. It is important to anticipate and identify mass effectinduced distortion of normal anatomy by large nodules and cysts (Video 11.1). A pre-procedure identification of critical structures is important for reducing the risk of complications.

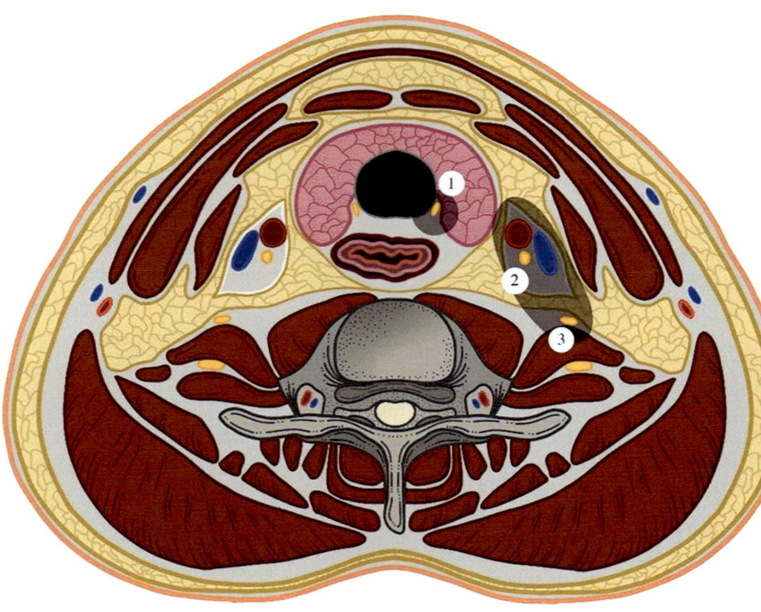

Fig. 11.1 Cross section anatomy of neck cadaver reconstruction: (1) Recurrent laryngeal nerve, esophagus and trachea, (2) Vagus, carotid artery and internal jugular vein, (3) Sympathetic ganglia

11.4 Embryological and Histological Aspects of Congenital and Acquired Neck Cysts

11.4.1 Congenital Cysts of the Neck

Congenital cysts are common at birth that include cysts of the thyroglossal duct, lymphoceles, and branchial cleft cysts. It is typical for congenital cysts to have an epithelial lining (Video 11.1). Thyroglossal duct cysts (TDC) are remnants of the embryological tract seen in 7–10% of general population and 25% of these cysts contain ectopic thyroid rests. Thyroglossal duct cysts manifest in children and young adults as asymptomatic swellings. They are less common in adults and may present with recurrent infection. The midline or just left of midline location of the cyst that moves with sticking out of the tongue is an important clinical clue indicating its attachment to the base of the tongue. The majority of these cysts are located below the hyoid bone and above the thyroid cartilage. Less commonly, they are located above the hyoid bone, base of the tongue, and very rarely located caudal to the thyroid gland. The prevalence of malignancy originating from thyroid rests within the TDC is approximately 1% [10]. In a series of 160 cases of TDC, there was a slight male preponderance, 70% reported history of recurrent infections, and 20% develop cutaneous fistula. Only one case of thyroid cancer was observed [11]. In another study, concomitant differentiated thyroid cancer was observed within the thyroid gland in about 60% of the subjects and 50% were multifocal [12]. Percutaneous ethanol injection of TGDC is an effective alternative to surgery [13] (Video 11.1).

11.4.2 Acquired Cysts of the Neck

The acquired cysts of the neck include thyroid cysts, postoperative cysts, chylous cysts (following thoracic duct injury), and cystic degeneration of metastatic malignant lymph nodes. The color of the aspirate can provide clues to the etiology of the cyst (Video 11.1). Acquired cysts are classified as either true cysts (chronic cysts with epithelial lining) or pseudocysts. Pseudo-cysts develop acutely following spontaneous hemorrhagic degeneration of solid nodules and are devoid of epithelial lining. Both benign and malignant thyroid nodules undergo acute hemorrhagic degeneration. Therefore, all cystic nodules should undergo ultrasound-guided (USG) aspiration and subjected to cytological analysis [3].

11.4.3 Thyroid Cysts and Cystic Thyroid Nodules

Although thyroid nodules are very common, only about 15–25% of the nodules are simple cysts or cystic thyroid nodules. Larger cysts (>4 cm) are less common and often yield insufficient or non-diagnostic cytology [3]. Malignancy is less common in cystic nodules compared to solid nodules [1, 3]. The majority of benign thyroid cysts and nodules are asymptomatic. About 15% of the solid nodules show progressive growth. Growth of benign nodules is common in younger (<45 years) subjects [14]. Complex cystic thyroid nodules are likely devoid of epithelial lining; especially those that develop acutely following cystic degeneration of solid thyroid nodules. These cysts respond well to simple aspiration with low chance of recurrence. The epithelialization of a cyst may play a role in the recurrence versus remission following aspiration alone. The introduction of a sclerosant such as 95% ethanol likely destroys this cellular lining, promoting adhesion leading to eventual obliteration of the cyst space. Partial recurrences result from incomplete obliteration of the cystic space. To date no study has evaluated the cyst histology for the presence or absence of epithelial lining and the risk of recurrence following aspiration or PEI.

11.5 Imaging Phenotypes of Cysts Based on the Architecture and Composition

Cystic degeneration within the thyroid nodules is not uniform and can assume one of the following patterns [15]:

1. Simple cyst. These cysts are thin-walled, uniloculated, with uniformly smooth walls, containing colloid of variable consistency. They often give rise to “snow globe” effect if the contents are thin with suspended particulates. The aspirate is usually straw colored (Fig. 11.2). Parathyroid cysts often mimic thyroid cysts.
2. Cysts with mural solid mass. These mural masses can be eccentric or concentric (Fig. 11.3).
3. Multiloculated cysts with or without solid masses which may contain vascular septa (Fig. 11.4).
4. Thick-walled cyst. These cysts often are either thick walled or develop a thick wall as the contents are aspirated. Therefore, this is a finding observed during or immediately fol-

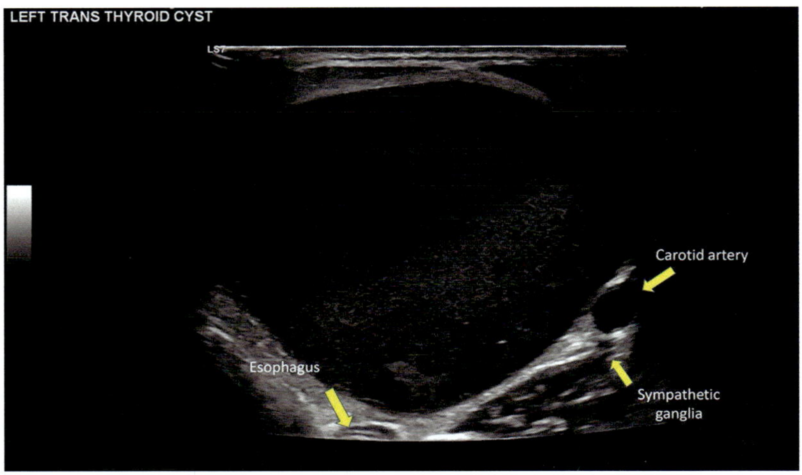

Fig. 11.2 Simple cyst with thin walls

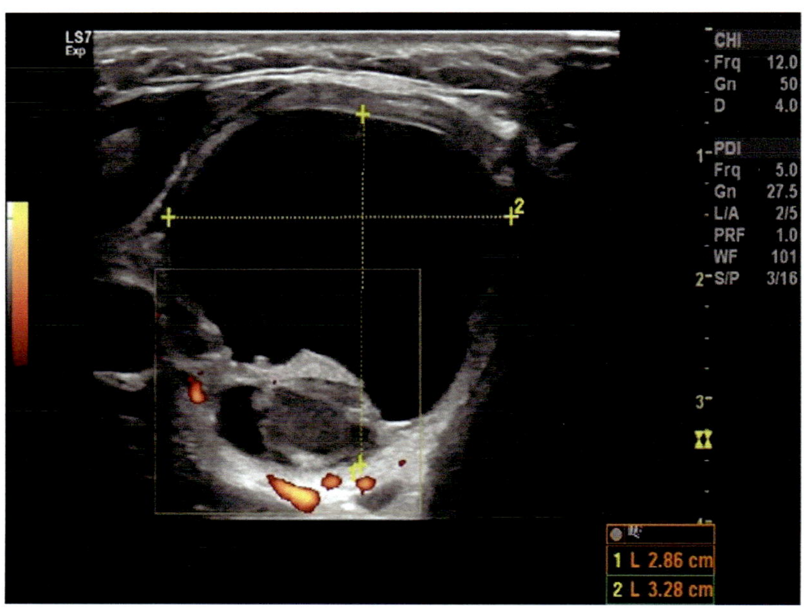

Fig. 11.3 Cyst with eccentric mural mass

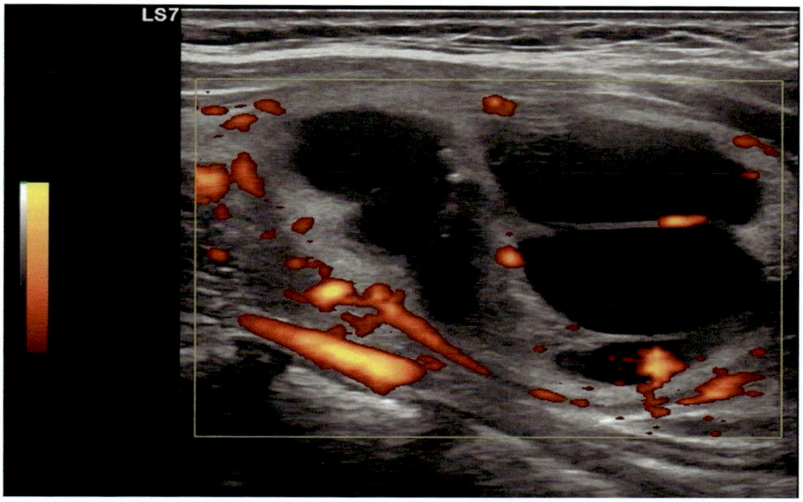

Fig. 11.4 Multiloculated cyst with vascular septum

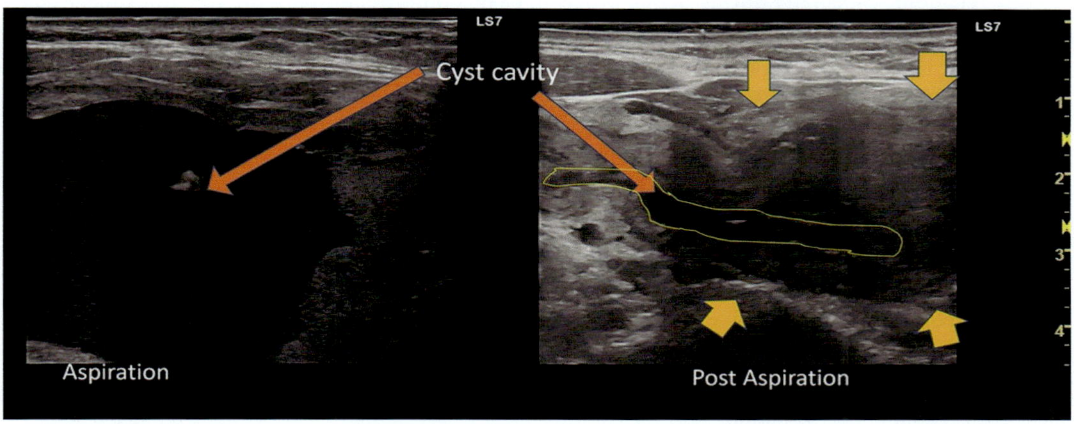

Fig. 11.5 Thick-walled cyst, concentric mural mass

lowing the aspiration of the fluid cyst content. The walls are vascular and are difficult to treat with PEI alone and may require additional RFA (Fig. 11.5).

11.6 Types of Sclerosing Agents

Over the past three decades, several organic and inorganic compounds were used to induce sclerosis of cysts and nodules. These agents include ethanol, talc, hydrochloric acid, inactivated bacteria, bleomycin, and tetracycline [16]. The most commonly used agent is 95% or greater purity of ethanol. The first reported use of ethanol as a sclerosing agent was by Rozman in 1989 [17]. A recent study used polidocanol, with results comparable to high purity ethanol. Polidocanol has anesthetic effects, therefore was associated with lesser pain [18]. Polidocanol is an alkyl polyglycol ether of lauryl alcohol with sclerosing, anesthetic, and potential antineoplastic properties. Following the intra-lesional administration, polidocanol (similar to ethanol) induces endothelial cell injury by disrupting calcium and nitric oxide pathways in the endothelium. This is followed by endothelial damage, platelets, and fibrin clot formation occluding the vessel [19]. Polidocanol is a relatively expensive compared to alcohol [18]. Therefore, for practical purposes, high purity ethanol is the preferred go-to agent for thyroid cyst ablation.

11.7 Anesthesia and Sedation for PEI and RFA

The routine use of infiltration anesthesia may not be necessary for FNA using 25 or 27 g needles with fewer (1–2) passes [20]. However, for chemical or thermal ablative therapies, lidocaine infiltration is required for optimal pain control. Some patients may require intravenous or oral sedation. US-guided infiltration of lidocaine up to and including the capsule using fine needles (30–25 G) is preferred. The most common practice is to administer lidocaine 1% in all patients not allergic to lidocaine. Patients report past history of tachycardia associated with lidocaine and epinephrine-mixed preparations as allergic reactions, especially during dental procedures. A detailed history avoids unnecessary withholding of 1% plain lidocaine in these patients. Some interventionists do not use any form of anesthesia for PEI. Monzani et al. used 20–22 g needles for treating autonomously functioning nodules without sedation or infiltration anesthesia. The authors reported that most patients complained of pain for 30–60 min following the procedure [21]. The administration of local anesthesia calms patients with the assurance that efforts are taken to curb the anticipated procedure-related pain. It reduces pain considerably with proper peri-capsular administration under guidance. This is particularly important when larger bore needles (22–14 G) are used for aspiration of thick cyst contents, for conducting core biopsy and during RFA. The administration of deep sedation or general anesthesia delays the recognition of recurrent laryngeal nerve injury and the application of rescue procedures. Oral pre-procedure administration of benzodiazepines reduces anxiety without causing sedation.

11.8 Percutaneous Ethanol Injection

Procedure and techniques involved in PEI of cystic thyroid nodule:

The general principles that apply to any percutaneous procedure including pre-procedure patient counseling, consenting, site identification, adherence to meticulous asepsis, and the administration of local anesthesia also apply to PEI. Even prior to the infiltration of local anesthesia, a detailed explanation and the anticipated sequence of the procedure in a reassuring manner can improve procedural success and patient tolerance. Allowing patients to speak normally or swallow during the procedure does not adversely affect the procedure. Detailed pre-procedure neck mapping of blood vessels and a mental "stock-taking" of the typical location of vital structures is very important to avoid complications (Fig. 11.1). The anterior jugular vein and other smaller branches of the external jugular veins course anterior to the thyroid gland. Due to easy compressibility with the transducer, they may go unnoticed during the introduction of the needle or electrode. Accidental injury of these smaller veins can cause nuisance bleeding during the entire intervention, even requiring premature termination of the procedure. It is good practice to relieve pressure on the transducer and map these veins before needle entry to avoid injury.

11.8.1 Efficacy and Outcomes of PEI for Thyroid Cysts and Cystic Nodules

Simple aspiration was first reported in 1966 by Crile [22]. The first use of ethanol for sclerosing recurrent thyroid cysts was reported by Rozman in 1989 [17]. Percutaneous ethanol injection is the most effective method to treat recurrent simple and complex thyroid cysts [5, 23–26]. A double blind controlled study by Bennedbaek et al. revealed alcohol to be superior to the inert saline injections. PEI resulted in 100% cyst volume reduction. It is notable to mention that the saline injections performed in the placebo arm resulted in 68% volume reduction despite being an inert substance [23]. Valcavi and Frasoldati reported a randomized study of 281 patients receiving simple aspiration vs PEI. A remarkable 86% cyst volume reduction was seen in the PEI group vs 7% in the aspiration-only group [27]. Zingrillo et al. used a fixed volume of alcohol injection,

2 mL of ethanol for cysts smaller than 20 mL cyst volume, 3 mL for 20–30 mL cysts, and 4 mL for larger cysts and reported good out comes [28, 29]. Suh et al. injected 50% of aspirated cyst volume but also removed the cyst content after 2–5 min of contact time with subsequent re-aspiration. The recurrence rate was 38.3%, 18.7% recurrence within 1 month, and 24.1% had delayed recurrences [30]. Re-aspiration of residual ethanol and cyst fluid content versus allowing natural absorption was addressed by Kim et al. Thirty patients in two groups were treated with removal of the cyst content after PEI vs allowing retention and gradual absorption with 93.3 and 96.7% effectiveness, respectively. Although there was no statistical difference between the groups, the procedure time for the re-aspiration group was much longer [15]. The main goal of PEI is to effectively aspirate the content completely without injuring the posterior or lateral wall of the cyst capsule and introduce alcohol prior to withdrawing the needle. The avoidance of bleeding within the cyst in turn improves the successfulness of PEI. Once bleeding occurs, the cyst can rapidly fill with blood until spontaneous tamponade ensues. Injecting alcohol under pressure increases the risk of leak of alcohol outside the thyroid capsule. If bleeding occurs it is best to avoid injection under pressure into a tensely cystic nodule. Complete aspiration of blood is often unsuccessful due to clotting, spontaneous liquefaction occurs over several days or weeks. Kim et al. compared the efficacy of PEI for cystic vs predominantly cystic nodules along with an analysis of factors that predict recurrence. Of the 217 nodules analyzed, the large and vascular, predominantly cystic nodules responded less well to PEI as compared to purely cystic nodules [31]. Del Prete et al. observed that out of the 98 cystic nodules with a mean volume of 35.3 mL almost all responded to PEI with very few recurrences at 9 years follow-up visit. Out of the 92 responders, only six subjects relapsed [32]. One factor reported as a predictor of success during PEI is the retention of alcohol within the cystic nodule. Rapid spontaneous clearance of alcohol by arterioles and draining veins are implicated in recurrence. The persistence of intra-nodular echo staining following PEI predicts a favorable outcome [6, 33].

11.8.2 Technical Aspects of PEI and Procedural Considerations

The goals of PEI is to reduce the risk of procedure induced intra-cystic bleeding and the extravasation of alcohol. One is to aspirate slowly with continuous on-screen monitoring of the needle tip and the other is to reposition the needle to avoid injury to the posterior capsule of the cyst. Extravasation of alcohol is prevented by inserting the needle through the isthmus (trans-isthmic approach). The cuff of isthmic thyroid tissue prevents extra-thyroidal leak upon withdrawal of the needle (Fig. 11.6). The other is to use the Z-track technique (Fig. 11.7). The Z-track method is adapted from the practice to prevent leak back of medication following intramuscular injections. The skin and the subcutaneous tissue are pulled before entry with the needle. Following aspiration and injection, the removal of the needle results in "spring back" of the tissue forming a natural "Z-track" [34]. In our experience, practicing either one of these two approaches reduces the risk of alcohol extravasation. It suffices to say that using the smallest bore needle to achieve complete emptying of the cyst content and

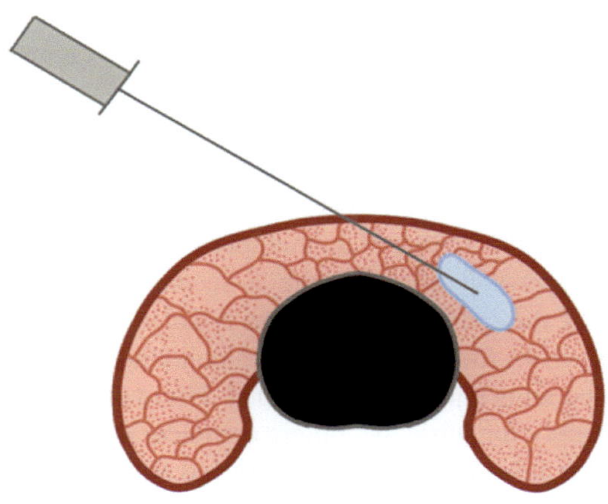

Fig. 11.6 Trans-isthmic needle insertion

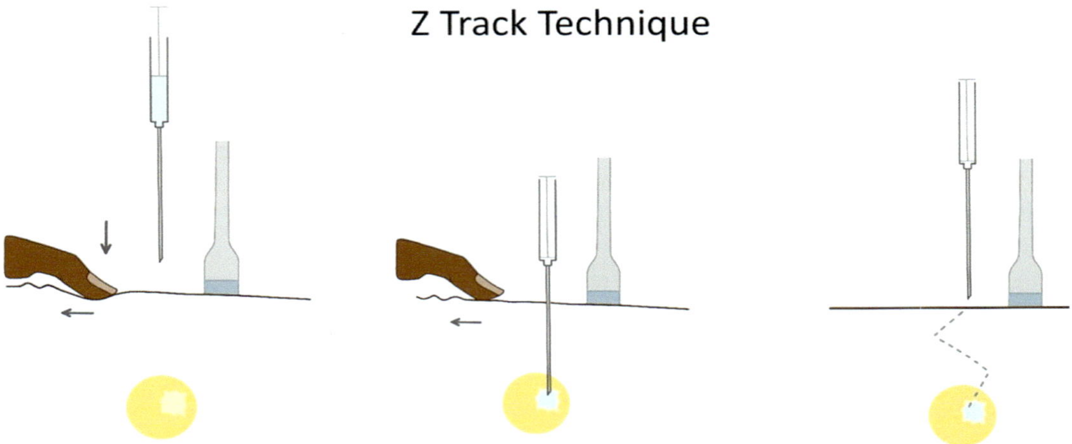

Fig. 11.7 Z-track technique

injection of alcohol also reduces risk of extravasation.

If the nodule contains vascular mural mass or vascular walls, taking care to avoid puncture or using soft-tip intravenous cannula can reduce risk of bleeding due to injury of the posterior wall. Fine bore cannulas (<18 G) tend to kink. Some cannulas are not sufficiently echogenic and therefore are difficult to visualize. Great care needs to be taken to avoid displacement of tip of the cannula or the needle tip from the cavity during the injection [15].

The ideal nodule for optimal outcomes to PEI is a pure or simple cyst, cysts with contents that can be aspirated easily using smaller gauge needles (20 G or smaller). Cystic nodules that collapse easily with floppy capsule respond well to PEI (Fig. 11.8). Those with vascular mural masses, thick-walled cyst or those cysts that appear to "re-form" a remnant nodule following aspiration respond less well to PEI [15]. Those cysts that contain very thick contents may be impossible to completely empty even with 14 G needles and often require a second procedure once the content becomes less viscid several days or weeks following the initial alcohol injection. If alcohol is injected into the thick viscid content to liquefy for subsequent more complete aspiration, then the volume should be reduced appropriately to reduce the risk of extravasation. Injecting alcohol into a tensely cystic nodule under pressure can lead to alcohol extravasation.

The typical volume of alcohol injection is variable and is dependent upon the completeness of aspiration and the absence of mural component. In general, 30–50% of the aspirated cysts content is replaced with 95% alcohol. If bleeding occurs during the procedure, it is very difficult to control it by direct pressure. Spontaneous tamponade usually results in most cases. Alcohol injection under pressure into tensely cystic recently bled nodule increases the risk of extravasation. A flow schematic for management of cystic nodules is described in Fig. 11.9.

11.8.3 PEI of Solid Benign Nodules and Toxic Adenomas

Thyroxine administration for preventing growth of benign thyroid nodule is no longer an accepted practice due to lack of efficacy and risks of iatrogenic hyperthyroidism [35, 36]. Alcohol injection is a cost-effective percutaneous therapy for benign thyroid nodules and toxic thyroid adenomas. It is particularly useful as an alternative therapy when a patient does not desire radioactive iodine or surgical intervention or if surgery is considered high risk due to comorbidities [6]. The availability of radiofrequency ablation holds

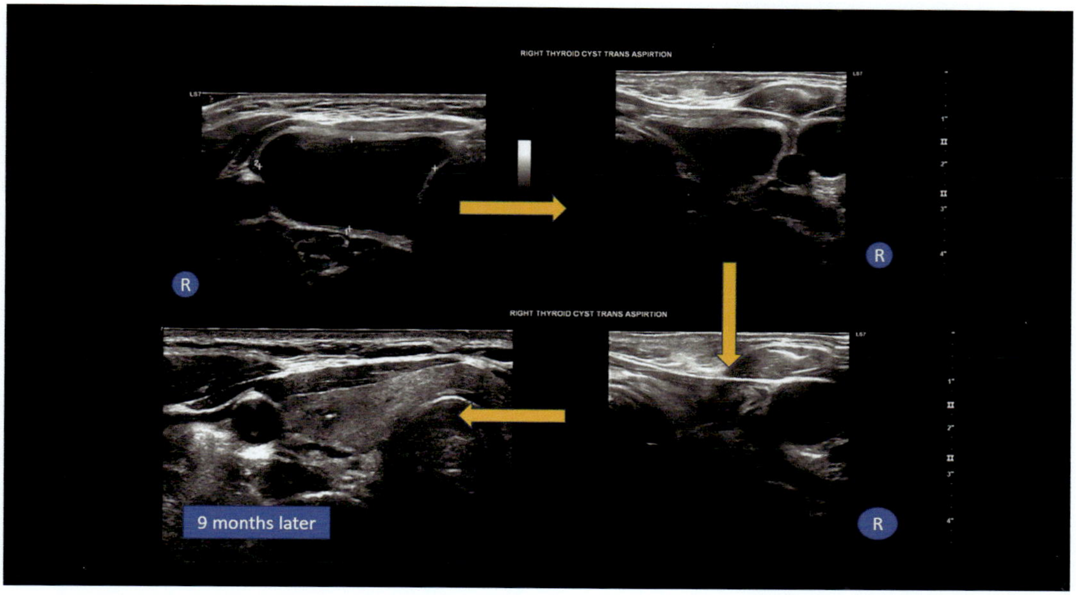

Fig. 11.8 Simple cyst with post PEI structural modification

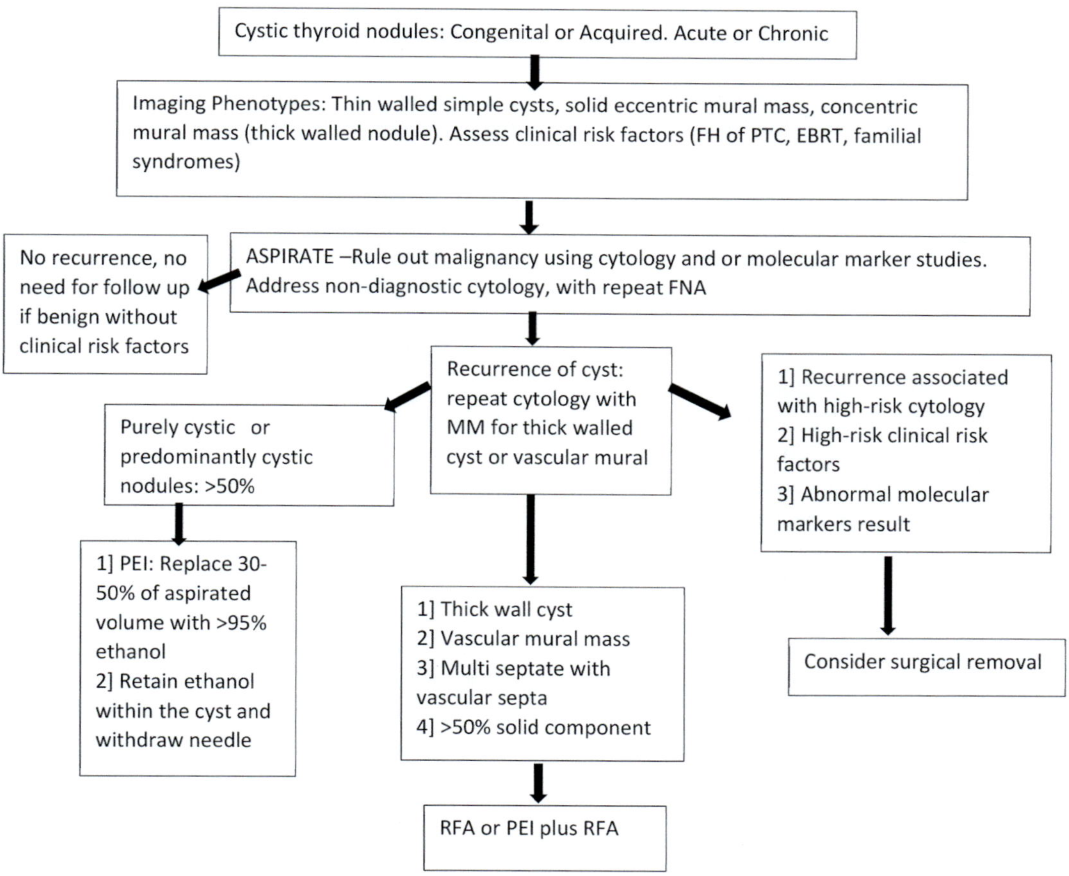

Fig. 11.9 Schematic flow chart for the evaluation and management of cystic thyroid nodules

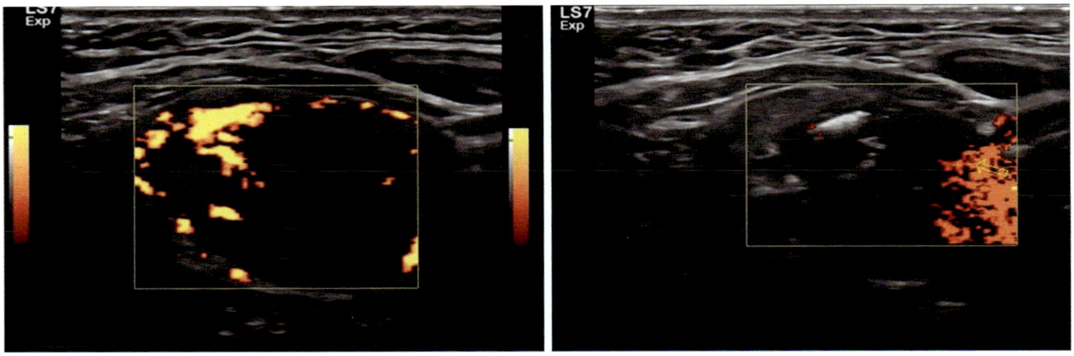

Fig. 11.10 Vascularity targeting of toxic adenoma

promise although limited head-to-head comparison studies between the two modalities have been conducted [7]. Alcohol ablation for solid nodules is relatively cumbersome compared to radiofrequency ablation due to multiple injections that are required over several sittings. However, it is cost-effective compared to RAI, surgery, and RFA, with very little equipment requirements. Earlier studies administered larger volume of alcohol injected into different parts of the nodules with variable results [37–39]. Vascularity targeting during PEI is an effective refinement of this procedure. Detailed power Doppler interrogation (PDI) is conducted on the entire nodule, and the vascularity of the nodule is mapped accurately. The procedure involves insertion of a 27 or 25 G needle attached to a preloaded 1–2 mL syringe with 95% ethanol, using a Z-track technique as close or into the largest blood vessel inside the capsule of the thyroid nodule. Toggling between power Doppler and B-mode will enable accurate placement of the needle close to or into the vasculature. Once satisfied with the positioning of the needle, alcohol is slowly injected under ultrasound guidance. A successful vascularity-targeted injection results in perfusion of alcohol into the blood vessel and will give the appearance of an arteriogram of the nodule. Vascular coagulation results in the instant development of echo staining within the intranodular vessels (Fig. 11.10) [40, 41]. The disappearance of blood flow by PDI predicts successful obliteration of vessels. Reestablishment of blood flow after transient reduction of flow usually occurs because of vascular spasm. Immediate reinjection improves outcomes if blood flow spontaneously resumes within 5–10 min after the initial injections. Vascular toxic adenomas can have multiple feeding vessels and may need careful injection into different blood vessels even in the same sitting. Intra-nodular edema and the appearance of echogenic areas and related acute coagulative changes associated with reduced blood flow by PDI (Fig. 11.10). Intra-nodular echo staining with absence of blood flow portends good outcome. Injecting the posterior aspects of the nodule first will avoid difficulty in visualizing the needle tip if anterior areas are injected first due to the development of echogenic coagulation zone [41]. Similarly, a caudal to cranial approach of injection may be applicable depending upon the positioning of the patient in relation to the operator, standing at the head end vs the respective sides of the patient.

11.8.4 PEI and RFA Combination Therapies for Complex Cystic Thyroid Nodules

Percutaneous ethanol injection combined with other modalities such as RFA, microwave ablation, laser ablation for the treatment of partially cystic nodules is necessary for optimal volume reduction in nodules refractory to PEI. Administering multiple modalities during the same sitting of therapeutic intervention can be technically challenging. Most percutaneous interventions can be tedious from the patient's perspective. Limited number of studies combining PEI and RFA or PEI and microwave therapy performed simultaneously appears safe and effective [33, 42, 43]. In one study, the three main factors that resulted in reduced efficacy of PEI/RFA for the treatment of complex cystic nodules includes the inability to aspirate thick gummy colloid, intra-cystic bleeding during the procedure and thick-walled nodules despite the aspiration of the cyst contents [44]. A different randomized clinical study by the same group compared the efficacy of RFA vs PE for predominantly cystic nodules. The volume reduction ratio (VRR) of the two groups, (RFA $n = 25$ and PEI 25) was comparable without evidence for superiority of RFA. The PEI cohort nodules were larger, yet the volume reduction was comparable (RFA VRR was 87% and PEI VRR 83%). The symptom improvement, cosmetic scores, and complication rates were comparable [33].

Combination treatment with RFA and PEI for predominantly cystic nodules (>50% cyst) has been well studied in small cohorts by Dr. Baek's group [33, 43–45]. The two possible combination or sequential treatment approaches are described below. One approach is to perform PEI for nodules with >50% cyst component initially and subsequently treat the solid portion with RFA. The other is to aspirate the cyst during a single session RFA and ablate the cyst cavity. The appearance of microbubbles within the collapsed cyst cavity indicates successful ablation.

Intra-cystic bleeding occurs because of injury to vascularized septa, mural masses, or the thick vascularized walls as the needle or electrode traverses the cyst cavity. Acute bleeding from the solid component can negate the efficacy of the procedures [44, 45]. Once bleeding occurs during the introduction of the electrode, it is virtually impossible to aspirate the clotted blood or apply pressure to arrest the bleeding. The bleeding vessel may be amenable to RAF with Doppler interrogation if the source of bleeding early during the procedure. Saline washing out of the cavity is often unsuccessful following acute procedure induced bleeding. One approach is to avoid entry into cyst cavity during RFA. Often times the solid component, which requires RFA is located distal to the cystic space in relation to the trans-isthmic entry of the electrode. Nodules with cystic component of <30% rarely require PEI. For nodules with larger cystic component (>50%), an alternate approach is to perform PEI a few weeks prior to conducting RFA to the solid portions. This approach provides an opportunity for the blood vessels on the walls of the cyst to sclerose prior to the RFA. In most patients, the cyst either completely disappears or it recurs partially. A partially recurred cyst is more manageable due to reduction of the original volume prior to the PEI. The predominantly cystic nodules are a heterogeneous group of nodules exhibiting different imaging phenotypes that responds variably to the different modalities of intervention. Therefore, not only patient selection is key, but also matching the modality of the treatment to the nodule phenotype is crucial for treatment success. In addition, the response to PEI and RFA can be variable among cystic nodules, often requiring multiple sequential interventions. A proper patient education regarding the need for multiple interventions reduces patient disappointment.

11.8.5 PEI of Thyroid Cancer Metastatic Lymphadenopathy

Micrometastasis (<2 mm) in cervical lymph nodes is seen in up to 90% of differentiated PTC patients with prophylactic neck dissection or by performing sensitive genetic analysis on the FNA specimens [46, 47]. Despite appropriate neck dissection during the initial thyroid surgery, intractable residual thyroid cancer metastasis and recurrence are common within the cervical lymph nodes. Reoperation of regional lymphadenopathy is associated with escalating surgical risks and does not guarantee durable remission [48]. The risk of injury to the recurrent laryngeal nerves (RLN) is relatively low with the initial surgery particularly in experienced hands [4]. In a large retrospective series of 1026 patients, the incidence of permanent RLN palsy was 1.1% for lobectomy and 4% for total thyroidectomy, the overall risk is about 1.8% [49]. The risk of recurrent laryngeal nerve injury with reoperation is as high as 10–20% [50]. Re-dissection of the central compartments also increases the risk of temporary and permanent hypoparathyroidism [51]. A sizable proportion of central and lateral compartment recurrences are stable or progress very slowly without imminent negative consequences. Therefore, watchful waiting is an option for most patients. In a study by Robenshtok et al., the vast majority (78%) of 166 patients with low-risk DTC remained stable without progression [52]. The 2015 ATA guidelines include watchful waiting as a management strategy [2]. However, patient acceptance of watchful waiting strategy is often low in practice. Percutaneous interventions such as PEI or RFA are acceptable alternative low-risk option.

11.8.6 The Procedure of PEI for Lymph Node Metastasis

The technique is similar to that of solid thyroid nodules. Smaller volumes of alcohol, as little as 0.1–0.25 cc may be sufficient depending upon the size of the metastatic lymph node. The posterior and caudal aspects of the nodule are injected initially. This optimizes the continuous visualization of the needle tip. Patients often described pain during injection particularly of lymph nodes likely due to capsular stretching. Slower injection reduces pain. Disappearance of vascularity predicts successful ablation [53].

11.8.6.1 Efficacy of PEI for Cervical Metastatic Differentiated Thyroid Cancer

The Mayo Clinic study by Lewis, 29 metastatic lymph nodes in 14 patients were treated with US-guided PEI. All treated lymph nodes decreased in mean volume from 492 mm^3 to 76 mm^3 after 12 months following the procedure. Lidocaine 1% infiltration was used in all patients and a few patients also received i.v. midazolam sedation. No complications were encountered. During the follow-up, 4 new lymph nodes were identified which were also treated with PEI [53].

Heilo et al. reported their outcomes on 69 patients in 2011. A total of 109 lymph nodes in 69 patients were ablated. Three patients were reassigned to surgery during the follow-up for disease progression. A total of 101 of the 109 lymph nodes responded to PEI (84%). The authors conclude that PEI is a safe alternative to surgical berry-picking following initial surgery [54].

A systematic and pooled analysis conducted in 2015 revealed the following findings. One thousand six hundred and seventeen patients with differentiated PTC were included in the analysis of which 168 patients (11%) underwent PEI (270 lesions) and 1449 patients (88.6%) underwent reoperation. Based on the pooled data analysis PEI was successful in 87.5% and surgery was successful in 94.8%. Pooled PEI-related risk of complications was 1.2 and 3.5% for surgery. The overall change in TG was not significant between the two modalities. The authors conclude that reoperation carries higher risks and PEI offers overall health care cost advantages [55]. While presenting the long-term outcome of their patients, the Mayo Clinic group made cost analysis comparing the two procedures. In 2002, the projected cost of PEI was $836 for a single procedure. This compares to $8000–12,000 for surgical neck exploration. The authors estimate a saving of $1.54 million by avoiding 40 neck re-explorations while avoiding concomitant surgical morbidity [56].

11.8.6.2 Patient Selection for PEI of Metastatic Lymphadenopathy

Indications for PEI of metastatic lymphadenopathy:

1. Proven small scale or isolated metastasis in patients who have received definitive surgery and radioactive iodine therapy.
2. Patients who have declined further surgeries.
3. Metastatic lymph nodes that are <2 cm in maximal dimension.
4. Elderly patients or patients with comorbidities precluding surgery.

5. As a palliative procedure for palpable metastatic adenopathy causing distress.

In general, the following are less than ideal situations for PEI or RFA of metastatic adenopathy:

1. Bulky lymphadenopathy.
2. Patients with progressive distant metastatic disease, who will require systemic TKI therapy.
3. Injection of ipsilateral level VI lymph node or thyroid bed disease in patients who have had prior contralateral RLN injury.
4. Bilateral or multi-compartment disease in younger patients.

11.9 Safety Policies

Adhering to institutional and strict procedure-suite safety policies reduces operator errors. Vials or ampoules containing similar appearing labels are best avoided in the procedure suite (image 2). Lidocaine and ethanol are clear and colorless liquids. Preloading both liquids in unlabeled syringes increases the risk of misadministration. Loading the respective fluids by the operator just prior to administration is a safer practice. Asking a third person to cross check during the procedure also eliminates medical errors.

11.10 Conclusions

PEI is effective for the treatment of predominantly cystic nodules compared to thermal ablations as an alternative to surgery. The equipment requirements are minimal. With careful patient selection, procedural morbidity is trivial. It also has significant cost advantages for patients and the health care systems. Partially cystic nodules may require sequential or concomitant administration of RFA for optimal volume reduction. Appropriate patient selection is important for PEI therapy of metastatic lymphadenopathy. Training and practice patterns vary considerably across different countries. Systematic training is lacking and policies to integrate training within postgraduate teaching programs is one solution.

References

1. Mazzaferri EL. Management of a solitary thyroid nodule. N Engl J Med. 1993;328(8):553–9. https://doi.org/10.1056/NEJM199302253280807.
2. Haugen BR, Alexander EK, Bible KC, Doherty GM, Mandel SJ, Nikiforov YE, et al. 2015 American Thyroid Association management guidelines for adult patients with thyroid nodules and differentiated thyroid cancer: the American Thyroid Association guidelines task force on thyroid nodules and differentiated thyroid cancer. Thyroid. 2016;26(1):1–133. https://doi.org/10.1089/thy.2015.0020.
3. de los Santos ET, Keyhani-Rofagha S, Cunningham JJ, Mazzaferri EL. Cystic thyroid nodules. The dilemma of malignant lesions. Arch Intern Med. 1990;150(7):1422–7. https://doi.org/10.1001/archinte.150.7.1422.
4. Bergenfelz A, Jansson S, Kristoffersson A, Mårtensson H, Reihnér E, Wallin G, et al. Complications to thyroid surgery: results as reported in a database from a multicenter audit comprising 3,660 patients. Langenbeck's Arch Surg. 2008;393(5):667–73. https://doi.org/10.1007/s00423-008-0366-7.
5. Gharib H, Hegedüs L, Pacella CM, Baek JH, Papini E. Clinical review: nonsurgical, image-guided, minimally invasive therapy for thyroid nodules. J Clin Endocrinol Metab. 2013;98(10):3949–57. https://doi.org/10.1210/jc.2013-1806.
6. Hahn SY, Shin JH, Na DG, Ha EJ, Ahn HS, Lim HK, et al. Korean Society of Thyroid Radiology (KSThR); Korean Society of Radiology. Ethanol ablation of the thyroid nodules: 2018 consensus statement by the Korean Society of Thyroid Radiology. Korean J Radiol. 2019;20(4):609–20. https://doi.org/10.3348/kjr.2018.0696.
7. Papini E, Monpeyssen H, Frasoldati A, Hegedüs L. 2020 European thyroid association clinical practice guideline for the use of image-guided ablation in benign thyroid nodules. Eur Thyroid J. 2020;9(4):172–85. https://doi.org/10.1159/000508484.
8. Hegedüs L, Frasoldati A, Negro R, Papini E. European thyroid association survey on use of minimally invasive techniques for thyroid nodules. Eur Thyroid J. 2020 Jul;9(4):194–204. https://doi.org/10.1159/000506513.
9. Ha EJ, Baek JH, Lee JH. Ultrasonography-based thyroidal and perithyroidal anatomy and its clinical significance. Korean J Radiol. 2015;16(4):749–66. https://doi.org/10.3348/kjr.2015.16.4.749.
10. Mazzaferri EL. Thyroid cancer in thyroglossal duct remnants: a diagnostic and therapeutic

dilemma. Thyroid. 2004;14(5):335–6. https://doi.org/10.1089/105072504774193140.
11. Hirshoren N, Neuman T, Udassin R, Elidan J, Weinberger JM. The imperative of the Sistrunk operation: review of 160 thyroglossal tract remnant operations. Otolaryngol Head Neck Surg. 2009;140(3):338–42. https://doi.org/10.1016/j.otohns.2008.12.002.
12. Pellegriti G, Lumera G, Malandrino P, Latina A, Masucci R, Scollo C, et al. Thyroid cancer in thyroglossal duct cysts requires a specific approach due to its unpredictable extension. J Clin Endocrinol Metab. 2013;98(2):458–65. https://doi.org/10.1210/jc.2012-1952.
13. Kim SM, Baek JH, Kim YS, Sung JY, Lim HK, Choi H, et al. Efficacy and safety of ethanol ablation for thyroglossal duct cysts. AJNR Am J Neuroradiol. 2011;32(2):306–9. https://doi.org/10.3174/ajnr.A2296.
14. Durante C, Costante G, Lucisano G, Bruno R, Meringolo D, Paciaroni A, et al. The natural history of benign thyroid nodules. JAMA. 2015;313(9):926–35. https://doi.org/10.1001/jama.2015.0956.
15. Kim DW, Rho MH, Kim HJ, Kwon JS, Sung YS, Lee SW. Percutaneous ethanol injection for benign cystic thyroid nodules: is aspiration of ethanol-mixed fluid advantageous? AJNR Am J Neuroradiol. 2005;26(8):2122–7.
16. Hegedüs L, Hansen JM, Karstrup S, Torp-Pedersen S, Juul N. Tetracycline for sclerosis of thyroid cysts. A randomized study. Arch Intern Med. 1988;148(5):1116–8. https://doi.org/10.1001/archinte.1988.00380050120018.
17. Jayesh SR, Mehta P, Cherian MP, Ilayaraja V, Gupta P, Venkatesh K. Efficacy and safety of USG-guided ethanol sclerotherapy in cystic thyroid nodules. Indian J Radiol Imaging. 2009;19(3):199–202. https://doi.org/10.4103/0971-3026.54879.
18. Gong X, Wang F, Du H, Chen X, Shi B. Comparison of ultrasound-guided percutaneous Polidocanol injection versus percutaneous ethanol injection for treatment of benign cystic thyroid nodules. J Ultrasound Med. 2018;37(6):1423–9. https://doi.org/10.1002/jum.14482.
19. PubChem. Bethesda, MD: National Library of Medicine (US), National Center for Biotechnology Information; 2004. PubChem Compound Summary for CID 656641, Polidocanol. https://pubchem.ncbi.nlm.nih.gov/compound/Polidocanol.
20. Kim DW, Rho MH, Kim KN. Ultrasound-guided fine-needle aspiration biopsy of thyroid nodules: is it necessary to use local anesthesia for the application of one needle puncture? Korean J Radiol. 2009;10(5):441–6. https://doi.org/10.3348/kjr.2009.10.5.441.
21. Monzani F, Caraccio N, Goletti O, Lippolis PV, Casolaro A, Del Guerra P, et al. Five-year follow-up of percutaneous ethanol injection for the treatment of hyperfunctioning thyroid nodules: a study of 117 patients. Clin Endocrinol. 1997;46(1):9–15. https://doi.org/10.1046/j.1365-2265.1997.d01-1752.x.
22. Crile G Jr. Treatment of thyroid cysts by aspiration. Surgery. 1966;59(2):210–2.
23. Bennedbaek FN, Hegedüs L. Treatment of recurrent thyroid cysts with ethanol: a randomized double-blind controlled trial. J Clin Endocrinol Metab. 2003;88(12):5773–7. https://doi.org/10.1210/jc.2003-031000.
24. Monzani F, Lippi F, Goletti O, Del Guerra P, Caraccio N, Lippolis PV, et al. Percutaneous aspiration and ethanol sclerotherapy for thyroid cysts. J Clin Endocrinol Metab. 1994;78(3):800–2. https://doi.org/10.1210/jcem.78.3.8126160.
25. Verde G, Papini E, Pacella CM, Gallotti C, Delpiano S, Strada S, et al. Ultrasound guided percutaneous ethanol injection in the treatment of cystic thyroid nodules. Clin Endocrinol. 1994;41(6):719–24. https://doi.org/10.1111/j.1365-2265.1994.tb02785.x.
26. Yasuda K, Ozaki O, Sugino K, Yamashita T, Toshima K, Ito K, et al. Treatment of cystic lesions of the thyroid by ethanol instillation. World J Surg. 1992;16(5):958–61. https://doi.org/10.1007/BF02067001.
27. Valcavi R, Frasoldati A. Ultrasound-guided percutaneous ethanol injection therapy in thyroid cystic nodules. Endocr Pract. 2004;10(3):269–75. https://doi.org/10.4158/EP.10.3.269.
28. Zingrillo M, Torlontano M, Ghiggi MR, D'Aloiso L, Nirchio V, Bisceglia M, et al. Percutaneous ethanol injection of large thyroid cystic nodules. Thyroid. 1996;6(5):403–8. https://doi.org/10.1089/thy.1996.6.403.
29. Zingrillo M, Torlontano M, Chiarella R, Ghiggi MR, Nirchio V, Bisceglia M, et al. Percutaneous ethanol injection may be a definitive treatment for symptomatic thyroid cystic nodules not treatable by surgery: five-year follow-up study. Thyroid. 1999;9(8):763–7. https://doi.org/10.1089/thy.1999.9.763.
30. Suh CH, Baek JH, Ha EJ, Choi YJ, Lee JH, Kim JK, et al. Ethanol ablation of predominantly cystic thyroid nodules: evaluation of recurrence rate and factors related to recurrence. Clin Radiol. 2015;70(1):42–7. https://doi.org/10.1016/j.crad.2014.09.008.
31. Kim YJ, Baek JH, Ha EJ, Lim HK, Lee JH, Sung JY, et al. Cystic versus predominantly cystic thyroid nodules: efficacy of ethanol ablation and analysis of related factors. Eur Radiol. 2012;22(7):1573–8. https://doi.org/10.1007/s00330-012-2406-5.
32. Del Prete S, Caraglia M, Russo D, Vitale G, Giuberti G, Marra M, et al. Percutaneous ethanol injection efficacy in the treatment of large symptomatic thyroid cystic nodules: ten-year follow-up of a large series. Thyroid. 2002;12(9):815–21. https://doi.org/10.1089/105072502760339398.
33. Baek JH, Ha EJ, Choi YJ, Sung JY, Kim JK, Shong YK. Radiofrequency versus ethanol ablation for treating predominantly cystic thyroid nod-

ules: a randomized clinical trial. Korean J Radiol. 2015;16(6):1332–40. https://doi.org/10.3348/kjr.2015.16.6.1332.
34. Hays D. Do it yourself the Z-track way. Am J Nurs. 1974;74(6):1070–1.
35. Gharib H, Mazzaferri EL. Thyroxine suppressive therapy in patients with nodular thyroid disease. Ann Intern Med. 1998;128(5):386–94. https://doi.org/10.7326/0003-4819-128-5-199803010-00008.
36. Bennedbaek FN, Nielsen LK, Hegedüs L. Effect of percutaneous ethanol injection therapy versus suppressive doses of L-thyroxine on benign solitary solid cold thyroid nodules: a randomized trial. J Clin Endocrinol Metab. 1998;83(3):830–5. https://doi.org/10.1210/jcem.83.3.4673.
37. Livraghi T, Paracchi A, Ferrari C, Bergonzi M, Garavaglia G, Raineri P, et al. Treatment of autonomous thyroid nodules with percutaneous ethanol injection: preliminary results. Work in progress. Radiology. 1990;175(3):827–9. https://doi.org/10.1148/radiology.175.3.2188302.
38. Goletti O, Monzani F, Caraccio N, Del Guerra P, Lippolis PV, Pucciarelli M, et al. Percutaneous ethanol injection treatment of autonomously functioning single thyroid nodules: optimization of treatment and short term outcome. World J Surg. 1992;16(4):784–9; discussion 789–90. https://doi.org/10.1007/BF02067387.
39. Lippi F, Ferrari C, Manetti L, Rago T, Santini F, Monzani F, et al. Treatment of solitary autonomous thyroid nodules by percutaneous ethanol injection: results of an Italian multicenter study. The Multicenter Study Group. J Clin Endocrinol Metab. 1996;81(9):3261–4. https://doi.org/10.1210/jcem.81.9.8784080.
40. Abraham D, Abraham NR. Nonsurgical treatment of thyroid cysts, nodules, thyroid cancer nodal metastases, and hyperparathyroidism: the role of percutaneous ethanol injection. In: Surgery of the thyroid and parathyroid glands; 2021. p. 472–8. https://doi.org/10.1016/B978-0-323-66127-0.00051-X.
41. Sharma A, Abraham D. Vascularity-targeted percutaneous ethanol injection of toxic thyroid adenomas: outcomes of a feasibility study performed in the USA. Endocr Pract. 2020;26(1):22–9. https://doi.org/10.4158/EP-2019-0329.
42. Su C, Liu YJ, Qian LX. Modified percutaneous ethanol injection method combined with microwave ablation for the treatment of symptomatic, predominantly cystic, benign thyroid nodules: a retrospective study of 201 cases. Int J Hyperth. 2021;38(1):995–1001. https://doi.org/10.1080/02656736.2021.1924407.
43. Yoon HM, Baek JH, Lee JH, Ha EJ, Kim JK, Yoon JH, et al. Combination therapy consisting of ethanol and radiofrequency ablation for predominantly cystic thyroid nodules. AJNR Am J Neuroradiol. 2014;35(3):582–6. https://doi.org/10.3174/ajnr.A3701.
44. Sung JY, Kim YS, Choi H, Lee JH, Baek JH. Optimum first-line treatment technique for benign cystic thyroid nodules: ethanol ablation or radiofrequency ablation? AJR Am J Roentgenol. 2011;196(2):W210–4. https://doi.org/10.2214/AJR.10.5172.
45. Sung JY, Baek JH, Kim KS, Lee D, Yoo H, Kim JK, et al. Single-session treatment of benign cystic thyroid nodules with ethanol versus radiofrequency ablation: a prospective randomized study. Radiology. 2013;269(1):293–300. https://doi.org/10.1148/radiol.13122134.
46. Qubain SW, Nakano S, Baba M, Takao S, Aikou T. Distribution of lymph node micrometastasis in pN0 well-differentiated thyroid carcinoma. Surgery. 2002;131(3):249–56. https://doi.org/10.1067/msy.2002.120657.
47. Arturi F, Russo D, Giuffrida D, Ippolito A, Perrotti N, Vigneri R, et al. Early diagnosis by genetic analysis of differentiated thyroid cancer metastases in small lymph nodes. J Clin Endocrinol Metab. 1997;82(5):1638–41. https://doi.org/10.1210/jcem.82.5.4062.
48. Burman KD. Treatment of recurrent or persistent cervical node metastases in differentiated thyroid cancer: deceptively simple options. J Clin Endocrinol Metab. 2012;97(8):2623–5. https://doi.org/10.1210/jc.2012-2480.
49. Wagner HE, Seiler C. Recurrent laryngeal nerve palsy after thyroid gland surgery. Br J Surg. 1994;81(2):226–8. https://doi.org/10.1002/bjs.1800810222.
50. Roh JL, Kim JM, Park CI. Central compartment reoperation for recurrent/persistent differentiated thyroid cancer: patterns of recurrence, morbidity, and prediction of postoperative hypocalcemia. Ann Surg Oncol. 2011;18(5):1312–8. https://doi.org/10.1245/s10434-010-1470-9.
51. Kim MK, Mandel SH, Baloch Z, Livolsi VA, Langer JE, Didonato L, et al. Morbidity following central compartment reoperation for recurrent or persistent thyroid cancer. Arch Otolaryngol Head Neck Surg. 2004;130(10):1214–6. https://doi.org/10.1001/archotol.130.10.1214.
52. Robenshtok E, Fish S, Bach A, Domínguez JM, Shaha A, Tuttle RM. Suspicious cervical lymph nodes detected after thyroidectomy for papillary thyroid cancer usually remain stable over years in properly selected patients. J Clin Endocrinol Metab. 2012;97(8):2706–13. https://doi.org/10.1210/jc.2012-1553.
53. Lewis BD, Hay ID, Charboneau JW, McIver B, Reading CC, Goellner JR. Percutaneous ethanol injection for treatment of cervical lymph node metastases in patients with papillary thyroid carcinoma. AJR Am J Roentgenol. 2002;178(3):699–704. https://doi.org/10.2214/ajr.178.3.1780699.
54. Heilo A, Sigstad E, Fagerlid KH, Håskjold OI, Grøholt KK, Berner A, et al. Efficacy of ultrasound-guided percutaneous ethanol injection treatment in

patients with a limited number of metastatic cervical lymph nodes from papillary thyroid carcinoma. J Clin Endocrinol Metab. 2011;96(9):2750–5. https://doi.org/10.1210/jc.2010-2952.
55. Fontenot TE, Deniwar A, Bhatia P, Al-Qurayshi Z, Randolph GW, Kandil E. Percutaneous ethanol injection vs reoperation for locally recurrent papillary thyroid cancer: a systematic review and pooled analysis. JAMA Otolaryngol Head Neck Surg. 2015;141(6):512–8. https://doi.org/10.1001/jamaoto.2015.0596.
56. Hay ID, Lee RA, Davidge-Pitts C, Reading CC, Charboneau JW. Long-term outcome of ultrasound-guided percutaneous ethanol ablation of selected "recurrent" neck nodal metastases in 25 patients with TNM stages III or IVA papillary thyroid carcinoma previously treated by surgery and 131I therapy. Surgery. 2013;154(6):1448–54; discussion 1454–5. https://doi.org/10.1016/j.surg.2013.07.007.

Radiofrequency Ablation (RA) of Benign Thyroid Nodules

12

Roberto Valcavi

12.1 Introduction

In this chapter, we will briefly look at the different thermal ablation techniques for benign thyroid nodules, assess the advantages and disadvantages of radiofrequency ablation (RFA), and highlight the importance of protecting adjacent nervous structures and in particular the recurrent laryngeal nerve (RLN) and external branch of superior laryngeal nerve (EBSLN). More specifically, we will look into the important aspects of RFA ablation procedures such as hydrodissection, including a rescue technique to avoid nerve damage, local anesthesia, and sedation. We will also discuss RFA guidelines, clinical settings, informed patient consent, and expected outcomes. Finally, we will consider the overall benefits to patients who undergo RFA procedures conducted on benign thyroid nodules, and we will suggest a training approach to become proficient in thyroid RFA.

Thyroid nodules are fairly widespread in the general population, with 4–7% being palpable [1], while the majority (up to 70%) are usually detected by ultrasound [2]. Year after year, an increasingly number of total thyroid surgeries mostly for benign nodules are performed worldwide [3, 4] and total thyroidectomy has been long considered the only safe and effective surgical option for patients suffering from thyroid nodules.

However, due to potential operating risks perceived by patients and the need for lifelong hormone supplementation, this option is currently being reassessed [5]. Even a hemithyroidectomy can be associated with the development of hypothyroidism. As reported by Ahn et al., this condition develops in 5.6–48.9% of patients who undergo a thyroid lobectomy, and this figure varies according to the follow-up period and strategy or the definition of hypothyroidism [6].

In fact, as thermal ablation procedures and in particular radiofrequency ablation (RFA) have become more advanced, they have been increasingly accepted as a viable alternative in thyroid nodule management, especially for patients with benign nodules [5, 7, 8]. Progress in high-resolution ultrasound (US) technology, which is used to visualize in real time the thyroid gland and nodule, hydrodissection, and needle electrode insertion and positioning, through the "moving shot" technique, has greatly contributed to the diffusion and acceptance of radiofrequency thyroid ablations.

Supplementary Information The online version contains supplementary material available at https://doi.org/10.1007/978-3-031-88229-6_12.

R. Valcavi (✉)
Department of Endocrinology, The Endocrine & Thyroid Clinic, Reggio Emilia, Italy

R. Valcavi et al. (eds.), *Thyroid Ablation*, https://doi.org/10.1007/978-3-031-88229-6_12

12.2 Thermal Ablation Technologies

Given a cytological diagnosis of a benign thyroid nodule (Bethesda Category II), usually evidenced by fine-needle aspiration (FNA), symptomatic patients now have an array of thermal ablation therapeutic options [5, 7, 8].

For large thyroid nodules, i.e., > 4 cm, the American Thyroid Association still suggests a total thyroidectomy [9], whereas European and Korean guideline recommendations suggest US-guided thermal ablation (TA) techniques as an alternative therapeutic option for the treatment of large symptomatic nodules [7, 8].

The various minimally invasive thermal ablation techniques are all based on the application of high temperatures which induce focal cellular apoptosis and subsequently coagulative necrosis [10, 11].

These include **RFA, laser ablation (LA), microwave ablation (MWA), and high-intensity focused ultrasound (HI-FU) ablation** which all apply heat to the nodule. However, they generate heat in differ ways.

During **RFA**, an electrode needle is inserted into the target lesion. High frequency alternating current causes frictional heating in the tissue as ions continuously realign themselves with the alternating direction of electrical current [11]. At temperatures above 60 °C, permanent hyperthermic cellular injury occurs, below this temperature, cellular damage is reversible [12]. At temperatures above 100 °C, cell desiccation and charring take place which increases impedance and reduces conduction in the tissue [11].

LA is performed using a diode laser as an energy source and optical fibers. As claimed by some authors, this thermal ablation technique achieves nodule volume reduction similar to RFA [8]. However, a systematic review published by Cho [13] found in a 3-year follow-up analysis that RFA was far superior to LA in terms of thyroid nodule Volume Reduction Rate (VRR) by almost 50%, with less regrowth and fewer successive surgeries. It has been suggested by Sim and Baek that lower regrowth is due to the ability of RFAs to more completely ablate nodule margins [14].

MWA generates an electromagnetic field creating wider ablation areas and higher temperatures. This thermal ablation technique could be more suitable in treating larger tumors [15]. However, the biggest drawback of MWAs is that they reach temperatures of up to 150 °C leading to tissue charring [16].

HI-FU is a novel ablation technique, based on the conversion of acoustic energy to thermal energy that can effectively shrink thyroid nodules. Although preliminary results are promising, further research with longer follow-up periods must be conducted [17].

Kim et al. (2006) first described RFA of benign thyroid nodules, and this technique has been increasingly adopted around the world [18, 19]. More recently, updated RFA guidelines have come to include indications beyond benign disease [2, 8, 19, 20].

12.2.1 Pros and Cons of Radiofrequency Ablation

The principal advantage of RFA is the preservation of a functional thyroid gland with no need to undergo lifelong thyroid hormone replacement therapy. In fact, while there may be a temporary post-operative thyroid dysfunction [21], long-term hypothyroidism is rare [22, 23].

Given that this is a minimally invasive procedure, there are also other numerous advantages such as no hospital admission, no need of incisions, hence absence of scars, no intubation for general anesthesia, no drainage tubes, fewer post-operative complications, minimal side effects, and faster recovery [24, 25].

It has been demonstrated while surgical resection and radiofrequency ablation are both effective treatments of thyroid nodules [26], RFAs are minimally invasive allowing a faster return to routine activities and greater quality of life [27]. Therefore, radiofrequency ablation should be considered a first-line treatment for benign thyroid nodules.

12.3 Recurrent Laryngeal Nerve Protection

Precaution must be taken to avoid damaging recurrent laryngeal nerves [28].

The recurrent laryngeal nerves (RLNs) are branches of the vagus nerve. The left RLN loops under aortic arch while the right RLN loops around right subclavian artery. Both RLNs run posterior to the thyroid gland in the tracheo-esophageal groove and enter the larynx at cricothyroid joint to innervate all intrinsic laryngeal muscles, except for the cricothyroid muscle which is innervated by the EBSLN which regulates voice projection and pitch.

RFA proceduralists should be aware that RLN has many anatomic variants [29]. In fact, in about 40% of cases, the RLN splits into two or more branches prior to entering the larynx. RLNs run posterior and medial to thyroid lobes in the so-called danger zone [19].

Thermal injury to RLN and EBSLN causes hoarseness of variable severity and phonation difficulties. Furthermore, damage to these nerves can cause laryngeal muscular weakness producing dysphagia and increasing the risk of aspiration [30].

Although many authors report that thermal damage to RLN and EBSLN is reversible over time [30], full recovery of voice quality and laryngeal intrinsic muscle strength is debatable. Hence, RLN and EBSLN thermal injuries during thyroid RFA should be absolutely avoided. If nervous thermal injury occurs in an RFA, a "rescue" procedure, which will be outlined later in this chapter, should be immediately applied.

Proper hydrodissections of nodule effectively protects nervous structures from the above-mentioned risks of thermal injury.

Due to its small diameter, RLN cannot be visualized by ultrasound. However, using US images, we can determine that RLN is positioned in the so-called danger area, posterior and medial to the thyroid lobe (Fig. 12.1).

12.3.1 Procedures for RLN Hydrodissection

Video 12.1 demonstrates an RFA procedure preceded by pericapsular local anesthesia. An injection of 10 mL, 2% lidocaine is performed under US assistance using a 25–27 G Chiba needle. Anterior hydrodissection and local anesthesia separate strap muscles and sternocleidomastoid muscle from nodule. If hydrodissection starts to diminish, which usually occurs within 15–20 min, a nonconductive solution of cold 5% dextrose (D5W) can be administered to restore hydrodissection volume.

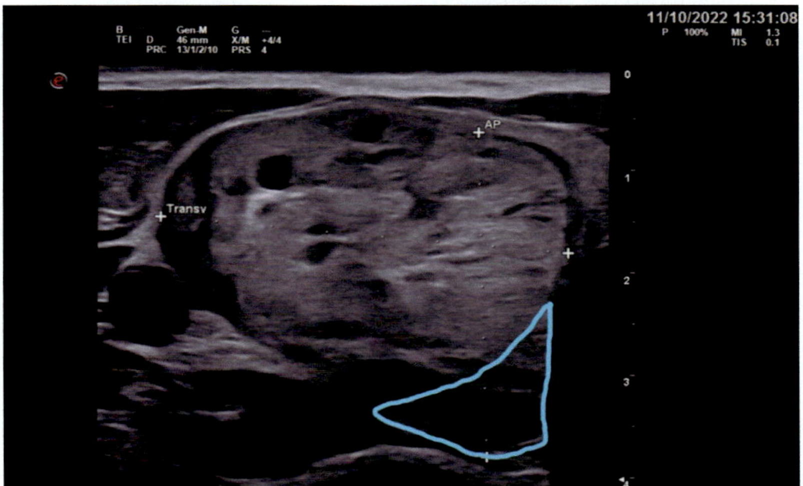

Fig. 12.1 US image of danger zone (blue outline)

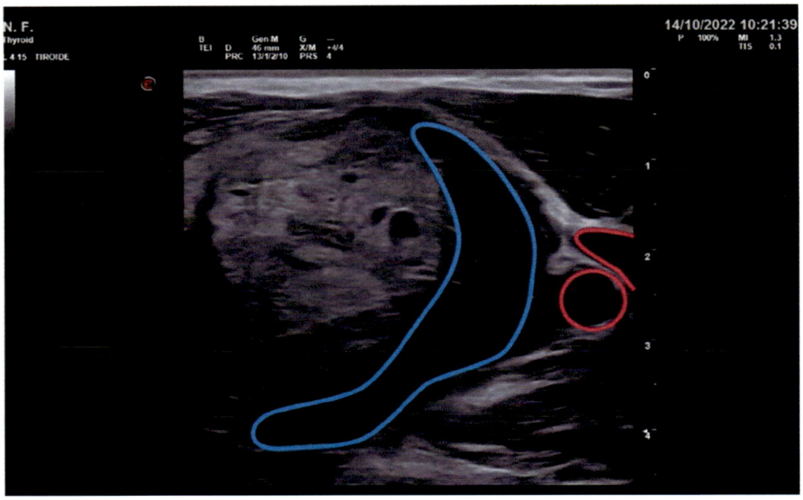

Fig. 12.2 Anterior and posterior hydrodissection merger (blue outline). Common carotid and internal jugular vein (red outline)

For posterior hydrodissection, 20–30 mL 5% cold (0–5 °C) D5W is administered. In Video 12.1, the posteriorly inserted needle tip is outlined by a red circle at 57″. Anterior and posterior hydrodissections merge, thus detaching the nodule from vital neck structures such as the common carotid artery and internal jugular vein (Fig. 12.2).

Superior hydrodissection protects EBSLN and middle cervical ganglion from damage by heating during RFA. The hydrodissection needle is inserted and advanced to the superior external margin of the nodule, and 10–20 mL cold D5W is administered until this margin is detached from the adjacent nervous structures (Video 12.2).

An alternative hydrodissection technique has been presented by Jeong and Baek [31]. In this procedure, a hydrodissection steel needle is inserted anteriorly, and fluid is injected until it also hydrodissects the posterior compartment. The hydrodissection needle is kept in position during the RFA procedure for continuous D5W infusion. At the same time, the RFA steel needle is inserted and activated.

This technique of continuous, large volume hydrodissection can certainly protect delicate structures surrounding the thyroid during an RFA procedure and might be beneficial in large thyroid nodule ablations as suggested by Ma et al. [32]. However, this approach imposes two risks: the first being the possibility of a voltaic arc due to electrical flux travelling from the ablation electrode needle tip to the hydrodissection steel needle; the second being difficulties in achieving and maintaining hydrodissection of posterior compartment because the hydrodissection needle could easily slide in or out of perithyroidal tissues during ablation.

In order to avoid the risk of voltaic arc, a silicone plastic catheter could be used instead of a steel needle. However, positioning this type of catheter in tracheoesophageal groove can be cumbersome, and the catheter could bend or kink.

In order to avoid these two risks, the hydrodissection steel needle should be withdrawn before applying RFA electric current. Instead, cold D5W should be injected when and as many times as necessary in order to maintain the protection zone between nodule and danger area during ablation.

Video 12.3 shows a repeated posterior hydrodissection in a partially ablated nodule, and retraction of the hydrodissection needle. After reestablishing RLN protection through a repeated hydrodissection, RFA can resume until ablation is completed. This technique permits a total nodule ablation, which is the ultimate goal of RFA [19].

12.3.2 Rescue Hydrodissection

A thorough knowledge of the function and position of the following RLN, EBSLN, vagus nerve, cervical sympathetic ganglion, cervical/brachial plexus, spinal accessory nerve, phrenic nerve is of clinical significance for early detection, prevention, and proper management of complications during RFA procedures. Symptoms of these complications include hoarseness, changes in voice projection, tone and pitch, tachycardia and abnormal heart rhythm, low blood pressure, and vomiting, Horner syndrome, arm numbness and paralysis, drooping shoulder, hiccups, etc. [33].

In the event of thermal damage to nerve structures, a direct injection of cold D5W is a simple and effective treatment that can result in rapid symptom resolution. More specifically, an RLN "rescue" procedure has been established if dysphonia occurs during thyroid RFA [34]. In fact, if hoarseness is detected during ablation, the procedure must be immediately stopped, and cold D5W should be injected into tracheoesophageal groove, as illustrated in Video 12.4. Injection of cold D5W usually mitigates thermal injury to RLN during RFA, and patient voice quality usually quickly returns to normal. Due to the serious repercussions of any nerve damage, RFA proceduralists should be familiar with this "rescue" procedure and have cold D5W on hand during all RFA procedures.

12.4 Guidelines for Radiofrequency Ablation

Respecting certain criteria and indications for RFA and thermal ablation in general is of utmost importance in order to guarantee a safe and efficient procedure and achieve desired outcomes; the first being the need to establish that the nodule is of a benign nature. Usually, two FNAs are performed to confirm this. For spongiform or cystic consistency nodules, some authors suggest only one benign biopsy and an US examination as an alternative assessment [5, 8, 19]. According to Korean Society of Thyroid Radiology, spongiform nodules, which are almost always benign [35], do not even require a FNA biopsy [19].

Although many guidelines do not state precise size limits for RFA, which can vary from 2 cm for the Korean Society of Thyroid Radiology [19] to 20 mL for Italian societies [20], larger nodules that often cause compressive and aesthetic concerns are particularly indicated for RFA procedures [5, 8, 19]. Other symptoms to take into consideration are dysphagia, globus sensation, positional discomfort, voice change, and shortness of breath [5, 8, 19]. Symptomatology differs dramatically from patient to patient and is also related to location of nodule as well as body habitus.

The decision to perform an RFA procedure depends on several factors, such as size and location of nodule, degree of perturbance, discomfort and voice compromission, and thyroid functionality. Proceduralists should discuss all these factors with patients in order to evaluate the correct therapeutic approach and outline the expected results of an agreed-upon treatment [36].

A well-delimited, thyroid nodule resulting in clearly observable symptoms is the most suitable type for an RFA procedure [37]. Other more complex diagnoses including multiple bilateral and substernal nodules are surely more complicated to treat. In any case, even if scientific literature endorsing RFA for these situations is scarce, some expert proceduralists sustain that RFA may be a safe and effective therapy for multiple bilateral [38] or substernal nodules [39].

For substernal nodules, a so-called iceberg technique consisting of a two/three-stage treatment has been proposed. In this technique, the cervical portion of nodule is ablated first. After a 6–12-month period, a volumetric reduction and retraction of the treated portion occur. This tissue retraction pulls the mediastinal (intrathoracic) component of nodule into cervical region, allowing the possibility of a second ablation. If the second RFA procedure fails to achieve a complete nodule ablation, successive procedures may be carried out until the nodule is totally ablated [40].

In any case, as RFA procedures become more advanced and refined, they will become more applicable for ablations of the above-mentioned diagnoses as well as for continuous growing of small nodules that may eventually lead to symptoms [25, 41].

When developing a patient–physician relationship, it is the responsibility of the proceduralist to interpret the clinical factors, evaluate patient expectations, and establish an appropriate treatment in order to achieve the maximum possible medical outcome. This is particularly important since, at present, there are no standard guidelines for selecting and evaluating patients for thyroid ablation.

The ultimate goal of any thyroid nodule therapy is to completely ablate the nodule and maintain/re-establish normal thyroid function or euthyroidism. However, achieving this goal is dependent on several issues, the most critical of which are the size and location of the nodule [41]. Patients with autonomously functioning thyroid nodules (AFTNs) may also be candidates for RFA [42, 43].

12.5 RFA Setting and Equipment

Up to now, RFA procedures have been carried out in operating rooms, outpatient day hospitals, or ambulatory clinics. These settings obviously offer different levels of patient protection and procedural options and incur different operational costs. Even if thyroid RFAs are carried out in vastly different settings, it is extremely important that certain medical and clinical criteria are met in order to satisfy these criteria. An optimal RFA environment suitable for thyroid ablation should include (Fig. 12.3):

- Ultrasound system with assorted probes including convex and linear probes
- Overhead monitor displaying ultrasound images
- Operating table with adjustable headrest
- Anesthetist cart with RF equipment, ECG monitor and defibrillator, aspirator, oxygen cylinder
- Operating throne with stabilizing back support and armrests

Due to technological advances especially in Artificial Intelligence (AI), US systems are being continuously further developed. For example, the multifrequency technology allows detailed visualization without the loss of resolution at different tissue depths. In addition, different probe configurations have vastly different features. In fact, linear probes, which are currently the standard for thyroid US imaging today, provide an adequate resolution with a limited visualization field. On the contrary, convex probes offer a wider visualization field, useful for larger and deeper nodules, although at lower resolutions.

The position of an overhead monitor is particularly important. As in videolaparoscopic surgery, the operator should look directly forward at a large overhead screen to facilitate eye-hand coordination (Fig. 12.4).

In addition, proceduralists should never stand while performing procedures rather they should sit on an operating throne with stabilizing back and armrests directly behind patient head, who is

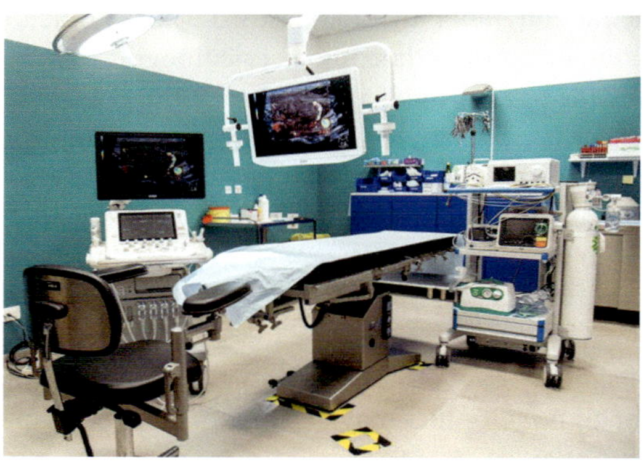

Fig. 12.3 Optimal RFA environment suitable for thyroid ablation

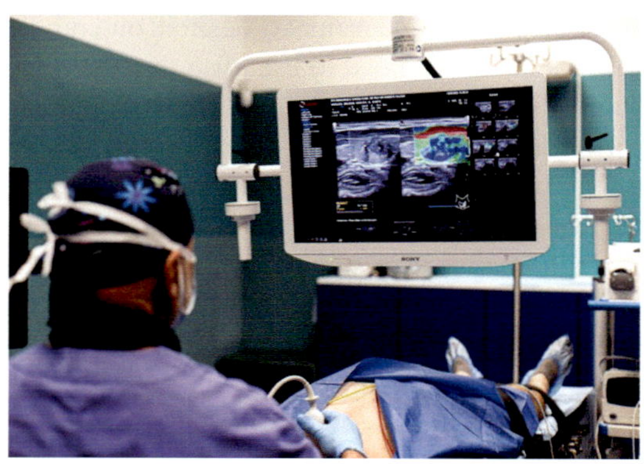

Fig. 12.4 Correct overhead position of monitor

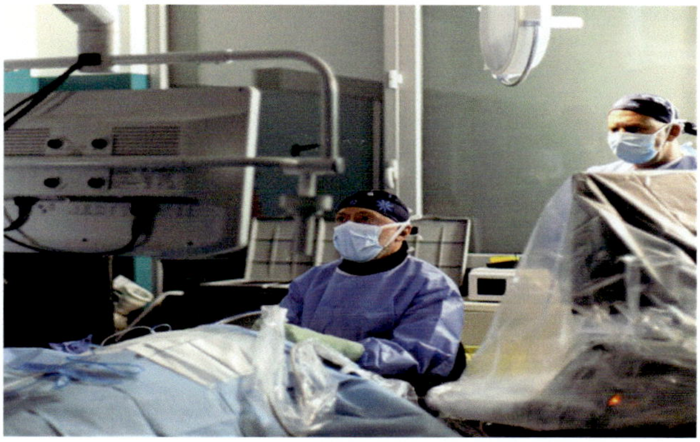

Fig. 12.5 RFA clinical setup. Proceduralist sits behind head of patient, looking directly at overhead monitor

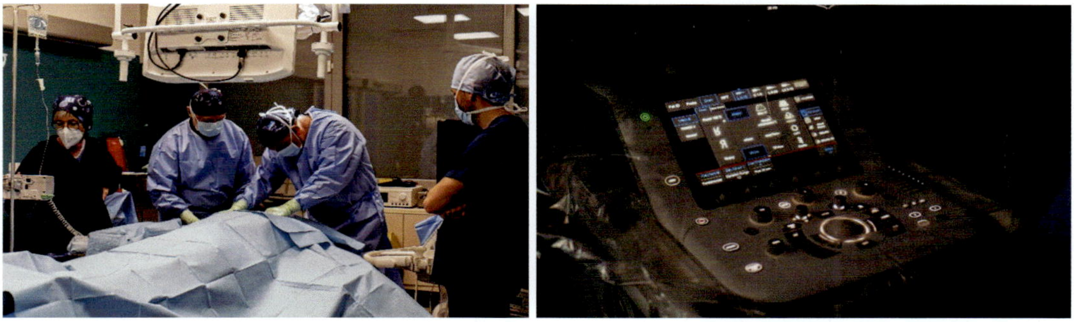

Fig. 12.6 Sterile field setup with extensive draping and ultrasound keyboard protected by a sterile cover

positioned with hyperextended neck on an adjustable operating table (Fig. 12.5).

RFAs are usually performed with local anesthesia and under sterile conditions (Fig. 12.6).

Sedation is advisable; however, general anesthesia is precluded since patients would be unable to communicate or produce vocal sounds during the procedure and therefore the proceduralist would be unable to detect any nerve damage.

12.6 Anesthesia and Sedation

RFA procedures are normally carried out under local anesthesia with 1–2% lidocaine except for extremely rare conditions of local anesthetic intolerance. About 1–2% mepivacaine could be an alternative anesthetic for longer ablation procedures. Anesthetic volume, based on body weight and renal function, must be calculated before administration.

Local anesthesia allows the patient to communicate with the proceduralist during the procedure and more importantly to produce vocal sounds demonstrating proper vocal cord movements indicating that no vocal nerves have been compromised.

In order to improve patient experience and mitigate pain, sedation and analgesia are advisable. Sedation is classified in three levels: minimal, moderate, and deep sedation (Table 12.1).

As previously stated, general anesthesia is not advisable because of patient inability to communicate with the proceduralist and produce vocal sounds to confirm vocal cord integrity.

In minimal sedation, patients respond normally to verbal stimulation and breathe spontaneously. Minimal sedation is obtained with the administration of oral benzodiazepines and can be carried out in a simple ambulatory clinic.

In moderate sedation, patients are partially sedated; however, they will still be able to pro-

Table 12.1 Sedation options for thyroid RFA

Description	Minimal sedation	Moderate sedation/ analgesia	Deep sedation/analgesia	General Anesthesia
Responsiveness	Normal response to verbal stimulation	Purposeful response to verbal or tactile stimulation	Purposeful response following repeated or painful stimulation	No response even with painful stimulus
Airway	Unaffected	No intervention required	Intervention may be required	Intervention often required
Spontaneous ventilation	Unaffected	Adequate	Maybe inadequate, O^2 supplementation	Frequently inadequate
Cardiovascular function	Unaffected	Usually maintained	Usually maintained	May be impaired
Drugs	Oral BZD alprazolam diazepam	i.v. midazolam/ flumazenil i.v. fentanyl/naloxone i.v. paracetamol/ NSAID	i.v. midazolam/flumazenil i.v. fentanyl/naloxone i.v. paracetamol/NSAID i.v.propofol	No need

duce vocal sounds upon request. Moderate sedation is achieved with a combined administration of i.v. midazolam and fentanyl.

Midazolam and fentanyl are preferred because they both have specific antagonists—flumazenil for the former and naloxone for the latter. All patients receive paracetamol as a follow-up to minimize post-operative pain.

Deep sedation is obtained with intravenous midazolam together with a 1-2 mg/kg/h. i.v. propofol infusion. In deep sedation with analgesia, patients have depressed consciousness with attenuation of reflexes and only respond to repeated and painful stimulation. Spontaneous breathing is sometimes inadequate, and oxygen supplementation may be needed. Unlike midazolam and fentanyl, propofol has no antagonists and must be gradually attenuated.

Many proceduralists follow a minimal sedation protocol under local anesthesia without the presence of an anesthetist. In this case, they can only perform simple routine ablations which limit their medical activity. Other clinics perform RFA procedures, where an anesthetist is not present but could be called in if a medical emergency occurs, usually within 15–20 min, so any immediate medical emergencies would have to be resolved by the RFA team.

In light of this shortcoming, it is suggested that RFAs are performed in an operating room setting with an anesthesiologist present. This obviously incurs additional costs, but it is well worth in terms of better patient management and protection against malpractice suits. Adopting a moderate sedation protocol combined with flexible fiberoptic laryngoscopy (FFL) and vocal cord ultrasound allows an excellent assessment of voice quality during ablation [44].

12.7 Ablation Procedure by RFA

After anesthesia has been administered and the hydrodissection needle has been withdrawn, the RFA needle electrode is inserted into the inferior portion of nodule, adjacent to the danger zone which has been isolated and protected by hydrodissection (Video 12.5).

Utilizing the so-called transisthmic approach, the needle is advanced through the thyroid isthmus into a thyroid nodule (Fig. 12.7). Entering the thyroid via the isthmus allows the creation of a buffer zone between the margin of the nodule and healthy thyroid tissue. This approach guarantees protection from skin burns and subcutaneous tissue overheating during ablation.

Ablation is initiated at the inferior part of nodule using the "moving shot" technique [18, 19]. Hyperechoic bubbles will appear around the electrode tip during ablation (Video 12.6).

Figure 12.8 shows a standard generator screen displaying several important parameters, such as

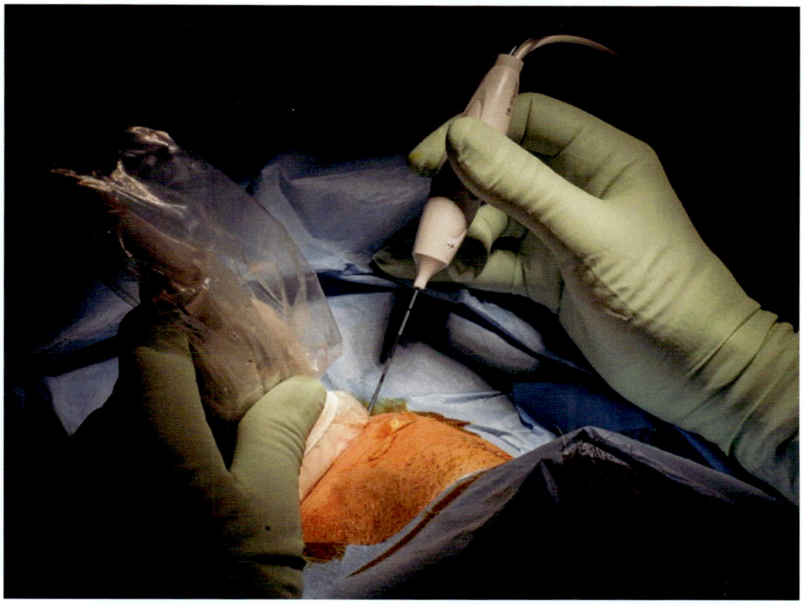

Fig. 12.7 Transisthmic approach for a left thyroid nodule ablation. The surgeon inserts an RFA needle electrode with the right hand, holding a Ultrasound linear probe with the left hand to visualize the needle. Hands must be interchanged when the nodule is in the right thyroid lobe. The patient's head is draped with blue surgical cloths

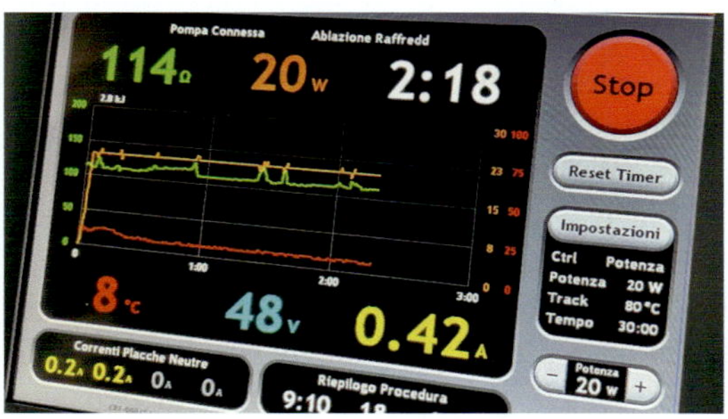

Fig. 12.8 Generator display

- Impedance (Ohms) which varies depending on tissue conductivity
- Power (Watts) which should be kept at a minimum to avoid tissue overheating and charring
- Duration of RFA (min/s)
- Temperature (C) of needle tip
- Tension (V)
- Current (Ampere)

Cooling the needle tip with cold saline is essential for dissipating heat inside the nodule. Circulating saline temperature is maintained at around 0 °C or even lower. However, when initially inserted, needle electrode temperature increases to 7–9 °C due to the temperature of surrounding tissue as seen in Fig. 12.8.

Using a standard exposed tip of 10 mm, the generator is initially set at a minimum value, i.e., 10–30 Watts and should never exceed 40. Using power settings higher than 40 Watts with an exposed tip of 10 mm runs the risk of boiling the liquid fraction of cells and carbonizing tissues.

Tissue temperature is measured by momentarily turning the circulation of saline coolant off and waiting 30–40 s until tissue temperature reaches and remains at a peak. This represents true tissue temperature during ablation. Tissue temperature readings should be taken at regular intervals during the procedure and should average around 60° which is optimal to obtain efficient tissue ablation [12]. Impedance peaks should be absolutely avoided as they are associated with excessive tissue heating and charring.

In order to visualize the needle electrode shaft, the ultrasound probe and needle must be perfectly aligned. Ablation starts at the lower portion of nodule, close to the danger zone, when hydrodissection protection of RLN is at a maximum (Video 12.7). As stated previously, this part of the nodule is ablated first before the hydrodissection diminishes, which usually lasts about 15–20 min and should be repeated if necessary. Ablation continues from the inferior portion to superior portion until the entire nodule has been ablated. For larger nodules, multiple needle electrode insertions and repositioning may be required to access superior portions of nodule.

Patients are usually moderately sedated so that they can respond to operator instructions and produce vocal sounds upon request. This is essential for monitoring vocal cord function and checking for any nerve damage especially to RLNs and EBSLNs.

Intraoperative Nerve Monitoring (IONM) is generally not feasible in thyroid RFA procedures because it requires intubation and general anesthesia [28]. Therefore, the gold standard for laryngeal motility assessment is Fiberoptic Fibro Laryngoscopy (FFL) [44].

FFL is preferably used for large and complex thyroid nodule ablations and for professional voice users such as singers, actors, and TV broadcasters where protection of RLNs and EBSLNs is of utmost importance. FFL is easily performed by an ENT specialist and well tolerated by patient.

FFL and vocal sounds produced by patient allow RLN and EBSLN assessment by visualizing of vocal cord symmetrical movements. Should vocal cord asymmetry appear during RFA, the procedure is immediately stopped and hydrodissection with cold D5W is performed. Video 12.8 shows how intraoperative FFL is performed. After moderate sedation and analgesia with fentanyl and midazolam, the endoscope is inserted and progressed until glottic plane. Through FFL monitoring, vocal cord symmetrical movements during calm breathing can be observed. A series of post-operative FFLs are performed on patients after RFAs in order to confirm normal vocal cord symmetric adduction during phonation and abduction during breathing.

In order to assess vocal cord function during an RFA procedure, patients are asked to produce vocal sounds. For instance, they are asked to pronounce "eee" at several intervals at different volumes and pitch. This, accompanied by US imaging, is an excellent technique to monitor normal symmetrical vocal cord movement.

Video 12.9 illustrates how to locate the vocal cords utilizing US and the thyroid cartilage notch as an anatomical reference. The glottic plane is about 5–11 mm below this notch which varies based on body size and gender. Contemporarily in Video 12.10, ultrasound images of vocal cords can be observed during the pronunciation of the "eee" sound. In order to alternatively monitor nodule ablation and vocal cord movements by US, the proceduralist must slide the probe back and forth from nodule to glottic plane.

Videos 12.11, 12.12, and 12.13 demonstrate ocal cord monitoring during an RFA procedure. In Video 12.11, the proceduralist asks the patient to pronounce "eee" while ablating the nodule and positioning the US probe over the glottic plane.

Video 12.12 shows US imaging of vocal cords moving symmetrically. The same movements can be observed by FFL in Video 12.13. Using these techniques provides thorough vocal cord monitoring and helps the proceduralist in detecting any foreseeable damage to adjacent nervous structures.

Post-operative therapy includes compression and ice for 30–60 min to minimize bruising and postprocedural hematoma (Fig. 12.9). Intravenous 1 g paracetamol infusion is administered to alleviate pain while 40 mg methylprednisolone is administered to reduce swelling and inflammation.

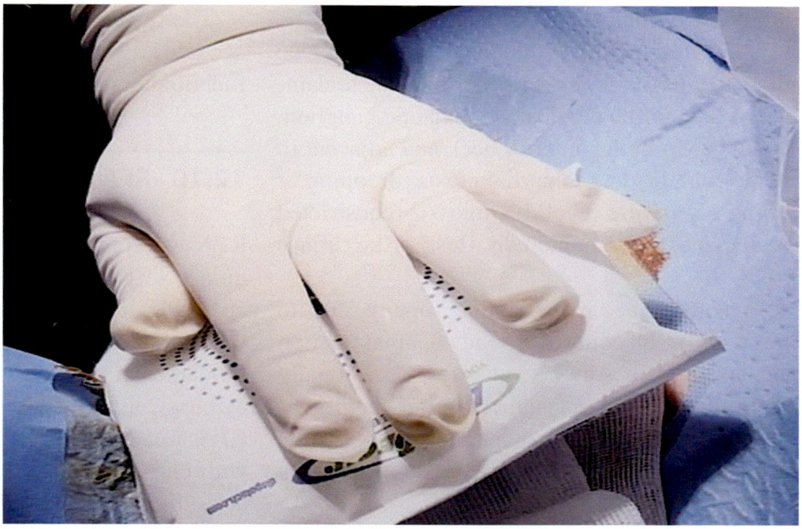

Fig. 12.9 Ice pack and pressure post-RFA procedure

Table 12.2 Post-RFA follow-up scheme

		Test						
Time	TSH	fT3	fT4	Ab TPO	Ab Tg	Tg	Tr Ab	Ultrasound
Day 1	√	√	√	√	√	If indicated	If indicated	√
Month 1	√	√	v	√	√	If indicated	If indicated	√
Month 6	√	If indicated	If indicated	√	√	If indicated	If indicated	√
Month 12	√	If indicated	If indicated	√	√	If indicated	If indicated	√
Year 2	√	If indicated	If indicated	√	√	If indicated	If indicated	√
Yearly	√	If indicated	If indicated	If indicated	If indicated	If indicated	If indicated	√

12.8 Informed Patient Consent

An informed patient consent is a fundamental component in determining the appropriate therapeutic strategy for dealing with thyroid ablative procedures.

For RFAs, as in any thyroid ablative procedure, patients should be fully informed of all clinical aspects such as therapeutic risks, recovery time, advantages and disadvantages, predictable outcomes, and limitations.

Specific to RFA, any discussion should center around the degree of expected volume reduction [14, 27] and possibility of regrowth for larger nodules [14] which may require additional RFAs or other therapies, perhaps even surgery.

Even if complications and recovery times are lower for RFA than for surgery [23], procedural risks and predictable outcomes should be presented and fully explained to the patient.

First among the risks and predictable outcomes is the fact that RFA often reduces but does not completely eliminate the nodule; therefore, the patient should be aware that a commitment to long-term follow-up treatment may be necessary.

Patients are always examined by ultrasound the day after RFA. Successive follow-ups are carried out at 1 month, 6 months, 1 year, and then yearly. During these follow-ups, thyroid function and antibodies are assessed. A typical follow-up scheme is seen in Table 12.2.

There is a series of infrequent but not negligible complications and side effects that should be explained to RFA patients [45, 46]. Among these, is the possibility of injury to neck nerves leading to various symptoms. These may include hoarseness, changes in voice projection, tone and pitch, tachycardia and abnormal heart rhythm, low blood pressure, vomiting, arm numbness and paralysis, drooping shoulder, hiccups, etc. [33, 34]. In addition, particular attention should be given to the risk of Horner syndrome due to damage of the middle cervical sympathetic ganglion, located deep in the anterior neck and adjacent to the thyroid, leading to partial ptosis (drooping or falling of upper eyelid), miosis (constricted pupil), and facial anhidrosis (loss of sweating) [45, 46].

In some rare cases, nodule rupture due to intranodular bleeding can lead to inflammation and swelling in soft neck tissues, occasionally requiring surgical management [47]. Other minor complications include hematomas, superficial skin burns, coughing, vomiting, and other globus sensations [30].

Operative- and post-operative pain and general discomfort in areas around the neck such as the ear, mouth, and teeth experienced during and after the procedure can be mitigated by administration of local anesthesia during the procedure and analgesics after the procedure.

Overall RFA is well tolerated by the patient.

12.9 Outcomes of RFA Procedures

RFA is a suitable alternative to surgery for benign thyroid nodules. Nodule shrinkage is gradual following ablation. Post-operative inflammation may increase nodule volume from 0 to 20% in the first week. Maximal volume reduction is obtained after the first 6 months. Smaller-volume reductions may continue for up to 2–3 years. A recent meta-analysis by Cesareo et al. [36] reported volume reduction rates of 64.5% at 6 months, 76.9% at 12 months, and 92.2% at 36 months.

Just as important but more difficult to quantify, RFA has been reported to be highly effective at reducing symptomatic issues and improving cosmetic aspects and quality of life in thyroid nodule patients [27, 49–51]. A study by Deandrea et al. [22] on 215 patients found an overall average VRR of 67%; however, nodules smaller than 10 mL achieved a greater reduction of 79% VRR at 1 year and 81% at 5 years.

The relation between nodule size and shrinkage rate is especially confirmed for autonomously functioning nodules [42, 43].

12.10 RFA Training

RFA is considered an advanced ultrasound-guided technique. In order to exploit RFA therapy, proceduralists and medical operators in general should be fully aware of the crucial and fundamental role of diagnosis with US and FNA cytology in determining suitability for thyroid RFA treatment. Operators should be familiar with clinical thyroidology, general, radiological, and ultrasound neck anatomy. A complete knowledge of nervous and vascular structures is fundamental. An understanding of sedation and local anesthesia is also required. Operators should also be able to carry out fine-needle aspiration cytology and core needle biopsy and be able to assess vocal cord movements by US and in some cases perform FFL.

Various educational bodies such as university medical schools, thyroid scientific associations, and individual expert practitioners may offer an array of RFA training opportunities. Training courses and programs sponsored and organized by the above-mentioned groups allow individuals to practice on phantom models in order to learn and perfect RFA techniques. One such phantom technique for thyroid RFA training is the soft-boiled quail egg model as used by the TNT Association in their RFA professional courses [52].

References

1. Dean DS, Gharib H. Epidemiology of thyroid nodules. Baillieres Best Pract Res Clin Endocrinol Metab. 2008;22(6):901–11. https://doi.org/10.1016/j.beem.2008.09.019.
2. Gharib H, Papini E, Garber JR, Duick DS, Harrell RM, Hegedus L, et al. American association of clinical endocrinologists, American college of endocrinology, and associazione Medici endocrinologi medical guidelines for clinical practice for the diagnosis and management of thyroid nodules—2016 update

appendix. Endocr Pract. 2016;22:1–60. https://doi.org/10.4158/ep161208.gl.
3. Meltzer C, Hull M, Sundang A, Adams JL. Association between annual surgeon total thyroidectomy volume and transient and permanent complications. JAMA. Otolaryngol Head Neck Surg. 2019;145(9):830. https://jamanetwork.com/journals/jamaotolaryngology/fullarticle/2739223.
4. Sosa JA, Hanna JW, Robinson KA, Lanman RB. Increases in thyroid nodule fine-needle aspirations, operations, and diagnoses of thyroid cancer in the United States. Surgery. 2013;154(6):1420–7. https://doi.org/10.1016/j.surg.2013.07.006.
5. Orloff LA, Noel JE, Stack BC Jr, Russell MD, Angelos P, Baek JH, et al. Radiofrequency ablation and related ultrasound-guided ablation technologies for treatment of benign and malignant thyroid disease: an international multidisciplinary consensus statement of the American Head and Neck Society Endocrine Surgery Section with the Asia Pacific Society of Thyroid Surgery, Associazione Medici Endocrinologi, British Association of Endocrine and Thyroid Surgeons, European Thyroid Association, Italian Society of Endocrine Surgery Units, Korean Society of Thyroid Radiology, Latin American Thyroid Society, and Thyroid Nodules Therapies Association. Head Neck. 2022;44(3):633–60. https://doi.org/10.1002/hed.26960.
6. Ahn D, Sohn JH, Jeon JH. Hypothyroidism following hemithyroidectomy: incidence, risk factors, and clinical characteristics. J Clin Endocrinol Metab. 2016;101(4):1429–36. https://doi.org/10.1210/jc.2015-3997.
7. Ha EJ, Chung SR, Na DG, Ahn HS, Chung J, Lee JY, et al. 2021 Korean thyroid imaging reporting and data system and imaging-based management of thyroid nodules: Korean society of thyroid radiology consensus statement and recommendations. Korean J Radiol. 2021;22(12):2094. https://doi.org/10.3348/kjr.2021.0713.
8. Papini E, Monpeyssen H, Frasoldati A, Hegedüs L. 2020 European thyroid association clinical practice guideline for the use of image-guided ablation in benign thyroid nodules. Eur Thyroid J. 2020;9(4):172–85. https://doi.org/10.1159/000508484.
9. Haugen BR, Alexander EK, Bible KC, Doherty GM, Mandel SJ, Nikiforov YE, et al. 2015 American thyroid association management guidelines for adult patients with thyroid nodules and differentiated thyroid cancer: the American thyroid association guidelines task force on thyroid nodules and differentiated thyroid cancer. Thyroid. 2016;26(1):1–133. https://doi.org/10.1089/thy.2015.0020.
10. Cheng Z, Liang P. Advances in ultrasound-guided thermal ablation for symptomatic benign thyroid nodules. Adv Clin Exp Med. 2020;29(9):1123–9. https://doi.org/10.17219/acem/125433.
11. Chu KF, Dupuy DE. Thermal ablation of tumours: biological mechanisms and advances in therapy. Nat Rev Cancer. 2014;14(3):199–208. https://doi.org/10.1038/nrc3672.
12. Kok HP, Cressman ENK, Ceelen W, Brace CL, Ivkov R, Grüll H, et al. Heating technology for malignant tumors: a review. Int J Hyperth. 2020;37(1):711–41. https://doi.org/10.1080/02656736.2020.1779357.
13. Cho SJ, Baek JH, Chung SR, Choi YJ, Lee JH. Long-term results of thermal ablation of benign thyroid nodules: a systematic review and meta-analysis. Endocrinol Metab (Seoul). 2020;35(2):339–50. https://doi.org/10.3803/enm.2020.35.2.339.
14. Sim JS, Baek JH. Long-term outcomes following thermal ablation of benign thyroid nodules as an alternative to surgery: the importance of controlling regrowth. Endocrinol Metab (Seoul). 2019;34(2):117. https://doi.org/10.3803/enm.2019.34.2.117.
15. Jin H, Fan J, Lu L, Cui M. A propensity score matching study between microwave ablation and radiofrequency ablation in terms of safety and efficacy for benign thyroid nodules treatment. Front Endocrinol (Lausanne). 2021;12:12. https://doi.org/10.3389/fendo.2021.584972.
16. Jin X, Feng Y, Zhu R, Qian L, Yang Y, Yu Q, et al. Temperature control and intermittent time-set protocol optimization for minimizing tissue carbonization in microwave ablation. Int J Hyperth. 2022;39(1):868–79. https://doi.org/10.1080/02656736.2022.2075041.
17. Kotewall N, Lang BHH. High-intensity focused ultrasound ablation as a treatment for benign thyroid diseases: the present and future. Ultrasonography. 2019;38(2):135–42. https://doi.org/10.14366/usg.18040.
18. Kim Y-S, Rhim H, Tae K, Park DW, Kim ST. Radiofrequency ablation of benign cold thyroid nodules: initial clinical experience. Thyroid. 2006;16(4):361–7. https://doi.org/10.1089/thy.2006.16.361.
19. Kim JH, Baek JH, Lim HK, et al. Guideline Committee for the Korean Society of Thyroid Radiology (KSThR) and Korean Society of Radiology. Thyroid radiofrequency ablation guideline: Korean Society of Thyroid Radiology. Korean J Radiol. 2017;19(4):632–55. https://doi.org/10.3348/kjr.2018.19.4.632.
20. Garberoglio R, Aliberti C, Appetecchia M, Attard M, Boccuzzi G, Boraso F, et al. Radiofrequency ablation for thyroid nodules: which indications? The first Italian opinion statement. J Ultrasound. 2015;18(4):423–30. https://doi.org/10.1007/s40477-015-0169-y.
21. Wang N, Zheng B, Wu T, Tan L, Lian Y, Ma Y, et al. Thyroid dysfunction following radiofrequency ablation for benign thyroid nodules: more likely to occur within one-week and in high-risk population. Int J Hyperth. 2021;38(1):1060–8. https://doi.org/10.1080/02656736.2021.1950849.
22. Deandrea M, Sung JY, Limone P, Mormile A, Garino F, Ragazzoni F, et al. Efficacy and safety of radiofrequency ablation versus observation for nonfunctioning benign thyroid nodules: a randomized controlled international collaborative trial.

Thyroid. 2015;25(8):890–6. https://doi.org/10.1089/thy.2015.0133.
23. Jung SL, Baek JH, Lee JH, Shong YK, Sung JY, Kim KS, et al. Efficacy and safety of radiofrequency ablation for benign thyroid nodules: a prospective multicenter study. Korean J Radiol. 2018;19(1):167. https://doi.org/10.3348/kjr.2018.19.1.167.
24. Kuo JH, McManus C, Lee JA. Analyzing the adoption of radiofrequency ablation of thyroid nodules using the diffusion of innovations theory: understanding where we are in the United States? Ultrasonography. 2022;41(1):25–33. https://doi.org/10.14366/usg.21117.
25. Jasim S, Patel KN, Randolph G, Adams S, Cesareo R, Condon E, et al. American association of clinical endocrinology disease state clinical review: the clinical utility of minimally invasive interventional procedures in the management of benign and malignant thyroid lesions. Endocr Pract. 2022;28(4):433–48. https://doi.org/10.1016/j.eprac.2022.02.011.
26. Che Y, Jin S, Shi C, Wang L, Zhang X, Li Y, et al. Treatment of benign thyroid nodules: comparison of surgery with radiofrequency ablation. AJNR Am J Neuroradiol. 2015;36(7):1321–5. https://doi.org/10.3174/ajnr.a4276.
27. Valcavi R, Tsamatropoulos P. Health-related quality of life after percutaneous radiofrequency ablation of cold, solid, benign thyroid nodules: a 2-year follow-up study in 40 patients. Endocr Pract. 2015;21(8):887–96. https://doi.org/10.4158/ep15676.or.
28. Sinclair CF, Téllez MJ, Peláez-Cruz R, Díaz-Baamonde A, Ulkatan S. Continuous neuromonitoring during radiofrequency ablation of benign thyroid nodules provides objective evidence of laryngeal nerve safety. Am J Surg. 2021;222(2):354–60. https://doi.org/10.1016/j.amjsurg.2020.12.033.
29. Randolph GW, Wu C-W, Dionigi G, Kamani D, Modi RR, Chiang F-Y, et al. The international RLN anatomic classification system. In: The recurrent and superior laryngeal nerves. Cham: Springer International Publishing; 2016. p. 125–38. https://doi.org/10.1007/978-3-319-27727-1_12.
30. Baek JH, Lee JH, Sung JY, Bae J-I, Kim KT, Sim J, et al. Complications encountered in the treatment of benign thyroid nodules with US-guided radiofrequency ablation: a multicenter study. Radiology. 2012;262(1):335–42. https://doi.org/10.1148/radiol.11110416.
31. Jeong SY, Baek JH, Chung SR, Choi YJ, Chung K-W, Kim TY, et al. Radiofrequency ablation of benign thyroid nodules: the value of anterolateral hydrodissection. Ultrasonography. 2023;42(3):432–9. https://doi.org/10.14366/usg.23017.
32. Ma Y, Wu T, Yao Z, Zheng B, Tan L, Tong G, et al. Continuous, large-volume hydrodissection to protect delicate structures around the thyroid throughout the radiofrequency ablation procedure. Eur Thyroid J. 2021;10(6):495–503. https://doi.org/10.1159/000519625.
33. Ha EJ, Baek JH, Lee JH. Ultrasonography-based thyroidal and perithyroidal anatomy and its clinical significance. Korean J Radiol. 2015;16(4):749. https://doi.org/10.3348/kjr.2015.16.4.749.
34. Chung SR, Baek JH, Choi YJ, Lee JH. Management strategy for nerve damage during radiofrequency ablation of thyroid nodules. Int J Hyperth. 2019;36(1):203–9. https://doi.org/10.1080/02656736.2018.1554826.
35. Kim JY, Jung SL, Kim MK, Kim T-J, Byun JY. Differentiation of benign and malignant thyroid nodules based on the proportion of sponge-like areas on ultrasonography: imaging-pathologic correlation. Ultrasonography. 2015;34(4):304–11. https://doi.org/10.14366/usg.15016.
36. Cesareo R, Egiddi S, Naciu AM, Tabacco G, Leoncini A, Napoli N, et al. Efficacy of radiofrequency and laser thermal ablation in solving thyroid nodule-related symptoms and cosmetic concerns. A systematic review and meta-analysis. Rev Endocr Metab Disord. 2022;23(5):1051–61. https://doi.org/10.1007/s11154-022-09743-8.
37. Lee M, Baek JH, Suh CH, Chung SR, Choi YJ, Lee JH, et al. Clinical practice guidelines for radiofrequency ablation of benign thyroid nodules: a systematic review. Ultrasonography. 2021;40(2):256–64. https://doi.org/10.14366/usg.20015.
38. Lang BHH, Fung MMH. Safety and efficacy of single-session radiofrequency ablation treatment for benign non-toxic multinodular goiter. World J Surg. 2022;46(7):1704–10. https://doi.org/10.1007/s00268-022-06527-8.
39. Chiang P-L, Lin W-C, Chen H-L, Luo S-D, Chen M-H, Chen W-C, et al. Efficacy and safety of single-session radiofrequency ablation for intrathoracic goiter: preliminary results and short-term evaluation. Int J Hyperth. 2021;38(1):976–84. https://doi.org/10.1080/02656736.2021.1942241.
40. Junior AR, Volpi EM, Schmid BP, Falsarella PM, Garcia RG. The iceberg technique: an innovative approach for radiofrequency ablation of diving thyroid nodules. Diagn Interv Radiol. 2023;29(4):628–31. https://doi.org/10.4274/dir.2022.221467.
41. Hussain I, Zulfiqar F, Li X, Ahmad S, Aljammal J. Safety and efficacy of radiofrequency ablation of thyroid nodules—expanding treatment options in the United States. J Endocr Soc. 2021;5(8):bvab110. https://doi.org/10.1210/jendso/bvab110.
42. Cesareo R, Palermo A, Pasqualini V, Manfrini S, Trimboli P, Stacul F, et al. Radiofrequency ablation on autonomously functioning thyroid nodules: a critical appraisal and review of the literature. Front Endocrinol (Lausanne). 2020;11:11. https://doi.org/10.3389/fendo.2020.00317.
43. Baek JH, Moon W-J, Kim YS, Lee JH, Lee D. Radiofrequency ablation for the treatment of autonomously functioning thyroid nodules. World J Surg. 2009;33(9):1971–7. https://doi.org/10.1007/s00268-009-0130-3.

44. Valcavi R, Gaino F, Novizio R, Mercante G. Vocal cord monitoring by flexible fiberoptic laryngoscopy during thyroid radiofrequency ablation. VideoEndocrinology. 2023;10(3):41–3. https://doi.org/10.1089/ve.2023.0012.
45. Lim JY, Kuo JH. Thyroid nodule radiofrequency ablation: complications and clinical follow up. Tech Vasc Interv Radiol. 2022;25(2):100824. https://doi.org/10.1016/j.tvir.2022.100824.
46. Issa PP, Cironi K, Rezvani L, Kandil E. Radiofrequency ablation of thyroid nodules: a clinical review of treatment complications. Gland Surg. 2024;13(1):77–86. https://doi.org/10.21037/gs-22-539.
47. Chung SR, Baek JH, Sung JY, Ryu JH, Jung SL. Revisiting rupture of benign thyroid nodules after radiofrequency ablation: various types and imaging features. Endocrinol Metab (Seoul). 2019;34(4):415. https://doi.org/10.3803/enm.2019.34.4.415.
48. Bernardi S, Giudici F, Cesareo R, Antonelli G, Cavallaro M, Deandrea M, et al. Five-year results of radiofrequency and laser ablation of benign thyroid nodules: a multicenter study from the Italian minimally invasive treatments of the thyroid group. Thyroid. 2020;30(12):1759–70. https://doi.org/10.1089/thy.2020.0202.
49. Jeong SY, Ha EJ, Baek JH, Kim TY, Lee Y-M, Lee JH, et al. Assessment of thyroid-specific quality of life in patients with benign symptomatic thyroid nodules treated with radiofrequency or ethanol ablation: a prospective multicenter study. Ultrasonography. 2022;41(1):204–11. https://doi.org/10.14366/usg.21003.
50. Jawad S, Morley S, Otero S, Beale T, Bandula S. Ultrasound-guided radiofrequency ablation (RFA) of benign symptomatic thyroid nodules—initial UK experience. Br J Radiol. 2019;92:20190026. https://doi.org/10.1259/bjr.20190026.
51. Cesareo R, Pasqualini V, Simeoni C, Sacchi M, Saralli E, Campagna G, et al. Prospective study of effectiveness of ultrasound-guided radiofrequency ablation versus control group in patients affected by benign thyroid nodules. J Clin Endocrinol Metab. 2015;100(2):460–6. https://doi.org/10.1210/jc.2014-2186.
52. Valcavi R, Gaino F, Mercante G. Soft-boiled quail egg: phantom model for thyroid radiofrequency ablation training. Video Endocrinol. 2023;10(4):29. https://doi.org/10.1089/ve.2023.002.

Radiofrequency Ablation for Autonomously Functioning Thyroid Nodules

13

Jules Aljammal and Juan Pablo Dueñas

13.1 Introduction

Thyroid nodules are quite common, with a prevalence of up to 60% in the general population when imaging is used [1]. In 1913, Henry Plummer was the first to describe toxic multinodular goiter (TMNG) and distinguish it from Graves' disease, and then in 1918, Emil Goetsch was the first to distinguish the subgroup of autonomous functioning thyroid nodule (AFTN) from TMNG [2]. Almost 10% of all thyroid nodules are AFTN [3]. They can be symptomatic either due to their size, location, or over secretion of thyroid hormone, approximately 75% of AFTN will have suppressed TSH [4].

Over the years, our understanding for AFTN has evolved, and new data suggest the lack of size cut off to predict thyroid nodule toxicity, as it has been reported that nodules as small as 0.8 mL or even smaller can exhibit toxicity [5].

This may indicate that different nodules have different capacities to oversecrete thyroid hormone related to internal factors, rendering some nodules to be more capable to make and release thyroid hormone compared to others, regardless of size. Conversely, even nodules with minimal thyroid hormone-producing capacity can become significant as they grow. It is noted that these nodules may gradually progress to subclinical hyperthyroidism and hyperthyroidism at a rate of approximately 4% per year, particularly in older patients, nodules with a maximum diameter exceeding 3 cm, and individuals residing in iodine-deficient areas [6].

AFTN is the third most common cause of hyperthyroidism, following Graves' disease and TMNG [7]. Different therapeutical strategies are employed to achieve biochemical control, including the use of antithyroid drugs, radioactive iodine (RAI), or surgery.

AFTNs necessitate definitive treatment; however, certain patients may not be suitable candidates for RAI or surgery, or these options may not always be acceptable to patients [8]. New technologies are now available, among these is ultrasound-guided radiofrequency ablation (RFA-US), a minimally invasive technique with promising efficacy in such cases [9]. Compared to RAI, RFA-US is particularly recommended for young patients due to its avoidance of radiation exposure and lower risk of hypothyroidism. And more importantly, studies have demonstrated that RFA-US achieves comparable max volume reduction (MVR) and higher biochemical control [10].

J. Aljammal (✉)
American Diplomat of Endocrinology and Metabolism, The Thyroid Clinic Utah, Salt Lake City, UT, USA
e-mail: Aljammal@thyroidclinicutah.com

J. P. Dueñas
Integral Endocrine Surgery Clinic, Medellín, Colombia
e-mail: jpduenas@cirendocrina.com

R. Valcavi et al. (eds.), *Thyroid Ablation*, https://doi.org/10.1007/978-3-031-88229-6_13

13.2 Indications and Background

Numerous scientific societies have proposed guidelines and recommendations addressing the indications of RFA-US for treating thyroid nodules. In fact, the Korean Society of Thyroid Radiology (KSThR) was the first organization to provide initial recommendations for this type of treatment. Currently, there are several statements from different organizations [11–19]. Some of these recommendations advocate thermal ablation for toxic or pre-toxic nodules, cautioning that larger AFTN (>20 mL) may exhibit reduced responsiveness [11, 12]. The majority of these guidelines suggest that RFA-US can be considered a safe alternative when primary treatment (such as surgery or RAI) is contraindicated [14, 16, 17, 20]. European guidelines [15], in particular, discourage the use of RFA-US as a first-line treatment for large AFTN and recommend it instead for young patients with small AFTN.

The first documented successful treatment of AFTN was by Deandrea et al., and they described treatment of 22 patients with hyperfunctioning thyroid nodule and 5 patients achieved euthyroid state [21]. Since that publication, an increasing number of studies have been published.

As part of the preprocedural evaluation of thyroid nodules, it is recommended to include the assessment of symptoms, cosmetic concerns, US examination, scintigraphy to confirm the presence of an AFTN, and at least one fine-needle aspiration cytology (FNAC) to evaluate for presence of malignancy, along with a comprehensive thyroid profile including evaluation for Graves' antibodies. The utilization of RFA-US in this context is expanding globally [22].

13.3 Outcomes

13.3.1 Predictors of Response

RFA-US has demonstrated both safety and effectiveness in attaining biochemical control in AFTN. Factors that may predict achieving a euthyroid state through this procedure include a small pretreatment nodule volume (<12 mL) [23], and achieving a volume reduction greater than or equal to 80% [24]. The rate of normalization of thyroid function is markedly higher in small nodules (86% compared to 45% in medium-sized nodules) [25].

In addition, AFTN capacity to oversecrete thyroid hormone may predict success as data show nodules with subclinical hyperthyroidism have higher success rate compared to nodules with overt hyperthyroidism [26], and full ablation of the AFTN leading to complete devascularization is essential to achieve that goal [21] (Fig. 13.1).

Amount of energy delivered was recently evaluated by Van der Meeren et al. [27]. Their study demonstrated that a cure was achieved in 91% of patients when >2.1 kJ/mL was delivered during RFA, in contrast to 44% when a lower amount of energy was administered, the study also noted that treatment to be three times more likely to be successful when treating single toxic adenoma compared to toxic multinodular goiter.

13.3.2 Efficacy

Numerous studies have described MVR in AFTN ranging from 36 to 99.5%, with a resolution of hyperthyroidism reported between 23 and 94.1% [9, 28, 29]. This variability is likely attributable to the initial size of the nodule, and technical methods are used. These studies have shown that euthyroid state is achievable for long term (Fig. 13.2).

Figure 13.2 represents progression of toxic nodule post RFA treatment with long-term follow-up.

Occasionally repeat treatment of large toxic thyroid nodules is needed (Fig. 13.3). The associated video link represents the first UG-RFA of the first treatment of this large toxic thyroid nodule.

Figure 13.3 represents left toxic adenoma needing two treatments to achieve normal thyroid function test.

Efficacy of RFA has been analyzed in few meta-analysis. The first review, conducted by Cesareo et al. [29], encompassed eight relevant studies focusing on RFA-US for autonomous or

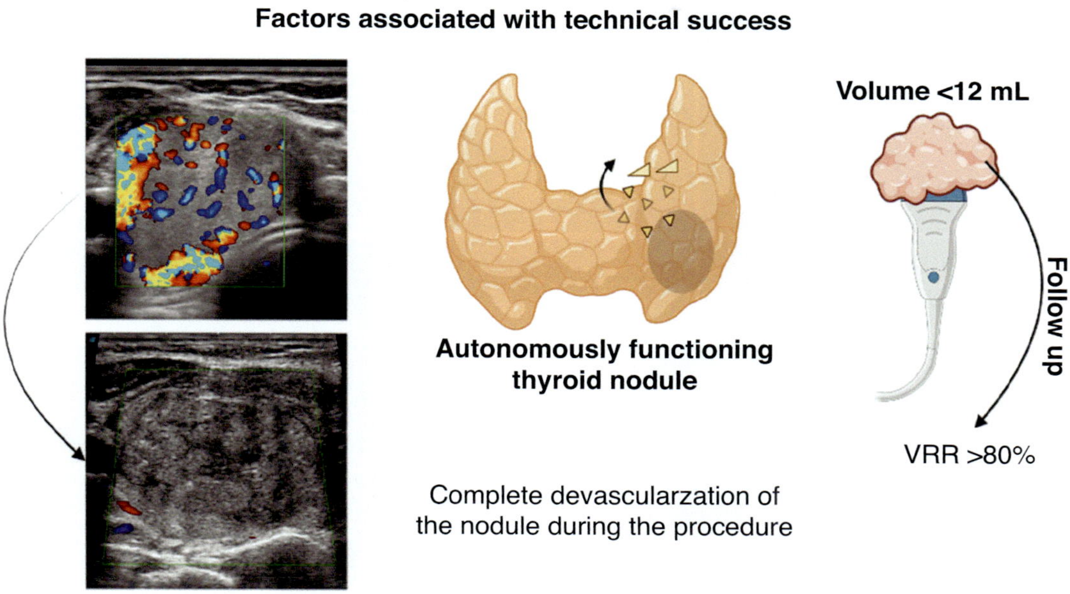

Fig. 13.1 Factors associated with technical success

toxic thyroid nodules. Among these, six studies had a prospective design, while two were retrospective. None of the included studies were clinical trials. The total number of AFTNs included in the analysis was 205, with a maximum follow-up period of 24 months.

It is worth noting that 37.5% of the studies, mainly early studies, employed a fixed electrode technique for RFA, which is not the current accepted technique (i.e., the moving shot technique). In the three studies using the fixed electrode technique, highest rate of achieving normal thyroid function was 53.5% with MVR of 77% at 12 months.

On the other hand, studies utilizing the moving shot technique achieved more than 80% TSH normalization and also reported MVR greater than 80% at 12 months. These findings highlight the possible impact of used technique on achieving biochemical control [30].

More recently Kim et al. [9] in their systematic review examined a total of 14 studies, with four of them utilizing laser ablation (LA) and ten utilizing RFA. Among the LA group, only one study achieved a TSH level in more than 80% of the cases, this study also achieved MVR greater than 80%. In contrast, among the ten studies in the RFA group, four of them achieved a normalized TSH level greater than 80% with MVR exceeding 70%. Notably, the ten studies included in the RFA group also encompassed the three studies that employed the fixed electrode technique, which were described and analyzed in the previous meta-analysis.

13.3.3 Safety

This procedure is considered safe, with retrospective studies indicating a lower risk of hypothyroidism [9]. This observation holds true for both surgical interventions [31] and RAI [10]. It is important to note that the risk of permanent hypothyroidism with RAI can be as high as 49%, and it may manifest several years after treatment [32].

Research on RFA has revealed a minimal risk of complications (2.7%), mostly restricted to temporary changes in voice, with no documented cases of post-procedural hypothyroidism or hypocalcemia [33]. Only a few isolated instances of complications have been found by systematic reviews addressing this outcome. One review documented that a patient experienced voice

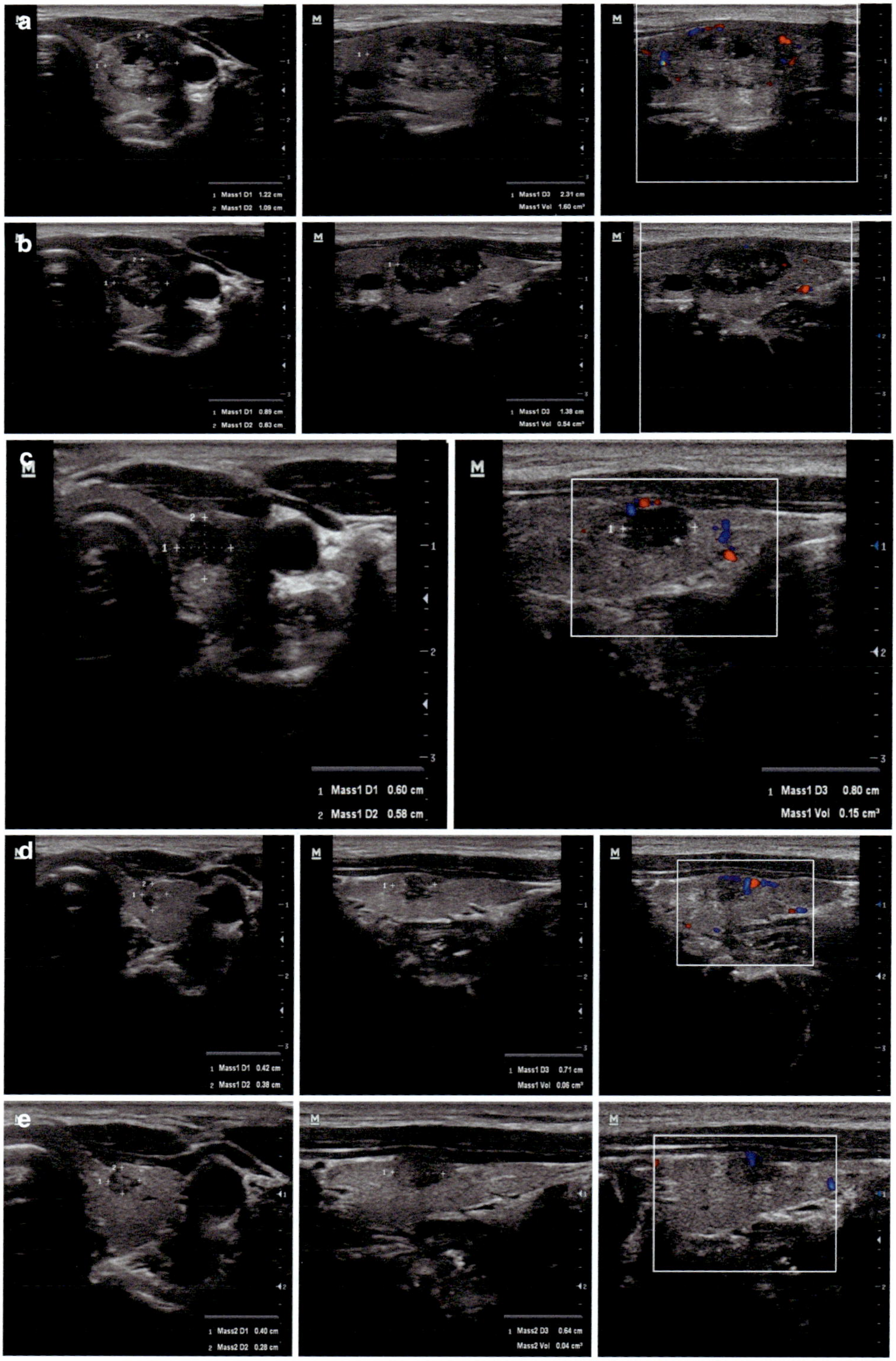

Fig. 13.2 (**a**) A 53-year-old female with toxic left thyroid nodule and atrial fibrillation, negative TSI, TRAB before treatment with localized uptake and scan, TSH level 0.17, FT4 level 1.01 initial volume 1.6 cc. (Courtesy of Jules Aljammal, MD). (**b**) Six weeks post ablation. TSH 0.67, FT4 1.0. (**c**) Six-month post ablation TSH 0.67, FT 0.95, 90% VR. (**d**) One year and half post ablation TSH 0.67, FT4 0.96, 96% VR. (**e**) Two years and half post ablation TSH 0.63, 97.5% VR

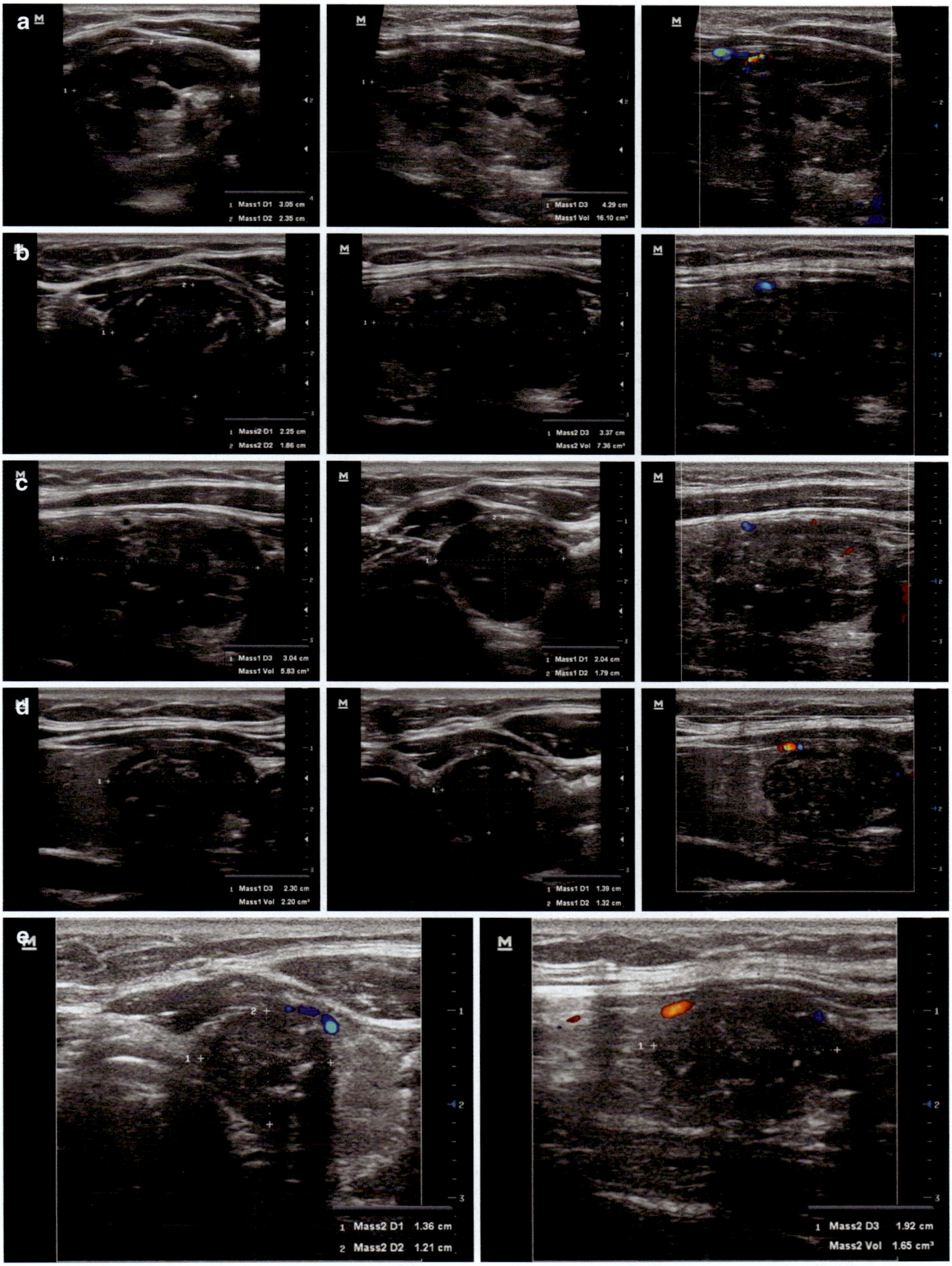

Fig. 13.3 (**a**) 33-year-old female with left toxic nodule, negative TRAB, localized activity on uptake on scan 24 h uptake 49%, TSH 0.007, FT4 1.32 initial volume 16.1 cc. (Courtesy of Jules Aljammal, MD). (**b**) Three months follow-up, TSH 0.009, FT4 0.97, 55% VR. (**c**) Six months follow-up, TSH 0.07, FT4 1.05, 64% VR, note persistent blood flow in the inferior portion of the nodule. (**d**) Six weeks follow-up post second treatment with RFA 8 months post first treatment, TSH 3.54, FT4 0.75, 86% VR. (**e**) Eight months follow-up post second RFA. TSH 2.34, FT4 0.96, 90% VR

changes that resolved within 1 month [9], while another review reported only one case of transient voice change and four cases of minor complications (out of 254 patients who underwent RFA, three experienced neck edema and one had a transient hematoma). These findings collectively support the favorable safety profile of the RFA procedure.

Table 13.1 provides a summary of the main studies conducted on RFA-US for the treatment of AFTNs.

Table 13.1 Main studies on RFA-US for AFTN

Author/year	Population/design	Results	Conclusions
Wang et al. [6] 2023	About 51 patients with AFTN confirmed by ^{99mTc}pertechnetate scintigraphy showing hot nodule with benign diagnoses in two separate FNA. The groups were separated into nontoxic and toxic, according to their thyroid function status Retrospective study	Median follow-up period of 18 months. 31 were nontoxic, and 20 toxic nodules before ablation. The MVR was 96.3% and 88.3% for the respective groups, while the rates of achieving euthyroid state were 93.5% and 75%. There were no significant differences observed in ablation technical efficacy between RFA (68.2%) and MWA (71.4%) ($p = 1.000$). However, it is worth noting that RFA was the chosen ablation technique in 86.3% of the included patients	Image-guided thermal ablation is efficacious and safe in treating AFTN, both nontoxic and toxic. It would be helpful to recognize nontoxic AFTN for treatment
Mauri et al. [35] 2022	About 361 patients treated with single thermal ablation for an AFTN Retrospective multicenter study	MVR was 58% at 6 months and 60% at 12 months. Antithyroid therapy was withdrawn in 32.5% of patients at 2 months, in 38.9% at 6 months, and in 41.3% at 12 months. A significant inverse relationship was observed in the rate of patients who withdrawn medical therapy based on nodule volume	Image-guided thermal ablation offers a further safe and effective therapeutic option in patients with AFTN. Clinical outcomes are more favorable in small AFTN
Vu et al. [28] 2022	Seventeen patients with AFTNs treated by RFA Prospective study	At 24 months after the procedure, the MVR was 95.65%. All 17 patients were restored euthyroid state	RFA was demonstrated as a safe and effective option for AFTN treatment
Kim et al. [9] 2021	About 411 patients with AFTNs treated by thermal ablation in 391 patients in 14 studies. Systematic review and meta-analysis	TSH normalization was achieved in 71.2% of patients, and the MVR was 69.4% at a mean follow-up period of 12.8 months. There was no significant difference in TSH normalization or MVR according to nodule volume	Thermal ablation is an effective and safe treatment method for patients with AFTNs. No patients experienced hypothyroidism or a life-threatening complication

(continued)

Table 13.1 (continued)

Author/year	Population/design	Results	Conclusions
Hussain et al. [26] 2021	About 24 patients with AFTN with overt hyperthyroidism or subclinical hyperthyroidism with symptoms and/or risk factors for adverse outcomes Retrospective, single center study	The MVR for nodules with an initial volume less than 5 mL was 75.2%, while for nodules larger than 20 mL was 50.4%. The thyroid function test showed significant improvement, although three patients were still taking methimazole at the last follow-up. Based on the baseline volume, euthyroid state was achieved in 100% of patients with nodules smaller than 10 mL, 66% for nodules between 10 mL and 20 mL, and 25% for nodules larger than 20 mL	The MVR had an inverse relationship with the volume of the nodule. It is especially effective for smaller AFTNs
Cappelli et al. [36] 2020	Seventeen patients with AFTN Retrospective	The mean pretreatment nodule volume was 7.2. The MVR was 39.5, 65, and 72.9% at 1, 6, 12 months, respectively. Euthyroid state was achieved in 94.1%. No major complications were observed	RFA-US is a clinically effective and safe treatment in patients with benign nodules with no difference between functioning and non-functioning lesions
Cervelli et al. [10] 2019	Twenty-two patients with 25 AFTN treated by RFA, and 25 patients treated by RAI (all patients were evaluated by thyroid scintigraphy) Retrospective	No statistical difference was found in MVR (68.4 vs. 76.4 after RAI and RFA, respectively). Restoration of euthyroid state was achieved in 72% of patients treated by RAI and in 90.9% treated by RFA	RFA was effective in all patients with no case of posttreatment clinical hypothyroidism; 20% of patients treated by RAI developed hypothyroidism
Cesareo et al. [29] 2019	About 205 AFTN treated by RFA. The time of follow-up ranged from 6 to 24 months. Systematic review and meta-analysis	The rate of patients with TSH normalization was 57%; with scintigraphy proven optimal response was 60%. The MVR at 1 year was 79%	Baseline nodules volume was associated with the rate of TSH normalization
Cesareo et al. [23] 2018	Twenty-nine patients with AFTN divided into two groups based on thyroid volume: 15 patients (<12 mL—Group A) and 14 patients (>12 mL—Group B); 24-month prospective single center open parallel-group trial	There was greater MVR and increase in TSH levels in group A compared with group B. The rate of responders at 24 months was 86% vs. 45% in group A and B, respectively	RFA was effective in achieving biochemical control in patients with small AFTNs

RFA-US ultrasound-guided radiofrequency ablation; *MWA* microwave ablation

13.4 Comparison with Alternative Treatments

Randomized trials comparing RFA with other modalities, such as surgery or RAI, are lacking. Studies directly comparing these treatments are limited. Cervelli et al. [10] assessed 22 patients with 25 nodules treated with a single session of RFA using the moving shot technique and compared the outcomes with 25 patients who underwent RAI. The features of both groups were similar, and there were no statistically significant differences in the posttreatment nodule volume reduction. However, RFA demonstrated effectiveness in all patients without any cases of posttreatment hypothyroidism, in contrast to RAI, where 5 out of 25 patients developed hypothyroidism.

In terms of surgery, a study by Che et al. [31] compared surgery to RFA in benign thyroid nodules, including some that were hyperfunctioning, the study revealed that both modalities are effective; however, RFA was linked to fewer complications, preservation of thyroid function, and reduced hospitalization days. Notably, the surgical group had a 71.5% rate of hypothyroidism, but the RFA group had 0% rate. It is important to note that the surgical procedures included lobectomy or total thyroidectomy. This presents a limitation, as using lobectomy alone would provide a more relevant basis for comparison [33].

A systematic review and comparative meta-analysis were recently carried out to assess the responses of RAI and RFA therapies in AFTN. The analysis included 23 studies, comprising 22 observational and only one randomized controlled trial involving a single session of RAI, with a total of 296 patients undergoing RFA and 1042 undergoing RAI. None of the studies directly compared both modalities. The authors concluded the superiority of RAI through indirect comparisons [34]. Unfortunately, this meta-analysis was not free of selection bias and suffered from the same limitation that each meta-analysis study suffers from, 8 of the 13 studies of RAI had less than 2 years follow-up, and some of those defined success by achieving hypothyroidism. Contrary to RFA studies that had significant heterogeneous population and success was defined with normalization and included half of studies that did not use moving shoot technique, it is not surprising that the validity of this meta-analysis is questioned.

13.5 Follow-Up

The goal of treatment of AFTN is to achieve clinical resolution of symptoms of hyperthyroidism and achieving normalization of thyroid function test and routine clinical follow-up with biochemical testing is essential.

When treatment is successful normalization of thyroid function test is expected in 4–6 weeks posttreatment with RFA-US with patient symptoms improving in the first few weeks.

Neck US at initial follow-up 6 weeks post ablation can be useful to calculate initial volume reduction and predict success, and treatment with ATDs if it was initiated before procedure can be discontinued if significant volume reduction and complete absence of vascular flow are achieved. Post-treatment surveillance for regrowth and recurrence should include appropriate clinical follow-up and serial imaging studies, performed at maximum 6-month intervals in the first year and potentially annually thereafter.

Additional imaging studies with thyroid scintigraphy can be considered when hyperthyroidism relapse occurs including additional work up to rule out other etiologies.

13.6 Conclusions

RFA-US is a potential technique for managing AFTNs and achieving biochemical control. Several studies have reported significant success in achieving control, with data suggesting up to 3 years in a maintained euthyroid state.

Currently, surgery and/or RAI are considered the first-line treatment options for AFTN. And RFA-US is considered as an alternative management approach, particularly for patients who have contraindications for surgery/RAI or when there is a strong preference for RFA-US.

In the authors' opinion, accumulating data suggests that RFA-US is non-inferior, and potentially superior, to RAI in attaining a euthyroid state. This, combined with its significantly lower complication rate compared to surgery and RAI, and the reduced cost relative to surgery in some healthcare systems, suggests a promising future where RFA-US may be considered a first-line treatment for benign AFTN.

References

1. Grani G, Sponziello M, Pecce V, Ramundo V, Durante C. Contemporary thyroid nodule evaluation and management. J Clin Endocrinol Metab. 2020;105:2869–83. https://doi.org/10.1210/clinem/dgaa322.
2. Hamburger JI. The autonomously functioning thyroid nodule: Goetsch's disease. Endocr Rev. 1987;8:439–47. https://doi.org/10.1210/edrv-8-4-439.
3. Hegedüs L. Clinical practice. The thyroid nodule. N Engl J Med. 2004;351:1764–71. https://doi.org/10.1097/00006527-199101030-00006.
4. Burch HB, Shakir F, Fitzsimmons TR, Jaques DP, Shriver CD. Diagnosis and management of the autonomously functioning thyroid nodule: the Walter reed army medical center experience, 1975-1996. Thyroid. 1998;8:871–80. https://doi.org/10.1089/thy.1998.8.871.
5. Goundan PN, Lee SL. Lack of a threshold size for autonomously functioning thyroid nodules that excludes hyperthyroidism. Endocr Pract. 2019;25:1263–7. https://doi.org/10.4158/EP-2019-0042.
6. Wang L, Wang P, Chen Z, Lin Y, Liu Y, Peng R, et al. Image-guided thermal ablation as a promising approach to both nontoxic and toxic autonomously functioning thyroid nodules. Acad Radiol. 2023;30:6–8. https://doi.org/10.1016/j.acra.2023.02.002.
7. Goichot B, Caron P, Landron F, Bouée S. Clinical presentation of hyperthyroidism in a large representative sample of outpatients in France: relationships with age, aetiology and hormonal parameters. Clin Endocrinol. 2016;84:445–51. https://doi.org/10.1111/cen.12816.
8. Pace-Asciak P, Russell JO, Shaear M, Tufano RP. Novel approaches for treating autonomously functioning thyroid nodules. Front Endocrinol (Lausanne). 2020;11:1–7. https://doi.org/10.3389/fendo.2020.565371.
9. Kim HJ, Cho SJ, Baek JH, Suh CH. Efficacy and safety of thermal ablation for autonomously functioning thyroid nodules: a systematic review and meta-analysis. Eur Radiol. 2021;31:605–15. https://doi.org/10.1007/s00330-020-07166-0.
10. Cervelli R, Mazzeo S, Boni G, Boccuzzi A, Bianchi F, Brozzi F, et al. Comparison between radioiodine therapy and single-session radiofrequency ablation of autonomously functioning thyroid nodules: a retrospective study. Clin Endocrinol. 2019;90:608–16. https://doi.org/10.1111/cen.13938.
11. Dietrich CF, Müller T, Bojunga J, Dong Y, Mauri G, Radzina M, et al. Statement and recommendations on interventional ultrasound as a thyroid diagnostic and treatment procedure. Ultrasound Med Biol. 2018;44:14–36. https://doi.org/10.1016/j.ultrasmedbio.2017.08.1889.
12. Kim J, Baek JH, Lim HK, Ahn HS, Baek SM, Choi YJ, et al. 2017 thyroid radiofrequency ablation guideline: Korean Society of Thyroid Radiology. Korean J Radiol. 2018;19:632–55.
13. Mauri G, Pacella CM, Papini E, Solbiati L, Goldberg SN, Ahmed M, et al. Image-guided thyroid ablation: proposal for standardization of terminology and reporting criteria. Thyroid. 2019;29:611–8. https://doi.org/10.1089/thy.2018.0604.
14. Dobnig H, Zechmann W, Hermann M, Lehner M, Heute D, Mirzaei S, et al. Radiofrequency ablation of thyroid nodules: "good clinical practice recommendations" for Austria: an interdisciplinary statement from the following professional associations: Austrian Thyroid Association (ÖSDG), Austrian Society for Nuclear Medicine and M. Wien Med Wochenschr. 2020;170:6–14. https://doi.org/10.1007/s10354-019-0682-2.
15. Papini E, Monpeyssen H, Frasoldati A, Hegedüs L. 2020 European thyroid association clinical practice guideline for the use of image-guided ablation in benign thyroid nodules. Eur Thyroid J. 2020;9:172–85. https://doi.org/10.1159/000508484.
16. Orloff LA, Noel JE, Stack BC, Russell MD, Angelos P, Baek JH, et al. Radiofrequency ablation and related ultrasound-guided ablation technologies for treatment of benign and malignant thyroid disease: an international multidisciplinary consensus statement of the American Head and Neck Society Endocrine Surgery Section with the Asia Pacific Society of Thyroid Surgery, Associazione Medici Endocrinologi, British Association of Endocrine and Thyroid Surgeons, European Thyroid Association, Italian Society of Endocrine Surgery Units, Korean Society of Thyroid Radiology, Latin American Thyroid Society, and Thyroid Nodules Therapies Association. Head Neck. 2022;44:633–60. https://doi.org/10.1002/hed.26960.
17. Ha EJ, Baek JH, Che Y, Chou YH, Fukunari N, Kim JH, et al. Radiofrequency ablation of benign thyroid nodules: recommendations from the Asian conference on tumor ablation task force—secondary publication. J Med Ultrasound. 2021;29:77–83. https://doi.org/10.4103/JMU.JMU_178_20.

18. Sinclair CF, Baek JH, Hands KE, Hodak SP, Huber TC, Hussain I, et al. General principles for the safe performance, training, and adoption of ablation techniques for benign thyroid nodules: an American Thyroid Association statement. Thyroid. 2023;33:1150–70. https://doi.org/10.1089/thy.2023.0281.
19. Lui MS, Patel KN. Current guidelines for the application of radiofrequency ablation for thyroid nodules: a narrative review. Gland Surg. 2024;13:59–69. https://doi.org/10.21037/gs-23-18.
20. Papini E, Pacella CM, Solbiati LA, Achille G, Barbaro D, Bernardi S, et al. Minimally-invasive treatments for benign thyroid nodules: a Delphi-based consensus statement from the Italian minimally-invasive treatments of the thyroid (MITT) group. Int J Hyperth. 2019;36:376–82. https://doi.org/10.1080/02656736.2019.1575482.
21. Baek JH, Moon WJ, Kim YS, Lee JH, Lee D. Radiofrequency ablation for the treatment of autonomously functioning thyroid nodules. World J Surg. 2009;33:1971–7. https://doi.org/10.1007/s00268-009-0130-3.
22. Jasim S, Patel KN, Randolph G, Adams S, Cesareo R, Condon E, et al. American Association of Clinical Endocrinology Disease State Clinical Review: the clinical utility of minimally invasive interventional procedures in the management of benign and malignant thyroid lesions. Endocr Pract. 2022;28:433–48. https://doi.org/10.1016/j.eprac.2022.02.011.
23. Cesareo R, Naciu AM, Iozzino M, Pasqualini V, Simeoni C, Casini A, et al. Nodule size as predictive factor of efficacy of radiofrequency ablation in treating autonomously functioning thyroid nodules. Int J Hyperth. 2018;34:617–23. https://doi.org/10.1080/02656736.2018.1430868.
24. Noel JE, Sinclair CF. Radiofrequency ablation for benign thyroid nodules. J Clin Endocrinol Metab. 2023;109:e12–7. https://doi.org/10.1210/clinem/dgad357.
25. Cesareo R, Palermo A, Pasqualini V, Manfrini S, Trimboli P, Stacul F, et al. Radiofrequency ablation on autonomously functioning thyroid nodules: a critical appraisal and review of the literature. Front Endocrinol (Lausanne). 2020;11:11. https://doi.org/10.3389/fendo.2020.00317.
26. Hussain I, Zulfiqar F, Li X, Ahmad S, Aljammal J. Safety and efficacy of radiofrequency ablation of thyroid nodules—expanding treatment options in the United States. J Endocr Soc. 2021;5:1–12. https://doi.org/10.1210/jendso/bvab110.
27. van der Meeren MMD, Joosten FBM, Roerink SHPP, Deden LN, Oyen WJG. Radiofrequency ablation for autonomously functioning nodules as treatment for hyperthyroidism: subgroup analysis of toxic adenoma and multinodular goitre and predictors for treatment success. Eur J Nucl Med Mol Imaging. 2023;50:3675–83. https://doi.org/10.1007/s00259-023-06319-9.
28. Vu DL, Pham MT, Nguyen VB, Le TM. Efficacy and safety of radiofrequency ablation for the treatment of autonomously functioning thyroid nodules: a long-term prospective study. Ther Clin Risk Manag. 2022;18:11–9. https://doi.org/10.2147/TCRM.S344464.
29. Cesareo R, Palermo A, Benvenuto D, Cella E, Pasqualini V, Bernardi S, et al. Efficacy of radiofrequency ablation in autonomous functioning thyroid nodules. A systematic review and meta-analysis. Rev Endocr Metab Disord. 2019;20:37–44. https://doi.org/10.1007/s11154-019-09499-8.
30. Muhammad H, Santhanam P, Russell JO. Radiofrequency ablation and thyroid nodules: updated systematic review. Endocrine. 2021;72:619–32. https://doi.org/10.1007/s12020-020-02598-6.
31. Che Y, Jin S, Shi C, Wang L, Zhang X, Li Y, et al. Treatment of benign thyroid nodules: comparison of surgery with radiofrequency ablation. Am J Neuroradiol. 2015;36:1321–5. https://doi.org/10.3174/ajnr.A4276.
32. Bolusani H, Okosieme OE, Velagapudi M, Parsons K, Lazarus JH. Determinants of long-term outcome after radioiodine therapy for solitary autonomous thyroid nodules. Endocr Pract. 2008;14:543–9. https://doi.org/10.4158/EP.14.5.543.
33. Podrat JL, Lee YK, Khadra HS. Efficacy of radiofrequency ablation for treatment of toxic thyroid nodules—a narrative review. Gland Surg. 2024;13:70–6. https://doi.org/10.21037/gs-22-644.
34. Giovanella L, Garo ML, Campenní A, Ovčariček PP. Radioiodine versus radiofrequency ablation to treat autonomously functioning thyroid nodules: a systematic review and comparative meta-analysis. Eur J Nucl Med Mol Imaging. 2024;51:2050. https://doi.org/10.1007/s00259-024-06625-w.
35. Mauri G, Papini E, Bernardi S, Barbaro D, Cesareo R, Feo P De. Image-guided thermal ablation in autonomously functioning thyroid nodules. A retrospective multicenter three-year follow-up study from the Italian Minimally Invasive Treatment of the Thyroid (MITT) Group; 2021.
36. Cappelli C, Franco F, Pirola I, Gandossi E, Marini F, Di Lodovico E, et al. Radiofrequency ablation of functioning and non-functioning thyroid nodules: a single institution 12-month survey. J Endocrinol Investig. 2020;43:477–82. https://doi.org/10.1007/s40618-019-01132-4.

14 Microwave Ablation for Benign Thyroid Nodules

Mattia Squarcia, Fernando Diego Choque Chavez, and Jie Yu

14.1 Benign Thyroid Nodules: Essentials

The 2023 European Thyroid Association defines a thyroid nodule as a lesion within the thyroid gland that is ultrasonographically distinct from the surrounding thyroid parenchyma [1]. Various investigations have revealed variable prevalence rates contingent upon the modality of detection. These rates range from 2 to 6% employing palpation, 19 to 35% through the utilization of ultrasound (US), and 8 to 65% when ascertained from autopsy records [2]. It is noteworthy that most of these nodular formations are benign, with the prevalence of cancer spanning from 1 to 15%, subject to the specific criteria employed for patient selection and evaluation [3].

Even though most thyroid nodules are benign (benign thyroid nodule, BTN) and remain asymptomatic, certain nodules may warrant treatment. Such treatment may be motivated by the presence of symptoms resulting from the compression of neighboring anatomical structures, such as the esophagus and trachea, or the development of subclinical or overt hyperthyroidism. Additionally, cosmetic concerns can also serve as a driving factor for treatment in certain cases. When treatment of a BTN is guaranteed, guidelines for thyroid nodules management recommend that surgical therapy and minimal invasive techniques (MIT) [1] or percutaneous ethanol injection (PEI) [1, 4] can be considered as management modalities.

Minimal invasive techniques include ethanol ablation (EA) and thermal ablation (TA). TA is a technique that includes microwave ablation (MWA), laser ablation (LA), radiofrequency ablation (RFA), and high-intensity focused ultrasound [1]. These techniques have been assessed for its efficacy and safety in treating BTNs in various studies [5–7] and currently are postulated as an alternative to surgery in certain clinical scenarios [1]. Regarding MWA, a growing body of research suggests that it is feasible, safe, effective, and efficient technique in the treatment of BTN [8–12].

14.1.1 Principles of Microwave Ablation

US-guided MWA represents a hyperthermic thermal ablation technique that, as previously mentioned, stands as one of the investigated percutaneous modalities in the treatment of BTNs. Much like other hyperthermal ablation techniques such as laser ablation (LA), radiofrequency ablation (RFA), and cryoablation, MWA shares the common objective of eliminating

M. Squarcia (✉) · F. D. C. Chavez
Hospital Clinic Barcelona, Barcelona, Spain
e-mail: squarcia@clinic.cat; choque@clinic.cat

J. Yu
Chinese People Liberation Army General Hospital, Beijing, China

R. Valcavi et al. (eds.), *Thyroid Ablation*, https://doi.org/10.1007/978-3-031-88229-6_14

tumor tissue by increasing the temperature within a defined target volume [13, 14].

This technique uses a specific range of electromagnetic energy, typically 915 MHz to 2.45 GHz, to generate heat and eliminate targeted tissue [13]. Microwave-induced heating is a consequence of dielectric hysteresis, known as rotation of dipoles. When electromagnetic energy is directed at tissue, polar molecules like water are induced to align with the electromagnetic field. However, due to the swift oscillations, these molecules cannot maintain alignment, resulting in the absorption of energy and subsequent tissue heating and irreversible coagulative tissue necrosis. Consequently, tissues with high water content are particularly susceptible to heating during MW ablation. In contrast to radiofrequency (RF) ablation, MW energy does not manifest as an electrical current but rather as a propagating electromagnetic field. This characteristic renders MW ablation valuable in tissues with poor electrical conductivity, such as previously ablated tissue. Furthermore, the ability of MW fields to overlap within tissue enables the simultaneous use of multiple applicators to create more extensive ablation [13–15].

Most MWA units consist of a microwave generator, a low-loss coaxial cable, and an internally cooled shaft antenna. The generator can produce 1–100 W of power at 2450 MHz, either in pulse or continuous mode. The antenna is specifically tailored for addressing superficial neck organ diseases, featuring a 16–18 G diameter, a 10 cm shaft, and a 3 mm narrow radiating segment at the antenna tip [13–16] (Fig. 14.1).

They have stainless steel shaft covered along their entire length with a double layer polytetrafluoroethylene coating. They are internally water-cooled antennas.

14.1.2 Patient Selection

The 2023 European Thyroid Association guidelines advocate the consideration of thermal ablation (TA) as a therapeutic option for managing solid BTNs that induce local symptoms, offering an alternative to surgical intervention.

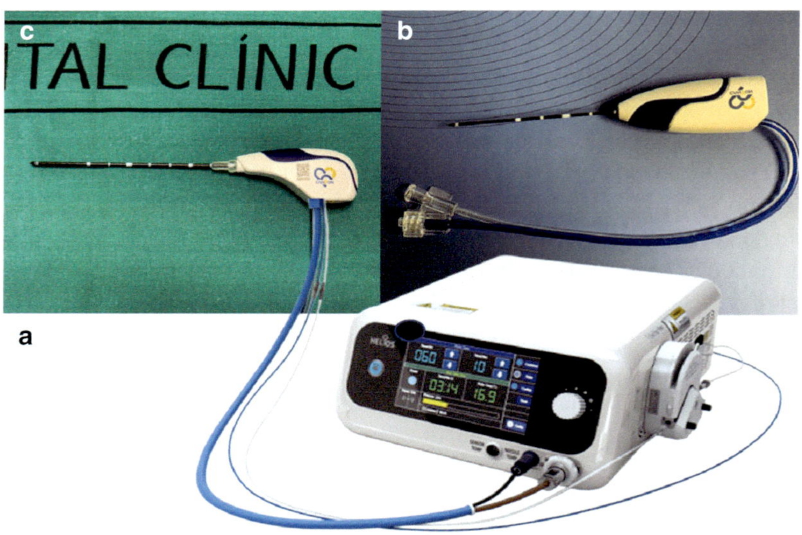

Fig. 14.1 Microwave ablation equipment consists of three main components: (**a**) microwave generator. The generator can produce 1–100 W of power in the form of pulses or continuous energy. Generator frequencies are generally 915 MHz or 2.45 MHz. (**b**) Coaxial cable. The distribution of electromagnetic energy from the generator to the antenna is done through a coaxial transmission cable. (**c**) Internally cooled antenna. Microwave antennas are the final and most critical component of the system, and they work to transfer energy to tissues. Dedicated microwave thyroid antenna has a 3 mm long active tip. They are short antennae, with a length 7 or 10 cm. They have sharp tip and are small diameter antennas of 16G (c1) or 18G (c2)

Additionally, TA is recommended for the treatment of cystic lesions that experience recurrence following ethanol ablation (EA). However, the guidelines do not provide specific recommendations regarding the choice of the TA technique to be employed [1]. On this manner, the 2020 European Thyroid Association Clinical Practice Guideline for the Use of Image-Guided Ablation in Benign Thyroid Nodules recommends MWA should currently be regarded as a secondary therapeutic option for patients who are unsuitable for or refuse other therapeutic ablation (TA) procedures. Additionally, it may be a suitable choice for individuals participating in structured clinical trials [17].

Established patient selection criteria for MWA in the treatment of BTNs remain lacking. Studies that evaluated this TA technique used different inclusion criteria. For instance, Luo et al. stipulated the following: BTNs confirmed via core-needle biopsy (CNB); nodules with a largest diameter larger than 3 cm; BTNs with a fluid component <80%, as seen with an ultrasound assessment; a normal serum free thyroxine (fT4) level and a corresponding normal or low thyrotropin (TSH) level; and no vocal cord immobility, as confirmed via a laryngoscope [8]. Wu et al. included patients with solid or predominantly solid nodules on ultrasound (solid component >75%), with complaints of pressure symptoms, throat constraint, and/or swallowing difficulty or esthetic problems, with benign cytology that means colloid and sheets of follicular cells without atypia, without a history of treatment and refused to surgery, and with normal thyroid function. Vorländer et al. considered mainly non-symptomatic thyroid nodules causing cosmetic concerns, symptomatic patients complaining of issues like swallowing difficulties, hoarseness, breathlessness, or pain, as well as those who declined surgery or had contraindications for it [18]. Cheng et al.'s criteria encompassed nodules with a maximal diameter not less than 2 cm, progressive growth, solid component exceeding 20%, symptomatic problems like neck pain, discomfort, foreign body sensation, or compressive symptoms, cosmetic concerns, clinical thyrotoxicosis, and hyperthyroidism stemming from autonomously functioning thyroid nodules (AFTNs), and no prior therapy [5]. Du et al. included benign nodules with a clear pathological result from CNB (Bethesda category: class II, benign), US without suspicious malignancy features, nodules with a longest diameter of ≥2 cm, large nodules (>4 cm in largest diameter) causing compressive, structural, or psychological symptoms, only a single nodule within the thyroid gland, patients who refused surgical treatment or couldn't tolerate it, and those with normal thyroid function [12].

In terms of exclusion criteria, there is also no consensus. Vorländer et al. applied exclusion criteria such as excessive thyroid volume with retrosternal growth including contiguous position to vessels, esophagus, trachea, or nerves; fine needle aspiration biopsy (FNAB) with cytological signs of follicular dysplastic proliferations; pathologic mismatch in 99mTc MIBI-scintigraphy as a sign of malignancy; and absence of symptoms [18]. Cheng et al. excluded patients with severe conditions, malignant or follicular thyroid neoplasms, those with prior thyroid surgery or medication, and individuals with vocal cord palsy contralateral to the target nodules [5]. Du et al. considered exclusion criteria including the absence of a clear pathological diagnosis or inaccurate CNB results (nondiagnostic or unsatisfactory; atypia of undetermined significance or follicular lesion of undetermined significance; follicular neoplasm or suspicion of a follicular neoplasm or specify if Hurthle cell type), pregnancy or lactation, severe coagulation disorders, severe heart or lung conditions impeding MWA tolerance, nodules accompanied by macrocalcifications (>1 cm), and infraclavicular goiters [12].

14.2 Preprocedural Evaluation

Preprocedural evaluation in most studies included a detailed physical examination, US examination, and laboratory test. Physical examination included estimation of symptom and cosmetic scores. Neck compression symptoms and dysphagia were evaluated with a visual analogue scale ranging from 0 to 10 and cosmetic scores

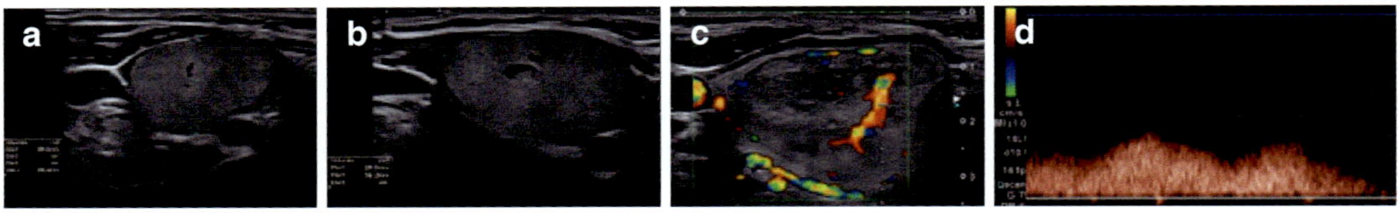

Fig. 14.2 MWA: Pretreatment assessment. Prior to microwave ablation, extensive ultrasound examination of the cervical and thyroid regions is routinely performed. Nodule volume, location, and echostructure are evaluated with b-mode ultrasound in the axial and sagittal plane (**a** and **b**). Color and pulsed Doppler are performed to evaluate intranodular vascularization prior to microwave ablation (**c** and **d**)

with a score ranging from 1 to 4: no palpable mass; palpable mass but no cosmetic problems; cosmetic problem on swallowing only or detected by an experienced physician; and a readily detected cosmetic problem [5, 10, 12]. In two studies, fiber laryngoscopy was performed on patients before MWA and on patients who complained of hoarseness or other symptoms related to nerve injury after MWA [5, 10]. US evaluation of the BNT includes location, length, width and depth, composition, echogenicity, margin, shape, echogenic foci, volume estimation, and blood flow evaluation with contrast-enhanced US (CEUS). Most studies evaluated nodule volume with the following formula: nodule volume $= \pi \times A \times B \times C \div 6$ (where A = the longest diameter; B, C = orthogonal diameters with A) [5, 8, 12] (Fig. 14.2).

Laboratory data included blood biochemistry analysis, a complete blood count, a blood coagulation test, and an assessment of thyroid function (including thyroid stimulating hormone, triiodothyronine, thyroxine, free triiodothyronine, and free thyroxine levels) and an electrocardiogram [5, 10, 19]. Anticoagulation and antiplatelet agents were temporarily omitted 5–7 days prior to the ablation and could be retaken after to the procedure [5].

14.3 Procedure

The procedure is typically performed with the patient in a supine position, with the neck being hyperextended, and with a venous catheter in the forearm where anesthesia is administered by anesthesiologist (typically propofol, 6–12 mg/kg/h). Patients' blood pressure, oxyhemoglobin saturation, and electrocardiogram are continuously monitored using a multiparametric monitor. Following the identification of the optimal puncture site, local anesthesia with 2% lidocaine is administered. Subsequently, a small incision, measuring less than 2 mm in length, is created. Of note, in cases where the thyroid nodule is situated in the upper or lower pole of the thyroid or near critical structures like the vagus nerve, trachea, or esophagus, hydrodissection can be considered to mitigate the risk of inadvertent injury. This technique involves the percutaneous introduction of a 21-gauge needle between the thyroid capsule adjacent to the target nodule and the neighboring structures. Subsequently, a solution of 0.9% saline is injected to create a separation between the thyroid and the surrounding structures (Fig. 14.3).

Moreover, if present, cystic component of the nodule can be aspirated with an 18 G percutaneous puncture needle. After that, guided by US, the disposable microwave antenna can be percutaneously inserted usually using a transisthmic approach into the nodule along its short axis, and the microwave therapeutic instrument is activated. A power output of 30–35 W is employed during the microwave ablation, with real-time ultrasound monitoring the changes in nodule echoes. The procedure followed the "moving-shot technique" with the extent of the ablation zone determined by alterations in echogenicity around the antenna. If the transient hyperechoic zone does not fully cover the entire nodule at one location, the antenna tip is adjusted, and other nodule portions are treated as necessary. The ablation is continued until the entire nodule is

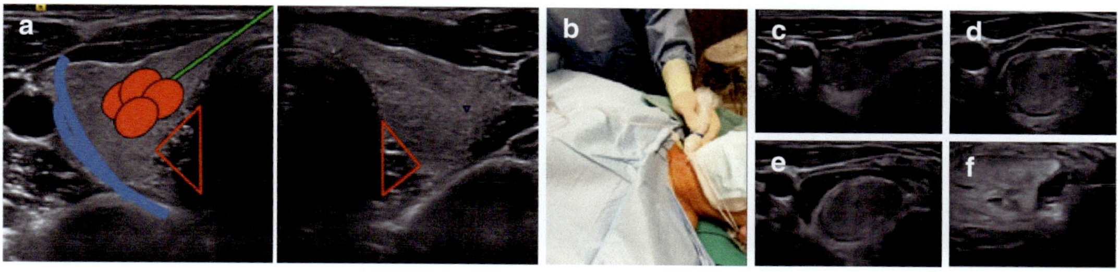

Fig. 14.3 MWA transisthmic approach and hydrodissection. Schematic representation of perithyroid hydrodissection and transisthmic approach (**a**). Pericapsular injection of local anesthetics is given prior to the procedure followed by hydrodissection. Photograph shows perithyroid saline injection through a percutaneous 18 G catheter (**b**). Axial ultrasound scan shows the presence of the 18 g catheter at the anterior pericapsular aspect of a right thyroid nodule (**c**). Axial ultrasound scan shows preprocedural perithyroid saline injection through a percutaneous 18 G catheter the distribution of 20 mL of saline solution between the thyroid nodule and perinodular structures (**d**) anterior pericapsular thyroidal saline injection separating thyroid nodule from precervical musculature and skin surface, (**e**) lateral pericapsular saline injection separating thyroid nodule from cervical neurovascular structures (common carotid artery, internal jugular vein, vagus nerve, and cervical sympathetic ganglions), (**f**) medial paratracheal saline injection separating thyroid nodule from the tracheal wall and the branches of the recurrent laryngeal nerve deeply located in the danger triangle

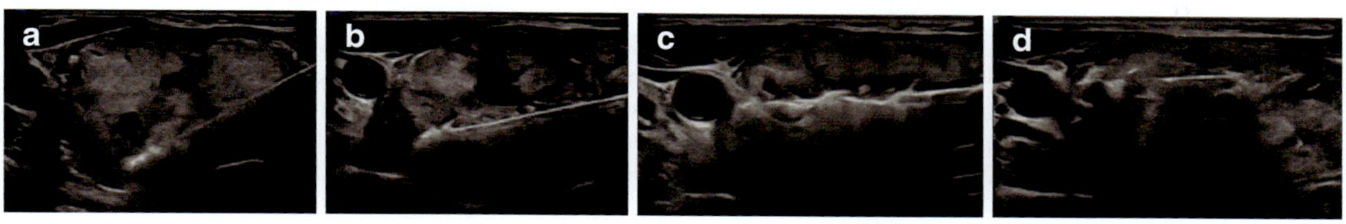

Fig. 14.4 MWA technique. Microwave ablation technique: Thyroid nodules are divided into multiple ablation units, and MW is performed unit by unit, moving the antenna (**a**). Microwave antenna is inserted using the transisthmic approach. The moving-shot technique with transisthmic approach permits visualization of the antenna in its entire length. Minimal exposure to heat of the "dangerous triangle" reduced risk of antenna position change when speaking or swallowing. A mixture of 0.9% lidocaine and physiological saline is infused into the surrounding thyroid capsule to achieve a "liquid-isolating region" (arrow), protecting the vital structures of the neck (carotid artery, trachea, esophagus, and nerve) from the thermal injury (blue area in **a**). The tip of the antenna is initially placed in the deepest position, and posterior to the nodule and ablation is started with 30 W. When an echogenic area appears, the electrode moves to an untreated area until the complete nodule is treated (**b**–**d**)

encompassed by the transient hyperechoic zone. In cases where a patient experiences intolerable pain during the ablation procedure, it is advisable to lower the power or temporarily cease the treatment for several seconds. The therapy should be concluded once the hyperechoic image completely envelops the nodule. It is essential to note, however, that certain areas of thyroid nodules situated in proximity to critical structures such as the recurrent laryngeal nerve and the esophagus may remain untreated [5, 10, 12, 19] (Fig. 14.4).

US evaluation is done after ablation to assess nodule location, size, texture, and their relationship with surrounding tissues. CEUS can be used to identify areas of non-enhancement, indicating coagulative necrosis resulting from MWA. In cases where the ablation range was deemed insufficient, signified by CEUS revealing contrast filling within the nodules, additional ablation can be carried out. After the procedure, mechanical compression is applied for 30 min to prevent bleeding or hematoma formation [5, 10, 12, 19] (Fig. 14.5).

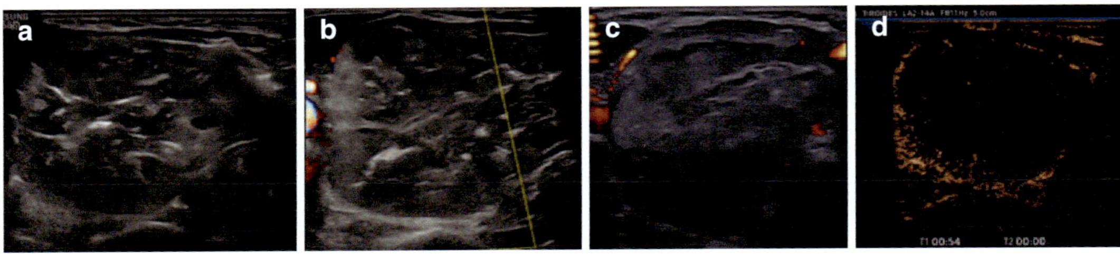

Fig. 14.5 Postprocedural ultrasound evaluation. Thyroid nodule MW ablation is considered completed when the entire nodule appears diffusely hypoechoic at b-mode ultrasound examination after hyperechoic images indicating extensive gas formation in the ablated are reabsorbed (**a**). Color Doppler, power Doppler, and contrast-enhanced ultrasound examination confirm the extensive nodular devascularization at the end of the procedure (**b**–**d**)

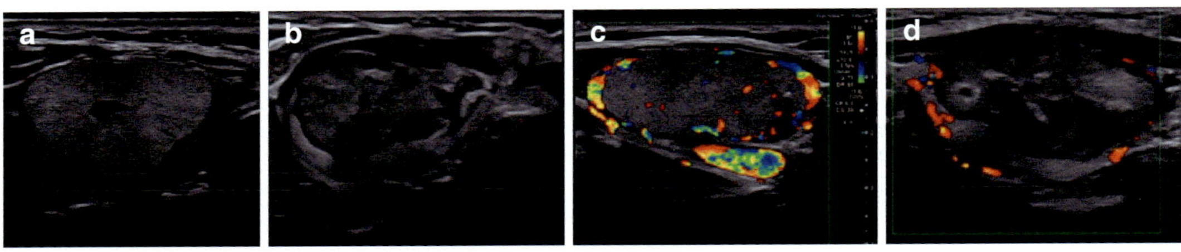

Fig. 14.6 US follow-up. During the follow-up nodule, volume and ecostructure are evaluated by b-mode ultrasound (a and b), and intranodular vascularization is evaluated by color Doppler examination (c and d). (a) Axial ultrasound image shows an isoechoic homogeneous right lobe thyroid nodule prior to MW ablation (**a**). Some nodule after MW ablation showing an extensive heterogeneous hypoechoic area, representing ablated area (**b**). Pre- and posttreatment ultrasound images of thyroid nodules demonstrating intranodular vascularity prior to treatment (**c**) and avascular treated nodule (**d**)

14.4 Follow-Up

Clinical and imaging assessments with US are performed at 1, 3, 6, 9, and 12 months after the procedure. Clinical assessment must include symptom evaluation using the scales previously mentioned and laboratory data used in pre-procedure assessment. It is mandatory to assess for complications and side effects immediately after the procedure and on each visit. On the other hand, US examination is used to assess changes in nodules volume, echogenicity, nodular vascularity, and BTN recurrence, defined as a nodule volume increase >50% over the smallest recorded volume. Nodule volume reduction rate (VRR) was calculated using the following equation: VRR (%) = 100 × (initial volume − final volume)/initial volume [5, 8, 12, 19] (Fig. 14.6).

14.5 Efficacy

A systematic review and meta-analysis included five cohorts, the VRRs at follow-up imaging were as follows: 53.9% (95% CI: 47.6–60.1%, I^2 = 92.8%) at 3 months, 74.9% (95% CI: 69.5–80.2%, I^2 = 88.5%) at 6 months, and 80.0% (95% CI: 76.6–83.5%, I^2 = 74.1%) at 12 months [20]. Another study that included 171 patients with 180 BTN treated with US-guided MWA showed that VRRs at the follow-up intervals of 1, 3, 6, 12, 24, and 36 months were recorded as 47.1%, 68.2%, 79.7%, 87.4%, 90.1%, and 93.2%, respectively. Of note, solid nodules showed significantly lower VRRs compared with the predominantly solid and predominantly cystic nodules at the 1-, 3-, and 6-month follow-ups [8] (Fig. 14.7).

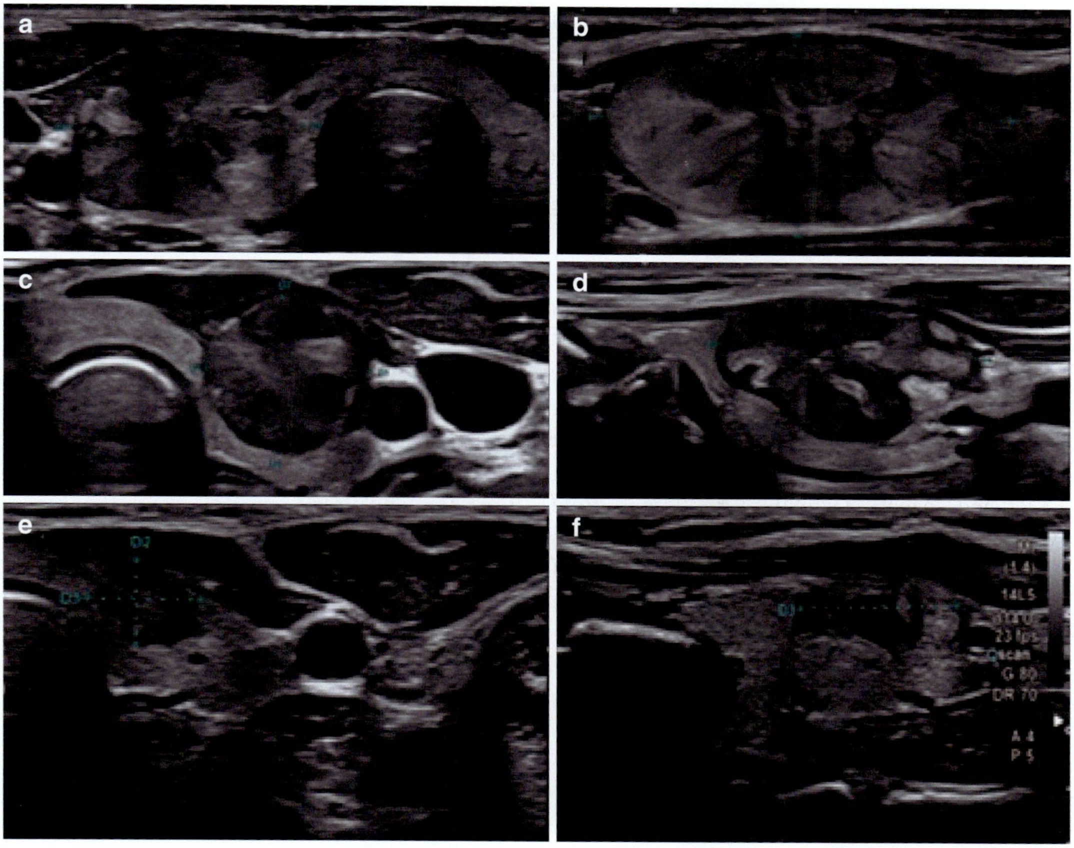

Fig. 14.7 Pretreatment b-mode left thyroid lobe ultrasound obtained immediately before MWA with the operator positioned behind the head of the patient as usual during left thyroid nodules treatment to allow transisthmic approach. The left side of the patient appears on the right side of the ultrasound image. Axial (**a**) and sagittal (**b**) b-mode ultrasound shows an 11 mL volume solid, heterogeneous left thyroid nodule. Three months post-MWA axial (**c**) and sagittal (**d**) b-mode follow-up ultrasound of the left thyroid lobe show a 3 mL left thyroid hypoechoic nodule with a volume of 3 mL and a volume reduction of 72%; 12 months post-MWA axial (**e**) and sagittal (**f**) b-mode follow-up ultrasound of the left thyroid lobe show a 0.6 mL hypoechoic left thyroid nodule with a volume reduction of 94%

Regarding clinical data, the previously cited systematic review and meta-analysis found significant decreases of symptomatic scores (SMD = 1.12, 95%CI: 0.38–1.87, p = 0.003; SMD = 1.45, 95%CI: 0.34–2.56, p = 0.011) and cosmetic scores (SMD = 0.94, 95%CI: 0.84–1.04, $p < 0.001$; SMD = 1.15, 95%CI: 0.83–1.47, $p < 0.001$ at the 6-month and 12-month follow-up [20]. Luo et al. observed that the reduction in nodule size corresponded to an enhancement in both cosmetic appearance and symptom relief. Prior to undergoing Microwave Ablation (MWA), 40.9% (70 out of 171) of the patients reported experiencing discomfort. However, this percentage significantly decreased to 17.5% (30 out of 171) 3 months following MWA. In addition, the prevalence of other symptoms exhibited noteworthy reductions: pre-MWA, 30.4% of patients expressed aesthetic concerns, which diminished to 15.2%; 13.5% of patients reported neck pressure, which decreased to 4.7%; the proportion of patients with difficulty swallowing decreased from 9.9% to 4.7%; and patients with a growing nodule size dropped from 5.2% to 1.8% at the

3-month post-MWA evaluation. Remarkably, all the aforementioned symptoms and cosmetic issues were fully resolved by the 12-month follow-up [8].

14.5.1 MWA vs. RFA

In a multicenter, prospective study conducted by Cheng et al., comparing microwave ablation (MWA) and radiofrequency ablation (RFA) for the treatment of benign thyroid nodules (BTN), it was demonstrated that both RFA and MWA proved to be effective and safe within the studied population. Nevertheless, the results concerning VRR and Mean Diameter Reduction Rate (MDRR) were notably superior in the RFA group at the 6-month mark and in subsequent follow-up assessments. In terms of clinical evaluation, both groups exhibited a substantial decrease in symptomatic and cosmetic scores and no statistically significant differences were observed between the two groups [5].

In a systematic review and meta-analysis conducted by Guo et al., a comparison was made between MWA and RFA for the treatment of BTNs. The study yielded the conclusion that both techniques proved effective; however, patients who underwent RFA demonstrated a higher VRRs at the 12-month mark (86.2% vs. 80.0%, p = 0.036). Based on these findings, it was inferred that RFA may yield superior long-term outcomes. Moreover, symptomatic and cosmetic scores decreased significantly after 6 and 12 months in both groups, and no statistically significant differences were observed between the two groups [20].

14.5.2 MWA vs. Surgery

In a prospective study involving 52 patients, the efficacy, tolerability, and cost-effectiveness of microwave ablation (MWA) were compared with those of thyroidectomy in the treatment of benign thyroid nodules (BTNs). The results revealed that MWA proved to be equally effective in managing non-active thyroid nodules, achieving a remarkable 92.4% reduction in nodule volume at the 12-month mark. Furthermore, symptoms associated with BTNs completely resolved in the MWA group, demonstrating non-inferiority when compared to the surgical cohort. In terms of cosmetic outcomes, no significant disparities were observed between the two groups, and both groups achieved excellent results. Both surgical interventions and MWA were deemed safe; however, MWA patients experienced fewer complications, shorter hospitalization, reduced surgical scar size, and shorter operative durations. Additionally, they reported improved overall and mental health. As for the reported complications, the study indicated that while complications were more frequent in the surgical group, there were no statistically significant differences between the two groups. Nevertheless, MWA outperformed surgery significantly in terms of hospitalization duration, surgical scar size, and operative time [21].

Another retrospective study was designed with the objective of assessing the safety and efficacy of microwave ablation (MWA) versus lobectomy for thyroid nodules larger than 4 cm. It demonstrated that MWA exhibits an efficacy profile comparable to surgery in terms of symptom and cosmetic score outcomes, as well as Volumetric Reduction Rate (VRR) with an average VRR of 90.5% at 12 months. Notably, MWA presents a superior safety profile, as evidenced by significantly lower frequencies of postoperative pain, hypothyroidism, hypocalcemia, surgical duration, hospitalization days, and incision size within the MWA group. Moreover, voice changes, hematomas, and surgical site infections were less frequent in the MWA group; however, no statistically significant differences were observed [22].

14.6 Complications

Major and minor complications have been recorded in the aftermath of MWA. Minor complications encompass pain radiating to the ear, shoulder, or teeth, minor instances of bleeding, hematoma, skin burns, hyperthyroidism, vomiting, and conditions such as transient Horner syn-

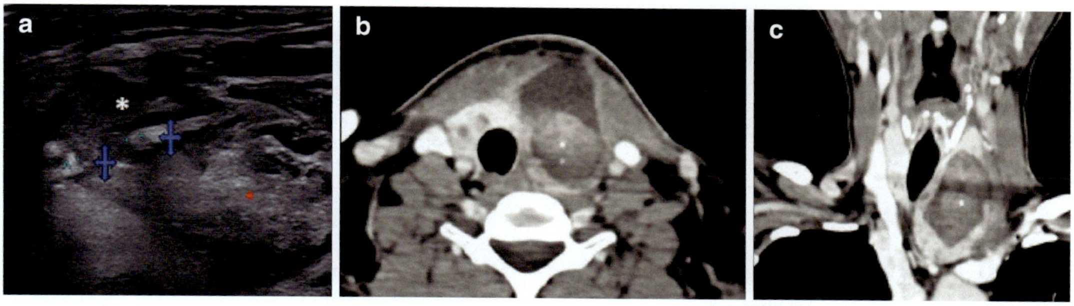

Fig. 14.8 Microwave ablation complications. Nodule rupture. (**a**) Axial ultrasound scan shows intranodular colliquation (*red asterisk*), the breakdown of the thyroid capsule (*between blue crosses*), and collection of the necrotic tissues into the cervical strap muscles (*). Nodule rupture observed at axial (**b**) and coronal (**c**) contrast-enhanced CT scan

drome, which typically normalized within 2 months, cough, and mild fever. Major complications that have been reported include transient alterations in voice quality, nodule rupture, formation of abscesses, vocal cord palsy, and nerve injury [5, 8, 10, 12]. Nonetheless, when compared to RFA, these complications do not exhibit statistically significant differences [5, 20] and, as previously mentioned, MWA has a better safety profile than surgery [21, 22] (Fig. 14.8).

14.7 Recurrence

In most studies, recurrence is defined as an increase of more than 50% in nodule volume within the total ablation area compared to the previous ultrasound examination [23, 24]. In a retrospective study involving 214 patients with 306 benign thyroid nodules (BTNs), recurrence was identified in 7 nodules (2.29%). Within the recurrence group, the initial maximum diameters and volumes were somewhat larger, though not statistically significant. Notably, the recurrence group exhibited a significantly higher energy-to-volume ratio compared to the non-recurrence group [23].

In another retrospective study involving 110 patients, recurrences were observed in 16 patients at the 12-month mark, with two of them undergoing repeat microwave ablation (MWA) due to unsatisfactory initial outcomes. The initial mean nodule volume in the 16 patients who experienced recurrence was 23.9 ± 12.5 mL, significantly larger than the initial median nodule volume of 11.6 ± 14.9 mL in the remaining 94 patients ($p < 0.01$). This study also revealed statistically significant differences between the nodular vascularity in the recurrence and non-recurrence groups. Additionally, the average energy deposited per milliliter of nodule volume demonstrated statistically significant differences between the two groups. A noteworthy finding was the higher frequency of nodules in close proximity to critical tissues in the recurrence group compared to the non-recurrence group (81.2% and 28.5%, respectively), a difference that also proved to be statistically significant [24].

These data suggests a greater amount of energy required to reduce the volume of 1 mL, a higher initial volume, proximity to important tissues, and higher vascularity of nodular tissue may be associated with a higher likelihood of recurrence.

14.8 Further Direction and Research

The future of MWA in the treatment of BTNs holds promise and ongoing development. In this manner, further prospective and multicentric clinical trials with more heterogeneous populations are needed. Also, long-term follow-up studies are necessary, so a more accurate estimation of recurrence can be accomplished. If MWA becomes more established, standardized guidelines and recommendations may be developed for its use in the management of BTNs.

14.9 Conclusion

MWA stands as a promising non-surgical technique for the treatment of BTNs. Actual evidence suggests that this TA technique is safe and effective. Also, it may offer advantages over surgery, including a reduced risk of complications such as scar formation, shorter hospitalization, and avoidance of general anesthesia, among others. Pre-procedure evaluation, procedure, and post-procedure follow-up are important for a successful treatment. However, further prospective studies focusing on longer follow-up and with more heterogeneous are needed to ascertain more definitively which patients might derive the greatest benefit from this treatment.

References

1. Durante C, Hegedüs L, Czarniecka A, Paschke R, Russ G, Schmitt F, et al. 2023 European Thyroid Association Clinical Practice Guidelines for thyroid nodule management. Eur Thyroid J. 2023;12(5):e230067. https://doi.org/10.1530/ETJ-23-0067.
2. Dean DS, Gharib H. Epidemiology of thyroid nodules. Best Pract Res Clin Endocrinol Metab. 2008;22(6):901–11. https://doi.org/10.1016/j.beem.2008.09.019.
3. Grussendorf M, Ruschenburg I, Brabant G. Malignancy rates in thyroid nodules: a long-term cohort study of 17,592 patients. Eur Thyroid J. 2022;11(4):e220027. https://doi.org/10.1530/ETJ-22-0027.
4. Haugen BR, Alexander EK, Bible KC, Doherty GM, Mandel SJ, Nikiforov YE, et al. 2015 American Thyroid Association Management Guidelines for adult patients with thyroid nodules and differentiated thyroid cancer: the American Thyroid Association Guidelines Task Force on Thyroid Nodules and Differentiated Thyroid Cancer. Thyroid. 2016;26(1):1–133. https://doi.org/10.1089/thy.2015.0020.
5. Cheng Z, Che Y, Yu S, Wang S, Teng D, Xu H, et al. US-guided percutaneous radiofrequency versus microwave ablation for benign thyroid nodules: a prospective multicenter study. Sci Rep. 2017;7(1):9554. https://doi.org/10.1038/s41598-017-09930-7.
6. Cui T, Jin C, Jiao D, Teng D, Sui G. Safety and efficacy of microwave ablation for benign thyroid nodules and papillary thyroid microcarcinomas: a systematic review and meta-analysis. Eur J Radiol. 2019;118:58–64. https://doi.org/10.1016/j.ejrad.2019.06.027.
7. Cho SJ, Baek JH, Chung SR, Choi YJ, Lee JH. Long-term results of thermal ablation of benign thyroid nodules: a systematic review and meta-analysis. Endocrinol Metab (Seoul). 2020;35(2):339–50. https://doi.org/10.3803/EnM.2020.35.2.339.
8. Luo F, Huang L, Gong X, Han Z, Liu F, Cheng Z, et al. Microwave ablation of benign thyroid nodules: 3-year follow-up outcomes. Head Neck. 2021;43(11):3437–47. https://doi.org/10.1002/hed.26842.
9. Yue W, Wang S, Wang B, Xu Q, Yu S, Yonglin Z, et al. Ultrasound guided percutaneous microwave ablation of benign thyroid nodules: safety and imaging follow-up in 222 patients. Eur J Radiol. 2013;82(1):e11–6. https://doi.org/10.1016/j.ejrad.2012.07.020.
10. Feng B, Liang P, Cheng Z, Yu X, Yu J, Han Z, et al. Ultrasound-guided percutaneous microwave ablation of benign thyroid nodules: experimental and clinical studies. Eur J Endocrinol. 2012;166(6):1031–7. https://doi.org/10.1530/EJE-11-0966.
11. Korkusuz H, Nimsdorf F, Happel C, Ackermann H, Grünwald F. Percutaneous microwave ablation of benign thyroid nodules. Functional imaging in comparison to nodular volume reduction at a 3-month follow-up. Nuklearmedizin. 2015;54(1):13–9. https://doi.org/10.3413/Nukmed-0678-14-06.
12. Du JR, Li WH, Quan CH, Wang H, Teng DK. Long-term outcome of microwave ablation for benign thyroid nodules: over 48-month follow-up study. Front Endocrinol (Lausanne). 2022;13:941137. https://doi.org/10.3389/fendo.2022.941137.
13. Ahmed M, Brace CL, Lee FT, Goldberg SN. Principles of and advances in percutaneous ablation. Radiology. 2011;258(2):351–69. https://doi.org/10.1148/radiol.10081634.
14. Knavel EM, Brace CL. Tumor ablation: common modalities and general practices. Tech Vasc Int Radiol. 2013;16(4):192–200. https://doi.org/10.1053/j.tvir.2013.08.002.
15. Cheng Z, Liang P. Advances in ultrasound-guided thermal ablation for symptomatic benign thyroid nodules. Adv Clin Exp Med. 2020;29(9):1123–9. https://doi.org/10.17219/acem/125433.
16. Mainini AP, Monaco C, Pescatori LC, De Angelis C, Sardanelli F, Sconfienza LM, et al. Image-guided thermal ablation of benign thyroid nodules. J Ultrasound. 2017;20(1):11–22. https://doi.org/10.1007/s40477-016-0221-6.
17. Papini E, Monpeyssen H, Frasoldati A, Hegedüs L. 2020 European thyroid association clinical practice guideline for the use of image-

guided ablation in benign thyroid nodules. Eur Thyroid J. 2020;9(4):172–85. https://doi.org/10.1159/000508484.
18. Vorländer C, David Kohlhase K, Korkusuz Y, Erbelding C, Luboldt W, Baser I, et al. Comparison between microwave ablation and bipolar radiofrequency ablation in benign thyroid nodules: differences in energy transmission, duration of application and applied shots. Int J Hyperth. 2018;35(1):216–25. https://doi.org/10.1080/02656736.2018.1489984.
19. Wu W, Gong X, Zhou Q, Chen X, Chen X. Ultrasound-guided percutaneous microwave ablation for solid benign thyroid nodules: comparison of MWA versus control group. Int J Endocrinol. 2017;2017:9724090. https://doi.org/10.1155/2017/9724090.
20. Guo DM, Chen Z, Zhai YX, Su HH. Comparison of radiofrequency ablation and microwave ablation for benign thyroid nodules: a systematic review and meta-analysis. Clin Endocrinol. 2021;95(1):187–96. https://doi.org/10.1111/cen.14438.
21. Zhi X, Zhao N, Liu Y, Liu JB, Teng C, Qian L. Microwave ablation compared to thyroidectomy to treat benign thyroid nodules. Int J Hyperth. 2018;34(5):644–52. https://doi.org/10.1080/02656736.2018.1456677.
22. Dong P, Wu XL, Sui GQ, Luo Q, Du JR, Wang H, et al. The efficacy and safety of microwave ablation versus lobectomy for the treatment of benign thyroid nodules greater than 4 cm. Endocrine. 2021;71(1):113–21. https://doi.org/10.1007/s12020-020-02338-w.
23. Xia B, Yu B, Wang X, Ma Y, Liu F, Gong Y, et al. Conspicuousness and recurrence related factors of ultrasound-guided microwave ablation in the treatment of benign thyroid nodules. BMC Surg. 2021;21(1):317. https://doi.org/10.1186/s12893-021-01312-1.
24. Wang B, Han ZY, Yu J, Cheng Z, Liu F, Yu XL, et al. Factors related to recurrence of the benign non-functioning thyroid nodules after percutaneous microwave ablation. Int J Hyperth. 2017;33(4):459–64. https://doi.org/10.1080/02656736.2016.1274058.

Active Surveillance in Micropapillary Cancer

15

Yasuhiro Ito, Akira Miyauchi, and Hossein Gharib

15.1 Introduction

Papillary thyroid carcinoma (PTC) measuring ≤10 mm in maximum diameter without invasion of surrounding vital organs, clinical node metastasis, or distant metastases is designated as low-risk papillary thyroid microcarcinoma (PTMC). In the past, PTMCs were incidentally detected in the thyroid specimens resected for benign thyroid diseases. Many autopsy studies on subject who died of non-thyroid diseases reported high incidences of latent thyroid carcinoma, most of which were small PTCs. Incidence of latent PTMCs measuring 3 mm or larger, which are detectable by ultrasound, were reported to be 3–5.2% of study subjects [1]. The incidences were more than 1000 times comparing with the prevalence of clinical thyroid carcinoma in Japanese women being reported at that time [1]. Recent development of ultrasound examination and of ultrasound-guided fine needle aspiration cytology (FNAC) has enabled us to detect and diagnose PTMC easily. Actually, Takebe et al. conducted a screening study for thyroid cancer using these techniques on women aged ≥30 years who visited his center for breast cancer screening and detected small thyroid carcinoma in 3.5% of them [2]. These findings on autopsy and clinical studies suggest that PTMC exists asymptomatically in very high incidences, and only a portion of the tumor grows and becomes clinical.

Based on the above findings, Akira Miyauchi at Kuma Hospital (Kobe, Japan) hypothesized that most PTMCs stay small, only a small minority grow and surgery for all PTMC patients may do more harm than good [1]. Of course, a minority of PTMCs will grow and become clinical. At that time (and even now), no pathological or molecular markers for cytological specimens were available to predict constant growth of PTMC. Miyauchi proposed that active surveillance (AS) is a reasonable strategy to select progressive cases and conversion surgery at the time of slight disease progression is not too late [1]. In October 1993, he proposed AS without immediate surgery (IS) as a management strategy for PTMC at a physicians' meeting at Kuma Hospital, and a prospective study of AS for PTMC was started after the approval by the physicians.

In 1995, 2 years later, the Cancer Institute Hospital (CIH, Tokyo, Japan) also initiated AS for PTMC and to date, favorable outcomes of AS for PTMC have been published from these institutions as described later. AS was adopted as a management option in the guidelines conducted by the Japan Association of Endocrine Surgeons/ Japanese Association of Thyroid Surgery (present

Y. Ito (✉) · A. Miyauchi
Department of Surgery, Kuma Hospital, Kobe, Hyogo, Japan
e-mail: ito01@kuma-h.or.jp; miyauchi@kuma-h.or.jp

H. Gharib
Endocrinology Division, Mayo Clinic College of Medicine, Rochester, MN, USA
e-mail: gharib.hossein@mayo.edu

R. Valcavi et al. (eds.), *Thyroid Ablation*, https://doi.org/10.1007/978-3-031-88229-6_15

the Japan Association of Endocrine Surgery) in 2010 and 2018 [3, 4], and by the American Thyroid Association (ATA) guidelines in 2015 [5]. After the publication of the ATA guidelines, several prospective studies were published also from many countries. In order to implement AS for PTMC, consensus statements from the Japan Association of Endocrine Surgeons and a position paper from the Japanese Thyroid Association were also published [6, 7].

15.2 Differences in Thyroid Carcinoma Incidence and Mortality

To date, researchers in several countries have reported significant discrepancies between overtime trends in thyroid cancer incidence and mortality [8–11]. In the United States, the incidence of thyroid carcinoma increased by 2.4-fold between 1973 and 2002 and by 2.9-fold between 1975 and 2009 [8, 9], while thyroid cancer mortality remained stable. They showed that the incidence of PTC measuring ≤20 mm, including PTMC, increased with time, while the incidences of larger PTCs remained almost stable. Therefore, they emphasized the possibility of over diagnosis and over treatment. In South Korea, the incidence of thyroid carcinoma increased as much as 15-fold between 1993 and 2011 mostly due to national screening program for thyroid cancer using ultrasound examination, while thyroid cancer mortality did not change and surgical complications increased [10]. Rapid increase in incidence but stable mortality of thyroid carcinoma was reported in many other countries, including Italy, France, England, Scotland, Australia, and Nordic countries [7, 11]. This could be because the widespread availability of ultrasound and ultrasound-guided FNAC enabled clinicians to detect and diagnose small thyroid carcinomas, leading to unnecessary surgeries for harmless small carcinomas.

15.3 How to Implement AS for PTMC

Having ultrasound technicians trained specifically for thyroid and neck is an absolute requirement for the safe implementation of AS. Otherwise, patients should be referred to other properly organized medical institutions. Of course, not all patients with PTCs ≤10 mm are suitable for AS.

In order to implement AS successfully, the following three domains should be carefully evaluated: tumor characteristics, patient characteristics, and medical team characteristics. Depending on the risk for AS, each of these is classified as ideal, appropriate, and inappropriate [12]. If some of these are inappropriate, managements other than AS should be considered. Tumor characteristics are mostly evaluated with ultrasound features (and CT scan occasionally), which is the key step for successful AS. Figure 15.1 indicates the representative cases that are ideal, appropriate, and inappropriate for AS. Table 15.1 indicates the contraindications of AS for PTMC.

Tumors having clinically high-risk features are strong candidates for IS. Performing IS should also be considered for tumors widely attached to the trachea and located in the course of the RLN. Especially, tumors attached to the trachea forming obtuse angles between their surfaces and those having no normal thyroid tissue with the course of the recurrent laryngeal nerve are strong candidates for IS [13]. Evidence is inadequate for AS for patients under age.

The ATA guidelines state that FNAC is not required for nodules ≤10 mm unless other signs or symptoms of high-risk malignancy are present [5]. However, we currently perform cytological examination for suspicious nodules ≥5 mm, because the guidelines published by the Japan Association of Breast and Thyroid Sonology recommend FNAC for suspicious thyroid nodules measuring ≥5 mm. Further, if we do not cytologically diagnose a nodule and do not tell the patient that he or she has PTMC, the patient

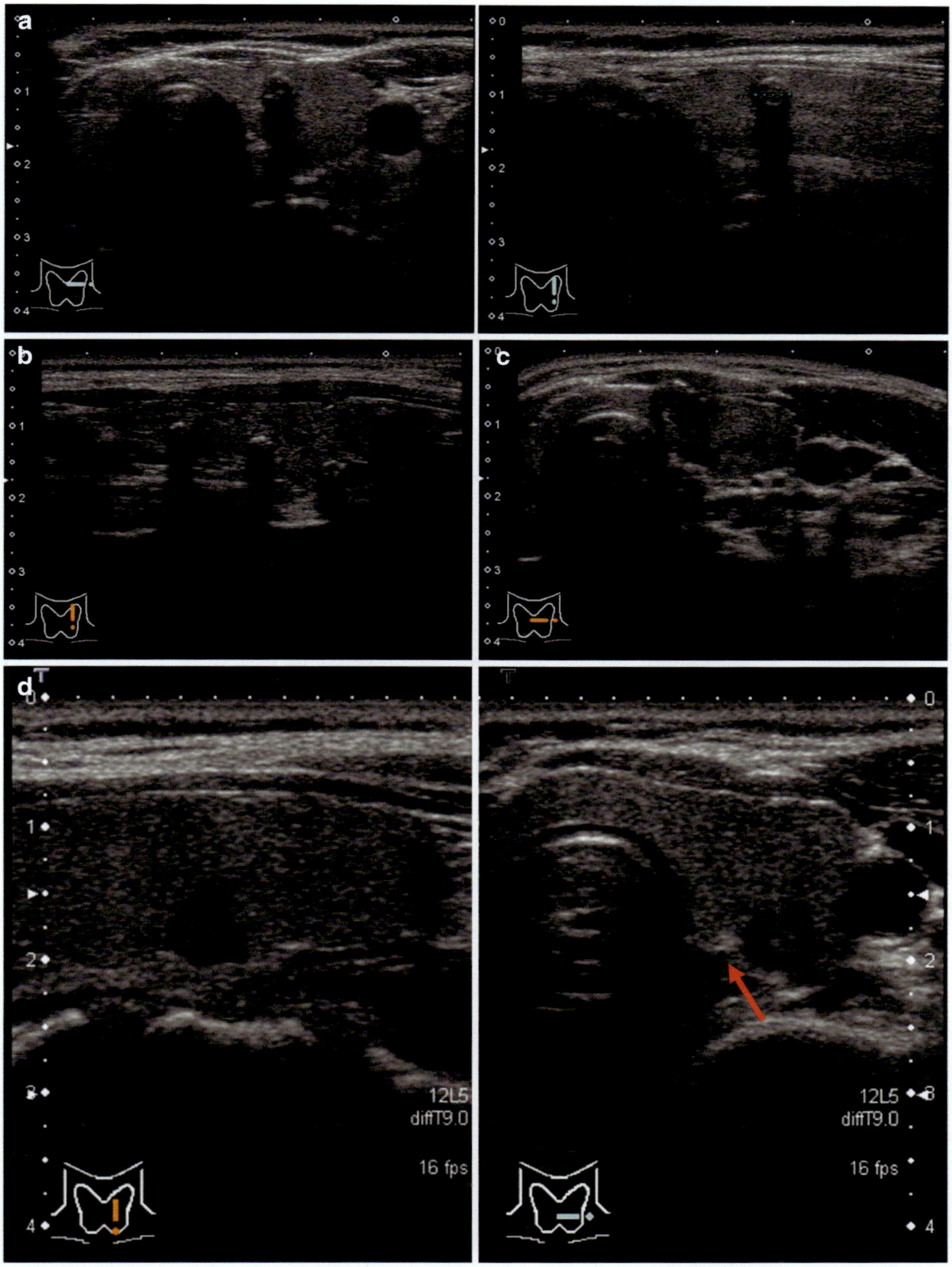

Fig. 15.1 Figure images of PTMC ideal, appropriate, and inappropriate for AS. (**a**) A 64-year-old woman. Solitary tumor surrounded by normal thyroid tissue (ideal). (**b**) A 67-year-old-woman. Multiple PTMC surrounded by thyroid tissue (appropriate). (**c**) A 41-year-old-woman. PTMC having minimal invasion to the thyroid capsule anteriorly (appropriate). (**d**) A 57-year-old-woman. Normal thyroid rim in the direction of the left recurrent laryngeal nerve (appropriate). (**e**) A 45-year-old-woman. Right recurrent laryngeal nerve at risk (inappropriate). (**f**) A 76-year-old-woman. PTMC forming acute angle with the trachea (appropriate). (**g**) A 70-year-old-woman. PTMC forming obtuse angle with the trachea (inappropriate). (**h**) A 70-year-old-woman. PTMC forming obtuse angle with the trachea (inappropriate). (**i**) A 48-year-old-woman. Metastatic lymph node metastasis is detected (inappropriate)

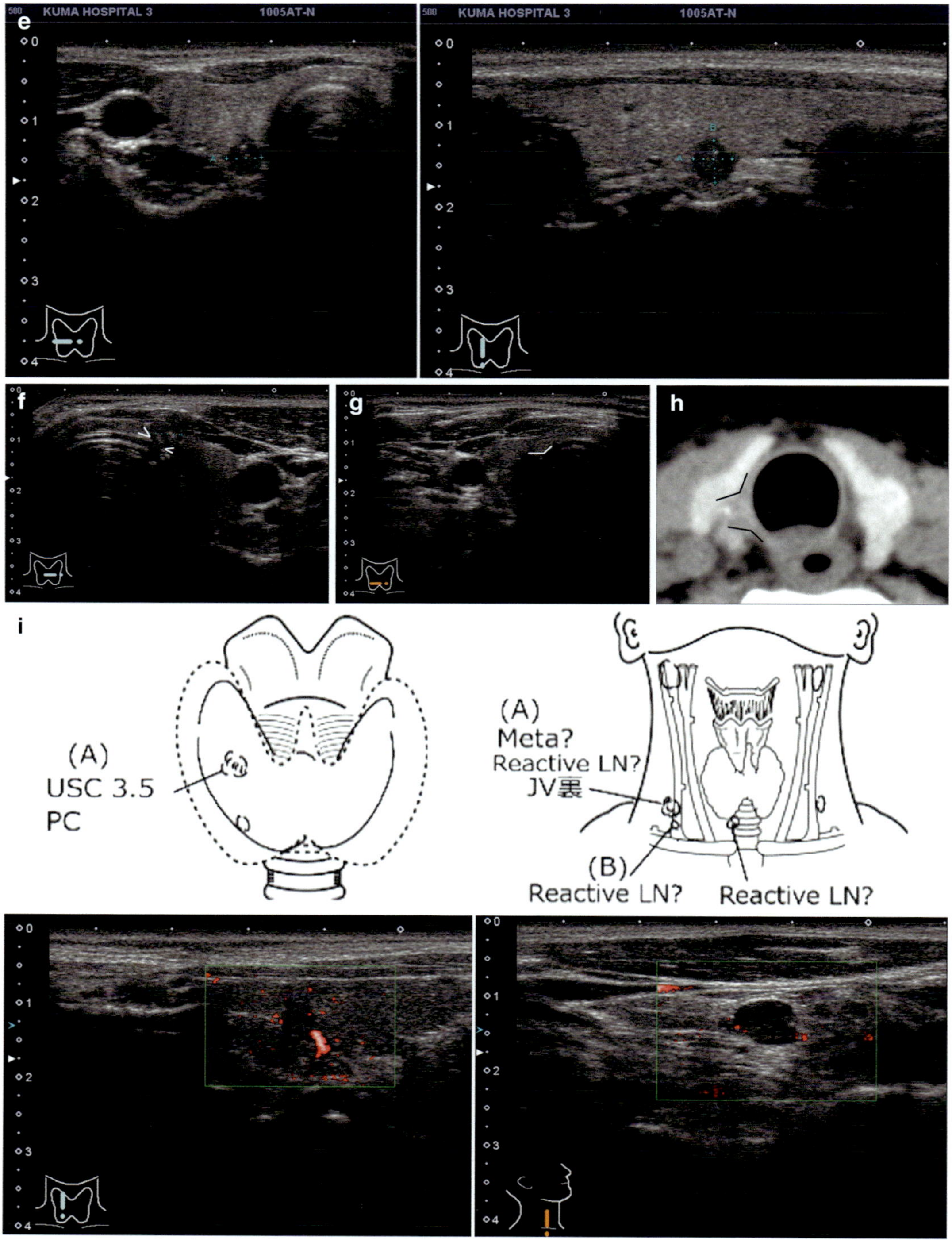

Fig. 15.1 (continued)

might see other physicians and they might perform FNAC and tell the patient, "You have thyroid cancer. Kuma Hospital failed to diagnose the cancer. You should undergo surgery immediately." This would be a terrible story for the patient and for us as well and such an unfortunate situation should be avoided.

Table 15.1 Contraindications for the AS of PTMC in patients 20 years or older

Types	Contraindications
Clinically high-risk features	1. Node metastasis or distant metastasis (very rare) detected on imaging studies 2. Signs or symptoms of invasion to the recurrent laryngeal nerve or trachea on imaging studies or fiberscope 3. High-grade malignancy on cytology (very rare)
A feature unsuitable for AS	Tumors having potential for invading the trachea or locating in the course of the recurrent laryngeal nerve

No adequate evidence available for patients younger than 20 years

In the past, after telling the result of cytology to patient with PTMC suitable for AS, we presented two options, AS and IS, equally, and asked him or her to select one. At present, however, we recommend AS as the preferred initial management, because of the accumulation of favorable data on AS. Figure 15.2 indicates how to manage PTMC patients.

Regarding a screening study to check distant metastasis, Kawano et al. reviewed 1000 consecutive patients with PTMC who underwent chest CT as a screening study before surgery and reported that none of them had metastatic lesions in the lung [14], indicating that distant metastasis in PTMC is indeed a very rare event. Therefore, we do not investigate distant metastasis using computer tomography (CT) or positron-emission tomography (PET)-CT.

Patients who chose AS are requested to visit our clinic 6 months later, and once a year thereafter. Patients are evaluated by ultrasound for tumor size change or new suspicious adenopathy.

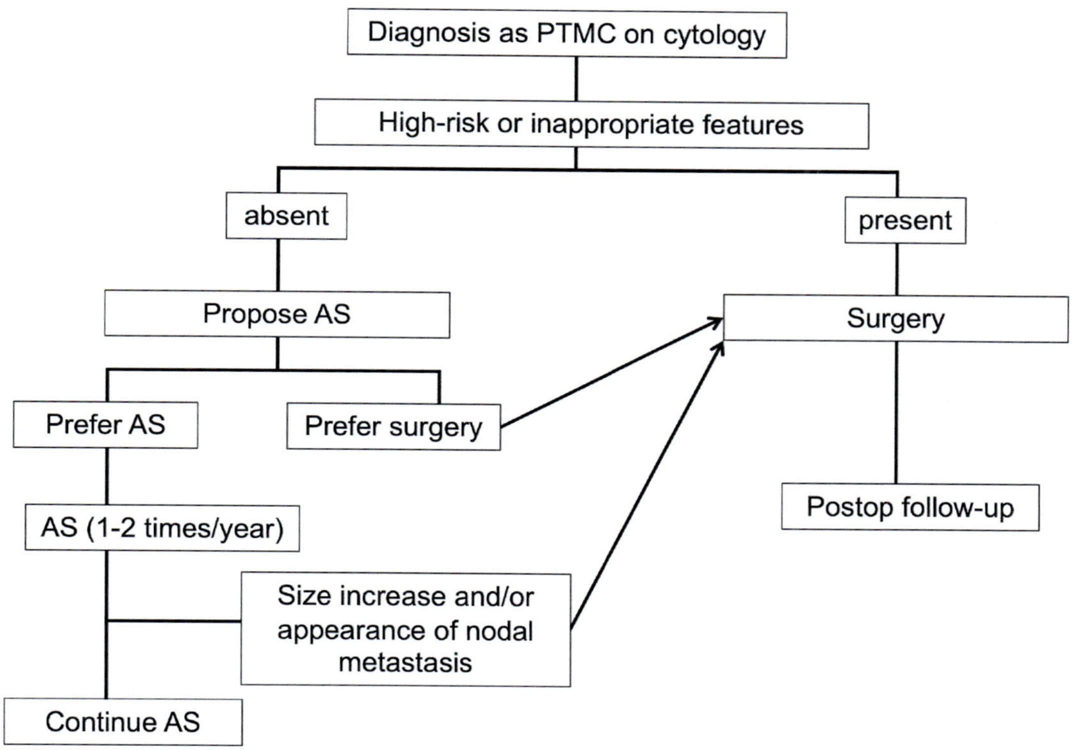

Fig. 15.2 Management flow chart for patients with PTMC

For suspicious lymph nodes, we perform FNAC together with measurement of thyroglobulin (Tg) level in the wash-out of the FNAC needles. If either of them is positive, we recommend conversion surgery (CS). Regarding the tumor size, we judge the tumor as enlarged when maximal diameter increases by ≥3 mm as compared with the reference size at diagnosis, which is defined as the mean of the first and second measurement to minimize observer variation [15]. However, if the tumor is not located at a risky location and the patient wishes to continue AS, we follow patient until tumor size reaches 13 mm or larger.

Between 1993 and 1997, only 30% of patients chose AS as their treatment of choice, but that number increased to 88% between 2014 and 2016 [16]. At present, around 95% of new patients choose AS (our unpublished data). Based on the accumulation of favorable data, physicians increasingly recommend AS with stronger confidence than before, which might explain the recent increase in the frequency of patients who opted AS.

15.4 Outcomes in Patients Who Underwent AS in Prospective Studies

To date, several prospective studies have been published regarding AS for small low-risk PTC, including PTMC. The first and second reports were published from Kuma Hospital in 2003 and 2010 [17, 18], and in 2010, CIH published its first report [19]; all of these demonstrated favorable outcomes of patients with AS. The outcomes of recent prospective studies are summarized in Table 15.2 [15, 20–29].

The most recent study from Kuma Hospital showed that 10- and 20-year tumor enlargement rates were 4.7% and 6.6%, respectively, and 10- and 20-year node metastasis appearance rates were 1.0% and 1.6%, respectively (Miyauchi et al. 2023). Nagaoka et al. at Nippon Medical School reported that 10- and 20-year enlargement rates were 9.9% and 18%, respectively, and 10- and 20-year node metastasis appearance rates were 1.4% and 3.9%, respectively [26]. None of

Table 15.2 Results of prospective studies of AS for small PTCs

Authors (Ref. number) (country)	Number of patients (tumors)	AS period	Definition of enlargement	Enlargement rate	Node metastasis appearance rate	Predictors of tumor enlargement	Predictors of node metastasis appearance
Ito et al. 2014 [20] (Japan)	1235 pts with PTMC	18–227 months (average 60 months)	Maximal diameter increased by ≥3 mm	5-year 4.9% 10-year 8.0%	5-year 1.7% 10-year 3.9%	Age <40 years	Age <40 years
Fukuoka et al. 2016 [21] (Japan)	384 pts with PTMC (480 tumors)	1–23 years (average 4.3 years)	Maximal diameter increased by ≥3 mm	5-year 6.3% 10-year 7.3%	0%	Age <50 years No/micro calcification Rich vascularization	Not listed
Tuttle et al. 2017 [22] (United States)	291 pts with low-risk PTC ≤1.5 cm	6–166 months (median 8.2 months)	1. Maximal diameter increased by ≥3 mm 2. Tumor volume increased by ≥50%	1. 2-year 2.5%, 5-year 12.1% 2. 2-year 11.5% 5-year 24.8%	0%	Age <50 years	Not listed
Oh et al. 2018 [23] (South Korea)	370 pts with PTMC	23.6–47.0 months (median 34.1 months)	1. Maximal diameter increased by ≥3 mm 2. Tumor volume increased by ≥50%	1. 3-year 3.2% 5-year 6.4% 2. 3-year 17.3% 5-year 36.2%	8.6%	Age <45 years	Not listed

(continued)

Table 15.2 (continued)

Authors (Ref. number) (country)	Number of patients (tumors)	AS period	Definition of enlargement	Enlargement rate	Node metastasis appearance rate	Predictors of tumor enlargement	Predictors of node metastasis appearance
Sanabria 2020 [24] (Colombia)	102 pts with low-risk PTC ≤1.5 cm	0.2–112 months (median 13.9 months)	1. Maximal diameter increased by ≥3 mm 2. Tumor volume increased by ≥50%	1. 2-year 10.2% 2. 2-year 23%	0%	Not listed	Not listed
Molinaro et al. 2020 [25] (Italy)	93 pts with low-risk PTC ≤1.3 cm	6–54 months (median 19 months)	1. Maximal diameter increased by ≥3 mm 2. Tumor volume increased by ≥50%	1. 2.2% 2. 16% (No time sequence analysis)	1.1% (No time sequence analysis)	Not listed	Not listed
Nagaoka et al. 2021 [26] (Japan)	571 pts with PTMC (718 tumors)	1–26 years (median 7.6 years)	Maximal diameter increased by ≥3 mm	10-year 9.9% 20-year 18.0%	10-year 1.4%, 20-year 3.9%	Age <40 years (either tumor enlargement or node metastasis appearance	
Tuttle et al. 2022 [27] (United States)	483 pts with low-risk PTC ≤1.5 cm	0.5–17 years (median 3.7 years)	1. Tumor volume increase >72% 2. Maximal diameter increase by >3 mm 3. Tumor volume increase >24%	1. 59 (12%), 5-year 15.9% 2. 472 (9%) 3. 64 (15.9%)	7 (1.4%) 5-year, 1.5%	None	None
Lee et al. 2022 [28] (South Korea)	755 pts with PTMC (Multicenter study)	Median 41.4 months (mean 41.4 ± 16.0)	Size increase ≥3 mm in one diameter, ≥2 mm in two diameters, or appearance of extrathyroid extension and node metastasis	2-year and 5-year progression rate, 5.3% and 14.2%		Age <30 years, male sex and tumor size ≥6 mm (independent predictors of progression)	
Ito et al. 2023 [15] (Japan)	2705 pts with PTMC	1–15.7 years (median 5.5 years)	Size increase ≥3 mm	5-year 3.0% 10-year 5.5% 15-year 6.2%	5-year 0.9% 10-year 1.1%, 15-year 1.1%	Age <40 years, high TSH level, tumor size ≥9 mm	Age <40 years, male sex
Miyauchi et al. 2023 [29] (Japan)	3222 pts with PTMC	1–29.3 years (median 7.3 years)	Size increase ≥3 mm	10-year 4.7% 20-year 6.6%	10-year 1.0% 20-year 1.6%,	Not listed	Not listed

AS active surveillance; *PTC* papillary thyroid carcinoma; *PTMC* papillary thyroid microcarcinoma; *pts* patients

the patients showed distant metastasis during AS or died of thyroid carcinoma. Favorable outcomes have also been demonstrated from other countries for small low-risk PTC.

15.5 Evaluation of Tumor Enlargement

In Japan, tumor enlargement is traditionally defined as size increase by ≥3 mm. This is because +/−2 mm was regarded as observer variation. However, Tuttle et al. set two definitions of tumor enlargement: a tumor diameter increase of ≥3 mm and a tumor volume increase of ≥50% [22]. They showed that the 5-year tumor volume increase ≥50% rate was 24.8%, which was much higher than tumor size ≥3 mm enlargement rate, at 12.1%. Based on this, they concluded that the serial measurement of tumor volumes might be useful for the early identification of tumors that will continue to grow. However, 1 mm increase of 7 mm tumor corresponds to 49% increase in tumor volume. We think that 50% increase in tumor volume is too sensitive to decide conversion surgery.

Miyauchi et al. studied tumor volume kinetics of PTMCs in 169 patients during AS calculating tumor volume doubling rate (TV-DR; an inverse of the tumor volume doubling time) and reported their TV-DR (/year) distributed from moderate growth (>0.5), slow growth (0.1–0.5), stable disease (−0.1–0.1), and clear decrease in tumor volume or regression (<−0.1) in 3%, 22%, 57%, and 17% of the patients, respectively [30]. This was the first report of spontaneous regression of structural disease of thyroid carcinoma in a large cohort of the patients. Miyauchi et al. also calculated the hypothetical TV-DR of PTMCs before presentation assuming that a single carcinoma cell measuring 10 μm was present at birth and grew at a constant growth rate and compared it with actual TV-DR observed during AS. They reported that, in most cases, tumor growth activity before presentation was higher than that during AS (Miyauchi et al. 2019), suggesting that growth activity of PTMC was rather rapid in its early phase but decreased along the way. Ito et al. demonstrated that TV-DR of PTMC significantly decreased after enlargement compared to before enlargement supporting the above report by Miyauchi et al. [31].

TV-DR can be calculated using a calculator that can be downloaded from the website of Kuma Hospital (https://www.kuma-h.or.jp/english/about/doubling-time-progression-calculator/), but otherwise it is difficult to calculate. Kuma Hospital, CIH, and Nippon Medical School have not experienced major failures such as anaplastic transformation or patients' mortality from thyroid carcinoma by adopting a ≥3 mm increase in maximal diameter as the definition of tumor enlargement for considering conversion surgery. Therefore, maximal diameter increase ≥3 mm is more practical and simpler than evaluating based on tumor volume increase. Another report from Italy also demonstrated that using a tumor size increase of ≥3 mm is better for performing AS for a long period [32].

Interestingly, Sasaki et al. investigated the difference in incidence of conversion surgery (CS) after AS with time by dividing the whole cohort of PTMC patients who chose AS based on the period of AS commencement into two periods: the first-half period (February 2005–November 2011) and the second-half period (December 2011–June 2017). They reported that the cumulative incidence of conversion surgery regardless of the reason for CS at 5 years decreased from 12.3% in the first-half period to 4.2% in the second-half period. This may be because the accumulation of favorable outcomes of this management strategy contributed to physicians' confidence and patients' trust and understanding of this disease [33].

15.6 Factors Associated with Progression of PTMC in AS

15.6.1 Age

As shown in Table 15.2, most prospective studies showed that young age at presentation was a strong predictor of tumor growth. Indeed, we demonstrated that PTMC in patients aged <40 years was more likely to enlarge and show appearance of lymph node metastasis than older patients, and on multivariate analysis, young age <40 years was an independent predictor of PTMC growth [15]. Interestingly, local recurrence was more likely to occur after surgery for PTMC patients <55 years than those ≥55 years [34], indicating that growth activity of PTMC in young patients is higher than that in old patients. This is in stark contrast to the well-known fact that the prognosis of clinical PTC is poorer in elderly patients than in young patients [35].

One may think that since PTMCs in young patients are more progressive than in old patients, IS is suitable for initial management in young patients. Miyauchi et al. estimated the lifetime probabilities of size increase based on the age decade-specific enlargement rates [36]. For patients in the 20s at presentation, the lifetime probability of tumor enlargement was estimated to be 48.6%. The incidence decreased with patient age; 25.3% in the 30s, 20.9% in the 40s, 10.3% in the 50s, 8.2% in the 60s, and 3.5% in the 70s. The lifetime probability of tumor enlargement in the 20s patients is high at 48.6%, but in other words, more than half of patients could avoid surgery. Since CS after slight progression is not technically difficult and, as described later, outcomes of patients who received CS are excellent, we think that young adult patients can also be candidates for AS.

15.6.2 Serum Thyroid-Stimulating Hormone (TSH) Level

To date, discrepant data have been published whether the TSH level is related to PTMC progression [37, 38]. In 2023, we demonstrated that low TSH level (less than the lower normal limit) was an independent negative predictor of tumor enlargement especially in young subset (age <40 years) [15]. Furthermore, Yamamoto et al. showed that patients who were started on levothyroxine during AS had significantly lower tumor growth activity after the administration than before the administration [39]. Administering levothyroxine to suppress TSH with mildly subnormal level while avoiding symptomatic hyperthyroidism might be useful for preventing tumor enlargement especially in young patients. Prospective studies are needed to further define this issue.

15.6.3 Ultrasound Findings

It was reported that, in PTMCs who underwent surgery, patients with multiple tumors were more likely to be positive for pathological lateral lymph node metastasis [40]. However, none of the prospective studies on AS showed that tumor multiplicity was related to tumor enlargement or novel node metastasis appearance (Table 15.2). If multiple tumors should undergo surgery, patients would usually receive total thyroidectomy, resulting in an increased incidence of recurrent laryngeal nerve damage and hypoparathyroidism. Therefore, AS would be better recommended for such patients. Fukuoka et al. showed that PTMCs negative for calcification or positive for rich vascularity are progressive [21], but they also showed that a consolidation of calcification and loss of vascularity occurred during AS, indicating that PTMCs can undergo AS regardless of the ultrasound findings of calcification and vascularity.

15.6.4 Pregnancy

It is known that pregnancy might cause enlargement of thyroid nodules because of the structural similarity between TSH and human chorionic gonadotropin, and thus, how to manage PTMC in young women who are possibly pregnant in the future is an important issue. In our series, only 4 tumors (8%) of the 50 patients showed size increase ≥3 mm during pregnancy [41]. Two of these underwent surgery after delivery, and no postoperative recurrences have been detected. The remaining two underwent continuous AS because their tumors did not continuously enlarge after delivery. Therefore, we think young women with PTMC can be candidates for AS.

15.7 Clinical Questions to Be Elucidated

15.7.1 Exploration of Cytological or Molecular Markers Predicting PTMC Progression

Hirokawa et al. reported that PTMCs surgically removed due to tumor enlargement had significantly higher Ki-67 labeling index than those without tumor enlargement [42]. However, Ki-67 labeling index cannot be evaluated on cytological specimens. Xing et al. demonstrated that *BRAF* and *TERT* mutations were strongly associated with poor prognosis in clinical PTC [43]. Ebina et al. also showed that *TERT* mutations independently predicted the poor disease-free survival and cause-specific survival of clinical PTCs [44]. However, in PTMC, *TERT* mutations were reported to be a very rare event and not associated with patients' prognosis [45, 46]. Therefore, at present, no markers can predict future progression of PTMC. Although very rare, PTMC can metastasize to distant organs. In our series, one of the 2424 IS patients developed pulmonary metastasis 12 years after surgery. One of the 3222 AS patients who underwent CS (because of patient's preference) after 2 years of AS developed pulmonary metastasis 12 years after diagnosis [29]. Their metastatic lesions did not accumulate radioactive iodine; however, they were alive (18.8 years and 18.4 years) after the initial diagnosis. The discovery of predictive molecular markers would be a great help to select potentially progressive PTMCs for immediate surgery and careful postoperative follow-up.

15.7.2 How Long Should as Be Continued?

It has been reported that the growth activity of PTMC significantly decreased in older patients. However, old age is a well-known prognostic factor for poor prognosis in clinical PTC (Ito et al. 2012), and if PTMC turned clinical, patients may suffer a dire prognosis. In the series of Tuttle et al., one of the 482 patients who underwent AS began to grow rather rapidly after AS for more than 4 years [27]. The patient underwent CS and was pathologically diagnosed as poorly differentiated carcinoma. In the series of medullary thyroid carcinoma, a few cases showing spontaneous increase of tumor growth activity have been reported [47], and a similar event may possibly be detected in PTC. Therefore, currently, we have to conclude that AS should be continued long term and as long as possible. We would like to remind readers that most patients who undergo surgery require lifetime follow-up and administration of levothyroxine.

15.8 Comparison Between AS and IS for PTMC

15.8.1 Prognosis

Postoperative prognosis for PTMC is reported to be favorable; 5- and 10-year lymph node recurrence-free survival rates, distant recurrence-free survival rates, and cause-specific survival rates were 99% and 99%, 100% and 100%, and 100% and 100%, respectively (Ito et al. 2012). Miyauchi et al. compared between the prognosis of PTMC patients who underwent AS and those received IS; 10- and 20-year lymph node metastasis occurrence/recurrence rates of AS and IS patients were 1.1% and 1.7%, and 0.4% and 0.7%, respectively (29. Lymph node metastasis occurrence rate in the AS group was very low, although slightly higher than node metastasis recurrence rate in the IS group. However, 10.3% of the IS group in this series underwent prophylactic lateral neck dissection at their initial surgery. Ten-year and 20-year remnant thyroid recurrence rates of the IS group patients who underwent hemithyroidectomy were 1.0% and 2.7%, respectively [29]. The proportion of the patients who underwent one or more surgeries was significantly higher in the IS group (100%) than in the AS group (12.3%) ($p < 0.01$). The proportion of the patients who underwent two or more surgeries was also significantly higher in the IS group (1.07%) than in the AS group (0.09%) ($p < 0.01$). Furthermore, overall mortality rate did not differ between the AS and IS group patients [33]. Taken together, the oncological outcomes of patients in the AS and IS groups are not meaningfully different, IS group underwent higher incidence of surgical intervention than AS group.

15.8.2 Unfavorable Surgical Events

Although surgery for PTMC is rather easy, Oda et al. showed that permanent vocal cord paralysis and permanent hypoparathyroidism occurred in 0.2% and 1.6% of their patients, respectively [48]. It is noteworthy that, in these series, surgery was done by experts for thyroid surgery. Recently, Sasaki et al. reviewed larger cohorts and confirmed that patients who underwent IS had significantly higher incidences of unfavorable events than patients who chose AS [49]. If patients had undergone surgery by non-experts, the incidence of unfavorable surgical events would have been much higher. This is an important issue when considering the significance of AS for PTMC, because such events would not have occurred in patients who chose AS over surgery.

15.8.3 CS After AS for PTMC Patients

A portion of patients undergo CS after AS for various reasons, e.g., progression of PTMC or coexisting thyroid or parathyroid diseases, change in patients' mind, and physicians' recommendation. Fujishima et al. reported that patients who underwent CS due to PTMC progression had larger tumors were more frequently positive for pathological node metastasis and had higher cell proliferating activity (as evaluated by the Ki-67 labeling index) than IS patients [50]. Despite those features, the postoperative prognosis of the two groups was similar. Thus, they suggested that AS and CS for progressive tumors efficiently selected the minority of PTMCs that truly require surgery. Further, Sasaki et al. showed that the incidence of unfavorable surgical events such as transient/permanent vocal cord paralysis and hypoparathyroidism did not significantly differ between patients who underwent CS after AS and those received IS [49]. These findings might warrant the validity of AS as the initial management for PTMCs.

15.8.4 Medical Costs

Discrepant results in regard to medical costs have been reported for foreign countries, because the costs for examinations, surgeries, and medical prescriptions differ significantly from country to country [51–54]. In Japan, most of clinical practices are performed under the national health insurance system. According to our calculation based on our clinical practice at Kuma Hospital, the total cost of immediate surgery and postoperative care for 10 years (including prescription medicines such as L-thyroxine) was USD $8437/person, which was 4.1 times the total cost of 10-year active surveillance ($2052/person) in the year 2017 [54].

15.8.5 Comparison of Quality of Life (QoL) Between Patients Treated with AS and IS

To date, only a few reports have been published about the QoL of patients who underwent AS and IS [55–59]. Their results are discrepant, but recent studies showed that patients under AS had a higher QoL than those who underwent IS, not only in terms of physical issues but also with respect to anxiety and other psychological challenges [55–58]. In this context, we suspect that the incidence and degree of various psychological issues in patients in the AS group are significantly dependent on the attitude of attending physicians. Specifically, patients would be less likely to worry about their illness if their physicians have confidence and conviction in recommending AS. Unfortunately, however, no reports have been published regarding the relationship between the emotional problems of PTMC patients and interactions with their physicians.

15.9 Conclusions

If appropriately implemented, AS is safe and beneficial management for PTMC patients when selected as the initial management.

References

1. Miyauchi A. Clinical trials of active surveillance of papillary microcarcinoma of the thyroid. World J Surg. 2016;40:516–22. https://doi.org/10.1007/s00268-015-3392-y.
2. Takebe K, Date M, Yamamoto Y. Mass screening for thyroid cancer with ultrasonography [in Japanese]. Karkinos. 1994;7:309–17.
3. Takami H, Ito Y, Okamoto T, Yoshida A. Therapeutic strategy for differentiated thyroid carcinoma in Japan based on a newly established guideline managed by Japanese Society of Thyroid Surgeons and Japanese Association of endocrine surgeons. World J Surg. 2011;35:111–21. https://doi.org/10.1007/s00268-010-0832-6.
4. Ito Y, Onoda N, Okamoto T. The revised clinical practice guidelines on the management of thyroid tumors by the Japan Associations of Endocrine Surgeons: core questions and recommendations for treatments of thyroid cancer. Endocr J. 2020;67:669–717. https://doi.org/10.1507/endocrj.EJ20-0025.
5. Haugen BR, Alexander EK, Bible KC, Doherty GM, Mandel SJ, Nikiforov YE, et al. 2015 American Thyroid Association management guidelines for adult patients with thyroid nodules and differentiated thyroid cancer: the American Thyroid Association guidelines task force on thyroid nodules and differentiated thyroid cancer. Thyroid. 2016;26:1–133. https://doi.org/10.1089/thy.2015.0020.
6. Sugitani I, Ito Y, Takeuchi D, Nakayama H, Masaki C, Shindo H, et al. Indications and strategy for active surveillance of adult low-risk papillary thyroid microcarcinoma: consensus statements from the Japan Association of Endocrine Surgery task force on management for papillary thyroid microcarcinoma. Thyroid. 2021;31:183–92. https://doi.org/10.1089/thy.2020.0330.
7. Horiguchi K, Yoshida Y, Iwaku K, Emoto N, Kasahara T, Sato J, et al. Position paper from the Japan thyroid association task force on the management of low-risk papillary thyroid microcarcinoma (T1aN0M0) in adults. Endocr J. 2021;68:763–80. https://doi.org/10.1507/endocrj.EJ20-0692.
8. Davies L, Welch HG. Increasing incidence of thyroid cancer in the United States, 1973–2002. JAMA. 2006;595:2164–7. https://doi.org/10.1001/jama.295.18.2164.
9. Davies L, Welch HG. Current thyroid cancer trends in the United States. JAMA Otolaryngol Head Neck Surg. 2014;140:317–22. https://doi.org/10.1001/jamaoto.2014.1.
10. Ahn HS, Kim HJ, Welch HG. Korea's thyroid-cancer "epidemic"—screening and overdiagnosis. N Engl J Med. 2014;371:1765–7.
11. Vaccarella S, Dal Maso L, Laversanne M, Bray F, Plummer M, Franceschi S. The impact of diagnostic changes on the rise in thyroid cancer incidence: a population-based study in selected high-resource countries. Thyroid. 2015;25:1127–36. https://doi.org/10.1056/NEJMp1409841.
12. Brito JP, Ito Y, Miyauchi A, Tuttle RM, Tuttle RM. A clinical framework to facilitate risk stratification when considering an active surveillance alternative to immediate biopsy and surgery in papillary microcarcinoma. Thyroid. 2016;26:144–9. https://doi.org/10.1089/thy.2015.0178.
13. Ito Y, Miyauchi A, Oda H, Kobayashi K, Kihara M, Miya A. Revisiting low-risk thyroid papillary microcarcinomas resected without observation: was immediate surgery necessary? World J Surg. 2016;40:523–8. https://doi.org/10.1007/s00268-015-3184-4.
14. Kawano S, Miyauchi A, Ito Y. Routine chest computed tomography at presentation does not identify distant metastasis in cT1aN0 papillary thyroid carcinoma. Thyroid. 2020;30:1620–4. https://doi.org/10.1089/thy.2020.0073.
15. Ito Y, Miyauchi A, Fujishima M, Noda T, Sano T, Sasaki T, et al. Thyroid-stimulating hormone, age, and tumor size are risk factors for progression during active surveillance of low-risk papillary thyroid microcarcinoma in adults. World J Surg. 2023;47:392–401. https://doi.org/10.1007/s00268-022-06861-x.
16. Ito Y, Miyauchi A, Kudo T, Oda H, Yamamoto M, Sasai H, et al. Trends in the implementation of active surveillance for low-risk papillary thyroid microcarcinomas at Kuma hospital: gradual increase and heterogeneity in the acceptance of this new management option. Thyroid. 2018;28:488–95. https://doi.org/10.1089/thy.2017.0448.
17. Ito Y, Uruno T, Nakano K, Takamura Y, Miya A, Kobayashi K, et al. An observation trial without surgical treatment in patients with papillary microcarcinoma of the thyroid. Thyroid. 2003;13:381–7. https://doi.org/10.1089/105072503321669875.
18. Ito Y, Miyauchi A, Inoue H, Fukushima M, Kihara M, Higashiyama T, et al. An observation trial for papillary thyroid microcarcinoma in Japanese patients. World J Surg. 2010;34:28–35. https://doi.org/10.1007/s00268-009-0303-0.
19. Sugitani I, Toda K, Yamada K, et al. Three distinctly different kinds of papillary thyroid microcarcinoma should be recognized: our treatment strategies and outcomes. World J Surg. 2010;34:1222–31. https://doi.org/10.1007/s00268-009-0359-x.
20. Ito Y, Miyauchi A, Kihara M, Higashiyama T, Kobayashi K, Miya A. Patient age is significantly related to the progression of papillary microcarcinoma of the thyroid under observation.

Thyroid. 2014;24:27–34. https://doi.org/10.1089/thy.2013.0367.

21. Fukuoka O, Sugitani I, Ebina A, Toda K, Kawabata K, Yamada K. Natural history of asymptomatic papillary thyroid microcarcinoma: time-dependent changes in calcification and vascularity during active surveillance. World J Surg. 2016;40:529–37. https://doi.org/10.1007/s00268-015-3349-1.
22. Tuttle RM, Fagin JA, Minkowitz G, Wong RJ, Roman B, Patel S, et al. Natural history and tumor volume kinetics of papillary thyroid cancers during active surveillance. JAMA Otolaryngol Head Neck Surg. 2017;143:1015–20. https://doi:10.1001/jamaoto.2017.1442
23. Oh HS, Ha J, Kim HI, Kim TH, Kim WG, Lin DJ, et al. Active surveillance of low-risk papillary thyroid microcarcinoma: a multi-center cohort study in Korea. Thyroid. 2018;28:1587–94. https://doi.org/10.1089/thy.2018.0263.
24. Sanabria A. Experience with active surveillance of thyroid low-risk carcinoma in a developing country. Thyroid. 2020;7:985–91. https://doi.org/10.1089/thy.2019.0522.
25. Molinaro E, Campopiano MC, Pieruzzi L, Matrone A, Agate L, Bottici V, et al. Active surveillance in papillary thyroid microcarcinomas is feasible and safe: experience at a single Italian center. J Elin Endocrinol Metab. 2020;105:e172–80. https://doi.org/10.1210/clinem/dgz113.
26. Nagaoka R, Ebina A, Toda K, Jikuzono T, Saitou M, Sen M, et al. Multifocality and progression of papillary thyroid microcarcinoma during active surveillance. World J Surg. 2021;45:2769–76. https://doi.org/10.1007/s00268-021-06185-2.
27. Tuttle RM, Fagin J, Minkowitz WR, Roman B, Patel S, et al. Active surveillance of papillary thyroid cancer: frequency and time course of the six most common tumor volume kinetic patterns. Thyroid. 2022;32:1337–45. https://doi.org/10.1089/thy.2022.0325.
28. Lee EK, Moon JH, Hwangbo Y, Ryu CH, Cho SW, Choi JY, et al. Progression of low-risk papillary thyroid microcarcinoma during active surveillance: interim analysis of a multicenter prospective cohort study of active surveillance on papillary thyroid microcarcinoma in Korea. Thyroid. 2022;32:1328–36. https://doi.org/10.1089/thy.2021.0614.
29. Miyauchi A, Ito Y, Fujishima M, Miya A, Onoda N, Kihara M, et al. Long-term outcomes of active surveillance and immediate surgery for adult patients with low-risk papillary thyroid microcarcinoma: 30-year experience. Thyroid. 2023;33:817–25. https://doi.org/10.1089/thy.2023.0076.
30. Miyauchi A, Kudo T, Ito Y, Oda H, Yamamoto M, Sasai H, et al. Natural history of papillary thyroid microcarcinoma: kinetic analyses on tumor volume during active surveillance and before presentation. Surgery. 2019;165:25–30. https://doi.org/10.1016/j.surg.2018.07.045.
31. Ito Y, Miyauchi A, Kudo T, Higashiyama T, Masuoka H, Miya A. Kinetic analysis of growth activity in enlarging papillary thyroid microcarcinomas. Thyroid. 2019;29:1765–73. https://doi.org/10.1089/thy.2019.0396.
32. Campopiano MD, Matrone A, Rago T, Scutani M, Prete A, Agete L, et al. Assessing mPTC progression during active surveillance: volume or diameter increase? J Clin Med. 2021;10:4068. https://doi.org/10.3390/jcm10184068.
33. Sasaki T, Miyauchi A, Ito Y, Kudo T, Kanemura N, Sano T, et al. Marked decrease over time in conversion surgery after active surveillance of low-risk papillary thyroid microcarcinoma. Thyroid. 2021;31:217–23. https://doi.org/10.1089/thy.2020.0319.
34. Ito Y, Miyauchi A, Fujishima M, Masuoka H, Higashiyama T, Kihara M, et al. Prognostic significance of patient age in papillary thyroid carcinoma with no high-risk features. Endocr J. 2022;69:1131–6. https://doi.org/10.1507/endocrj.EJ22-0056.
35. Ito Y, Kudo T, Kobayashi K, Miya A, Ichihara K, Miyauchi A. Prognostic factors for recurrence of papillary thyroid carcinoma in the lymph nodes, lung, and bone: analysis of 5,768 patients with average 10-year follow-up. World J Surg. 2012;36(6):1274–8. https://doi.org/10.1007/s00268-012-1423-5.
36. Miyauchi A, Kudo T, Ito Y, Oda H, Sasai H, Higashiyama T, et al. 2018 estimation of the lifetime probability of disease progression of papillary microcarcinoma of the thyroid during active surveillance. Surgery. 2018;163:48–52. https://doi.org/10.1016/j.surg.2017.03.028.
37. Sugitani I, Fujimoto Y, Yamada K. Association between serum thyrotropin concentration and growth of asymptomatic papillary thyroid microcarcinoma. World J Surg. 2014;38:673–8. https://doi.org/10.1007/s00268-013-2335-8.
38. Kim HI, Jang HW, Ahn HS, Ahn S, Park SY, Oh YL, et al. High serum TSH level is associated with progression of papillary thyroid microcarcinoma during active surveillance. J Clin Endocrinol Metab. 2018;103:446–51. https://doi.org/10.1210/jc.2018-00530.
39. Yamamoto M, Miyauchi A, Ito Y, Fujishima M, Sasaki T, Kudo T. Active surveillance outcomes of patients with low-risk papillary thyroid microcarcinoma according to levothyroxine treatment status. Thyroid. 2023;33:1182–9. https://doi.org/10.1089/thy.2023.0046.
40. Ito Y, Tomoda C, Uruno T, Takamura Y, Miya A, Kobayashi K, et al. Papillary microcarcinoma of the thyroid: how should it be treated? World J Surg. 2004;28:1115–21. https://doi.org/10.1007/s00268-004-7644-5.
41. Ito Y, Miyauchi A, Kudo T, Ota H, Yoshioka K, Oda H, et al. 2016 effects of pregnancy on papillary microcarcinomas of the thyroid re-evaluated in the entire patient series at Kuma hospital. Thyroid. 2016;26(1):156–60.https://doi.org/10.1089/thy.2015.0393.

42. Hirokawa M, Kudo T, Ota H, Suzuki A, Miyauchi A. Pathological characteristics of low-risk papillary thyroid microcarcinoma with progression during active surveillance. Endocr J. 2016;63:805–10. https://doi.org/10.1507/endocrj.EJ16-0097.
43. Xing M, Liu R, Liu X, Murugan AK, Zhu G, Zeiger MA, et al. 2BRAF V600E and TERT promoter mutations cooperatively identify the most aggressive papillary thyroid cancer with highest recurrence. J Clin Oncol. 2014;32:2718–25. https://doi.org/10.1200/JCO.2014.55.5094.
44. Ebina A, Togashi Y, Baba S, Sato Y, Sakata S, Ishikawa M, et al. *TERT* promoter mutation and extent of thyroidectomy in patients with 1-4 cm intrathyroidal papillary carcinoma. Cancers (Basel). 2020;12:2115. https://doi.org/10.3390/cancers12082115.
45. Yabuta T, Matsuse M, Hirokawa M, Yamashita S, Mitsutake N, Miyauchi A. TERT promoter mutations were not found in papillary thyroid microcarcinomas that showed disease progression on active surveillance. Thyroid. 2017;27:1206–7. https://doi.org/10.1089/thy.2016.0645.
46. De Biase D, Gandolfi G, Ragazzi M, Eszlinger M, Sancisi V, Gugnoni M, et al. TERT promoter mutations in papillary thyroid microcarcinoma. Thyroid. 2015;25:1013–9. https://doi.org/10.1089/thy.2015.0101.
47. Miyauchi A, Kudo T, Kihara M, Oda H, Ito Y, Miya A. Spontaneous deceleration and acceleration of growth rate in medullary thyroid carcinomas suggested by changes in calcitonin doubling times over long-term surveillance. World J Surg. 2019;43:504–12. https://doi.org/10.1007/s00268-018-4789-1.
48. Oda H, Miyauchi A, Ito Y, Yoshioka K, Nakayama A, Sasai H, et al. Incidence of unfavorable events in the management of low-risk papillary microcarcinoma of the thyroid by active surveillance versus immediate surgery. Thyroid. 2016;26:150–5. https://doi.org/10.1089/thy.2015.0313.
49. Sasaki T, Miyauchi A, Fujishima M, Ito Y, Kudo T, Noda T, et al. Comparison or postoperative unfavorable events in patients with low-risk papillary thyroid carcinoma: immediate surgery versus conversion surgery following active surveillance. Thyroid. 2023;33:186–91. https://doi.org/10.1089/thy.2022.0444.
50. Fujishima M, Miiyauchi A, Ito Y, Kudo T, Noda T, Sano T, et al. Active surveillance is an excellent management technique for identifying patients with progressive low-risk papillary thyroid microcarcinoma requiring surgical treatment. Endocr J. 2023;70:411–8. https://doi.org/10.1507/endocrj.EJ22-0559.
51. Lin JF, Jonker PKC, Cunich M, Sidhu SB, Delbridge LW, Glover AR, et al. Surgery alone for papillary thyroid microcarcinoma is less costly and more effective than long term active surveillance. Surgery. 2020;167:110–6. https://doi.org/10.1016/j.surg2019.05.078.
52. Kim K, Choi JY, Kim SJ, Lee EK, Lee YK, Ryu JS, et al. Active surveillance versus surgery for low-risk papillary thyroid microcarcinoma patients in South Korea: a cost-minimization analysis from the MAeSTro study. Thyroid. 2022;32:648–56. https://doi.org/10.1089/thy.2021.0679.
53. Lang BH, Wong CK. A cost-effectiveness comparison between early surgery and non-surgical approach for incidental papillary thyroid microcarcinoma. Eur J Endocrinol. 2015;173:367–75.
54. Oda H, Miyauchi A, Ito Y, Sasai H, Masuoka H, Yabuta T, et al. Comparison of the costs of active surveillance and immediate surgery in the management of low-risk papillary microcarcinoma of the thyroid. Endocr J. 2017;64:59–64. https://doi.org/10.1507/endocrj.EJ16-0381.
55. Yoshida Y, Horiuchi K, Okamoto T. Patients' view on the management of papillary thyroid microcarcinoma: active surveillance or surgery. Thyroid. 2020;30:681–7. https://doi.org/10.1089/thy.2019.0420.
56. Jeon MJ, Lee YM, Sung TY, Han M, Shin YW, Kim WG, et al. Quality of life in patients with papillary thyroid microcarcinoma managed by active surveillance or lobectomy: a cross-sectional study. Thyroid. 2019;29:956–62. https://doi.org/10.1089/thy.2018.0711.
57. Moon JH, Ryu CH, Cho SW, Choi JY, Chung EJ, Hah JH, et al. Effect of initial treatment choice on 2-year quality of life in patients with low-risk papillary thyroid microcarcinoma. J Clin Endocrinol Metab. 2021;106:724–35. https://doi.org/10.1210/clinem/dgaa889.
58. Nakamura T, Miyauchi A, Ito Y, Ito M, Kudo T, Tanaka M, et al. Quality of life in patients with low-risk papillary thyroid microcarcinoma: active surveillance versus immediate surgery. Endocr Pract. 2020;26:1451–7. https://doi.org/10.4158/EP-2020-0201.
59. Kazusaka H, Sugitani I, Toda K, Sen M, Saito M, Nagaoka R, et al. Patient-reported outcomes in patients with low-risk papillary thyroid carcinoma: cross-sectional study to compare active surveillance and immediate surgery. World J Surg. 2022;47:1190–8. https://doi.org/10.1007/s00268-022-06786-5.

16 Radiofrequency Ablation for Papillary Thyroid Microcarcinoma

Mattia Squarcia, Fernando Diego Choque Chavez, and Roberto Valcavi

16.1 Introduction

Papillary thyroid carcinoma (PTC) is the most common subtype of thyroid malignant neoplasm. PTCs measuring 1 cm or less were defined by the World Health Organization (WHO) as papillary thyroid microcarcinoma (PTMC) [1]. According to most guidelines, surgery is the primary therapy for PTC [2, 3]. However, thyroid surgery's significant morbidities, such as hypothyroidism, hypoparathyroidism, and laryngeal nerve impairment, are worth noting in a context where patients with PTMC have a disease-specific survival that exceeds 99% after 10 years of follow-up [4, 5]. In this sense, two strategies have been postulated as substitutes for treatment de-escalation for patients with low-risk PTMC, aiming to reduce surgery-associated morbidity: active surveillance (AS) [2, 3, 6] and thermal ablation [7–9]. Thermal ablation, a technique that includes microwave ablation (MWA), laser ablation (LA), and radiofrequency ablation (RFA), has been assessed for its efficacy and safety in treating benign thyroid nodules [10–12] and recurrent PTC [13–16]. However, the application of thermal ablation as a primary therapeutic tool for low-risk PTMCs remains controversial. In light of this, multiple clinical trials have evaluated the use of thermal ablation for treating low-risk PTMCs [7, 8, 17–19], reassuring its efficacy and safety in selected patients. Moreover, the 2017 Korean RFA guidelines and Italian opinion statement presented the potential therapeutic role of RDA ablation in primary thyroid cancer in patients with high surgical risk or who refuse surgery [20, 21].

The forthcoming chapter will center on RFA as a treatment modality for PTMC, elucidating key aspects encompassing RFA principles, efficacy, safety, procedural methodologies, complications, and the subsequent follow-up.

16.1.1 Papillary Thyroid Microcarcinoma Essentials

Papillary thyroid carcinoma (PTC) is the most common subtype of thyroid malignant neoplasm. PTCs measuring 1 cm or less were defined by the World Health Organization (WHO) as papillary thyroid microcarcinoma (PTMC) and may or may not have lymph node (LN) metastasis [1, 22]. Papillary carcinomas may present as solitary or multifocal lesions within the thyroid gland, and PTMC is usually found incidentally. These tumors are often close to the thyroid capsule, can exhibit well-defined or encapsulated characteristics, and may exhibit fibrosis and calcification,

M. Squarcia (✉) · F. D. C. Chavez
Hospital Clinic Barcelona, Barcelona, Spain
e-mail: squarcia@clinic.cat; choque@clinic.cat

R. Valcavi
Department of Endocrinology, The Endocrine & Thyroid Clinic, Reggio Emilia, Italy

R. Valcavi et al. (eds.), *Thyroid Ablation*, https://doi.org/10.1007/978-3-031-88229-6_16

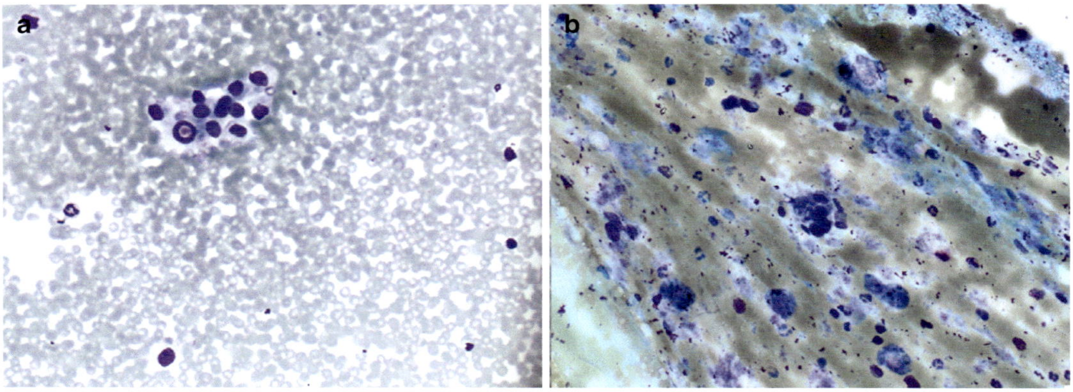

Fig. 16.1 FNA of thyroid nodules. (**a**) Cytologic specimen demonstrating a blood-based smear in which a group of follicular cells with irregular nuclei is observed with the presence of a nuclear pseudoinclusion compatible with Bethesda class VI cytology. (**b**) Cytologic specimen of a malignant Bethesda VI. In the center of the image, there is a group of large cells, with lighter nuclei, pseudoinclusions, and nuclear molding compatible with papillary carcinoma

often displaying cystic features. Diagnosis always hinges upon microscopic examination [1, 23] (Fig. 16.1).

Epidemiology of PTC and PTMC has changed over the years. The incidence of PTC increased from 8 to 14.9 per 100,000, reached a state of stability, and subsequently exhibited a reduction to 13.5 per 100,000 by 2018 [24, 25]. Regarding risk factors for PTMC, radiation exposure and family history of a thyroid cancer syndrome (familial polyposis, Carney complex, multiple endocrine neoplasia type 2—MEN2, Werner syndrome, or Cowden syndrome, may increase risk of thyroid cancer) have been reported [1, 26–29]. In terms of prognosis, PTMC has an indolent nature and has a favorable outcome. Only a limited subset of patients—specifically those with distant metastases, extensive tumor invasion into the airway, nerves, or major neck vessels, or individuals aged over 55 at diagnosis—are predisposed to adverse outcomes [30, 31]. Moreover, patients with PTMC have a disease-specific survival that exceeds 99% after 10 years of follow-up [4, 5].

Thyroidectomy is the first-line treatment for PTMC as endorsed by guidelines [2, 3, 32]. Nevertheless, it carries risks such as hypothyroidism, hypoparathyroidism, and laryngeal nerve impairment and can result in overtreatment. In this sense, two strategies have been postulated as substitutes for treatment de-escalation for patients with low-risk PTMC, aiming to reduce surgery-associated morbidity: active surveillance (AS) [2, 3, 6] and thermal ablation [7–9] (Fig. 16.2).

In case of AS, ultrasound examination must confirm absence of tumor progression during the follow-up. Prior to thermal ablation, US-guided evaluation of the location of the lesion and its relationship to thyroid capsule and perithyroid structures is mandatory to plan the treatment. AS is performed with ultrasound performed every 6 months for 1–2 years and then annually in cases of PTC of ≤1 cm without concerning LN [32]. If appropriately applied, AS of low-risk PTMC constitutes a secure management approach, yielding favorable outcomes and maintaining quality of life with cost-effectiveness [32, 33]. Nonetheless, factors such as ensuring proper compliance, educating both patients and physicians, and evaluating the psychological impact of this approach, which can lead to heightened patient anxiety and distress, need to be considered [34].

On the contrary, thermal ablation stands as a therapeutic modality encompassing MWA, LA, and RFA. Its effectiveness and safety have been subject to evaluation in the management of benign thyroid nodules [10–12] and recurrent PTC [13–16]. Nevertheless, the utilization of

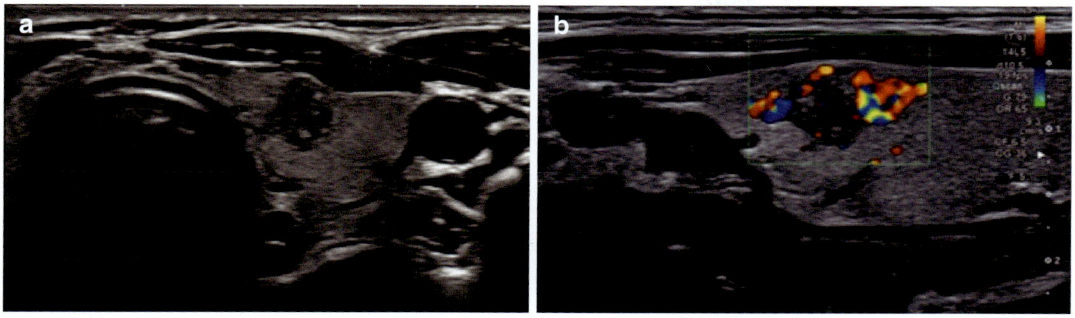

Fig. 16.2 (**a**) Axial b-mode ultrasound of the left thyroid lobe demonstrates the presence of a solid, hypoechoic, taller than width infracentimetric nodule presenting punctiform hyperechoic spots indicating microcalcification. (**b**) Sagittal Color Doppler examination showing intranodular and peripheral vascularization

thermal ablation as a therapeutic intervention for low-risk PTMCs has sparked controversy and lacks endorsement in the guidelines delineated by the National Comprehensive Cancer Network (NCCN) for thyroid carcinoma and the American Thyroid Association (ATA) [2, 32]. In consideration of this, numerous studies have evaluated the application of thermal ablation in the treatment of low-risk PTMCs, providing reassurance regarding its efficacy and safety within specific patient cohorts [7, 8, 17–19]. Additionally, the 2017 Korean RFA guidelines and Italian opinion statement have outlined the plausible therapeutic role of RFA ablation in cases of primary thyroid cancer, particularly for patients with elevated surgical risks or those who opt against surgery [20, 21].

16.2 Principles in Radiofrequency Ablation (RFA)

Ultrasound (US)-guided radiofrequency ablation (RFA) stands as one of the extensively investigated percutaneous modalities. In the domain of thyroid lesions, it emerges as a non-surgical and minimally invasive therapeutic alternative. Analogous to MWA, LA, and cryoablation, RFA similarly seeks to accomplish thermal ablation of lesions and eradicate malignant cells within a designated target volume [35, 36].

RFA setup creates a simple electrical circuit formed by a generator, cabling, electrodes, and tissues as the resistive element. Generator provides power generation, control, and user interface. Regarding electrodes, the majority of radiofrequency ablation (RFA) systems predominantly function within a monopolar configuration, facilitated through the incorporation of two distinct electrodes: interstitial electrodes and dispersive electrodes, the latter also identified as ground pads. The interstitial electrode assumes the role of administering energy to the tumor, resulting in the establishment of a region characterized by intensified current density and localized heating. The dispersive electrode serves the purpose of finalizing the electrical circuit path and disperses energy over a large surface area, a fact that is intended to reduce the risk of thermal injury to the skin [35, 36]. There are also bipolar systems. They utilize two interstitial electrodes, oscillating current between them, either within the same or separate applicators. This configuration confines current flow to enhance tissue heating between the electrodes, while limiting cooling effects from heat sinks [35]. Finally, the resistive elements of the circuit are the tissues. Due to its intrinsic electrical impedance, tissues are poor electricity conductors, and current passage incites ionic agitation and the subsequent generation of heat via Joule effect. During the process, tissues that are located closer to an electrode are subject to more efficient heating, while peripheral areas acquire heat through thermal conduction [36].

The heating of the target lesion causes a variety of tissue changes in the lesion and around it [37]. The lesion ablated is thought to have three zones: the central zone that is near the electrode and undergoes coagulative necrosis, the peripheral zone which undergoes apoptosis or recovers from reversible injury, and the surrounding tissue that is unaffected by ablation [38].

Like other hyperthermal ablation techniques, i.e., MWA and LA, RFA induces cell death through both direct and indirect mechanisms. Direct cellular harm transpires across various tiers, spanning subcellular to tissue levels, and hinges on factors such as the extent and rate of thermal energy application, as well as the thermal susceptibility of the targeted tissue. Direct mechanisms include cell membrane collapse, protein denaturation, and DNA polymerase and mitochondrial dysfunction [38, 39]. Indirect or delayed cellular damage induces cell damage through apoptosis, vascular damage causing ischemia and ischemia-reperfusion injury, and stimulation of an immune response through releasing lysosomal contents that are released during tumor necrosis [38].

16.2.1 RFA Procedure for PTMC

Patient selection criteria for RFA in the treatment of PTMC are not well established. In a prospective study, Zhang et al. included patients with PTMC confirmed by US-guided CNB, no extrathyroidal invasions, no LN metastasis on imaging studies, no metastases beyond the neck, no history of neck irradiation, and patients who had medical contraindications for surgery or refused surgery. This study excluded patients with PTMC close to the danger triangle (within 5 mm distance from the trachea-esophageal groove), patients with aggressive histological PTMC, pregnant woman, patients with severe heart failure, liver failure, renal failure, coagulation disorder, conscious disturbance or neck extension disorder that could not tolerate RFA, cardiac pacemaker implantation, and contralateral vocal cord paralysis [19]. In another study, Lim et al. used similar inclusion and exclusion criteria; nevertheless, the study included patients with tumors in the danger triangles [8]. Based on these studies and in a recent systematic review and meta-analysis, patients with contraindications for thyroid surgery or refuse surgery with PTMC confirmed by US and FNA or core needle biopsy, without LN metastases, without extrathyroidal extension on US before RFA may be considered for RFA. It is important to note that it is recommended to exclude patients with aggressive histologic variants, extrathyroidal extension, and LN metastases. Contraindications for RFA (pregnant woman, coagulation disorder, severe heart failure, liver failure, and renal failure) should be considered, and in each case, a team-based assessment of the risks and benefits should guide the decision-making process.

The pre-procedure assessment should include a complete blood count, coagulation panel, thyroid function assessments, and a thorough examination of factors impacting the coagulation cascade. Discontinuation of clopidogrel should transpire over 7–10 days, warfarin over 3–5 days, and heparin within a window of 4–6 h. Administration of heparin may be initiated 2–6 h post-RFA, warfarin on the evening after the procedure, while aspirin or clopidogrel can be resumed on the subsequent day. Nevertheless, decisions should prioritize risk-benefit balance [20].

Just before the RFA procedure, it is recommended to determine tumor locations and its relationship with critical structures such as nerves, esophagus, and trachea. Using Doppler US to assess blood vessels around the PTMC is also recommended since avoiding them during the procedure may help to prevent hemorrhage [8, 19] (Fig. 16.3).

Procedure goes as follows. After US-guided administration of local anesthesia at the puncture site and around the thyroid capsule, hydrodissection technique with injection of 5% dextrose using a 20 gauge needle may be used to prevent thermal injury. If PTMC is located near to the danger triangle (within 5 mm distance from the tracheo-esophageal groove), hydrodissection may also help to prevent lesions in this space. After that, a trans-isthmic approach is used to approach the lesion. Once at the lesion, ablation process starts with an initial RFA power that can range from 15 to 40 W, depending on the size of the electrode tip. RFA power can be increased in

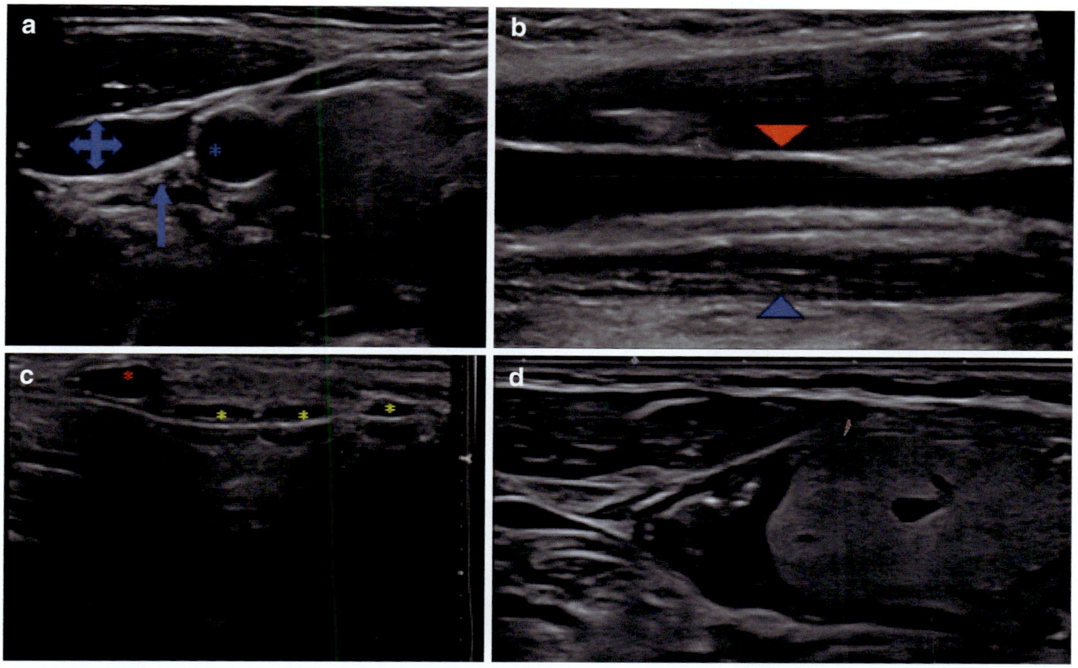

Fig. 16.3 Relevant anatomical cervical structures are depicted in B-mode neck ultrasound. Vagus nerve (*blue arrow*), common carotid artery (*blue asterisk*), and internal jugular vein (*blue star*) (**a**) are observed in B-mode axial US at the level of the right thyroid lobe. Esophagus (*blue arrow head*) and and internal jugular vein (*red arrow head*) (**b**) are observed in B-mode sagittal US. Anterior ring of the cricoid cartilage (*red asterisk*) and tracheal rings (*yellow asterisks*) are observed in B-mode sagittal US. Perithyroid hydrodissection is performed by injecting 5% dextrose solution prior to RFA to protect perithyroid structures (**c**) before Anterior ring (**d**) before Perithyroid hydrodissection

5–10 W if no transient hyperechoic zone is not seen at the electrode tip within 5–10 s. After completing the ablation of the tumor and to prevent marginal recurrence, at least 2 mm of normal thyroid tissue can be ablated [8, 20].

Post-procedure evaluation should encompass symptom assessment, sign evaluation, and ultrasound examination of the ablated zone. Long-term follow-up protocols lack clear establishment. In a study by Lim et al., ultrasound follow-up was conducted at 1 week, 2-, 6-, and 12-months post-procedure, followed by subsequent evaluations every 6 to 12 months. US assessment included evaluation of tumor volume, and its largest diameter and the development of new tumors and LN metastasis were monitored. All patients underwent contrast-enhanced neck CT at 2- and 4-years post-ablation for assessing LN metastases. Additionally, thyroid function was tested immediately after ablation, as well as at 2-, 6-, and 12-months post-ablation [8]. Zhang et al. employed ultrasound and clinical assessments at 1, 3, 6, and 12 months, followed by biannual evaluations. The study included contrast-enhanced US (CEUS) to detect the largest diameter and volume of ablation and to screen for recurrence [19]. RFA ablations of tumor recurrence can be performed, and any LN suspicious of metastases should be further studied.

16.3 Efficacy and Safety of RFA in PTMC

16.3.1 Efficacy of RFA

Three systematic reviews and meta-analyses found that RFA is an effective therapy to manage PTMCs. First, Van Dijk et al., involving 1770 patients across 15 studies, showed that 79% of

PTMC patients achieved complete tumor disappearance at the end of follow-up (Figs. 16.4 and 16.5).

Among the remaining 21% without complete disappearance, only 7 patients (0.4%) had confirmed residual PTMC through fine-needle aspiration (FNA). The overall tumor progression rate was 1.5% (26 patients), with 0.4% (7 patients) showing residual PTMC in the ablation area, 0.9% (15 patients) developing new PTMC in the thyroid gland, and 0.2% (4 patients) developing LN metastases during follow-up. No distant metastases were observed. The combined proportion of tumor progression was 1% (95% CI: 0–1%), without significant heterogeneity (I^2 = 4.9%; P = 0.38). Patients with tumor progression underwent additional RFA sessions (n = 25), and one patient initiated AS [40]. Tong et al. found similar results in another meta-analysis, a complete disappearance demonstrated a pooled proportion of 76.2% (95% CI: 50.0–95.4%; I^2 = 97.1%) [41]. Choi et al. depicted a pooled proportion for complete disappearance of 65.2% (95% CI: 24.3–100%; I^2 = 100%) [9] (Fig. 16.6).

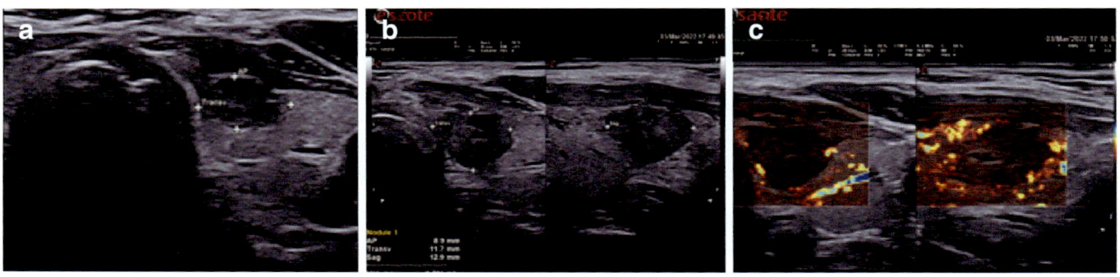

Fig. 16.4 RFA of unifocal PTMC. B-mode axial ultrasound of the left thyroid lobe demonstrates the presence of a 7-mm markedly hypoechogenic nodule (**a**). FNA revealed Bethesda class VI cytology. No adenopathy was observed at cervical ultrasound examination. Hence, RFA procedure, as an alternative to total thyroid surgery, was proposed. The patient accepted this proposal. Postprocedural B-mode axial ultrasound of the left thyroid lobe demonstrates the presence of the dark shadow of the ablated tumor including a 2–4 mm safety ring to eliminate any malignant cell infiltration into surrounding healthy tissues (**b**). MicroV Doppler mode shows a complete devascularization of the tumor and safety ring (**c**)

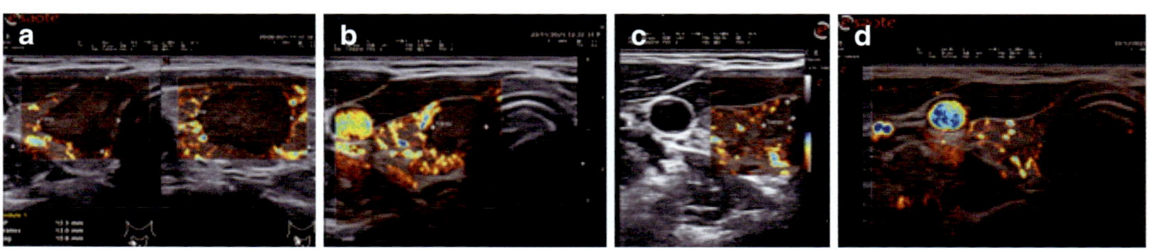

Fig. 16.5 Unifocal PTMC postprocedural US follow-up. Same nodule as depicted in Fig. 16.4. One day after RFA percutaneous treatment, the extension of the ablation is evident as a marked hypoechoic area (**a**). During the follow-up at 1 month, 6 months, and 1 year, (**b–d**) a steady and remarkable reduction in size of the ablated area is evident, until its complete disappearance

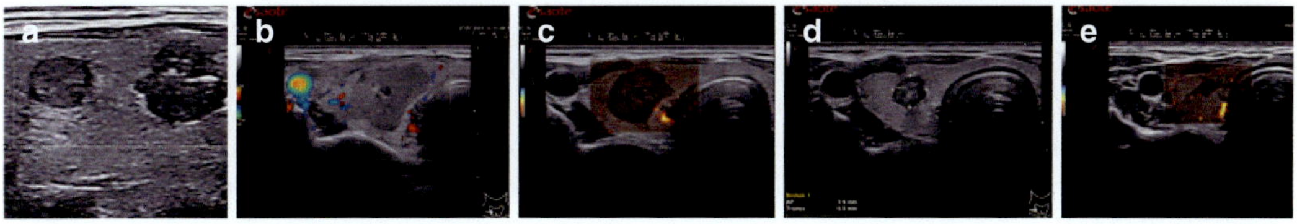

Fig. 16.6 Multifocal PTCM RFA and follow-up. Two markedly hypoechoic right lobe nodules of about 7 and 10 mm in diameter were detected. No satellite lymph nodes were found. B-mode axial ultrasound of the right thyroid lobe demonstrates the presence of two markedly hypoechoic right lobe nodules of about 7 and 10 mm in diameter (**a**). FNA revealed Bethesda class VI cytology in both nodules. No adenopathy was observed at cervical ultrasound examination. The patient was proposed a total thyroid surgery. The patient refused, seeking an alternative option. Hence, RFA procedure, as an alternative to total thyroid surgery, was proposed. The patient accepted this proposal. One day after RFA percutaneous treatment, the extension of the ablation is evident as a marked hypoechoic area (**b**). During the follow-up at 1 month (**c**), 6 months (**d**) a steady and remarkable reduction in size of the ablated area is evident. At 1 year US follow-up, there is still a remnant of the ablated area due to extent of initial ablation (**e**)

16.3.2 RFA Compared with MWA and LA

Two meta-analyses compared RFA, MWA, and LA for treating PTMC. Tong et al. observed a greater proportion of complete disappearance after RFA in comparison to the other two therapeutic modalities. The combined proportions of complete disappearance were 76.2% (95% CI: 50.0–95.4%; I^2 = 97.1%) for RFA, 62.9% (95% CI: 19.7–96.6%; I^2 = 98.5%) for MWA, and 57.3% (95% CI: 13.0–95.4%; I^2 = 95.6%) for LA. However, the differences were not statistically significant. The study also indicated a lower local recurrence after RFA in comparison to MWA and LA, yet these differences lacked statistical significance. Of note, no distant metastasis were reported in any of the studies [41]. Choi et al. found similar results. The pooled proportions of complete disappearance were 65.2% (95% CI: 24.3–100%; I^2 = 100%) for RFA, 56.5% (95% CI: 16.3–96.7%; I^2 = 99%) for MWA, and 48.7% (95% CI: 2.1–95.4%; I^2 = 95%) for LA [9].

Regarding local recurrence and distant metastasis, the previously cited meta-analysis reported that post-RFA local recurrence (0.01%) is lower than MWA (0.85%) and LA (1.87%), though lacking statistical significance [41]. Superiority of RFA over MWA and LA in terms of efficacy may be attributable to moving-shot technique, which allows multidimensional ablation of the entire tumor.

16.3.3 RFA Compared with Surgery

It has been mentioned before that surgery is the standard treatment for patients with PTMC. Nevertheless, there are studies that showed that RFA had similar efficacy when compared to surgery when compared to surgery. A retrospective study reported no significant differences were found in the disease progression (4.5% vs. 3.8%, P = 1.000), LN metastases (2.3% vs. 3.8%, P = 1.000), persistent lesion (2.3% vs. 0%, P = 0.272), and recurrence-free survival rates (97.7% vs. 96.2%, P = 0.673) in the RFA and surgery group. The outcomes of RFA and surgery group were comparable between RFA and surgery for unilateral multifocal PTMC. This study also reported that the complication rate in the surgery group was 7.5%, whereas none on the RFA-treated patients experienced any complications [42]. Tao li did a systematic review and network meta-analysis to evaluate the safety and efficacy of thermal ablation and surgery for PTMC. The study concluded that similar efficacy profiles between RFA, LA, MWA, and surgery exist [43]. Another retrospective study showed that among 218 patients with PTMC in the isthmus, RFA might be not inferior to total thyroidectomy in terms of rate of recurrence and LN metastases. Moreover, surgical time, blood loss, hospital stays, and treatment costs were higher in patients that underwent total thyroidectomy. Regarding quality of life, the study used the thyroid carcinoma-specific questionnaire of quality of life (THYCA-QOL) during the follow-up. The THYCA-QOL score of the RFA group was significantly higher than in the thyroidectomy group ($p < 0.001$) which led to a better quality of life [44].

16.4 Complications and Safety of RFA

Evidence suggests that RFA is a safe procedure. It is also well-tolerated, and rates of complications are low [8, 40]. Complications reported are pain, voice changes, and changes in thyroid function. On a systematic review and meta-analysis that included 15 studies (a total of 1770 patients), major complications occurred in only three patients: 2 voice changes that resolved spontaneously after 2 months and 1 temporary cardiac arrhythmia. Regarding minor complications, 20 patients experienced post-procedural pain, 14 patients transient voice changes that resolved 1 month, 5 patients had skin burns, 4 patients had hematomas, 1 patient had transient hypoparathyroidism, and 1 patient had fever. The pooled proportion of total complication rate was 2% (95% CI, 1–3%), with moderate heterogeneity between studies ($I^2 = 60.9\%$; $P < 0.001$). The pooled proportion of major complication rate was 0% (95% CI, 0–1%), showing no heterogeneity between studies ($I^2 = 0.00\%$; $P = 0.99$) [40]. Similar findings were observed on another meta-analysis by Tong, where major (voice hoarseness and hypothyroidism) and minor complications (pain, bleeding, and skin burn) were reported after RFA with overall pooled proportions of 1.7% (95% CI: 0.1–4.5%; $I^2 = 0.0\%$) [41]. Moreover, the pooled proportion of major complications after RFA was 2.6% (95% CI: 0–5.1%; $I^2 = 0.0\%$) in another meta-analysis [9].

16.5 Future Directions and Challenges

The future of RFA in PTMC is likely to be influenced by several factors. In the present, multiple studies have suggested that RFA is a safe and efficient method to treat PTMC in selected patients. Long-term follow-up studies will be necessary to determine whether RFA for treating PTMC is associated with clinical long-term benefits. Moreover, it will be important to design multicenter studies that include more heterogeneous populations and more defined protocols.

16.6 Conclusions

In summary, RFA stands as a viable, safe, and effective treatment for selected patients with PTMC. Along with AS, it may represent an alternative for patients who refuse to surgery or have risks that contraindicate surgery. Pre-procedure, procedure, and post-procedure follow-up are important for a successful procedure. However, further studies focused on evaluating more heterogeneous populations and with prospective designs are needed to understand better the impact of RFA on patients' quality of life over longer periods of follow-up.

References

1. LiVolsi VA. Papillary thyroid carcinoma: an update. Mod Pathol. 2011;24:S1–9. https://doi.org/10.1038/modpathol.2010.129.
2. Haugen BR, Alexander EK, Bible KC, Doherty GM, Mandel SJ, Nikiforov YE, et al. 2015 American Thyroid Association management guidelines for adult patients with thyroid nodules and differentiated thyroid cancer: the American Thyroid Association guidelines task force on thyroid nodules and differentiated thyroid cancer. Thyroid. 2016;26(1):1–133. https://doi.org/10.1089/thy.2015.0020.
3. Durante C, Hegedüs L, Czarniecka A, Paschke R, Russ G, Schmitt F, et al. 2023 European thyroid association clinical practice guidelines for thyroid nodule management. Eur Thyroid J. 2023;12(5):e230067. https://doi.org/10.1530/ETJ-23-0067.
4. Van Velsen EFS, Stegenga MT, van Kemenade FJ, Kam BLR, van Ginhoven TM, Visser WE, et al. Comparing the prognostic value of the eighth edition of the American joint committee on cancer/tumor node metastasis staging system between papillary and follicular thyroid cancer. Thyroid. 2018;28(8):976–81. https://doi.org/10.1089/thy.2018.0066.
5. Kuo EJ, Roman SA, Sosa JA. Patients with follicular and Hurthle cell microcarcinomas have compromised survival: a population level study of 22,738 patients. Surgery. 2013;154(6):1246–53; discussion 1253–4. https://doi.org/10.1016/j.surg.2013.04.033.

6. Ito Y, Miyauchi A, Oda H. Low-risk papillary microcarcinoma of the thyroid: a review of active surveillance trials. Eur J Surg Oncol. 2018;44(3):307–15. https://doi.org/10.1016/j.ejso.2017.03.004.
7. Jeong SY, Baek JH, Choi YJ, Chung SR, Sung TY, Kim WG, et al. Radiofrequency ablation of primary thyroid carcinoma: efficacy according to the types of thyroid carcinoma. Int J Hyperth. 2018;34(5):611–6. https://doi.org/10.1080/02656736.2018.1427288.
8. Lim HK, Cho SJ, Baek JH, Lee KD, Son CW, Son JM, et al. US-guided radiofrequency ablation for low-risk papillary thyroid microcarcinoma: efficacy and safety in a large population. Korean J Radiol. 2019;20(12):1653–61. https://doi.org/10.3348/kjr.2019.0192. Erratum in: Korean J Radiol. 2020;21(4):510.
9. Choi Y, Jung SL. Efficacy and safety of thermal ablation techniques for the treatment of primary papillary thyroid microcarcinoma: a systematic review and meta-analysis. Thyroid. 2020;30(5):720–31. https://doi.org/10.1089/thy.2019.0707.
10. Sim JS, Baek JH. Long-term outcomes following thermal ablation of benign thyroid nodules as an alternative to surgery: the importance of controlling regrowth. Endocrinol Metab (Seoul). 2019;34(2):117–23. https://doi.org/10.3803/EnM.2019.34.2.117.
11. Mauri G, Nicosia L, Della Vigna P, Varano GM, Maiettini D, Bonomo G, et al. Percutaneous laser ablation for benign and malignant thyroid diseases. Ultrason Seoul Korea. 2019;38(1):25–36. https://doi.org/10.14366/usg.18034.
12. Yue W, Wang S, Yu S, Wang B. Ultrasound-guided percutaneous microwave ablation of solitary T1N0M0 papillary thyroid microcarcinoma: initial experience. Int J Hyperth. 2014;30(2):150–7. https://doi.org/10.3109/02656736.2014.885590. Erratum in: Int J Hyperth. 2022;39(1):229.
13. Chung SR, Baek JH, Choi YJ, Lee JH. Longer-term outcomes of radiofrequency ablation for locally recurrent papillary thyroid cancer. Eur Radiol. 2019;29(9):4897–903. https://doi.org/10.1007/s00330-019-06063-5.
14. Yang Z, Yan L, Xiao J, Li W, Li X, Li Y, et al. Long-term results of radiofrequency ablation for locally recurrent papillary thyroid carcinoma. Int J Hyperth. 2023;40(1):2191912. https://doi.org/10.1080/02656736.2023.2191912.
15. Lim HK, Baek JH, Lee JH, Kim WB, Kim TY, Shong YK, et al. Efficacy and safety of radiofrequency ablation for treating locoregional recurrence from papillary thyroid cancer. Eur Radiol. 2015;25(1):163–70. https://doi.org/10.1007/s00330-014-3405-5.
16. Kim JH, Yoo WS, Park YJ, Park DJ, Yun TJ, Choi SH, et al. Efficacy and safety of radiofrequency ablation for treatment of locally recurrent thyroid cancers smaller than 2 cm. Radiology. 2015;276(3):909–18. https://doi.org/10.1148/radiol.15140079.
17. Teng DK, Li HQ, Sui GQ, Lin YQ, Luo Q, Fu P, et al. Preliminary report of microwave ablation for the primary papillary thyroid microcarcinoma: a large-cohort of 185 patients feasibility study. Endocrine. 2019;64(1):109–17. https://doi.org/10.1007/s12020-019-01868-2.
18. Ji L, Wu Q, Gu J, Deng X, Zhou W, Fan X, et al. Ultrasound-guided percutaneous laser ablation for papillary thyroid microcarcinoma: a retrospective analysis of 37 patients. Cancer Imaging. 2019;19(1):16. https://doi.org/10.1186/s40644-019-0204-x.
19. Zhang M, Luo Y, Zhang Y, Tang J. Efficacy and safety of ultrasound-guided radiofrequency ablation for treating low-risk papillary thyroid microcarcinoma: a prospective study. Thyroid. 2016;26(11):1581–7. https://doi.org/10.1089/thy.2015.0471.
20. Kim JH, Baek JH, Lim HK, Ahn HS, Baek SM, Choi YJ, et al. 2017 thyroid radiofrequency ablation guideline: Korean Society of Thyroid Radiology. Korean J Radiol. 2018;19(4):632–55. https://doi.org/10.3348/kjr.2018.19.4.632.
21. Garberoglio R, Aliberti C, Appetecchia M, Attard M, Boccuzzi G, Boraso F, et al. Radiofrequency ablation for thyroid nodules: which indications? The first Italian opinion statement. J Ultrasound. 2015;18(4):423–30. https://doi.org/10.1007/s40477-015-0169-y.
22. WHO Classification of Tumours Online. 2023. https://tumourclassification.iarc.who.int/welcome/.
23. Lloyd RV, Buehler D, Khanafshar E. Papillary thyroid carcinoma variants. Head Neck Pathol. 2011;5(1):51–6. https://doi.org/10.1007/s12105-010-0236-9.
24. Powers AE, Marcadis AR, Lee M, Morris LGT, Marti JL. Changes in trends in thyroid cancer incidence in the United States, 1992 to 2016. JAMA. 2019;322(24):2440–1. https://doi.org/10.1001/jama.2019.18528.
25. Deng Y, Li H, Wang M, Li N, Tian T, Wu Y, et al. Global burden of thyroid cancer from 1990 to 2017. JAMA Netw Open. 2020;3(6):e208759. https://doi.org/10.1001/jamanetworkopen.2020.8759.
26. Kitahara CM, Schneider AB. Epidemiology of thyroid cancer. Cancer Epidemiol Biomarkers Prev. 2022;31(7):1284–97. https://doi.org/10.1158/1055-9965.EPI-21-1440.
27. Schneider AB, Sarne DH. Long-term risks for thyroid cancer and other neoplasms after exposure to radiation. Nat Clin Pract Endocrinol Metab. 2005;1(2):82–91. https://doi.org/10.1038/ncpendmet0022.
28. Pal T, Vogl FD, Chappuis PO, Tsang R, Brierley J, Renard H, et al. Increased risk for nonmedullary thyroid cancer in the first degree relatives of prevalent cases of nonmedullary thyroid cancer: a hospital-based study. J Clin Endocrinol Metab. 2001;86(11):5307–12. https://doi.org/10.1210/jcem.86.11.8010.
29. Hemminki K, Eng C, Chen B. Familial risks for nonmedullary thyroid cancer. J Clin Endocrinol Metab. 2005;90(10):5747–53. https://doi.org/10.1210/jc.2005-0935.
30. Momesso DP, Tuttle RM. Update on differentiated thyroid cancer staging. Endocrinol Metab Clin N Am. 2014;43(2):401–21. https://doi.org/10.1016/j.ecl.2014.02.010.

31. Tuttle RM, Haugen B, Perrier ND. Updated American joint committee on cancer/tumor-node-metastasis staging system for differentiated and anaplastic thyroid cancer (eighth edition): what changed and why? Thyroid. 2017;27(6):751–6. https://doi.org/10.1089/thy.2017.0102.
32. Haddad RI, Bischoff L, Ball D, Bernet V, Blomain E, Busaidy NL, et al. Thyroid carcinoma, version 2.2022, NCCN clinical practice guidelines in oncology. J Natl Compr Cancer Netw. 2022;20(8):925–51. https://doi.org/10.6004/jnccn.2022.0040.
33. Sugitani I, Ito Y, Takeuchi D, Nakayama H, Masaki C, Shindo H, et al. Indications and strategy for active surveillance of adult low-risk papillary thyroid microcarcinoma: consensus statements from the Japan Association of Endocrine Surgery Task Force on Management for Papillary Thyroid Microcarcinoma. Thyroid. 2021;31(2):183–92. https://doi.org/10.1089/thy.2020.0330.
34. Davies L, Roman BR, Fukushima M, Ito Y, Miyauchi A. Patient experience of thyroid cancer active surveillance in Japan. JAMA Otolaryngol Head Neck Surg. 2019;145(4):363–70. https://doi.org/10.1001/jamaoto.2018.4131.
35. Knavel EM, Brace CL. Tumor ablation: common modalities and general practices. Tech Vasc Interv Radiol. 2013;16(4):192–200. https://doi.org/10.1053/j.tvir.2013.08.002.
36. Ahmed M, Brace CL, Lee FT, Goldberg SN. Principles of and advances in percutaneous ablation. Radiology. 2011;258(2):351–69. https://doi.org/10.1148/radiol.10081634.
37. Dobrinja C, Bernardi S, Fabris B, Eramo R, Makovac P, Bazzocchi G, et al. Surgical and pathological changes after radiofrequency ablation of thyroid nodules. Int J Endocrinol. 2015;2015:576576. https://doi.org/10.1155/2015/576576.
38. Chu KF, Dupuy DE. Thermal ablation of tumours: biological mechanisms and advances in therapy. Nat Rev Cancer. 2014;14(3):199–208. https://doi.org/10.1038/nrc3672.
39. Nikfarjam M, Muralidharan V, Christophi C. Mechanisms of focal heat destruction of liver tumors. J Surg Res. 2005;127(2):208–23. https://doi.org/10.1016/j.jss.2005.02.009.
40. Van Dijk SPJ, Coerts HI, Gunput STG, van Velsen EFS, Medici M, Moelker A, Peeters RP, et al. Assessment of radiofrequency ablation for papillary microcarcinoma of the thyroid: a systematic review and meta-analysis. JAMA Otolaryngol Head Neck Surg. 2022;148(4):317–25. https://doi.org/10.1001/jamaoto.2021.4381.
41. Tong M, Li S, Li Y, Li Y, Feng Y, Che Y. Efficacy and safety of radiofrequency, microwave and laser ablation for treating papillary thyroid microcarcinoma: a systematic review and meta-analysis. Int J Hyperth. 2019;36(1):1278–86. https://doi.org/10.1080/02656736.2019.1700559.
42. Yan L, Zhen Y, Li Y, Li X, Xiao J, Jing H, et al. Five-year outcome between radiofrequency ablation vs. surgery for unilateral multifocal papillary thyroid microcarcinoma. J Clin Endocrinol Metab. 2023;108(12):3230–8. https://doi.org/10.1210/clinem/dgad360.
43. Li T, Lu B, Zhang Y, Sun Y. Meta-analysis of the application effect of different modalities of thermal ablation and surgical treatment in papillary thyroid microcarcinoma. Dis Markers. 2022;2022:9714140. https://doi.org/10.1155/2022/9714140.
44. Song Q, Gao H, Ren L, Tian X, Lan Y, Yan L, et al. Radiofrequency ablation versus total thyroidectomy in patients with papillary thyroid microcarcinoma located in the isthmus: a retrospective cohort study. Int J Hyperth. 2021;38(1):708–14. https://doi.org/10.1080/02656736.2021.1916625.

17 Microwave Ablation for Micropapillary Thyroid Cancer

Lin Zheng and Ping Liang

17.1 Introduction

Although papillary thyroid microcarcinomas (PTMCs) are relatively indolent, most patients prefer treatment rather than active surveillance because of anxiety about cancer [1]. However, surgery may lead to more harm than benefit due to surgery-related complications, such as permanent recurrent laryngeal nerve injury, inadvertent hypoparathyroidism [2], cosmetic problems, and lifelong need for thyroid hormone replacement [3, 4], which might not be accepted by all patients. Thermal ablation provides an intermediate option for patients with advantages of minimally invasive and low cost [5]. Studies have reported promising results of thermal ablation in the treatment of PTMC, and it is considered an alternative to surgery [6–8]. Compared to radiofrequency ablation (RFA), microwave ablation (MWA) can provide large regions of coagulative necrosis with short treatment period. This chapter describes the technique, results, and the feasibility of ultrasound-guided percutaneous MWA for PTMCs.

L. Zheng · P. Liang (✉)
Chinese People's Liberation Army General Hospital, Beijing, China

17.2 Mechanism

High-frequency electromagnetic energy generated by a microwave power generator is transferred through a coaxial cable as an antenna into surrounding tissues to cause a rise in temperature to 60 °C or above, which leads to protein denaturation and coagulative necrosis [9]. MWA offers many of the benefits of RFA and has several other theoretical advantages that may increase its effectiveness in the treatment of tumors. The potential benefits of microwave technology include consistently higher intratumoral temperatures, larger tumor ablation volumes, faster ablation times, ability to use multiple applicators, improved convection profile, optimal heating of cystic masses, and less procedural pain. In addition, microwave ablation does not require the placement of grounding pads [10].

17.3 Inclusion Criteria and Exclusion Criteria

Inclusion criteria for MWA of micropapillary thyroid cancer are as follows: (1) solitary suspicious thyroid nodule diameter of 1 cm or less detected by US; (2) no US and/or CT detected lymph node metastasis or distant metastasis; (3) papillary thyroid carcinoma pathologically confirmed by fine-needle aspiration or core-needle biopsy but without histopathologically or immunohistochemically proven aggressive histological

R. Valcavi et al. (eds.), *Thyroid Ablation*, https://doi.org/10.1007/978-3-031-88229-6_17

types, according to the WHO classification of thyroid tumors; (4) patients refuse clinical observation; and (5) patients refuse operative resection or have surgical contraindication.

The exclusion criteria are as follows: (1) tumors with US-apparent extrathyroidal extension, multicentricity, or participants with coexisting malignancies such as medullary carcinoma, (2) abnormal contralateral vocal cord, and (3) patients with severe coagulation disorders and severe cardiac or pulmonary disease.

17.4 Patient Preparation

Written informed consent should be obtained from each patient.

Preoperative US and/or contrast-enhanced US (CEUS) examination is important for characterizing the nodule and evaluating the surrounding anatomical structures and cervical lymph nodes. Pathological results of the nodule need to be confirmed before ablation by fine-needle aspirations or core-needle biopsies.

Laboratory tests usually include complete blood count, coagulation test, and thyroid function tests. Imaging studies usually include chest radiography and bilateral vocal cords laryngofiber scope examination. Anticoagulation medications should be suspended for at least a week before MWA.

17.5 Equipment

The MWA system consists of an MWA generator and a Teflon-coated, internally cooled microwave antenna, which is usually capable of producing 1–100 W of power at 2450 MHz. The needle antenna has a diameter of 1.6 mm and a 10 cm shaft. A narrow radiating segment of 3 mm is embedded on the shaft, 3 mm away from the tip for 2450 MHz applicator.

17.6 MWA Procedures

Patients are placed in the supine position with hyperextended neck during the procedure, and a venous catheter is inserted in a forearm vein. A multiparametric monitor is connected to the patient monitoring blood pressure, pO2, and electrocardiogram. Lidocaine (1%) is performed subcutaneously on the puncture site for local anesthesia.

The trans-isthmic approach method is usually adopted for MWA. The antenna is inserted from the isthmus to the targeted tumor. The entire length of the antenna can be visualized under the US view (Fig. 17.1).

A power output of 20–50 W is recommended during MWA. The fixed antenna technique may result in a round ablation zone and is used in cases in which a single insertion and ablation are planned. Moving-shot technique, which means dividing the tumor into multiple small conceptual ablation units and performing ablation unit by unit, by moving the antenna tip, can be applied in cases in which multiple ablations are planned for the target tumor. The antenna tip is initially positioned in the deepest portion of the tumor to prevent visual disturbance caused by echogenic bubbles (Fig. 17.2). When a transient hyperechoic area appears, microwave power is decreased, and the antenna tip is moved. The ablation is terminated when the hyperechoic area covers the entire tumor and extends for at least 2 mm from the original tumor margin. During the procedure, the participants are intermittently asked to speak to monitor the phonation.

If the tumor is close to critical structures such as the anterior muscle, carotid artery, recurrent laryngeal nerve, trachea, or esophagus, hydrodissection technique is needed before ablation. A 21-gauge core needle is inserted between the tumor and adjacent critical structures. Normal saline is injected continuously to achieve a safe distance of at least 5 mm to prevent thermal injury (Fig. 17.3).

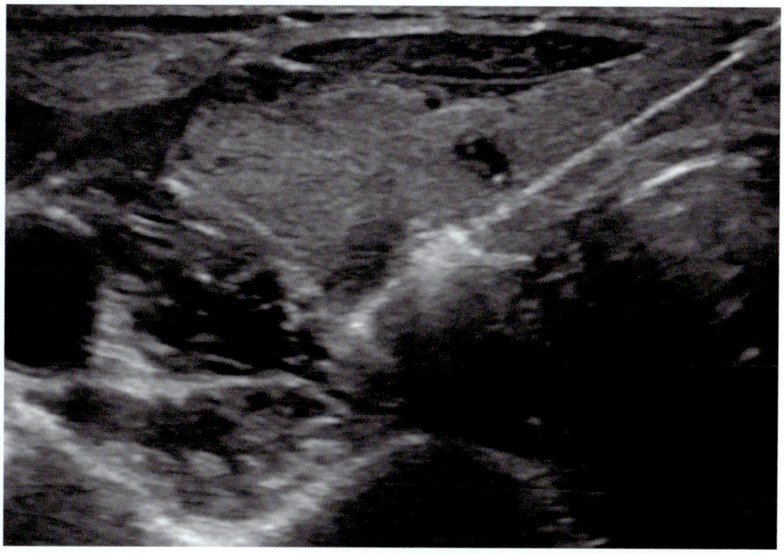

Fig. 17.1 Images of a 77-year-old man with PTMC located in the left gland of thyroid. The antenna was inserted from the isthmus to the targeted tumor. The entire length of the antenna can be visualized under the US view

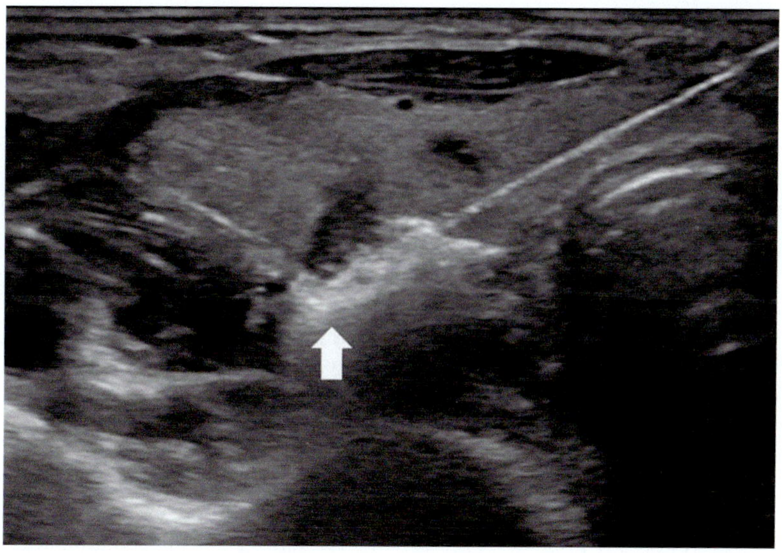

Fig. 17.2 Image of the procedure of hydrodissection performed on a 77-year-old man with PTMC located in the left gland of thyroid. A 21-gauge core needle was inserted between the tumor and adjacent tissue. Normal saline is injected continuously as isolating fluid to achieve a safe distance to prevent thermal injury of the recurrent laryngeal nerve (*white arrow*)

Fig. 17.3 Image of the procedure of microwave ablation performed on a 77-year-old man with PTMC located in the left gland of thyroid. The antenna tip was initially positioned in the deepest portion of the tumor to prevent visual disturbance caused by echogenic bubbles (*white arrow*)

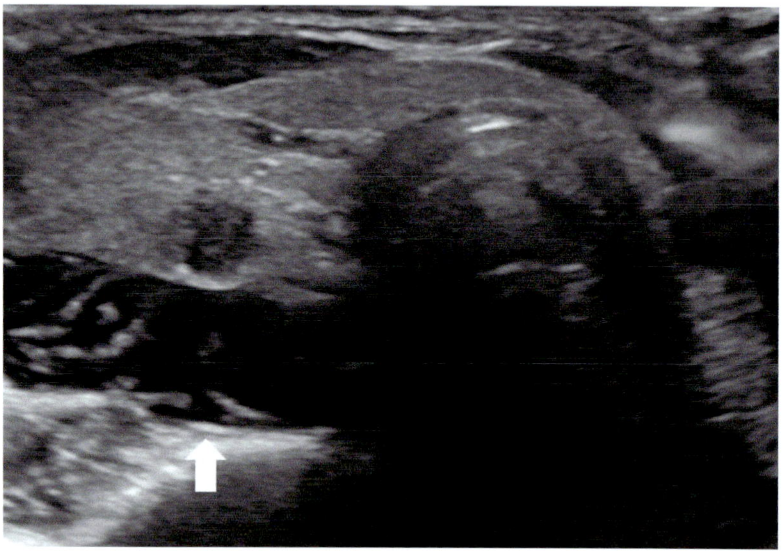

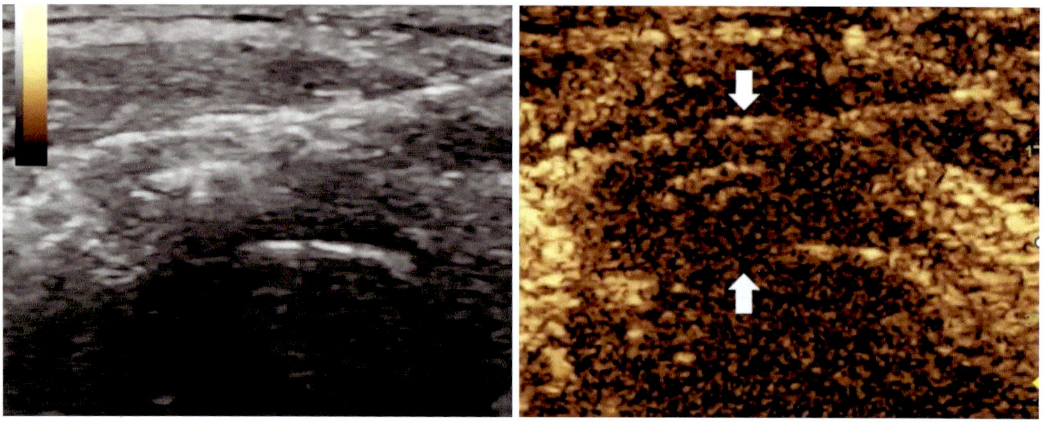

Fig. 17.4 Image of the contrast-enhanced US performed on a 77-year-old man with PTMC immediately after microwave ablation evaluating the treatment outcome. The absence of enhancement in the tumor on contrast-enhanced US indicated the complete necrosis of the tumor (*white arrows*)

Application of an ice bag during ablation may prevent skin burns at the electrode puncture site. At the end of the procedure, all patients remain under observation for 30 min to monitor potential complications. An ice bag is compressed on the neck for 2 h to prevent bleeding.

17.6.1 Technical Success Assessment

CEUS would be performed to confirm the completeness of the ablation. Technical success is defined as absence of enhancement in the tumor on contrast-enhanced US immediately after ablation (Fig. 17.4). Additional ablation would be performed immediately if residual enhancement is present inside the ablation zone or if the extended ablation zone is less than 2 mm.

17.6.2 Treatment Efficacy Assessment and Follow-Up

TSH is advised to be suppressed in a range of 0.5–1 mU/L with levothyroxine in 5 years after treatment to reduce the risk of recurrence.

Patients are evaluated with thyroid ultrasound at 1 day and the 1, 3, 6, and 12 months in the first year after ablation, every 6 months the second year and every 12 months thereafter. The US examination is acquired to assess the changes of MWA-induced lesions (the ablation area), including the size, vascularity, and echogenicity. The thyroid functional examinations, such as fT3, fT4, TSH, are also evaluated at each follow-up. CEUS is performed 6 months and 12 months after ablation to verify the effectiveness of the treatment. The effectiveness of ablation is defined as the absence of enhancement in any areas of the original tumor. CT of the neck and chest is performed annually to monitor for distant metastases.

Biopsy would be performed for imaging-suspected tumor recurrence or lymph node metastasis. Additional ablation or surgical resection would be performed for unsuccessfully treated or recurrent tumors based on the request of patients.

17.6.3 Complication Assessment

Side effects and minor complications of MWA for thyroid tumor include a mild sensation of heat in the neck or slight pain, vasovagal reaction, choking and coughing, slight fever not more than 37.5 °C, mild bleeding or hematoma, vomiting, and skin burn. The possible major complications of MWA for thyroid tumor include hoarse voice, abscess formation, hypothyroidism, and brachial plexus injury.

Various technical tips for avoiding complications during ablation of thyroid tumor can be adopted. For example, thermal injury to the recurrent laryngeal nerve may be prevented by hydrodissection and the moving-shot technique. Hematoma can usually be controlled by compression of the neck and the use of hemagglutinin drugs. Hoarseness usually improves gradually within 6 months after ablation.

17.6.4 Treatment-Related Clinical Research

In terms of treatment efficacy, according to a prospective study of *Yue* on MWA for PTMC with a follow-up period of approximately 37 months after treatment, no participants developed local tumor recurrence while 0.88% (1 of 119) developed lymph nodes metastasis, and the volume of ablation area decreased from 1.27 ± 0.87 ml to 0.01 ± 0.04 ml, 78.1% participants (89 of 114) showed complete resolved at the latest US examination [11]. In another study of *Han* with a follow-up period of approximately 34 months after treatment, 0.47% patients (6 of 1278) developed local tumor recurrence and 0.78%patients (10 of 1278) developed lymph nodes metastasis [12].

In terms of treatment related complications, *Yue* reported 6.7% (8 of 119) hoarse voice, 3.4% (4 of 119) labored breathing and coughing, and 0.8% (1 of 119) subcutaneous hematoma when performing MWA for PTMC, which recovered 1 week to 3 months after ablation; mild sensation of heat and slight pain in the neck were experienced by most patients, but no one needed procedure to stop [11]. In the article of *Han*, the overall complication rate was 1.41% (18 of 1278), including 1.10% (14 of 1278) hoarse voice, 0.16% (2 of 1278) choking cough, 0.08% (1 of 1278) infections, and 0.08% (1 of 1278) hematoma, which recovered 1–6 month after MWA [12].

17.7 Tumor in Particular Location

According to the literature, MWA is a safe and effective treatment for PTMCs located in isthmus, close to the capsule or with minimal capsular invasion [13, 14].

For PTMC located in isthmus, *Cao* reported 100% (34 of 34) technique success and 70.6% (24 of 34) complete tumor disappears rate on US examination with no local tumor occurrence or

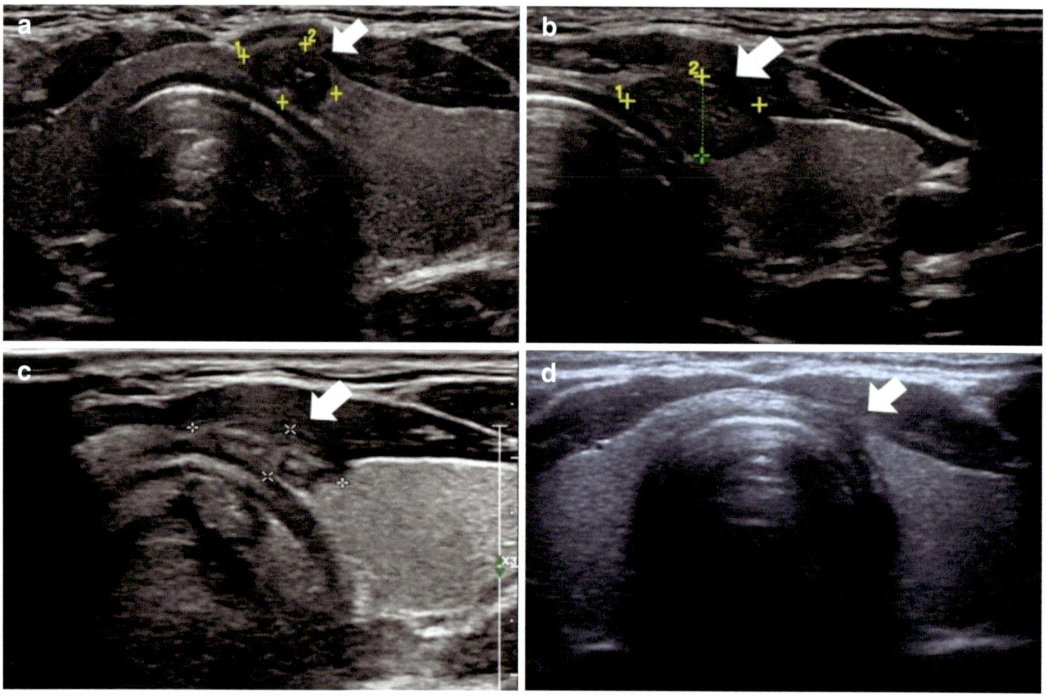

Fig. 17.5 Images of a 30-year-old man with PTMC located in the isthmus of thyroid. (**a**) Preablation US image of the tumor (*white arrow*) located in isthmus. (**b**) Image of the ablation zone 1 months after ablation (*white arrow*). (**c**) Image of the ablation zone 6 months after ablation (*white arrow*). (**d**) The ablation area had almost disappeared 1 year after ablation (*white arrow*)

lymph nodes metastasis approximately 17 months after MWA, and no complications recorded [13]. *Zheng* reported 100% (21 of 21) technique success and 31.8% (7 of 21) complete tumor disappearance rate on US examination with no local tumor occurrence or lymph nodes metastasis during approximately 3 years follow-up period and no complications recorded (Fig. 17.5) [14].

In a prospective study on MWA for PTMC with US-detected capsular invasion, *Zheng* reported 99% (82 of 83) technique success excepted one case of hydrodissection failure [15]. In those with and those without capsular invasion, comparable complications incidence rates occurred (1% [one of 82] vs 3% [11 of 378], $P = 0.38$), and no evidence of differences was found in disease progression (2% [1 of 82] vs 1% [4 of 378]; $P = 0.82$) or tumor shrinkage (mean, 97% ± 8 [SD] vs 96% ± 13; $P = 0.58$) with a mean follow-up period of 20 months (Fig. 17.6) [15]. In a retrospective study on MWA for PTMC close to the capsule, *Wu* reported 100% (106 of 106) technique success with 5.7% (6 of 106) complication of light voice changes, 70.0% (71of 106) tumor disappeared completely, and 1.9% (2 of 106) patients developed lymph node metastasis or new tumors during the follow-up period of 25 months.

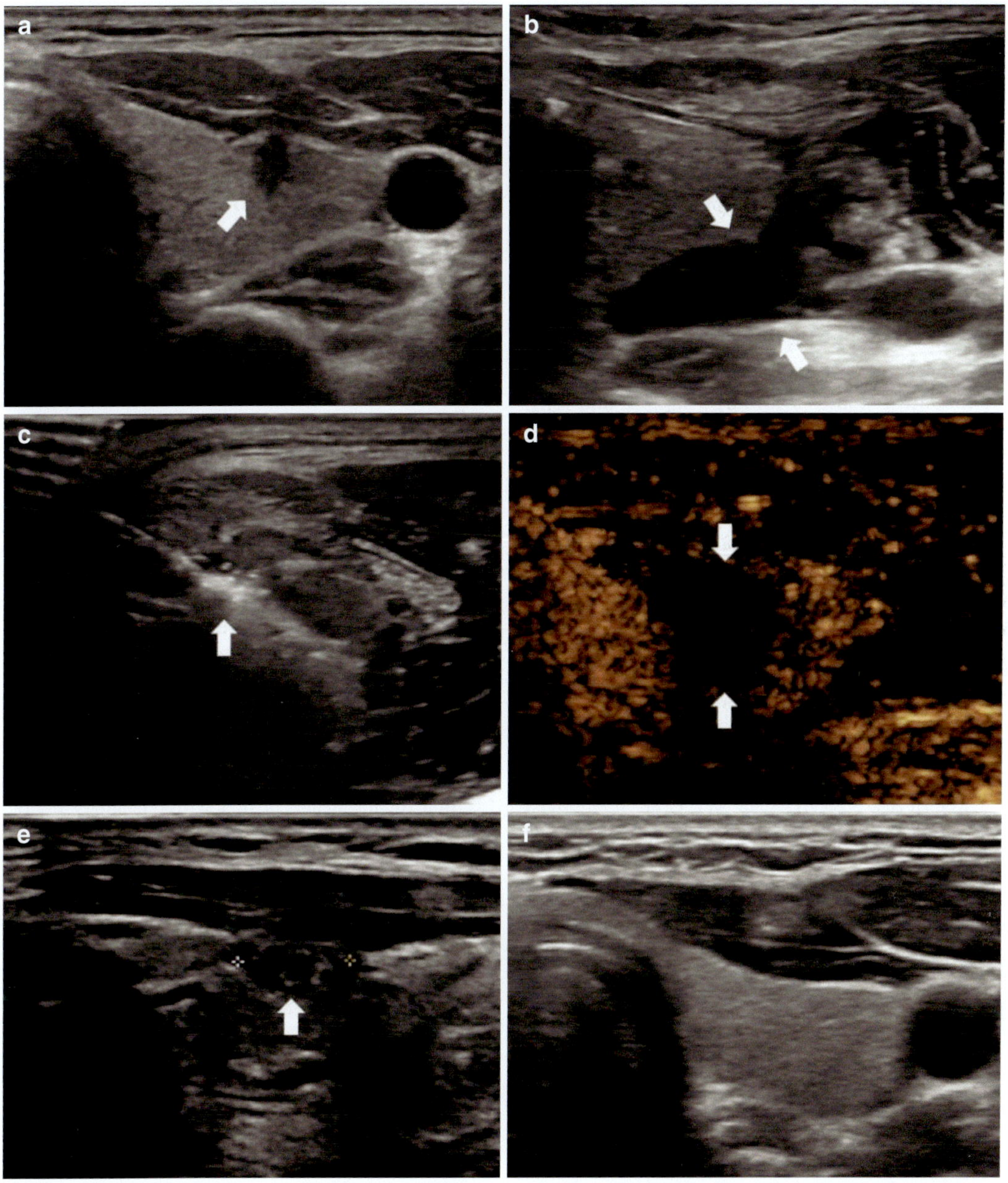

Fig. 17.6 Images of a 46-year-old woman with PTMC presented minimal invasion of the capsule in the left lobe of the thyroid. (**a**) Preablation US image of the tumor with capsular invasion (*white arrow*). (**b**) The hydrodissection technique (*white arrows*) was used to protect the carotid artery and vagus nerve. (**c**) Hyperechoic pattern in the tumor during the ablation procedure (*white arrow*). (**d**) Postablation contrast-enhanced US image shows no enhancement in the tumor area (*white arrows*). (**e**) Image of the ablation zone 6 months after ablation (*white arrowheads*). (**f**) The ablation area had almost disappeared 1 year after ablation

17.8 Conclusion

MWA is a safe and effective alternative technique for micropapillary thyroid cancer. It is important to maximize efficacy and minimize complications. Its efficacy can be maximized by complete necrosis of thyroid tumor, which is essential in order to effectively eliminate the tumor. Consideration of possible complications and available preventative techniques is important to minimize complications. However, the current literatures have limitations, so prospective random control studies with large sample and long-term follow-up period are necessary to determine the efficacy, safety, cost/benefit balance, and quality of life.

References

1. Yoshida Y, Horiuchi K, Okamoto T. Patients' view on the management of papillary thyroid microcarcinoma: active surveillance or surgery. Thyroid. 2020;30(5):681–7. https://doi.org/10.1089/thy.2019.0420.
2. Kazaure HS, Zambeli-Ljepovic A, Oyekunle T, Roman SA, Sosa JA, Stang MT, et al. Severe hypocalcemia after thyroidectomy: an analysis of 7366 patients. Ann Surg. 2021;274(6):e1014–21. https://doi.org/10.1097/SLA.0000000000003725.P.
3. Choi KW, Kim Y, Fava M, Mischoulon D, Na EJ, Kim SW, et al. Increased morbidity of major depressive disorder after thyroidectomy: a Nationwide population-based study in South Korea. Thyroid. 2019;29(12):1713–22. https://doi.org/10.1089/thy.2019.0091.
4. Sethukumar P, Ly D, Awad Z, Tolley NS. Scar satisfaction and body image in thyroidectomy patients: prospective study in a tertiary referral Centre. J Laryngol Otol. 2018;132(1):60–7. https://doi.org/10.1017/S0022215117002158.
5. Cho SJ, Baek JH, Chung SR, Choi YJ, Lee JH. Thermal ablation for small papillary thyroid cancer: a systematic review. Thyroid. 2019;29(12):1774–83. https://doi.org/10.1089/thy.2019.0377.
6. Cao XJ, Yu MA, Zhu YL, Qi L, Cong ZB, Yan GZ, et al. Ultrasound-guided thermal ablation for papillary thyroid microcarcinoma: a multicenter retrospective study. Int J Hyperth. 2021;38(1):916–22. https://doi.org/10.1080/02656736.2021.1936218.
7. Zhang M, Tufano RP, Russell JO, Zhang Y, Zhang Y, Qiao Z, et al. Ultrasound-guided radiofrequency ablation versus surgery for low-risk papillary thyroid microcarcinoma: results of over 5 years' follow-up. Thyroid. 2020;30(3):408–17. https://doi.org/10.1089/thy.2019.0147.
8. Ywata de Carvalho A, Kohler HF, Gomes CC, Vartanian JG, Kowalski LP. Predictive factors for recurrence of papillary thyroid carcinoma: analysis of 4,085 patients. Acta Otorhinolaryngol Ital. 2021;41(3):236–42. https://doi.org/10.14639/0392-100X-N1412.
9. Huang H, Zhang L, Moser MAJ, Zhang W, Zhang B. A review of antenna designs for percutaneous microwave ablation. Phys Med. 2021;84:254–64. https://doi.org/10.1016/j.ejmp.2021.03.010.
10. Simon CJ, Dupuy DE, Mayo-Smith WW. Microwave ablation: principles and applications. Radiographics. 2005;25(Suppl 1):S69–83. https://doi.org/10.1148/rg.25si055501.
11. Yue WW, Qi L, Wang DD, Yu SJ, Wang XJ, Xu HX, et al. US-guided microwave ablation of low-risk papillary thyroid microcarcinoma: longer-term results of a prospective study. J Clin Endocrinol Metab. 2020;105(6):dgaa128. https://doi.org/10.1210/clinem/dgaa128.
12. Han ZY, Dou JP, Zheng L, Che Y, Yu MA, Wang SR, et al. Safety and efficacy of microwave ablation for the treatment of low-risk papillary thyroid microcarcinoma: a prospective multicenter study. Eur Radiol. 2023;33(11):7942–51. https://doi.org/10.1007/s00330-023-09802-x.
13. Cao XJ, Zhao ZL, Wei Y, Peng LL, Li Y, Wu J, et al. Microwave ablation for papillary thyroid cancer located in the thyroid isthmus: a preliminary study. Int J Hyperth. 2021;38(1):114–9. https://doi.org/10.1080/02656736.2021.1880028.
14. Zheng L, Liu FY, Yu J, Cheng ZG, Yu XL, Dong XC, et al. Thermal ablation for papillary thyroid microcarcinoma located in the isthmus: a study with 3 years of follow-up. Future Oncol. 2022;18(4):471–80. https://doi.org/10.2217/fon-2021-0463.
15. Zheng L, Dou JP, Han ZY, Liu FY, Yu J, Cheng ZG, et al. Microwave ablation for papillary thyroid microcarcinoma with and without US-detected capsule invasion: a multicenter prospective cohort study. Radiology. 2023;307(3):e220661. https://doi.org/10.1148/radiol.220661.

Laser Ablation of Thyroid Nodules

18

Roberto Negro

18.1 Device and Technique

Laser is the acronym of "Light Amplification by Stimulated Emission of Radiation." Laser is a collimated and monochromatic energy that is delivered into small targets through optical fibers [1]. Common primary sources are laser diode or neodymium–yttrium aluminum garnet, which produce optical wavelengths of 820 nm or 1064 nm. When laser light hits the target, a local increase of temperature occurs, causing permanent damages such as coagulative necrosis (46–100 °C) and tissue carbonization/vaporization (100–110 °C). The tissue damage depends on many factors such as the amount of energy released, the application time, and the composition of the nodule [2]. When treating thyroid nodules with laser, one or more optical fibers are inserted at a 10-mm distance from each other, usually along the longitudinal axis, into the target nodule through thin and flexible 21-gauge needles. A 300 μm diameter plane-cut quartz optical fiber is inserted and advanced up to the introducer needle tip, so that 5 mm active tip is in direct contact with the target tissue (Fig. 18.1).

The heat-induced changes of the tissue are visible through the appearance of hyperechoic signals due to the formation of gas microbubbles [3] (Fig. 18.2).

In vivo studies on swine models demonstrated that delivering 1400 J induces an ablation area of 0.57 mL, but delivering 1800 J induces an ablation area of 1.12 mL, showing that the energy delivered plays a pivotal role in tissue damage [4]. Common protocols are based on a mean power of 3–5 W, for a total energy delivery of 1200–1800 J for every illumination. After the first illumination, the fiber(s) can be pulled back by 10–15 mm. The backward re-positioning ("pull back") of the fiber optics during the procedure allows the destruction of large portions of the thyroid nodule (Fig. 18.3).

Globally, to obtain a satisfactory ablation, it is suggested to deliver 400–500 J/mL of thyroid nodule [5]. Before laser ablation, a comprehensive assessment of the target lesion is needed (size, shape, and spatial relations with adjacent organs). Local anesthesia is generally used, preferably with a conscious sedation, depending on patient anxiety and operator preference. The procedure is performed in an outpatient setting and requires 15–30 min [6].

R. Negro (✉)
Department of Experimental Medicine, University of Salento, Lecce, Italy

Division of Endocrinology, "V. Fazzi" Hospital, Lecce, Italy

R. Valcavi et al. (eds.), *Thyroid Ablation*, https://doi.org/10.1007/978-3-031-88229-6_18

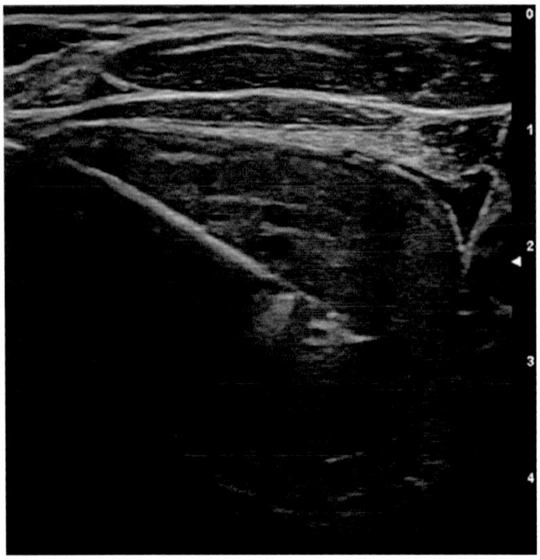

Fig. 18.1 The tip of the needle is inserted in the lower part of the nodule

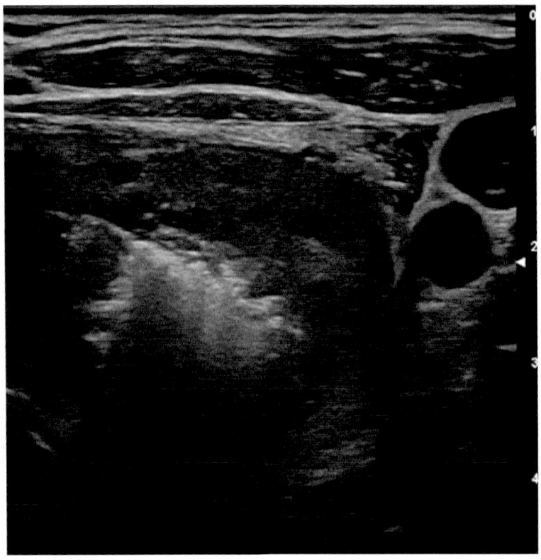

Fig. 18.2 Laser energy released in the lower part of the nodule

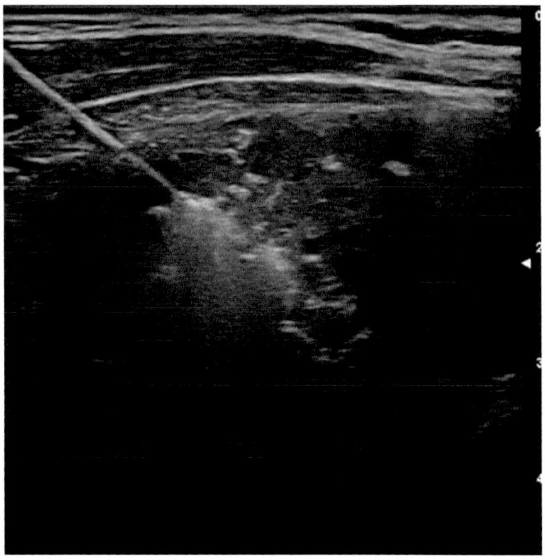

Fig. 18.3 Laser energy released in the upper part of the nodule

18.2 Clinical Studies in Benign Nonfunctioning Thyroid Nodules

The first feasibility study for the use of laser in thyroid nodules was published more than 20 years ago by Pacella et al. [7]. The tissue damage induced by laser treatment was histologically assessed in 18 resected thyroid glands and in 2 volunteers before thyroidectomy for large autonomously functioning nodules. Few years later, the same group published a series of 20 patients who refused surgery or were ineligible for surgery for benign thyroid nodule inducing local symptoms of compression. Thermal treatment obtained a 64% reduction at 6 months (from 24 to 10 mL) [8].

Since then, many studies confirmed the clinical efficacy of this technique. In 2007, for the first time, a randomized controlled trial compared clinical and ultrasound changes induced in thyroid nodules by laser ablation vs follow-up or levothyroxine (LT4) suppressive therapy. Results showed that laser-treated patients obtained a significant nodule reduction at 6 and 12 months (by about 43%), while a nonsignificant nodule shrinkage was observed in LT4-treated group, and a nonsignificant volume increase was observed in untreated group. As a consequence, an improvement of local symptoms was registered in 81.2% of laser treated patients while no complications were noted [9]. Another pivotal study was published by Valcavi et al. who evaluated 122 laser-treated patients with a 3-years follow-up [10]. The authors showed a stable reduction of thyroid nodules by about 50% and demonstrated that small nodules shrink more that large ones. Also, a regrowth above baseline volume was observed in 9% of cases. Symptoms improved in 73.0%, were unchanged in 22.9%, and worsened in 4.1%. Cosmetic signs improved in 71.3%, were unchanged in 23.8%, and worsened in 4.9%. The rate of complications was very low, as just 2 patients (1.6%) experienced transients voice change with vocal cord motility recovery after 6–10 weeks; no significant changes in thyroid function or autoimmunity were observed. Another investigation that is worth to be cited is a multicenter randomized study that evaluated 200 patients assigned to laser treatment or follow-up [11]. At 3 years follow-up, nodules (6–17 mL) increased by 25% in the untreated group while reduced by 57% with a reduction >50% in 67.3% of cases in the laser-treated group. As a consequence, significant amelioration in local symptoms and cosmetic signs were observed.

A confirmation of the clinical efficacy of laser also came from a meta-analysis evaluating 12 studies of radiofrequency-treated patients and 12 studies of laser-treated patients. Results showed an 87% reduction at 3 years for radiofrequency and a 44% reduction for laser [12]. In a multicenter retrospective study, the rates of technique efficacy, regrowth, and retreatment were evaluated in 406 patients treated with either radiofrequency or laser with a follow-up of 5 years [13]. Radiofrequency and laser significantly reduced benign thyroid nodule volume, and this reduction was generally maintained for 5 years. Technique efficacy (defined as a reduction ≥50% after 1 year from the treatment) was achieved in 85% in the radiofrequency group and in 63% in the laser group. Regrowth occurred in 28% of patients (20% in the radiofrequency and 38% in the laser group). In the majority of cases, further treatment was not required as only 18% of patients were retreated (12% in the radiofrequency and 24% in the laser group). In a propensity score matching analysis, radiofrequency obtained a 75% volume reduction ratio vs 56% of laser, with radiofrequency being associated with a lower risk of regrowth. Both thermal ablation techniques resulted in a clinically significant and long-lasting volume reduction of benign thyroid nodules. The longest follow-up study was the one done by Gambelunghe et al. who evaluated 171 laser-treated patients for 10 years [14]. Technique efficacy was achieved in 92% of patients at 1 year, and median nodule volume significantly decreased from 16.7 to 5.0 mL at 1 year (volume reduction ratio of 68%). The benefit of the treatment was durable with a volume reduction ratio of 59% after 10 years. The authors did not observe any case of nodule regrowth >50% at 1 year, although such cases did occur after 4 years ($n = 3$; 1.7% of the overall cohort) and after 7 years ($n = 8$; 4.7%). The largest and most prolonged effect was observed in patients with nodules <15 mL. Treatment was well tolerated, with only minor, transient complications of fever and local pain, and 98% of patients willing to recommend the treatment. The same Gambelunghe published the results of 24 patients suffering from very large nodules (mean nodule volume 138 mL, ranging from 102 to 289 mL) [15]. Patients underwent 1–3 laser sessions within 12 months, with the majority (75%) having 2 sessions. At 1 year, technique efficacy was achieved in 75% of patients, with a volume reduction ratio at 1 year of 81%. At 4-year follow-up, median VRR was 80%. Only 2 patients had nodule regrowth >50% and went to surgery. No major complications were observed (transient fever in 12% and mild-to-moderate pain in 8%.) The above-mentioned results showed that LA is able to obtain long-term benefits also in very large nodules.

As the main scope of thermal ablation is to obtain a significant shrinkage of nodule volume and to offer a valid alternative to surgery, the occurrence of regrowth (≥50% increase compared with the previous smallest volume at ultrasound examination) has to be considered an undesirable event [16]. In the cited paper by Bernardi et al., nodules submitted to LA had regrowth in 38% of cases and those with a higher probability of regrowth were those larger than 15 mL [13]. A much lower rate of regrowth (7.3%) was observed by Gambelunghe which occurred more frequently in nodules larger than 25 mL [14]. From data of the literature, it is clear that the larger is the nodule, the higher is the chance of regrowth. This is due to the fact that usually large nodules receive a smaller amount of energy per ml in respect to small-medium nodules. This in turn means that a significant part of a large nodule is left untreated and that the untreated part is prone to regrow [17]. Other than nodule volume and energy delivered, another important point is represented by the nodule composition. As already demonstrated by the study of Valcavi, solid nodules are more prone to regrow in respect do spongiform nodules [10]. This notion has been subsequently confirmed by a 4-year follow-up study by Negro et al. This retrospective investigation clearly demonstrated that solid nodules shrink less than spongiform and tend to regrow. On the contrary, spongiform nodules obtain a significant volume reduction ratio that steadily reaches 75% [18].

The above-mentioned data of the literature demonstrate that 500 J/mL is the targeted energy to deliver and that the ideal nodule candidate for a successful laser ablation is a spongiform nodule with a volume less than 15 mL [5, 13, 18].

18.3 Clinical Studies in Toxic Adenoma

A toxic adenoma (TA) is a monoclonal, autonomously functioning thyroid nodule that produces supraphysiological amounts of thyroid hormones resulting in the suppression of serum TSH [19]. While the standard treatments for TA are traditionally represented by radioiodine (RAI) or surgery, the advent of thermal ablation offered a new potential option for this disease, with the aim of ablating the hyperfunctioning tissue and consequent reduction of thyroid hormone production.

One of the first investigations examining the use of laser ablation in TA was published by Døssing et al. [20]. The authors in a randomized prospective study compared a single radioiodine dose and a single laser therapy session in 29 nodules. The baseline volume was about 11 mL which reduced in both arms by about 45%. Euthyroidism was achieved in 100% of iodine-treated patients vs 50% in laser-treated patients (energy delivered: about 200 J/mL). Later on, Gambelunghe treated with a single session 82 TAs having a mean volume of 12 mL [21]. In this 3-year follow-up study, nodules reduced by 58%, and methimazole was suspended in 100% of patients with nodules <5 mL and in 28.5% in nodules >25 mL, demonstrating that when the nodule is small and it is completely ablated the suprafisiologic production of thyroid hormone is totally prevented. A relevant multicenter Italian study retrospectively evaluated the clinical outcomes of thermal ablation in 361 patients with TA, followed for 3 years [22]. Nodules were treated with laser in 243/361 cases (67.3%) and with radiofrequency in 118 cases (32.7%). Results showed that nodule volume was significantly reduced at all time points by about 60%. Serum TSH values significantly increased, and anti-thyroid therapy was withdrawn in 41.3% at 12 months. A significant difference in the rate of patients who withdrawn medical therapy at 12 months was registered between small (<10 mL) (74%), medium (49%), and large (>30 mL) nodules (19%). Patients who attained serum TSH normalization at 12 months maintained TSH values within normal limits until the 3-year control. Moreover, radiofrequency resulted in a significantly higher nodule volume reduction compared to laser while no significant difference was observed between the two techniques for serum TSH changes and drug therapy reduction or withdrawal. So, even if radiofrequency appeared to obtain a higher volume reduction, functional parameters were similar between the two techniques.

The above-mentioned investigations pointed out that laser ablation offers a safe and effective therapeutic option in patients with TA and that may be preferably used for small TAs; the incomplete ablation of large nodules allows that the untreated part continues to produce thyroid hormones and tends to regrow due to its monoclonal nature. In this field, two studies explored the efficacy of a combination treatment, i.e., laser plus radioiodine for large TAs that are usually addressed to surgery. In the first study, 15 patients were treated with radioiodine alone and 15 with combination treatment [23]. Results showed that combination treatment obtained at 24 months with a volume reduction rate of about 70% vs 47% of radioiodine alone; moreover, the combination treatment group needed a lower amount of radioiodine and demonstrated a more rapid amelioration of local symptoms, demonstrating that laser followed by radioiodine may be a valid alternative to surgery. Another study addressed the feasibility of combining laser and radioiodine vs lobectomy in large TAs (>20 mL) with a calculated therapeutic activity exceeding 600 MBq [24]. Patients randomly received laser + RAI or lobectomy. Six months after laser + RAI nodules reduced by 68% and patients in both arms of treatment experienced a similar improvement in health-related quality of life (HRQoL). The rate of subclinical hypothyroidism was similar in both groups (about 15%). Then, the study demonstrated that for patients with a large TA, the combination of laser + RAI is a feasible alternative to surgery. Similar to surgery, laser+RAI resolves the mechanical discomfort induced by nodule pressure and effectively treats hyperthyroidism. This procedure also avoids the potential complications associated with surgery while guaranteeing a similar HRQoL benefit.

As a conclusion, data of the literature show that laser ablation is an alternative option to RAI especially in small TAs and is an alternative option to surgery in large TAs if laser is used in combination with RAI. Putative categories of patient who may benefit from laser in treatment in TAs are those who refuse surgery and RAI, pregnant or lactating woman, and women who plan pregnancy in order to avoid RAI administration.

References

1. Papini E, Bizzarri G, Pacella CM. Percutaneous laser ablation of benign and malignant thyroid nodules. Curr Opin Endocrinol Diabetes Obes. 2008;15:434–9. https://doi.org/10.1097/MED.0b013e32830eb89a.
2. Mauri G, Cova L, Monaco CG, Sconfienza LM, Corbetta S, Benedini S, et al. Benign thyroid nodules treatment using percutaneous laser ablation (PLA) and radiofrequency ablation (RFA). Int J Hyperthermia. 2017;33:295–9. https://doi.org/10.1080/02656736.2016.1244707.
3. Mauri G, Gennaro N, Lee MK, Baek JH. Laser and radiofrequency ablations for benign and malignant thyroid tumors. Int J Hyperthermia. 2019;36:13–20. https://doi.org/10.1080/02656736.2019.1622795.
4. Ridouani F, Tuttle RM, Ghosn M, Li D, Wong RJ, Fagin JA, et al. Ultrasound-guided percutaneous laser ablation of the thyroid gland in a Swine model: comparison of ablation parameters and ablation zone dimensions. Cardiovasc Intervent Radiol. 2021;44:1798–806. https://doi.org/10.1007/s00270-021-02915-0.
5. Gambelunghe G, Fede R, Bini V, Monacelli M, Avenia N, D'Ajello M, et al. Ultrasound-guided interstitial laser ablation for thyroid nodules is effective only at high total amounts of energy: results from a three-year pilot study. Surg Innov. 2013;20:345–50. https://doi.org/10.1177/1553350612459276.
6. Papini E, Monpeyssen H, Frasoldati A, Hegedüs L. 2020 European Thyroid Association clinical practice guideline for the use of image-guided ablation in benign thyroid nodules. Eur Thyroid J. 2020;9:172–85. https://doi.org/10.1159/000508484.
7. Pacella CM, Bizzarri G, Guglielmi R, Anelli V, Bianchini A, Crescenzi A, et al. Thyroid tissue: US-guided percutaneous interstitial laser ablation-a feasibility study. Radiology. 2000;217:673–7. https://doi.org/10.1148/radiology.217.3.r00dc09673.
8. Papini E, Guglielmi R, Bizzarri G, Pacella CM. Ultrasound-guided laser thermal ablation for treatment of benign thyroid nodules. Endocr Pract. 2004;10:276–83. https://doi.org/10.4158/EP.10.3.276.
9. Papini E, Guglielmi R, Bizzarri G, Graziano F, Bianchini A, Brufani C, et al. Treatment of benign cold thyroid nodules: a randomized clinical trial of percutaneous laser ablation versus levothyroxine therapy or follow-up. Thyroid. 2007;17:229–35. https://doi.org/10.1089/thy.2006.0204.
10. Valcavi R, Riganti F, Bertani A, Formisano D, Pacella CM. Percutaneous laser ablation of cold benign thyroid nodules: a 3-year follow-up study in 122 patients. Thyroid. 2010;20:1253–61. https://doi.org/10.1089/thy.2010.0189.

11. Papini E, Rago T, Gambelunghe G, Valcavi R, Bizzarri G, Vitti P, et al. Long-term efficacy of ultrasound-guided laser ablation for benign solid thyroid nodules. Results of a three-year multicenter prospective randomized trial. J Clin Endocrinol Metab. 2014;99:3653–9. https://doi.org/10.1210/jc.2014-1826.
12. Trimboli P, Castellana M, Sconfienza LM, Virili C, Pescatori LC, Cesareo R, et al. Efficacy of thermal ablation in benign non-functioning solid thyroid nodule: a systematic review and meta-analysis. Endocrine. 2020;67:35–43. https://doi.org/10.1007/s12020-019-02019-3.
13. Bernardi S, Giudici F, Cesareo R, Antonelli G, Cavallaro M, Deandrea M, et al. Five-year results of radiofrequency and laser ablation of benign thyroid nodules: a multicenter study from the Italian minimally invasive treatments of the thyroid group. Thyroid. 2020;30:1759–70. https://doi.org/10.1089/thy.2020.0202.
14. Gambelunghe G, Stefanetti E, Avenia N, De Feo P. Percutaneous ultrasound-guided laser ablation of benign thyroid nodules: results of 10-year follow-up in 171 patients. J Endocr Soc. 2021;5:bvab081. https://doi.org/10.1210/jendso/bvab081.
15. Gambelunghe G, Ristagno S, Stefanetti E, Avenia N, De Feo P. Ultrasound-guided laser ablation of very large benign thyroid nodules: 4-year, retrospective follow-up in 24 patients. Int J Hyperthermia. 2022;39:217–21. https://doi.org/10.1080/02656736.2022.2025923.
16. Mauri G, Pacella CM, Papini E, Solbiati L, Goldberg SN, Ahmed M, et al. Image-guided thyroid ablation: proposal for standardization of terminology and reporting criteria. Thyroid. 2019;29:611–8. https://doi.org/10.1089/thy.2018.0604.
17. Negro R, Trimboli P. Thermal ablation for benign, non-functioning thyroid nodules: a clinical review focused on outcomes, technical remarks, and comparisons with surgery. Electromagn Biol Med. 2020;39:347–55. https://doi.org/10.1080/15368378.2020.1809448.
18. Negro R, Salem TM, Greco G. Laser ablation is more effective for spongiform than solid thyroid nodules. A 4-year retrospective follow-up study. Int J Hyperthermia. 2016;32:822–8. https://doi.org/10.1080/02656736.2016.1212279.
19. Hamburger JI. Evolution of toxicity in solitary non-toxic autonomously functioning thyroid nodules. J Clin Endocrinol Metab. 1980;50:1089–93. https://doi.org/10.1210/jcem-50-6-1089.
20. Døssing H, Bennedbaek FN, Bonnema SJ, Grupe P, Hegedüs L. Randomized prospective study comparing a single radioiodine dose and a single laser therapy session in autonomously functioning thyroid nodules. Eur J Endocrinol. 2007;157:95–100. https://doi.org/10.1530/EJE-07-0094.
21. Gambelunghe G, Stefanetti E, Colella R, Monacelli M, Avenia N, De Feo P. A single session of laser ablation for toxic thyroid nodules: three-year follow-up results. Int J Hyperthermia. 2018;34:631–5. https://doi.org/10.1080/02656736.2018.1437931.
22. Mauri G, Papini E, Bernardi S, Barbaro D, Cesareo R, De Feo P, et al. Image-guided thermal ablation in autonomously functioning thyroid nodules. A retrospective multicenter three-year follow-up study from the Italian Minimally Invasive Treatment of the Thyroid (MITT) Group. Eur Radiol. 2022;32:1738–46. https://doi.org/10.1007/s00330-021-08289-8.
23. Chianelli M, Bizzarri G, Todino V, Misischi I, Bianchini A, Graziano F, et al. Laser ablation and 131-iodine: a 24-month pilot study of combined treatment for large toxic nodular goiter. J Clin Endocrinol Metab. 2014;99:E1283–6. https://doi.org/10.1210/jc.2013-2967.
24. Negro R, Greco G. Quality of life and outcomes in patients with a large toxic adenoma undergoing laser ablation plus radioiodine vs lobectomy. Int J Hyperthermia. 2019;36:191–5. https://doi.org/10.1080/02656736.2018.1549335.

HIFU Ablation of Thyroid Nodules

19

Mohamed Fawzi, Safaa ElMandouh, Ahmed Said Badr, Alaa Eid Elbanna, and Micheal Ezzat Narouz

19.1 Introduction

Thyroid nodules are growths or lumps that can form in or on the thyroid gland, which is located in the neck [1]. According to medical research, thyroid nodules are a relatively common occurrence. Studies have shown that up to 68% of people who are considered to have a normal thyroid gland may have thyroid nodules that can be visualized using ultrasound [2]. Factors that may increase the risk of developing thyroid nodules or thyroid cancer include a family history of thyroid disease, exposure to radiation, iodine deficiency or excess, and certain genetic conditions [3].

In fact, the majority of thyroid nodules are benign (non-cancerous) and do not require immediate treatment. Nonetheless, it is important for individuals who have been diagnosed with thyroid nodules to undergo regular monitoring and evaluation to ensure that any changes in the size or appearance of the nodules are promptly detected [4].

The first crucial step in diagnosing thyroid nodules involves assessing the patient's medical history and identifying any predisposing factors. This is followed by conducting a thorough ultrasound scan of the neck, with a specific focus on the thyroid gland (Fig. 19.1). This enables a

M. Fawzi (✉) · S. ElMandouh · A. S. Badr · A. E. Elbanna · M. E. Narouz
Radiology Department, National Hepatology and Tropical Medicine Research Institute, Cairo, Egypt

R. Valcavi et al. (eds.), *Thyroid Ablation*, https://doi.org/10.1007/978-3-031-88229-6_19

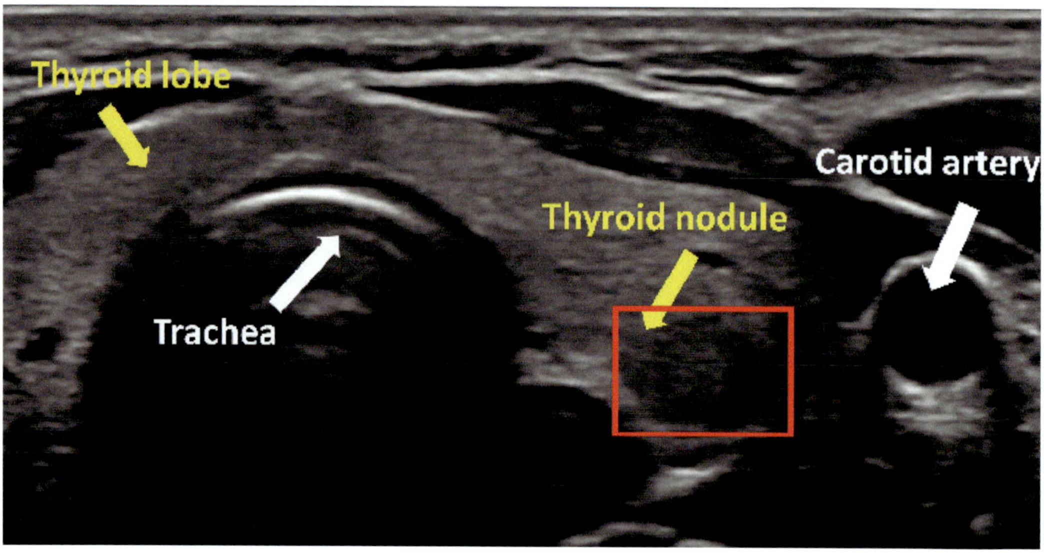

Fig. 19.1 Annotated ultrasound image for some neck structures and right thyroid lobe with a nodule detected within. (Note. Adapted from "Automated Thyroid Nodule Detection from Ultrasound Imaging Using Deep Convolutional Neural Networks," by F. Abdolali, J. Kapur, J.L. Jaremko, M. Noga, A.R. Hareendranathan, and K. Punithakumar, 2020, Comput Biol Med, 122, p. 103871. (https://www.sciencedirect.com/science/article/abs/pii/S0010482520302262). CC BY-NC-ND 4.0 [5]. Reused with written permission)

comprehensive evaluation of the size and characteristics of the nodule, which is essential for determining the likelihood of malignancy and the need for a biopsy. To accurately assess the risk of malignancy, various sonographic scoring systems, such as the highly regarded thyroid imaging reporting and data systems, can be utilized [6].

The treatment approach for thyroid nodules depends on the underlying cause of the condition and the severity of the symptoms. In some cases, watchful waiting with periodic monitoring may be recommended, particularly for small or asymptomatic cases. However, if the nodule is causing symptoms or affecting the patient's quality of life, treatment options may include medication, surgery, or other interventions (Fig. 19.2; [7]). Traditionally, surgery has been the primary treatment for thyroid nodules. However, advances in medical technology and techniques have led to a greater emphasis on minimally invasive treatment modalities, particularly for benign nodules [8].

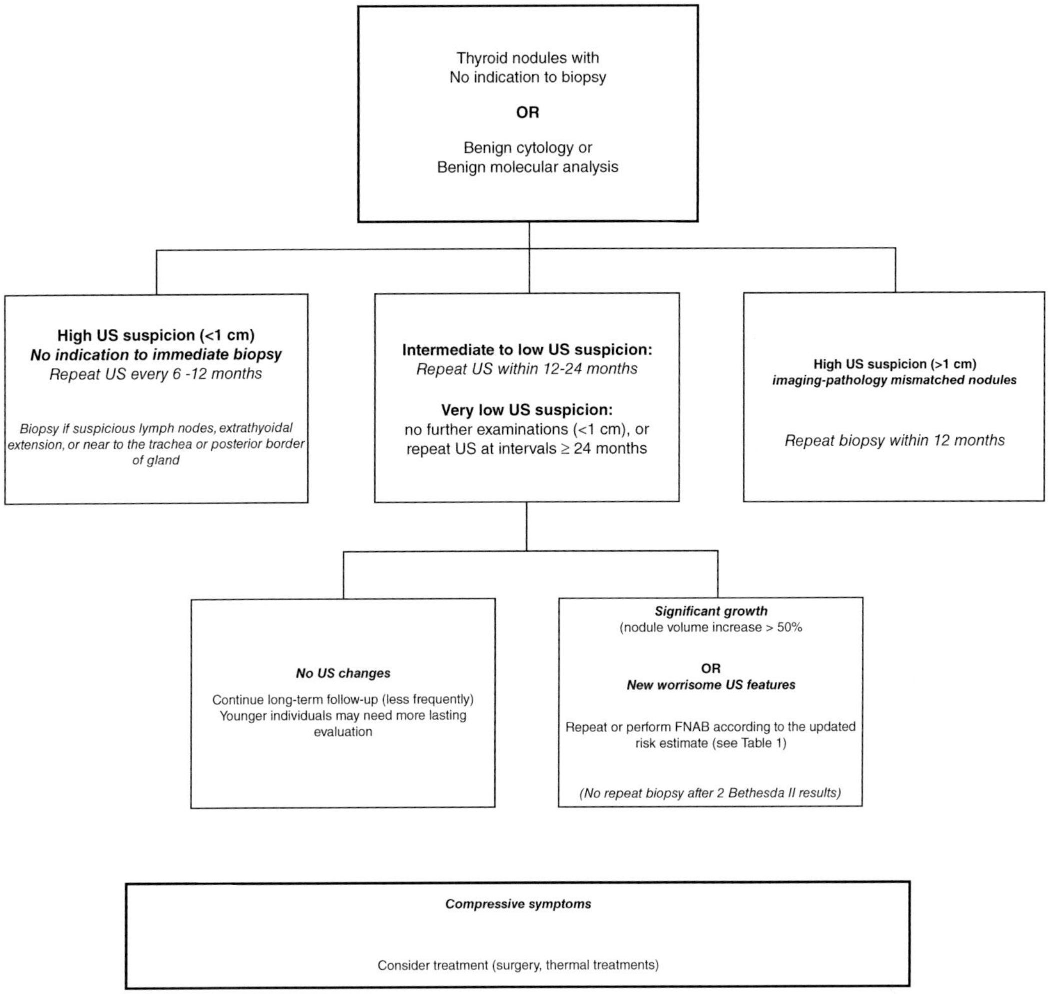

Fig. 19.2 Suggested management and follow-up for thyroid nodules. (Note. Adapted from "Contemporary Thyroid Nodule Evaluation and Management," by G. Grani, M. Sponziello, V. Pecce, V. Ramundo, and C. Durante, 2020, J Clin Endocrinol Metab, 105(9), pp. 2869-2883. https://academic.oup.com/jcem/article/105/9/2869/5850848. CC BY-NC-ND 4.0 [6]. The figure is reused under the terms of the creative commons CC BY license)

19.2 HIFU Technology Overview

HIFU is a non-invasive or minimally invasive medical treatment that uses focused ultrasound waves to heat and destroy targeted tissue (Fig. 19.3). It has been applied to address a range of clinical conditions, including some types of cancer, uterine fibroids, and prostate diseases. It is a treatment option that does not require incisions or anesthesia in most cases [9]. During the procedure, an ultrasound probe is used to focus the sound waves on the targeted tissue. The tissue is heated to a temperature that destroys the cells while leaving surrounding healthy tissue unharmed. The destroyed tissue is then gradually absorbed and eliminated by the body's natural processes. Compared to traditional surgery or radiation therapy, HIFU is generally considered a safer and less invasive treatment option. It can result in fewer side effects, less pain, and faster recovery times. However, it may not be suitable for all patients or all medical conditions [10].

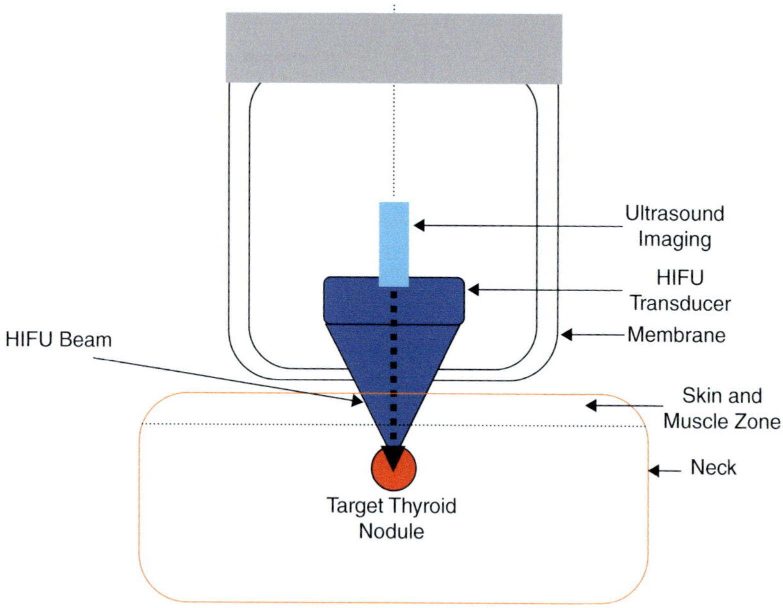

Fig. 19.3 Illustrated diagram for thyroid nodule ablation using HIFU therapy

For symptomatic benign thyroid nodules, HIFU presents a promising alternative to surgical interventions like thyroidectomy or radioactive iodine treatment, which entail considerable surgical risks, potential loss of thyroid function, high financial burden, and a requirement for general anesthesia. As a minimally invasive thermal ablation therapy, HIFU can circumvent these challenges and offer a more favorable outcome for patients with thyroid nodules. Its aims to target and destroy the tissue that makes up the nodule without damaging surrounding healthy tissue, with the goal of reducing its size or eliminating it altogether. This can potentially relieve symptoms and prevent further growth of the nodule [11].

HIFU causes focused injury by two components (thermal and mechanical) without needle puncture or skin penetration. Thermal injury is caused by maintaining high temperatures within the target area. When the temperature reaches 56 °C or above, proteins in the area are denatured and coagulative necrosis occurs in a matter of seconds. When the temperature reaches this level, the water present in the body's tissues begins to vaporize, leading to the formation of microbubbles within the targeted area. On the other hand, mechanical injury leads to cavitation. Cavitation is a phenomenon in which bubbles form and grow within the targeted area. As these bubbles repeatedly expand and collapse, they cause mechanical harm to the neighboring cells, known as popcorn effect. This type of damage can ultimately cause irreversible cell death through processes involving the coagulation and breakdown of cellular structures [12].

19.3 HIFU Procedure for Benign Thyroid Nodules

19.3.1 Patient Selection

HIFU ablation aims to inhibit the growth of autonomously functioning thyroid nodules, while also restoring normal thyroid function, achieving a significant reduction in the volume of the nodules. The treatment is particularly suitable for patients who are not candidates for surgery or who prefer a non-invasive alternative.

In order to achieve a successful outcome, it is imperative to implement specific technical measures, such as ensuring that the targeted nodule must be accessible in both transverse and longitudinal dimensions. Additionally, the depth of the nodule beneath the skin's anterior surface should be less than 17 mm, and there should be no

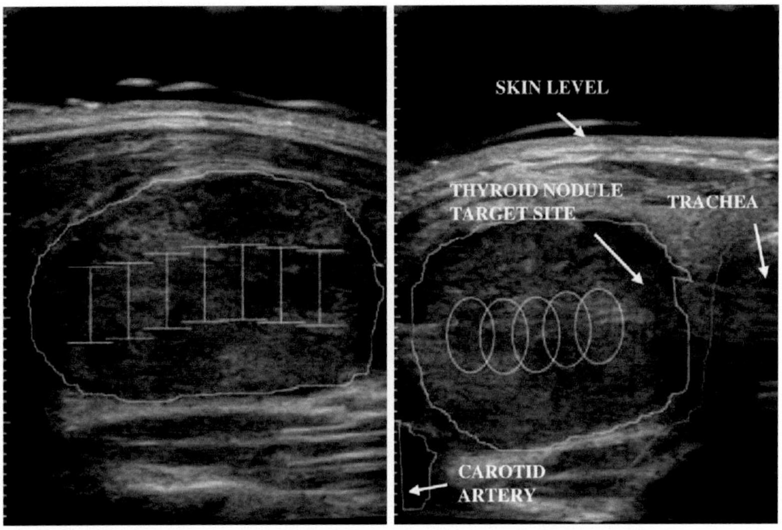

Fig. 19.4 Planning for thyroid nodule ablation using HIFU device. (Note. Adapted from "Horner's Syndrome During High-Intensity Focused Ultrasound Ablation for a Benign Thyroid Nodule," by A. Ben Hamou and H. Monpeyssen, 2021, AACE Clin Case Rep, 7(3), pp. 164-168. https://pubmed.ncbi.nlm.nih.gov/34095479/#:~:text=Conclusion%3A%20HS%20is%20a%20rare,but%20further%20investigation%20is%20needed. CC BY-NC-ND 4.0 [13]. Reused with written permission)

obstruction from the collarbone that interferes with the HIFU unit's movements. Nodule size should be greater than 10 mm in all directions but less than or equal to 35 mm. Furthermore, it is important to ensure the absence of intraocular macrocalcifications that could potentially interfere with the HIFU treatment (Fig. 19.4).

Qualifying criteria for HIFU treatment typically include being over the age of 18, having solitary or dominant thyroid nodules that are predominantly solid with cystic components making up less than 30% of its volume, and having all signs of malignancy excluded. Additionally, the vocal cords must be freely moving during laryngoscopy. Finally, vulnerable neck parts such as the carotid artery, trachea, sympathetic nervous system, and recurrent laryngeal nerve should be absent along the beam pathway (Fig. 19.5). To ensure the safety and efficacy of the procedure, these specific inclusion and technical criteria must be followed.

Exclusion criteria for HIFU thyroid treatment typically include nodules located near precarious neck parts such as the carotid artery, trachea, sympathetic nervous system, and recurrent laryngeal nerve. Additionally, subjects with a history of malignancy or radiotherapy on the neck, pregnancy, sensitivity, or contraindications related to intravenous sedation are typically excluded. These criteria are established to ensure the safety and well-being of the participant and to minimize potential complications. Patients must be informed about the procedure, the anticipated outcomes and adverse events, the post-treatment monitoring period, and the number of treatments required and must provide written informed consent before proceeding.

19.3.2 Patient Preparation

Pre-procedural ultrasound scan is essential for the assessment of the attributes of thyroid nodules, the adjacent structures, and the treatment settings. Additionally, the examiner should also estimate the distance between the skin and the front surface of the nodule and evaluate the nodule's composition and echogenicity both before and after treatment. Generally, the size of the nodule is determined by its three dimensions: length, width, and depth. The nodule's volume can then be calculated using these dimensions.

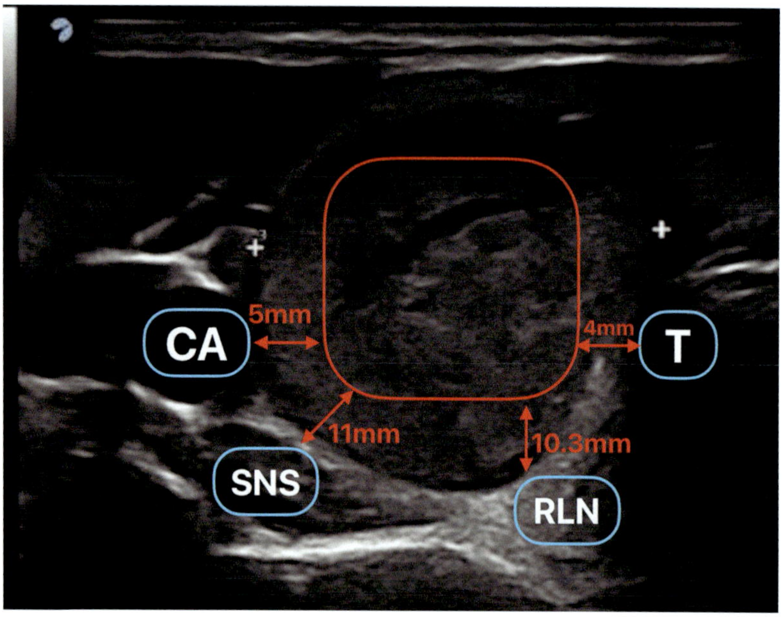

Fig. 19.5 Vulnerable structures such as the carotid artery, trachea, and recurrent laryngeal nerve should be absent along the beam pathway by taking the presented safety margins into consideration. *CA* carotid artery, *RLN* recurrent laryngeal nerve, *SNS* sympathetic nervous system, *T* trachea

The Doppler pattern within the nodule can also be categorized based on previous definitions, including type 0 (no flow), type I (patchy and uneven flow), type II (increased but patchy flow), and type III (hypervascular flow pattern showing homogeneous distribution). To verify the type of the nodule, a fine-needle biopsy and histopathology examination are required and nodules with Bethesda II are indicated for treatment. This is a crucial procedure for distinguishing between benign and malignant nodules.

Before treatment, all patients should undergo indirect laryngoscopy to evaluate the vocal cord and ensure its mobility. Patient symptoms can be assessed using a 0–10 cm visual analog scale, and the esthetic discipline can be categorized using a 1–4 grade scale indicating the degree of visibility and palpability of the nodule, with grade 1 indicating no palpable nodule, grade 2 indicating a palpable but not visible nodule, grade 3 indicating a visible nodule on swallowing, and grade 4 indicating a readily visible nodule. Thyroid function, autoimmunity, and serum calcitonin levels are commonly monitored.

19.3.3 HIFU Ablation Device and Procedure

The ablation procedure is performed entirely under the guidance of ultrasound imaging. Currently, there is a commercially available device that has been approved for the purpose of ablating thyroid nodules. This device was known as EchoPulse® (Theraclion SA, Malakoff, France [14]). And it has an updated version named Beamotion software (Theraclion SA, France). This equipment, generally, consists of several components (Fig. 19.6). The main component is the energy generator, which generates high-intensity ultrasound waves that are used for ablation. The visualization and treatment unit contains the imaging transducer and the HIFU transducer. The imaging transducer produces real-time ultrasound images of the thyroid gland allowing the operator to visualize the nodule and surrounding structures during the treatment. The HIFU transducer produces high-intensity ultrasound waves that are focused on the targeted nodule to ablate it. The skin-cooling device is used to prevent skin

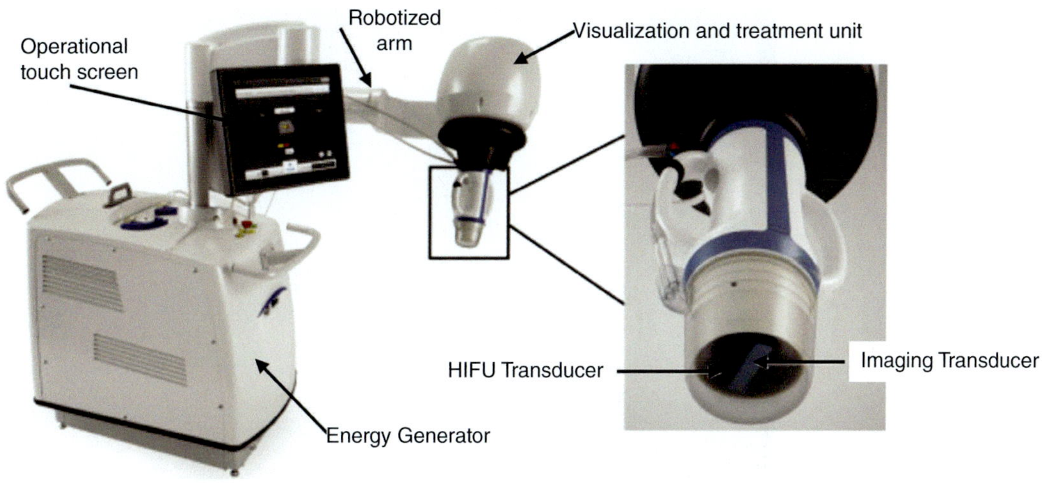

Fig. 19.6 Major component of US-HIFU device. (Note. Adapted from "Extracorporeal Treatment with High Intensity Focused Ultrasound of an Incompetent Perforating Vein in a Patient with Active Venous Ulcers," by A. Obermayer, J.F. Aubry, and N. Barnat, 2021, EJVES Vasc Forum, 50, pp. 1-5. (https://www.sciencedirect.com/science/article/pii/S2666688X20300782). CC BY-NC-ND 4.0 [15]. Reused with a written permission)

burns during the HIFU treatment by cooling the skin surface around the treatment area. Finally, the touch screen interface provides an intuitive and user-friendly interface for the operator to plan and execute the HIFU treatment [16].

During the procedure, the patient is positioned comfortably on a treatment table, and the HIFU equipment is adjusted to the appropriate settings. Then, the operator applies a conductive gel to the patient's skin and places the treatment head on the skin surface. To ensure more safety, the operator highlights vital surrounding structures on the screen, such as the trachea, carotid artery, and laryngeal nerve. The targeted nodule is then adjusted to be within the treatment zone, which has a depth of 5–30 mm below the skin surface (Fig. 19.7).

After adjusting the nodule on the screen, the device divides the target nodule into treatment voxels automatically. The standard size of each voxel is 7.3 mm in depth and 5 mm in width. The ablation process starts by sending an 8-s pulse for each voxel, and then the beam stops for 20–30 of cooling time before moving to the next sequential voxel (Fig. 19.8). A balloon filled with liquid at 10 °C is placed at the tip of the treatment head to cool the skin during the procedure and to prevent skin burns.

In every patient, the initial HIFU pulse was administered at a constant intensity of 45 watts per site. This intensity was continued for subsequent pulses only if the patient was comfortable. However, in cases where the patient experienced any discomfort, the intensity of the following pulses was adjusted based on the patient's ability to tolerate the treatment, with the range of intensity varying from 19 to 35 watts per site [18].

The duration of the procedure is measured in minutes and is calculated as the time between the first and last pulse. Typically, it takes around 30–45 min to perform the necessary treatment on a 3-cm nodule using a beam. However, when dealing with larger nodules that have a volume greater than 30 mL, it may be necessary to use two or more consecutive treatments in order to fully ablate the nodule.

During HIFU ablation, greyscale changes in ultrasound imaging can indicate successful treatment of thyroid nodules (Fig. 19.9). These

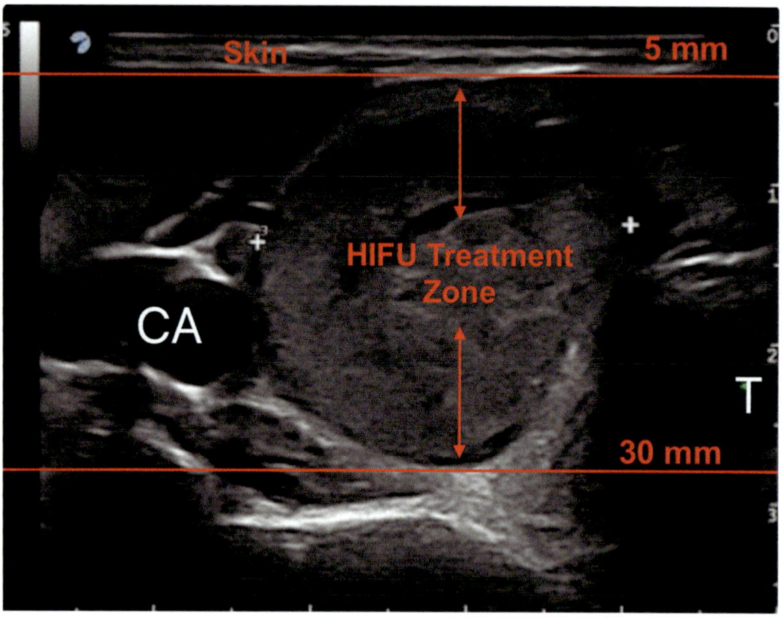

Fig. 19.7 HIFU treatment zone

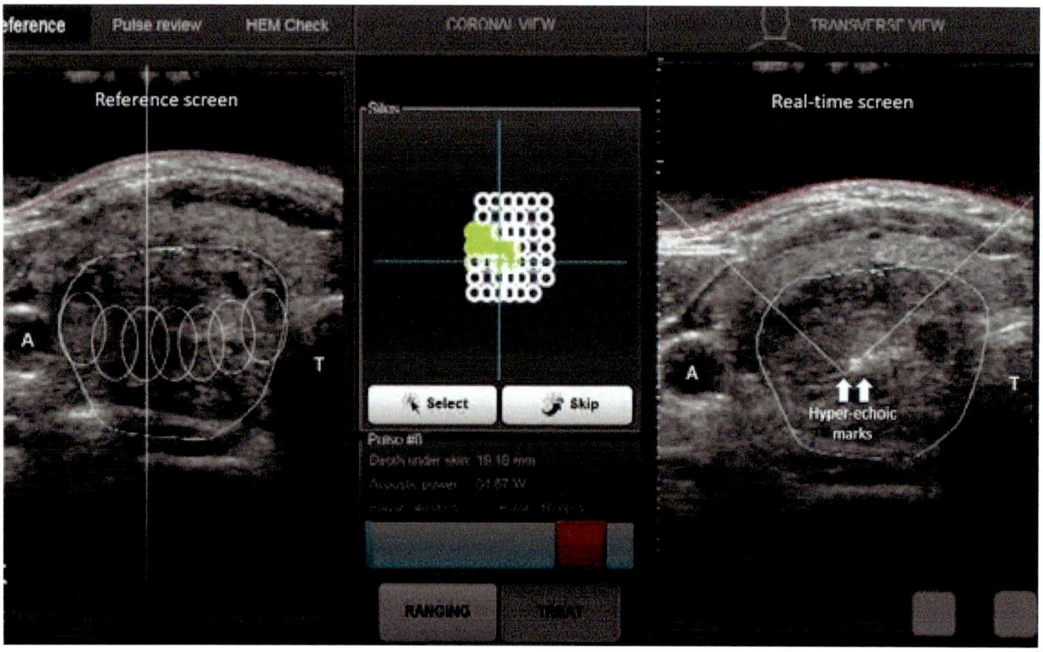

Fig. 19.8 HIFU treatment voxels of the targeted thyroid nodule. (Note. Adapted from "High intensity focused ultrasound (HIFU) ablation of benign thyroid nodules—a systematic review," by B.H.H. Ang and A.L.H. Wu, 2017, J Ther Ultrasound, 5, p. 11. https://journals.sagepub.com/doi/pdf/10.1186/s40349-017-0087-3. CC BY 4.0 [17]. The figure is reused under the terms of the creative commons CC BY license)

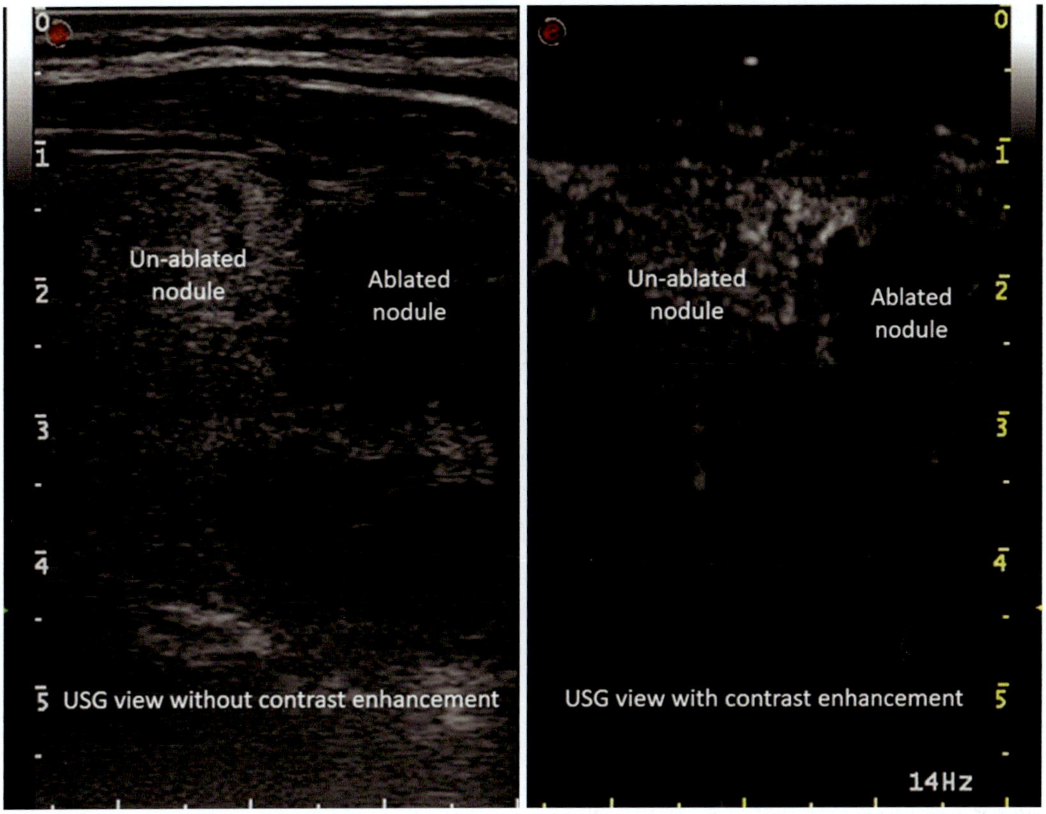

Fig. 19.9 Ultrasound image with and without contrast enhancement displaying the difference between ablated and unabated thyroid nodules using HIFU therapy. (Note. Adapted from "High intensity focused ultrasound (HIFU) ablation of benign thyroid nodules—a systematic review," by B.H.H. Ang and A.L.H. Wu, 2017, J Ther Ultrasound, 5, p. 11. https://journals.sagepub.com/doi/pdf/10.1186/s40349-017-0087-3. CC BY 4.0 [17]. The figure is reused under the terms of the creative commons CC BY license)

changes can include a hypoechoic or darkened appearance of the treated area, which may indicate tissue necrosis or cell death. The treated area may also become heterogeneous or have irregular borders due to tissue damage. In addition, the presence of microbubbles (Fig. 19.10) within the treated area on contrast-enhanced ultrasound imaging can indicate successful ablation. However, it is important to note that these changes may not be apparent immediately after treatment and may require follow-up imaging to confirm treatment success.

A motion detector that used lasers was installed to immediately suspend the energy delivery during ablation if the patient is moved or swallowed. Also, it is essential to monitor the patient's vital signs during the procedure. It is common to apply 1% lidocaine as a local anesthetic around the thyroid gland before the procedure, but a recent study has reported that a minimum level of pulse energy can be used for effective ablation of thyroid nodules without the need for local anesthesia [19].

19.3.4 Post-procedural Care

After receiving HIFU treatment, patients are typically transferred to a recovery room and monitored for up to 2 h. During this time, an ice pack is applied to the targeted area of the neck to alleviate discomfort and swelling associated with the

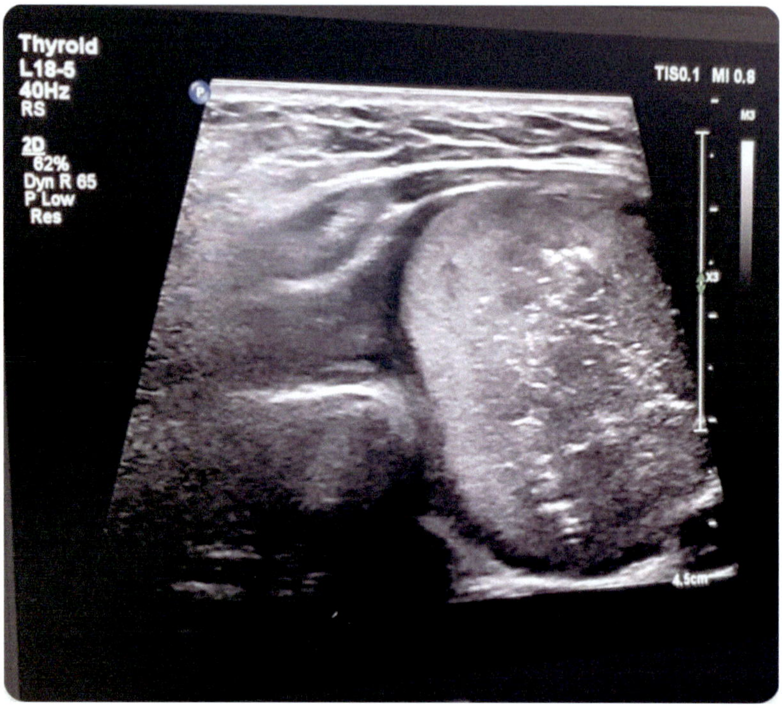

Fig. 19.10 Ultrasound image of thyroid nodule showing successful signs of ablations using HIFU therapy

treatment. After a 2–3 h recovery period, the patient can resume an oral diet. If no adverse events occur, the patient can be discharged. If the patient experiences voice changes or swallowing difficulties after the procedure, an indirect laryngoscopy should be arranged 24 h later to evaluate the vocal cords thoroughly.

Follow-up US imaging is a crucial part of monitoring patients after HIFU treatment for thyroid nodules. The frequency and duration of follow-up US may vary depending on the nodule size, characteristics, and patient's needs. The first follow-up is usually after 1–3 months to check the size and echogenicity of the treated area. Subsequent follow-ups may be at 6 months, 1 year, or 2 years post-treatment or as recommended by the doctor.

During follow-up, the treated area is assessed for volume reduction, changes in echogenicity, and vascularity. A significant reduction in the nodule size, a decrease in vascularity, and changes in echogenicity can indicate successful treatment. However, some nodules may not respond to treatment or may show signs of recurrence, requiring further evaluation or treatment.

Patients may also undergo laboratory tests to evaluate thyroid function and monitor for adverse events or complications related to the HIFU treatment. Follow-up US is essential for long-term monitoring after HIFU treatment for thyroid nodules to ensure treatment effectiveness and detect any potential complications or recurrence.

19.4 Efficacy and Safety Concerns

19.4.1 Efficacy

The pioneering study of HIFU ablation was conducted by Esnault et al. [20], who examined 25 patients with nodular goiter, comprising 5 men and 20 women aged between 25 and 82 years. Two weeks prior to surgery, all patients underwent HIFU treatment, and the excised specimens were histologically examined. Clear necrosis was observed in 10 patients' thyroid nodules following HIFU treatment, while cavitation was observed in the other cases. According to the study, HIFU treatment can induce various types of lesions in thyroid nodules, including coagulative necrosis, fibrotic scars, thrombosis, and cysts. The use of a gradually increasing HIFU pulse acoustic energy allowed for the creation of lesions suitable for histological examination.

Another study by Kovatcheva et al. [21] investigated the efficacy of HIFU in treating benign solid thyroid nodules. The study included 20 patients with euthyroid nodular goiter, and US assessments were conducted at various time points (1 and 3 months) after a single HIFU ablation session. This study found some patients experienced temporary enlargement of treated nodules, while most patients showed a significant reduction in nodule volume from 1 month to 3 months after HIFU treatment.

Another study evaluated the efficacy of HIFU therapy for benign thyroid nodules at a 24-month follow-up [22]. The applied median power used 42 W/site corresponding to 263 J/site as median energy. The results of the study suggest that HIFU treatment can be an effective non-invasive option for reducing benign thyroid nodules by more than 40% within 1 year.

Another German study addressed the efficacy of HIFU with a main focus on the influence on thyroid profile, variables impacting successful procedure, and nodule size [23]. This study recruited patients over a 5-year period with a total cohort of 75 nodules (72 patients). The results showed that HIFU treatment is an effective non-invasive option for reducing the size of thyroid nodules at all follow-up points. However, for preablative nodules <3 mL and >3 mL, the reduction in volume was not significant. The study highlights the importance of selecting appropriate parameters for efficient HIFU treatment, such as treating solid nodules and utilizing general anesthesia. Furthermore, the study demonstrates that HIFU therapy does not significantly affect thyroid hormones, with a very low reversible complication rate reaching 3.8%.

A recent systematic review [24] comprehensively evaluated the efficacy and safety of high-intensity HIFU in the treatment of benign thyroid nodules. It included the published articles from 1990 to 2021. Totally, this review analyzed 9 studies. The results of the meta-analysis were based on only 6 studies, showing that HIFU treatment was associated with a pooled estimate of a significant volume reduction rate along the time points of follow-up (3, 6, and 24 months). No adverse events were reported; however, no study reported total dissolution of the targeted nodule. The reported rates of Horner syndrome, vocal cord paralysis, and voice hoarseness were minimal and transient.

19.4.2 Safety Concerns

HIFU treatment for thyroid nodules has shown high efficacy and low complication rates, making it a promising non-invasive option [25]. However, safety concerns associated with HIFU remain, including the risk of vocal cord paresis, unintentional skin burns, and changes in thyroid function.

19.4.2.1 Vocal Cord Paralysis (VCP)

VCP is a potential complication associated with HIFU treatment for thyroid nodules. VCP occurs when one or both vocal cords become partially paralyzed, resulting in changes in voice quality and difficulty speaking or breathing. This is due to the affection of the left recurrent laryngeal nerve. This typically happens when the targeted nodule sits near the tracheoesophageal groove where the nerve runs [26]. The risk of VCP can be minimized by using appropriate treatment parameters, such as limiting the amount of energy delivered to the target tissue, precise targeting of the nodule, and monitoring of vocal cord function during the procedure. Also, it is crucial to have a minimum safe distance of 1.1 cm between the tracheoesophageal groove and beam focus. Additionally, the use of intraoperative nerve monitoring can help detect early changes in vocal cord function during the procedure and enable timely intervention to prevent further damage. While the incidence of VCP following HIFU treatment for thyroid nodules is relatively low [24], it is important to inform patients of this potential risk and monitor them closely for any signs of vocal cord dysfunction. In the rare cases where VCP does occur, most patients recover full vocal cord function within several months, although some may require ongoing treatment and rehabilitation.

19.4.2.2 Unintentional Skin Burns and Damage of Nearby Structures

Unintentional skin burns are another potential complication of HIFU treatment [24]. Their occurrence is related to various factors such as inappropriate treatment parameters, inadequate cooling, and poor patient selection. These burns can occur if the beam focus overshoots or undershoots the target tissue. In this situation, the heat delivered through HIFU could damage the skin or surrounding neck structures. The incidence is extremely rare when precautions have been taken. Therefore, appropriate patient selection, proper treatment planning, and skilled execution are essential to minimize the risk of skin burns. Also, the balloon filled with liquid at 10 °C attached to the treatment head plays a pivotal role in preventing these burns. Additionally, intraoperative monitoring of skin temperature and thorough attention to the patient's movements and heat delivery dynamics.

19.4.2.3 Changes in Thyroid Function

HIFU treatment for thyroid nodules has been reported to have minimal effects on thyroid function [24]. However, some studies have reported transient changes in thyroid hormone levels after the procedure, including a slight increase in serum thyroxine (T4) levels and a decrease in thyroid-stimulating hormone (TSH) levels [23, 27].

These changes in thyroid function are believed to be due to the thermal effects of HIFU on the thyroid gland, which may cause transient thyroid cell damage and inflammation. However, the extent and duration of these changes in thyroid function are generally mild and self-limiting and of little clinical significance [27].

Overall, the effects of HIFU treatment on thyroid function are generally minimal and transient. Nonetheless, it is important to monitor thyroid function closely in patients undergoing HIFU treatment for thyroid nodules, particularly those with pre-existing thyroid conditions. Follow-up monitoring of thyroid hormone levels after the procedure can help ensure that any changes in thyroid function are detected and managed appropriately.

19.5 Limitations and Future Implications

Despite its promising results, HIFU ablation for thyroid nodules still has several limitations and challenges that need to be addressed. One of the most significant drawbacks is the limited treatment capability for larger or deeper nodules due to the current HIFU device's maximum depth of penetration. This restriction may limit the applicability of HIFU to a subset of patients with smaller and more superficial nodules, and alternative treatments may be required for those with larger or deeper nodules.

Another limitation of HIFU is the lengthy treatment time required for complete ablation of the target tissue. Compared to other ablation techniques such as RFA, microwave ablation, or LA, HIFU treatment times are significantly longer, which may increase the risk of complications such as skin burns and patient discomfort. Therefore, the development of more efficient and faster HIFU devices is necessary to improve treatment outcomes and reduce the risk of adverse events.

Furthermore, there is a lack of long-term data on the efficacy of HIFU ablation for thyroid nodules. While initial studies have shown promising results, longer follow-up periods are necessary to determine the durability of the treatment effects and the rate of nodule recurrence. Additionally, factors affecting HIFU efficacy, such as operator experience, energy delivery, and tumor characteristics, need to be further explored to optimize treatment outcomes.

Lastly, the initial cost of HIFU treatment is higher than that of other ablation techniques, which may limit its availability to patients in certain regions or healthcare settings. However, as the technology continues to evolve, it is expected that the cost of HIFU treatment will decrease over time, making it more accessible to a broader range of patients.

In addition to its potential therapeutic applications, HIFU ablation also has significant potential as a diagnostic tool for thyroid nodules. Recent studies have shown that HIFU elastography, a technique that measures tissue elasticity, can help differentiate benign from malignant thyroid nodules with high accuracy [28]. This noninvasive technique offers a safe and effective alternative to conventional biopsy procedures and may be particularly useful in patients who are not ideal candidates for biopsy due to medical comorbidities or other factors.

Another area of research is focused on optimizing energy delivery during HIFU ablation. Recent technological advancements, such as the use of nanodroplets, have shown promising results in enhancing the ablation capacity of HIFU while reducing the risk of collateral damage to healthy tissue. This approach may enable shorter treatment times and more efficient energy delivery, improving treatment outcomes and reducing the risk of adverse events.

Furthermore, ongoing research is exploring the use of HIFU ablation in combination with other therapeutic modalities, such as chemotherapy or immunotherapy, to enhance treatment efficacy. Preclinical studies have shown that combining HIFU with chemotherapy can significantly enhance drug delivery to the target tissue, improving treatment outcomes. Additionally, combining HIFU with immunotherapy may enhance the immune response to cancer cells, improving the overall efficacy of the treatment approach.

Moreover, it would be worthwhile to conduct studies that compare HIFU treatment with other techniques such as laser, radiofrequency, and microwave ablation. Such studies would provide valuable insights into the relative effectiveness, safety, and long-term outcomes of these different techniques. By comparing the advantages and limitations of each technique, healthcare providers can make more informed decisions about which treatment option is most appropriate for each patient. These studies could also help to identify areas for improvement and innovation in the field of thyroid nodule treatment. Overall, a comparative analysis of HIFU with other techniques could enhance our understanding of the best approaches to managing thyroid nodules.

19.6 Conclusion

In conclusion, HIFU is a safe and effective treatment option for thyroid nodules. And it is a rapidly evolving technology that has significant potential for the management of other thyroid conditions. While vocal cord paresis and changes in thyroid function are potential complications, they are rare and typically self-limiting. Careful monitoring of skin changes and attention to safety distances can minimize the risk of complications. With proper patient selection and careful technique, HIFU can provide a safe and effective alternative to surgery for patients with symptomatic thyroid nodules. While several limitations and challenges remain, ongoing research and development efforts, as well as multidisciplinary collaboration, patient education, cost-effectiveness analysis, and standardized regulatory approval and reimbursement policies, are necessary to fully realize the potential benefits of this treatment modality for patients with thyroid nodules.

References

1. Welker MJ, Orlov D. Thyroid nodules. Am Fam Physician. 2003;67(3):559–66.
2. Haugen BR. 2015 American Thyroid Association management guidelines for adult patients with thyroid nodules and differentiated thyroid cancer: what is new and what has changed? Cancer. 2017;123(3):372–81.
3. Fan L, Tan L, Chen Y, Du C, Zhu M, Wang K, et al. Investigation on the factors that influence the prevalence of thyroid nodules in adults in Tianjin, China. J Trace Elem Med Biol. 2018;50:537–42.
4. Gharib H, Hegedüs L, Pacella CM, Baek JH, Papini E. Clinical review: nonsurgical, image-guided, minimally invasive therapy for thyroid nodules. J Clin Endocrinol Metab. 2013;98(10):3949–57.
5. Abdolali F, Kapur J, Jaremko JL, Noga M, Hareendranathan AR, Punithakumar K. Automated thyroid nodule detection from ultrasound imaging using deep convolutional neural networks. Comput Biol Med. 2020;122:103871.
6. Grani G, Sponziello M, Pecce V, Ramundo V, Durante C. Contemporary thyroid nodule evalu-

ation and management. J Clin Endocrinol Metab. 2020;105(9):2869–83.
7. Trimboli P, Castellana M, Sconfienza LM, Virili C, Pescatori LC, Cesareo R, et al. Efficacy of thermal ablation in benign non-functioning solid thyroid nodule: a systematic review and meta-analysis. Endocrine. 2020;67(1):35–43.
8. Cho SJ, Baek JH, Chung SR, Choi YJ, Lee JH. Long-term results of thermal ablation of benign thyroid nodules: a systematic review and meta-analysis. Endocrinol Metab. 2020;35(2):339–50.
9. Maloney E, Hwang JH. Emerging HIFU applications in cancer therapy. Int J Hyperthermia. 2015;31(3):302–9.
10. Liu L, Wang T, Lei B. High-intensity focused ultrasound (HIFU) ablation versus surgical interventions for the treatment of symptomatic uterine fibroids: a meta-analysis. Eur Radiol. 2022;32(2):1195–204.
11. Chung SR, Baek JH, Suh CH, Choi YJ, Lee JH. Efficacy and safety of high-intensity focused ultrasound (HIFU) for treating benign thyroid nodules: a systematic review and meta-analysis. Acta Radiol. 2020;61(12):1636–43.
12. Mearini L. High intensity focused ultrasound, liver disease and bridging therapy. World J Gastroenterol. 2013;19(43):7494–9.
13. Ben Hamou A, Monpeyssen H. Horner's syndrome during high-intensity focused ultrasound ablation for a benign thyroid nodule. AACE Clin Case Rep. 2021;7(3):164–8.
14. ECHOPULSE—Theraclion [Internet]. [cited 2023 Jul 26]. https://www.theraclion.com/products/echopulse/.
15. Obermayer A, Aubry JF, Barnat N. Extracorporeal treatment with high intensity focused ultrasound of an incompetent perforating vein in a patient with active venous ulcers. EJVES Vasc Forum. 2021;50:1–5.
16. Kotewall N, Lang BHH. High-intensity focused ultrasound ablation as a treatment for benign thyroid diseases: the present and future. Ultrasonography. 2019;38(2):135–42.
17. Lang BHH, Wu ALH. High intensity focused ultrasound (HIFU) ablation of benign thyroid nodules—a systematic review. J Ther Ultrasound. 2017;5:11.
18. Pałyga I, Pałyga R, Młynarczyk J, Kopczyński J, Góźdź S, Kowalska A. The current state and future perspectives of high intensity focused ultrasound (HIFU) ablation for benign thyroid nodules. Gland Surg. 2020;9(Suppl 2):S95–104.
19. Trimboli P, Bini F, Marinozzi F, Baek JH, Giovanella L. High-intensity focused ultrasound (HIFU) therapy for benign thyroid nodules without anesthesia or sedation. Endocrine. 2018;61(2):210–5.
20. Esnault O, Franc B, Ménégaux F, Rouxel A, De Kerviler E, Bourrier P, et al. High-intensity focused ultrasound ablation of thyroid nodules: first human feasibility study. Thyroid. 2011;21(9):965–73.
21. Kovatcheva RD, Vlahov JD, Stoinov JI, Zaletel K. Benign solid thyroid nodules: US-guided high-intensity focused ultrasound ablation-initial clinical outcomes. Radiology. 2015;276(2):597–605.
22. Trimboli P, Pelloni F, Bini F, Marinozzi F, Giovanella L. High-intensity focused ultrasound (HIFU) for benign thyroid nodules: 2-year follow-up results. Endocrine. 2019;65(2):312–7.
23. Vorländer C, Fischer A, Korkusuz H. High intensity focused ultrasound in the therapy of benign thyroid nodules-first German bicentric study with long-term follow-up. Endocrine. 2022;77(1):112–20.
24. Cheong CWS, Au JXY, Lim MY, Fu EW, Li H, Gan JY. The efficacy and safety of high-intensity focused ultrasound in the treatment of benign thyroid nodules: a systematic review and meta-analysis from 1990 to 2021. Ann Acad Med Singap. 2022;51(2):101–8.
25. Lang BHH, Woo YC, Chiu KWH. Two-year efficacy of single-session high-intensity focused ultrasound (HIFU) ablation of benign thyroid nodules. Eur Radiol. 2019;29(1):93–101.
26. Korkusuz H, Fehre N, Sennert M, Happel C, Grünwald F. Volume reduction of benign thyroid nodules 3 months after a single treatment with high-intensity focused ultrasound (HIFU). J Ther Ultrasound. 2015;3:4.
27. Lang BHH, Woo YC, Chiu KWH. High-intensity focused ablation (HIFU) of single benign thyroid nodule rarely alters underlying thyroid function. Int J Hyperthermia. 2017;33(8):875–81.
28. Mauri G, Nicosia L, Xu Z, Di Pietro S, Monfardini L, Bonomo G, et al. Focused ultrasound: tumour ablation and its potential to enhance immunological therapy to cancer. Br J Radiol. 2018;91(1083):20170641.

20 Microwave Ablation of Malignant Thyroid Tumors

Giovanni Mauri, Yujie Ren, and Shuhang Xu

The morbidity and mortality of papillary thyroid carcinoma have increased worldwide during the recent 30 years [1]. Ultrasonography (US) and US-guided aspiration have helped uncover more cases of papillary thyroid microcarcinoma (PTMC), a major subtype of thyroid carcinoma [2]. In the past decades, surgery has been practiced in all the patients with thyroid carcinoma, regardless of size, location, and pathology. Indeed, the low mortality of papillary thyroid carcinoma (PTC) has been noticed, so a concern of overtreatment has been proposed. Active surveillance (AS) has been practiced at some centers, proving that the progression of PTMC is slow enough to be controlled with conservative efforts, rather than surgery.

Previous studies have shown that PTMC progresses slowly. In Japan, 340 PTMC patients at Kuma Hospital were followed up over a mean period of 74 months (range 18–187). Of them, 6.4% and 15.9% showed an increase of PTMC size by more than 3 mm during 5- and 10-year follow-up, respectively; 1.4% and 3.4% showed novel nodal metastasis during the two periods, respectively [3]. A multi-center research from South Korea showed a low risk of PTMC enlargement. During a median follow-up of 32.5 months, the maximal diameter of PTMC increased by more than 3 mm in 3.5% [4]. Delayed surgery for PTMC has been proved to be not associated with higher risk of structural recurrent/persistent disease compared to immediate surgery [5]. However, the anxiety of deterioration is still the most important reason for surgery. In a meta-analysis including four Asian populations (two in Japan, one in South Korean, and one in North American), PTMC enlargement and LNM were not reasons for delayed operation in the Asia [6]. Therefore, image-guided minimally invasive strategies have been designed to treat PTMC through preventing either PTMC progression or surgery. Increasing evidence demonstrates that thermal ablations, including laser ablation (LA), radiofrequency ablation (RFA), and microwave ablation (MWA), have achieved satisfactory results in the treatment of low-risk papillary thyroid carcinoma (PTC), particularly PTMC. Furthermore, thermal ablation has also been demonstrated to be a safe and effective alternative to surgery for the treatment of recurrent PTC and metastatic lymph node, especially in patients who are ineligible for surgery.

G. Mauri
European Institute of Oncology, Milan, Italy

Y. Ren · S. Xu (✉)
Jiangsu Province Hospital on Integration of Traditional Chinese and Western Medicine, Nanjing, China

R. Valcavi et al. (eds.), *Thyroid Ablation*, https://doi.org/10.1007/978-3-031-88229-6_20

20.1 Principles in MWA Application

20.1.1 Physics of Microwaves

Microwave has a frequency ranging from 900 to 2450 MHz. The water molecule (H_2O) has a polar form and asymmetric charges. Electromagnetic radiation has electric charge as well. The "wave" represents the electric charge flipping between positive and negative poles. The molecule flips in a very high speed whenever interacting an oscillating electric charge. Vigorous friction between water molecules raises the temperature of water. In this way, electromagnetic microwaves can heat the tissue and induce cellular death via coagulation necrosis [7]. Microwaves penetrate through materials with low electrical conductivity, such as lung, bone, and dehydrated or charred tissue. Irreversible injury occurs in cells heated to 46 °C for 60 min and becomes more severe as the temperature rises. Microwaves can produce extremely high (>150 °C) temperatures [8]. Compared with RFA, MWA relies predominately on direct heating, rather than thermal conductance. MWA can be used for faster and larger ablation zone, with less sensitive to the heat sink effect and the perfusion mediated cooling [9].

20.1.2 Procedure of MWA

The patient is placed in the supine position, with the neck extended. Local anesthesia is performed to relieve discomfort during operation. As appropriated, hemocoagulase is injected to reduce bleeding during the procedure [10]. Normal saline is injected surrounding the thyroid capsule to form a liquid barrier against thermal injury (Figs. 20.1 and 20.2). A 16-G [10–15] or 17-G [14, 16, 17] short needle is used for skin puncture. A 19-G needle is a new instrument [18]. The microwave antenna is percutaneously inserted into tumors. A "multidimensionally fixed needle ablation" method is used for small nodules (≤10 mm in diameter) to acquire the sufficiently necrotic zone. The output power is usually set to be 20–30 W [11–14, 16, 17], sometimes 35–50 W (Fig. 20.1) [10, 15, 18]. Using contrast-enhanced US, the margin of target ablation area is allowed to exceed the tumor edge by 5 mm [10, 12, 16, 17], to avoid marginal residue and recurrence. During ablation the operator should inquire about symptoms and vocalizations from time to time. Postoperative compression of ice should be done immediately to prevent bleeding and reduce swelling. During 0.5–1 h after MWA, some possible complications are monitored, such as voice change, skin burns, tracheal injury, and esophageal perforation.

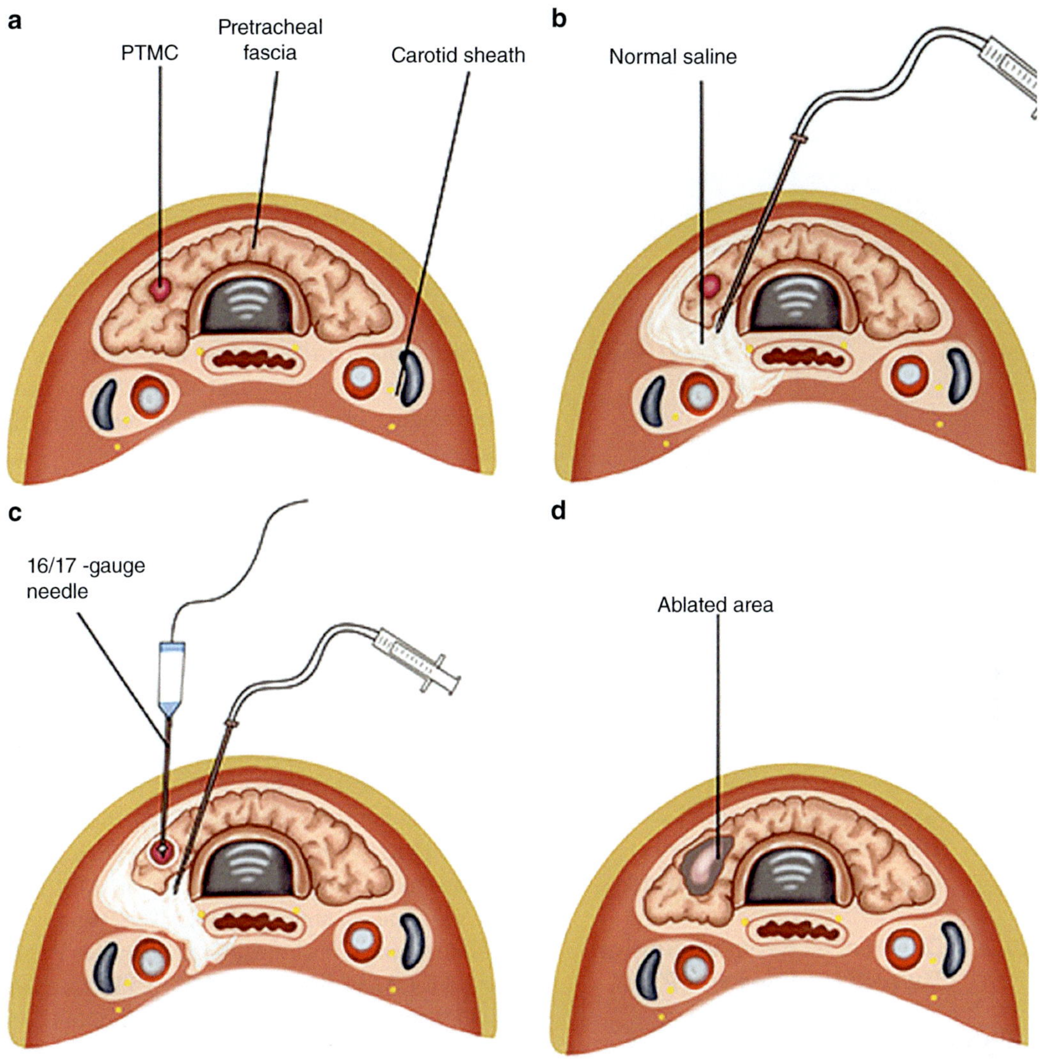

Fig. 20.1 Schematic diagram of microwave ablation for papillary thyroid microcarcinoma. (**a**) Anatomical structure of neck. The carotid sheath with sympathetic chain behind contains common carotid artery, internal jugular vein, and vague nerve. Pretracheal fascia contains thyroid, trachea, esophagus, and recurrent nerve. (**b**) Normal saline is injected as the spacer fluid to separate the normal tissues from the ablated area. (**c**) The target area should exceed the tumor edge to avoid marginal residue and recurrence. (**d**) An extended ablated area is shown. PTMC, papillary thyroid microcarcinoma

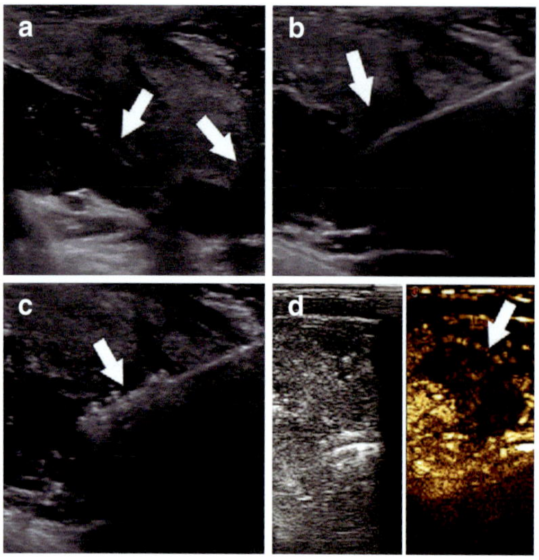

Fig. 20.2 Ultrasonographic imaging of MWA. (**a**) Hydrodissection is to build up a barrier against thermal injury to protect normal tissues; (**b**) The microwave antenna is percutaneously inserted into PTMC lesion; (**c**) The power puts out with tissue degeneration; (**d**) Contrast-enhanced ultrasonography after ablation with a filling defect. *MWA* microwave ablation, *PTMC* papillary thyroid carcinoma

20.2 Treatment of Papillary Thyroid Microcarcinomas

20.2.1 Differences Between Benign Thyroid Nodules and PTMC

20.2.1.1 Treatment Goals

The treatment goals vary according to the pathology of thyroid nodules. For PTMC, MWA aims to completely ablate cancer lesion; for benign thyroid nodules (BTN), MWA aims to reduce volume and alleviate compression-caused symptoms. MWA is suitable for those who are at low risk of microcarcinoma without any lymph node metastasis (LNM). Before MWA treatment, it is extremely crucial to rule out the possibility of PTMC metastasis.

20.2.1.2 Techniques

Moving shot technique is used to eliminate benign nodular tissues; however, it is unsuitable for PTMC. The probe is fixed in one or more dimensions to prevent needle seeding in the treatment of PTMC, called multidimensionally fixed ablation [14]. BTN should be treated with moderate MWA to prevent carbonation, while PTMC should be treated with strong MWA to ensure a complete ablation of tumor cell. Generally, the margin of ablation area exceeds the border of PTMC to kill possible tumor cells, but this does not suit benign nodules. The hydrodissection technique is the most common method to build up a thermal barrier against thermal injury for both benign nodules and PTMC. Adequate surrounding space should be reserved during the extended ablation of PTMC.

20.2.1.3 Volume Reduction Rate

MWA decreases the volume of benign or malignant thyroid nodules. A meta-analysis [19] showed that the pooled proportion of volume reduction rate (VRR) is 63%. The VRR is 75% for benign thyroid nodules and 59% for PTMC. In our center, the VRR of benign nonfunctioning thyroid nodules is 81.31% at 12 months after MWA [20]. It seems that MWA is more effective in reducing the volume of benign thyroid nodules than PTMC. VRR shows difference arising from ablated area and delivery energy in MWA for PTMC and benign nodules. The pattern of volume change is a little different between PTMC and BTN. The volume of PTMC rapidly increases in short term, with a VRR of $-1770.85 \pm 2161.54\%$ at 1 month after operation, then after 6 months follow-up slowly reduces to the same size as that before operation [13]. The increase of volume is more likely related to the extended ablation. Otherwise, the volume of benign nodules increases rarely, except for some solid nodules that may swell 1 month after ablation [21, 22].

20.2.1.4 Thyroid Function

There are no significant differences in thyroid function throughout a 12-month follow-up in patients with benign nodules [22, 23]. Thyroglobulin level increases significantly within 24 h after ablation, then decreases during a 3-month follow-up, even below the initial level [24]. Thyroid function shows no difference at one month after MWA [12, 13], and no hypothyroidism appears after MWA for PTMC [11, 14, 16–18, 25]. We have also found transient thyrotoxicosis with suppressed serum thyrotropin level and elevated free thyroxine level within 24 h after ablation. It may result from cell lysis and tissue destruction upon thermal assault. However, a minority of patients suffer from hypothyroidism at our center, which may be associated with the use of iodinated contrast media (ICM) for computed tomography (CT) scan to exclude metastasis before MWA.

20.2.1.5 Supplementary Ablation

Liu et al. [22] have found that 11% of BTN require twice MWA, while 2% require thrice MWA to achieve complete inactivation. Currently, it is recommended to supplement an ablation for residual tissues at post-treatment 3–6 months. The efficacy of supplementary MWA has not been reported in detail. It is assumed that the efficacy of secondary MWA is weaker than the first, like RFA [26]. Supplementary ablation has been used for tumor recurrence and LNM [17, 18]. However, caution should be given to recurrence and MWA-related complications in repeated MWA for PTMC.

20.2.1.6 Follow-Up

To follow-up patients receiving MWA with both BTN and PTMC, thyroid US can be performed at 1, 3, 6, and 12 months, subsequently every 6 or 12 months after ablation. The strategy should be stricter in PTMC than BTN. The US is mainly used to evaluate the size of ablated areas. Otherwise, core-needle biopsy (CNB) is applied to check residual carcinoma tissue at 3 or 6 months after MWA according to the volume of ablated area. CT scan is also conducted in follow-up for PTMC, but their time points remain unstandardized, mostly at 1 year after ablation. Thyroid function is commonly monitored within 6 months after MWA. Other ablation-related complications such as pain, hoarseness, and hypoparathyroidism also need attention.

20.2.2 Efficacy of MWA

The tumor shrinks and even disappears after MWA (Fig. 20.3). All the study found no residual tumor after MWA. The volume firstly increases sharply, then decreases slowly. VRR shows obvious heterogeneity but consistent regularity among studies. One study shows that the volume decreases just at

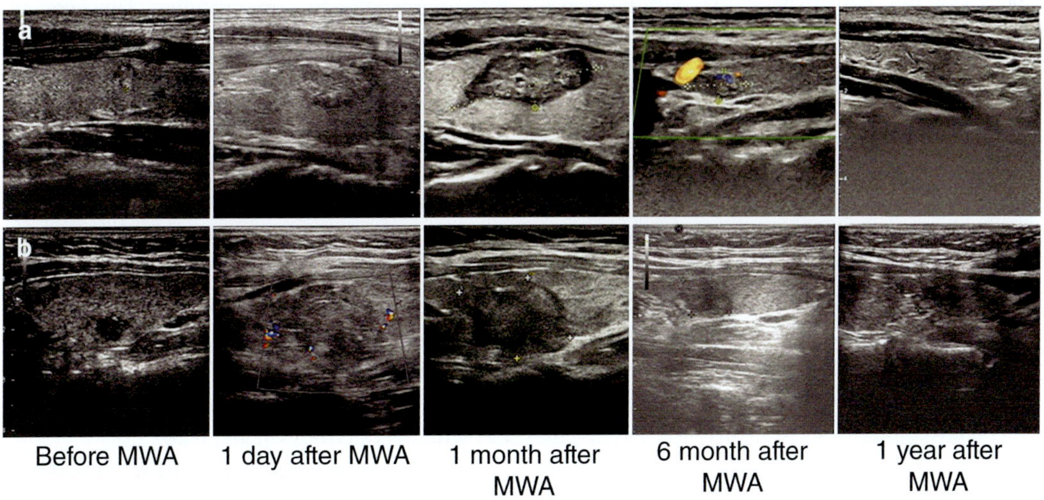

Fig. 20.3 Dynamic change of ablated PTMC in ultrasonography after MWA. (**a**) Male, 31 years old; ablated area disappeared at 1 year after MWA. (**b**) Female, 17 years old; VRR was −36% at 1 year. *PTMC* papillary thyroid carcinoma, *MWA* microwave ablation

1 month after MWA [14], meanwhile more studies [12, 13, 16] show the same result even at 12 months after MWA. These studies show that the VRR can reach to 98% at 1-year follow-up [14, 18] or 3-year follow-up [12, 13]. The volumes at 1, 3, 6, 12, and 18 months display a significant decreasing trend, but not significantly afterwards [16].

The number of disappeared PTMC also varies among studies. Only 16.67% completely disappear in Li's study [16] using 30 W MWA, compared to 97.56% in Teng's research using 20 W MWA [11] and 22.2% in Yue's using 40 W MWA [10]. It seems that the efficacy of 20 W MWA is better than that of 30 W or 40 W MWA. But a research using 30 W MWA [14] reveals that 78.1% (89/114) disappear completely and 15.8% (18/114) leave needle tracks or crevice echo only. One study including 185 patients shows that the complete absorption rate increases over the follow-up (8.3%, 33.0%, 60.2%, 80.1%, 83.5%, 84.0%, and 84.5%, respectively) [13]. Considering the various ablation time and volume, the results are more possibly associated with total energy and delivery energy rather than ablation power.

20.2.3 Safety of MWA

MWA is a safe method for PTMC from the available researches. Pain, especially a burning sensation, is common during MWA. Toothache [12, 13], earache [13], labored breathing, and cough [14] also appear during MWA and relieve after MWA. Hematoma [13, 14, 18] and hoarseness [10, 12–14, 16, 18] are major complications. Hoarseness, which is more frequent than hematoma, is always transient and disappears within 2–3 months. No other serious complications have been reported, including skin burns, local infection, or damage to vital structures of the neck (esophagus, trachea, spinal accessory nerves, sympathetic ganglion, and phrenic nerves).

The possibility of local recurrence and distant metastasis is low. Two studies have reported LNM. Li et al. [17] have found five lymph node metastatic recurrences during 0.5–3.6 years of follow-up and two PTMC recurrences during 3.0–3.7 years of follow-up among 161 patients after MWA. Totally, 95.8% (161/168) of patients experience no recurrence during 1–5 years of follow-up. Yue et al. [14] have reported one (0.88%) cervical LNM at 26 months after MWA. A new nodule (0.5%) is diagnosed as papillary thyroid cancer by FNA at the 1-month follow-up and treated with secondary ablation [13]. Both supplementary ablation and delayed surgery can be applied to prevent progression without increasing mortality risk.

20.2.4 MWA Compared with RFA, LA

A meta-analysis [25, 27] shows a higher proportion of PTMC disappear after RFA than that after MWA and LA, and significant between-study heterogeneity in all ablation modalities. RFA, MWA, and LA reduce nodule volume significantly. RFA achieves the highest VRR (99.3%), followed by MWA (95.3%) and LA (88.6%) [27]. MWA achieves a higher pooled standard mean difference of tumor volume than RFA and LA [25]. However, no significant differences are found in the proportion of disappeared nodules, VRR, and standard mean difference of tumor volume.

The 16-gauge or 17-gauge antenna is often applied in MWA, 21-gauge antenna in LA, and 18-gauge antenna in RFA [28]. The size of antenna may correspond to complications. However, no statistical differences are found in overall and major complications caused by three modalities [27]. The complications are rare in all ablation modalities. The pooled proportions of overall complications are 0.6%, 5.6%, and 2.6% in LA, MWA, and RFA, and those of major complications are 0%, 2.5%, and 0%, respectively [27]. Although LA has the lowest complication rate, no statistical significance is observed. MWA is mainly complicated with voice hoarseness and bleeding, RFA with voice hoarseness and hypothyroidism (occasionally with pain, bleeding and skin burns), and LA with hypothyroidism and pain [25].

The recurrence rate after RFA (0.01%) is lower than those after MWA (0.85%) and LA (1.87%), but without statistical differences [25]. No distant metastasis occurs during the follow-up period in all studies.

20.2.5 MWA Compared with Surgery

There is no statistically significant difference in recurrence, LNM, and disease-free survival between surgery and MWA for PTMC. It is worth noting that 4.2% (7/168) and 4.2% (6/143) of patients developed LNM and PTMC recurrence in MWA and surgery groups, respectively, with similar recurrence rates in the neck. The mean disease-free survival is 1702 days in MWA group compared with 2001 days in surgery group. No statistically significant difference lies in the 5-year disease-free survival between MWA group (95.8%) and surgery group (95.5%) [17].

More complications are found in surgery group than in MWA group. Complication rates of surgery and MWA are 43.5% (including dysphagia, transient and permanent hoarseness, transient hypoparathyroidism, hematoma, postoperative hyperthyroidism, and transient and permanent hypothyroidism) and 4.3% (transient hoarseness), respectively [16]. On the other side, the mean length of stay, cost, mean blood loss, surgical incision number, operative time, and complication incidence in MWA group are less than those in surgery group [15, 16]. The quality of life and physical function after MWA are better than that after surgery. Meanwhile, WMA shows advantages of stress response. The stress response of patients in surgery group is stronger than that in MWA group, as shown by their higher levels of C-reaction protein, interleukin-6, and tumor necrosis factor-α at 24 h after operation [15].

All patients in surgery group receive thyroid hormone replacement to maintain euthyroid function or suppress serum thyrotropin to reduce the risk of recurrence. There is no consensus about whether patients undergoing MWA should receive thyrotropin suppression. In some cases, levothyroxine is given after MWA [10–12]. A meta-analysis [25] shows insignificant heterogeneity in recurrence rate between studies about thyrotropin suppression. So far, the efficacy of thyrotropin suppression for PTMC patients after MWA has been seldom studied.

20.3 T1bN0M0 PTC

The efficacy and safety of thermal ablation in the treatment of T1bN0M0 PTC are equivalent to T1a. A favorable efficacy and local tumor control of RFA as an initial treatment of selected patients with T1N0M0 PTC were demonstrated. Cao et al. [29] conducted a multi-center retrospective study to compare the therapeutic effects of MWA and RFA in the treatment of T1bN0M0 PTC. During the average follow-up period of 24.9 months, 61.6% of the tumors disappeared completely. In total, the LNM rate was 0.6%, the new tumor rate was 1.2%, the total complication rate was 5.2%, and none of the complications were life-threatening. There was no significant difference in tumor disappearance and complication rate between the two groups. Both MWA and RFA are considered to be treatment modalities for T1N0M0 PTC, with MWA possibly being more advantageous in the treatment of larger nodules and thorough treatment. Wang et al. [30] compared the two treatment methods for VRR 2 years after T1bN0M0 PTC and discovered that the "tumor volume" of the MWA group was greater than that of the RFA group in the short term after treatment, but after a long-term follow-up, both subgroups showed good VRR, and the difference was not statistically significant ($P > 0.05$). The difference in the short-term increase of the "tumor volume" of the ablation zone is primarily due to the different ablation principles. At the last follow-up point, the VRR was 93.47%, and the disease progress rate was 2.8%. For newly observed or recurrent tumors, all patients received secondary TA, while patients with lymph node metastases mostly undergo open surgery.

The efficacy of MWA and surgery through propensity score matching was compared [31]. After 2 years of follow-up, the disease progression rates of MWA and surgical treatment of T1a PTC were 3.4% and 3.8%, respectively ($P = 0.89$), and the disease progression rates of T1b PTC were 6.8% and 5.0%, respectively

($P = 0.72$). There was no significant difference between MWA and surgery in the treatment of T1N0M0 PTC, but the tumor disappeared earlier in T1a than in T1b, and the disappearance rate was higher.

Generally, the existing evidence supports that ultrasound-guided thermal ablation for T1aN0M0 and T1bN0M0 PTC has similar efficacy and safety. Thermal ablation is a safe and effective alternative to surgery for the treatment of T1bN0M0 PTC, especially in patients who are ineligible for surgery or refusal to undergo it.

20.4 Recurrent Thyroid Cancer

The standard treatment for locally recurrent thyroid cancer is surgery, but for those patients who have undergone neck dissection, reoperation may be a challenge, which makes patients at risk of higher incidence of complications. Thermal ablation is considered as a non-surgical treatment option for locally recurrent thyroid cancer.

Many studies have proved the effectiveness and safety of thermal ablation in the treatment of local recurrent PTC. Yue et al. [32] included 17 patients with 23 recurrent lesions for MWA treatment. The mean VRR was 47 ± 12%, 70 ± 33%, and 91 ± 14% at the 3, 6, and 18 months follow-up visit, respectively (all $P < 0.05$). During follow-up, except for one patient who had a new recurrent tumor (≤5 mm) in the lateral aspect of the neck (level IV), no patient had a recurrence at the treatment site. Therefore, thermal ablation is an acceptable treatment for local recurrent thyroid cancer, which is used to treat patients who are not suitable for surgery or refuse surgery.

20.5 Metastatic Lymph Nodes

The American Thyroid Association guidelines recommend PTC treatment as the surgical removal of choice for the neck LNM but given the risk of reoperation. Postoperative fibrosis leads to tissue adhesion and anatomical changes, thereby increasing the risk of complications [33]. Reoperation also presents technical challenges because small and medium-sized lymph node metastases are difficult to be identified during surgery. Therefore, it is of great significance to find a minimally invasive technique to replace surgical resection for LNM.

Teng et al. [34] included 11 patients in total with 24 cervical lymph nodes (LNs) diagnosed with CMLN from PTC underwent MWA at a power of 20 W. During the mean follow-up period of 32 months (range 18–42 months), the mean Tg was significantly decreased and all LNs disappeared. The mean VRR of the LNs was 38.43 ± 20.29%, 75.20 ± 17.20%, 95.45 ± 8.60%, 99.34 ± 2.85%, and 100% in 1, 3, 6, 12, and 18 months after MWA, respectively. No new recurrent lesions or distant metastases were detected. Yet there are some details the authors highlight in MWA treatment regarding multiple lesions, smaller and deeper LNs should be ablated first and the procedure of hydrodissection for small LNs should be accurate to inject the fluid around the LNs. A meta-analysis shows that the average VRR of CLNM treated by thermal ablation is 91.28%, the complete disappearance rate is 63.3%, the recurrence rate is 7.8%, and the incidence of major complications is 0.3%, all of which are non-life-threatening voice changes [35]. Thermal ablation is an effective and safe alternative treatment for PTC metastatic lymph nodes.

However, there are also some controversial documents. The results of Zhang et al. [36] showed that the VRR was 88.4% at the last follow-up, the incidence of major complications was 4.0%, and the major complication rate after LNM ablation in the central region was 12.0%. Among the 20 patients with nerve injury, 19 cases were located in the central area, 1 case was located in the superior lateral area of the clavicle, the other 4 cases had skin burns, and 1 case had hematoma. Almost all the serious complications came from the central area. Further research is needed on the control of ablation complications of LNM in the central region, but ultrasonography-guided thermal ablation is still a promising treatment method, especially for patients with high surgical risk or refusing cooperation.

20.6 Conclusion

In conclusion, MWA is effective and safe in the treatment for selected patients with low-risk PTC, recurrent PTC, and metastatic lymph node as an alternative option for clinicians and patients. High risk features should be ruled out before MWA for patients with PTMC, such as younger age, multifocality, and capsular invasion, LNM, etc. Informed consent of patients should be completed prior to any non-surgical treatment. Regular follow-up to identify any LNM and tumor residual after thermal ablation is also needed. The curative effects of various ablation modalities deserve further exploration.

References

1. Deng Y, Li H, Wang M, Li N, Tian T, Wu Y, Xu P, Yang S, Zhai Z, Zhou L, et al. Global burden of thyroid cancer from 1990 to 2017. JAMA Netw Open. 2020;3(6):e208759.
2. Lim H, Devesa SS, Sosa JA, Check D, Kitahara CM. Trends in thyroid cancer incidence and mortality in the United States, 1974-2013. JAMA. 2017;317(13):1338–48.
3. Ito Y, Miyauchi A, Inoue H, Fukushima M, Kihara M, Higashiyama T, Tomoda C, Takamura Y, Kobayashi K, Miya A. An observational trial for papillary thyroid microcarcinoma in Japanese patients. World J Surg. 2010;34(1):28–35.
4. Oh HS, Ha J, Kim HI, Kim TH, Kim WG, Lim DJ, Kim TY, Kim SW, Kim WB, Shong YK, et al. Active surveillance of low-risk papillary thyroid microcarcinoma: a multi-center cohort study in Korea. Thyroid. 2018;28(12):1587–94.
5. Jeon MJ, Kim WG, Kwon H, Kim M, Park S, Oh HS, Han M, Sung TY, Chung KW, Hong SJ, et al. Clinical outcomes after delayed thyroid surgery in patients with papillary thyroid microcarcinoma. Eur J Endocrinol. 2017;177(1):25–31.
6. Cho SJ, Suh CH, Baek JH, Chung SR, Choi YJ, Chung KW, Shong YK, Lee JH. Active surveillance for small papillary thyroid cancer: a systematic review and meta-analysis. Thyroid. 2019;29(10):1399–408.
7. Simon CJ, Dupuy DE, Mayo-Smith WW. Microwave ablation: principles and applications. Radiographics. 2005;25(Suppl 1):S69–83.
8. Ahmed M, Brace CL, Lee FT Jr, Goldberg SN. Principles of and advances in percutaneous ablation. Radiology. 2011;258(2):351–69.
9. Kim C. Understanding the nuances of microwave ablation for more accurate post-treatment assessment. Future Oncol. 2018;14(17):1755–64.
10. Yue W, Wang S, Yu S, Wang B. Ultrasound-guided percutaneous microwave ablation of solitary T1N0M0 papillary thyroid microcarcinoma: initial experience. Int J Hyperthermia. 2014;30(2):150–7.
11. Teng D, Li W, Du J, Wang H, Yang D, Wu X. Effects of microwave ablation on papillary thyroid microcarcinoma: a five-year follow-up report. Thyroid. 2020;30(12):1752–8.
12. Teng D, Sui G, Liu C, Wang Y, Xia Y, Wang H. Long-term efficacy of ultrasound-guided low power microwave ablation for the treatment of primary papillary thyroid microcarcinoma: a 3-year follow-up study. J Cancer Res Clin Oncol. 2018;144(4):771–9.
13. Teng DK, Li HQ, Sui GQ, Lin YQ, Luo Q, Fu P, Du JR, Jin CX, Wang H. Preliminary report of microwave ablation for the primary papillary thyroid microcarcinoma: a large-cohort of 185 patients feasibility study. Endocrine. 2019;64(1):109–17.
14. Yue WW, Qi L, Wang DD, Yu SJ, Wang XJ, Xu HX, Wang SR. US-guided microwave ablation of low-risk papillary thyroid microcarcinoma: longer-term results of a prospective study. J Clin Endocrinol Metab. 2020;105(6):dgaa128.
15. Xu B, Zhou NM, Cao WT, Gu SY. Comparative study on operative trauma between microwave ablation and surgical treatment for papillary thyroid microcarcinoma. World J Clin Cases. 2018;6(15):936–43.
16. Li J, Liu Y, Liu J, Qian L. Ultrasound-guided percutaneous microwave ablation versus surgery for papillary thyroid microcarcinoma. Int J Hyperthermia. 2018;34(5):653–9.
17. Li J, Liu Y, Liu J, Yang P, Hu X, Qian L. A comparative study of short-term efficacy and safety for thyroid micropapillary carcinoma patients after microwave ablation or surgery. Int J Hyperthermia. 2019;36(1):640–6.
18. Zhou W, Ni X, Xu S, Zhang L, Chen Y, Zhan W. Ultrasound-guided laser ablation versus microwave ablation for patients with unifocal papillary thyroid microcarcinoma: a retrospective study. Lasers Surg Med. 2020;52(9):855–62.
19. Cui T, Jin C, Jiao D, Teng D, Sui G. Safety and efficacy of microwave ablation for benign thyroid nodules and papillary thyroid microcarcinomas: a systematic review and meta-analysis. Eur J Radiol. 2019;118:58–64.
20. Chen M, Xu SH, Xu Y, Wang YL, Chu XQ, Liu C. Safety and ultrasonographic morphologic analysis of ultrasound-guided percutaneous microwave ablation on benign nonfunctioning thyroid nodules. Int J Endocrinol Metab. 2019;39(5):294–7, 301.
21. Yue W, Wang S, Wang B, Xu Q, Yu S, Yonglin Z, Wang X. Ultrasound guided percutaneous microwave ablation of benign thyroid nodules: safety and imaging follow-up in 222 patients. Eur J Radiol. 2013;82(1):e11–6.

22. Liu YJ, Qian LX, Liu D, Zhao JF. Ultrasound-guided microwave ablation in the treatment of benign thyroid nodules in 435 patients. Exp Biol Med (Maywood). 2017;242(15):1515–23.
23. Zhi X, Zhao N, Liu Y, Liu JB, Teng C, Qian L. Microwave ablation compared to thyroidectomy to treat benign thyroid nodules. Int J Hyperthermia. 2018;34(5):644–52.
24. Heck K, Happel C, Grunwald F, Korkusuz H. Percutaneous microwave ablation of thyroid nodules: effects on thyroid function and antibodies. Int J Hyperthermia. 2015;31(5):560–7.
25. Tong M, Li S, Li Y, Li Y, Feng Y, Che Y. Efficacy and safety of radiofrequency, microwave and laser ablation for treating papillary thyroid microcarcinoma: a systematic review and meta-analysis. Int J Hyperthermia. 2019;36(1):1278–86.
26. Bernardi S, Giudici F, Cesareo R, Antonelli G, Cavallaro M, Deandrea M, Giusti M, Mormile A, Negro R, Palermo A, et al. Five-year results of radiofrequency and laser ablation of benign thyroid nodules: a multicenter study from the Italian Minimally Invasive Treatments of the Thyroid Group. Thyroid. 2020;30(12):1759–70.
27. Choi Y, Jung SL. Efficacy and safety of thermal ablation techniques for the treatment of primary papillary thyroid microcarcinoma: a systematic review and meta-analysis. Thyroid. 2020;30(5):720–31.
28. Chen J, Cao J, Qiu F, Huang P. The efficacy and the safety of ultrasound-guided ablation therapy for treating papillary thyroid microcarcinoma. J Cancer. 2019;10(21):5272–82.
29. Cao XJ, Liu J, Zhu YL, Qi L, Liu G, Wang HL, Wang ZH, Zhou Y, He JF, Guo JQ, et al. Efficacy and safety of thermal ablation for solitary T1bN0M0 papillary thyroid carcinoma: a multicenter study. J Clin Endocrinol Metab. 2021;106(2):e573–81.
30. Wang MH, Liu X, Wang Q, Zhang HW. Safety and efficacy of ultrasound-guided thermal ablation in treating T1aN0M0 and T1bN0M0 papillary thyroid carcinoma: a meta-analysis. Front Endocrinol (Lausanne). 2022;13:952113.
31. Wei Y, Niu WQ, Zhao ZL, Wu J, Peng LL, Li Y, Yu MA. Microwave ablation versus surgical resection for solitary T1N0M0 papillary thyroid carcinoma. Radiology. 2022;304(3):704–13.
32. Yue W, Chen L, Wang S, Yu S. Locoregional control of recurrent papillary thyroid carcinoma by ultrasound-guided percutaneous microwave ablation: a prospective study. Int J Hyperthermia. 2015;31(4):403–8.
33. Luster M, Aktolun C, Amendoeira I, Barczynski M, Bible KC, Duntas LH, Elisei R, Handkiewicz-Junak D, Hoffmann M, Jarzab B, et al. European perspective on 2015 American Thyroid Association management guidelines for adult patients with thyroid nodules and differentiated thyroid cancer: proceedings of an interactive international symposium. Thyroid. 2019;29(1):7–26.
34. Teng D, Ding L, Wang Y, Liu C, Xia Y, Wang H. Safety and efficiency of ultrasound-guided low power microwave ablation in the treatment of cervical metastatic lymph node from papillary thyroid carcinoma: a mean of 32 months follow-up study. Endocrine. 2018;62(3):648–54.
35. Tang W, Tang X, Jiang D, Zhang X, Wang R, Niu X, Zang Y, Zhang M, Wang X, Zhao C. Safety and efficacy of thermal ablation for cervical metastatic lymph nodes in papillary thyroid carcinoma: a systematic review and meta-analysis. Front Endocrinol (Lausanne). 2022;13:967044.
36. Zhang X, Ni T, Zhang W. Ultrasonography-guided thermal ablation for cervical lymph node metastasis of recurrent papillary thyroid carcinoma: is it superior to surgical resection? Front Endocrinol (Lausanne). 2022;13:907195.

Side Effects and Complications in Thyroid Radiofrequency Ablation

21

Roberto Novizio and Roberto Valcavi

21.1 Introduction

Thyroid radiofrequency ablation is an effective, well-tolerated, and safe therapeutic strategy for the treatment of thyroid nodules with low complication rate when performed by skilled operators [1]. Traditionally, complications have been divided into "major complications" and "minor complications.. According to the Society of Interventional Radiology, major complications are defined as ones that, if left untreated, might threaten the patient's life, lead to substantial morbidity or disability, or result in a lengthened hospital stay. All other complications are considered minor [2]. Focusing on radiofrequency ablation of benign thyroid nodules, the overall complication rate is less than 5%, while the major complication rate is less than 2%. Complication rates are very different when it comes to malignant thyroid nodules, reaching an overall frequency of about 10%, with 7% of major complications. In different studies, different complication rates (percentages) are reported, probably due to differences in techniques used, instruments, but also different experiences of the operators and volumes of procedures performed [3–5]. Moreover, the procedure setting, under local anesthesia in ambulatory setting or under general anesthesia in operating room, can impact side effects and complications rates.

For practicality reasons, a different type of sorting can be adopted, based on the timing of onset of the complication, in relation to the intervention. Complications are sorted out in three categories: intra-operative complications, immediate post-operative complications, and periprocedural/delayed complications [6]. Intra-operative side effects occur during the procedure such as intense pain, intranodular or pericapsular bleeding, vasovagal reaction, and intense cough. Immediate post-operative side effects occur 24–48 h after the procedure such as swelling, cutaneous burn, transient laryngeal dysfunction, permanent laryngeal dysfunction, brachial plexus injury, and Horner's syndrome. Periprocedural side effects occur within 30 days after the procedure, while delayed side effects such as bruise, fever, nodule rupture, and nodule colliquation occur after 30 days. This way of classifying side effects enhances the signs and symptoms to focus on during different phases of patient recruitment, procedure execution, and follow-up, allowing the better tailoring of countermeasures to prevent them (Fig. 21.1).

In this study, we explore the various intra-operative complications, immediate post-operative complications, and periprocedural/delayed complications associated with thyroid RFA, along with potential management strategies.

R. Novizio (✉)
Volunteer Consultant Endocrinologist, A. Cardarelli Hospital, Naples, Italy

R. Valcavi
Department of Endocrinology, The Endocrine & Thyroid Clinic, Reggio Emilia, Italy

R. Valcavi et al. (eds.), *Thyroid Ablation*, https://doi.org/10.1007/978-3-031-88229-6_21

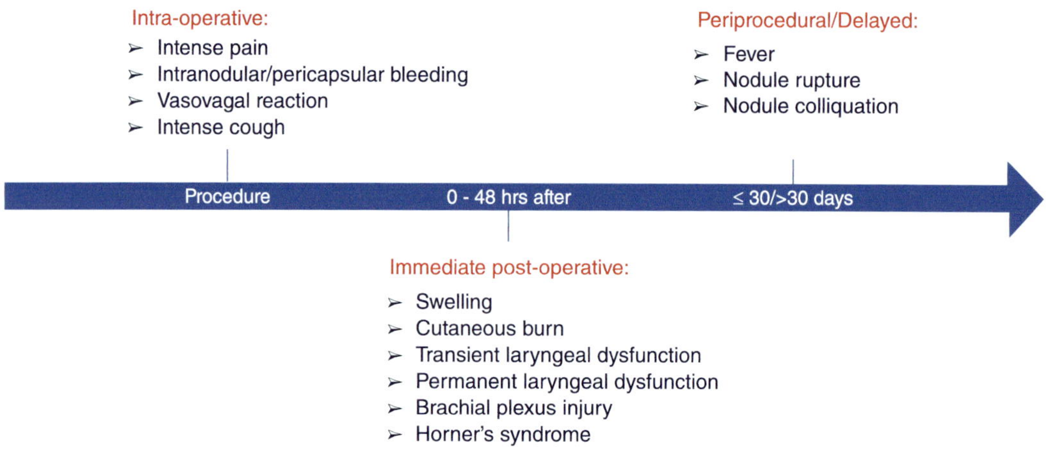

Fig. 21.1 Temporal sorting or possible side effects and complications during and after thyroid thermal ablation

21.2 Side Effects

21.2.1 Intra-operative

Side effects such as intense pain, intranodular or pericapsular bleeding, vasovagal reaction, and intense cough occur during the procedure.

21.2.1.1 Intense Pain

Pain is the most common complaint during procedures. Incidence rates ranges from 2 to 17.5%. To minimize the discomfort, local anesthesia with lidocaine 2% is generally performed in ambulatory setting. Since sensory nerves are present in the thyroid capsule but not inside the gland, pericapsular anesthesia is sufficient. Lidocaine has a rapid action onset, allowing for an almost immediate starting of the procedure. However, it is also associated with a rapid dissolution of the effect. A subsequent infiltration with ropivacaine diluted with physiological solution can help to get a prolonged anesthetic effect.

Pain is generally referred from the patient at the entrance point of the needle or diffusely in the anterior part of the neck. Occasionally, pain can radiate around the neck, spreading to gonial angle, ear, shoulder, or teeth. While almost all patients experience mild-to-moderate pain, few patients suffer intense intra-operative pain that can require medications such as intravenous paracetamol and methylprednisolone, or even the interruption of the procedure [4].

Pain and intense pain rates during procedure decrease to 0% if the procedure is performed in operating room setting under general anesthesia [7]. This advantage is discussed since some authors consider pain as an early detector of complications.

21.2.1.2 Intranodular or Pericapsular Bleeding

The incidence of intranodular bleeding is about 7.5%, while 2.5% for pericapsular bleeding. In general, bleeding can be detected by ultrasound as a rapidly expanding hypoechoic or anechoic signal. Intranodular bleeding generally occurs during needle insertion, possibly with an enlargement of the target nodule. Pericapsular bleeding tends to be evident at the end of the procedure as a thin anechoic layer, probably due to tissue needle-related stress. Most of the time hemorrhages are asymptomatic. Hematomas can be prevented by stopping medications associated with hemorrhage risk for one or more days based on the type of drugs before RFA. Mild pressure can help in limiting the progression of pericapsular bleeding, while immediate RF ablation after needle insertion into the nodule prevents and reduces the intranodular bleeding by vessel coagulation. Hematoma completely disappears after 1 or 2 weeks. Although there are no cases described in literature of life-threatening hemorrhages, it is necessary to evaluate progression of the hematoma during and after procedure, since massive forms can cause airway obstruction requiring emergency surgery [8].

21.2.1.3 Vasovagal Reaction

Vagus nerve stimulation can trigger the activation of parasympathetic nervous system, with cardiovascular symptoms such as bradycardia or hypotension, bronchospasm, vomiting, and defecation. Vasovagal reaction occurs in about 2% of procedures, but most of the time symptoms are mild. These symptoms can last up to 15 min and usually the recovery is spontaneous. It is important to stop the procedure until the complete recovery. This reaction is associated with nodule nearby the vascular bundle of the neck since vagus nerve is usually located between the common carotid artery and internal jugular vein but may also be located adjacent to the thyroid gland [9]. Anesthesiologic assistance with atropine administration, in operating room setting, could be precious for severe reactions [4, 8].

21.2.1.4 Intense Cough

Troublesome cough has been reported in up to 5% of cases treated in ambulatory setting. It can last up to 1 minute. It does not seem to be associated with any injury to trachea or larynx, but the simple movement of the needle into the thyroid gland seems to tickle cough reflex. Powering off and repositioning of the needle can favor a faster recovery [4, 7, 8].

21.2.2 Immediate Post-operative

Side effects such as swelling, cutaneous burn, transient laryngeal dysfunction, permanent laryngeal dysfunction, brachial plexus injury, and Horner's syndrome occur 24–48 h after the procedure.

21.2.2.1 Swelling

Due to difficulties in quantifying it, there is inconsistency in the reported incidence of swelling during or after RFA in different studies. Moderate swelling is quite common and can be detected in up to 10% of cases in ambulatory setting [7]. A minimal amount of transient edema surrounding thyroid parenchyma immediately after RFA is not evitable. Most of the time, no symptoms occur, and no treatment is needed, so that it can even be not reported as a side effect unless pressure symptoms take place. Airways are not affected. Administering intravenous methylprednisolone reduces swelling rate to 0.95%. In our center, the protocol is administering intravenous methylprednisolone 40 mg in bolus during the procedure, with anesthesiologic assistance. Cases of post-ablation painful swelling have been reported. This complication disappeared completely in 12 days with oral anti-inflammatory treatment [9].

21.2.2.2 Cutaneous Burn

Cutaneous burn is damage to the skin caused by heat. Few cases of first-grade skin burn are described in literature, presenting with skin redness and mild pain. One case of first-degree skin burn occurred in our center (Fig. 21.2). Patient recovered in few days without specific treatment. Another case of higher-grade post-RFA skin burn is described, caused by a use of an active tip needle next to the skin. The patient recovered in one month, after topical gentamicin sulfate hyaluronic acid on the skin burn for the first week, activated charcoal cloth with silver for the second week, and a collagen wound dressing for another

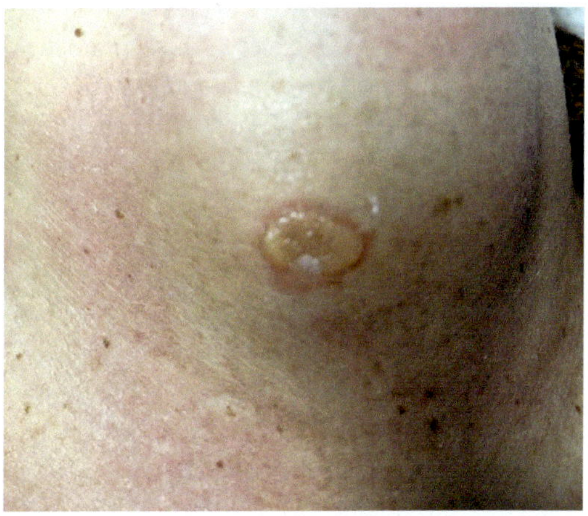

Fig. 21.2 Radiofrequency ablation-induced first-degree skin burn, 24 h after the treatment

2 weeks after surgical debridement of the wound. The skin burn recovered 1 month later [10, 11].

In thyroid RF ablation, only skin burn at the electrode puncture site has been reported, but another type of skin burn has been observed in liver RF ablation, at the sites of pad attachment. In thyroid RF ablation, the risk of burns at the pad attachment site is relatively low because RF energy in the thyroid is lower (30–120 W) than in the liver.

21.2.2.3 Transient and Permanent Laryngeal Dysfunction

Laryngeal dysfunction is a major complication, scaring both for the patient and the physician. Impairment of the recurrent laryngeal nerve due to heating entails paralysis of all intrinsic muscles of the larynx, except for cricothyroid muscles (innervated by the superior laryngeal nerve). The proposed mechanisms of nerve dysfunction include RFA-induced thermal injury of the recurrent laryngeal nerve, lidocaine injection nearby the nerve, stretching of the nerve over a hematoma, post-hemorrhage inflammation, and fibrosis around the nerve. Voice changes and hoarseness can be found during the procedure or immediately after ablation. Most of time voice change is transient, affecting about 5% of patients in ambulatory setting. Most patients recover spontaneously after few months without special treatments. Laryngoscopic evaluation can help in objectifying the vocal cord paralysis. Phoniatric re-education and prednisone cycles may be useful in accelerating the recovery. An accurate evaluation of neck anatomy and nodule position is paramount before RFA. Generally, recurrent laryngeal nerve is located in the tracheoesophageal groove, while the vagus nerve is located between the carotid artery and internal jugular vein. Maintaining at least 3 mm of distance between the tip of the electrode needle and the "dangerous triangle" helps in avoiding injuries. Moreover, when treating ablation units nearby the nerve is necessary, hydrodissection between the nodule and dangerous triangle is useful in protecting the nodule [1]. Hydrodissection consists in using dextrose 5% at 5 °C injected in between the danger zone and ablating target area. Saline is not recommended as it contains ions and is not electrically inert. In our center, we perform a first infusion of dextrose 5% before treating the in-danger target area and, when needed, a second infusion after ablation is performed ("*rescue*" hydrodissection). Encouraging the patient to communicate throughout the procedure is useful to check out in case danger to recurrent laryngeal nerve. Operating room management of thyroid RFA decreased the incidence of laryngeal dysfunction, probably due to general sedation that allows physician to operate without movement interferences precisely targeting the ablating area. However, it makes trickier to check patient's voice during procedure [7].

21.2.2.4 Brachial Plexus Injury

Very few cases have been reported. The brachial plexus provides nerve supply to the skin and muscles of the arms. Its lancing can cause numbness and decreased sensation in fingers. Keeping the electrode in thyroid gland during ablation, respecting the trans-isthmic approach and the retracting back moving shoot techniques minimize this risk [12]. Spinal accessory nerve (SAN) injury has been described, with patient complaining about limitation of abduction of the shoulder joint or drooping of the shoulder. In described cases, patients spontaneously recovered after few months.

21.2.2.5 Horner's Syndrome

Horner's syndrome is characterized by damage to the cervical sympathetic nervous trunk system, which can no longer counterbalance the action of the parasympathetic. Prevailing of parasympathetic nervous system entails enophthalmos, ptosis, miosis, and anhidrosis of the face. The cause is the damage of the middle cervical sympathetic ganglion (mCSG), located bilaterally at the inferior third of the thyroid gland, laterally to the common carotid artery, often wrongly identified as a lymph node at US examination. In cases described, Horner's syndrome occurs immediately after ablation, probably due to heating damage of the mCSG. One case of Horner's syndrome occurred in our center. Patient recovered in 1 month after a course of steroids treatment.

21.2.3 Periprocedural/Delayed

Periprocedural side effects occur within 30 days after the procedure, while delayed side effects such as bruise, fever, nodule rupture, and nodule colliquation occur after 30 days.

21.2.3.1 Bruise

Skin bruising in the electrode insertion area may appear 3–5 days after the procedure and persist up to 5 weeks. Immediate compression and ice pack use after RFA reduced this side effect from 5 to 1.59% of patients in our center.

21.2.3.2 Fever

Fever can occur after thyroid RFA in about 5–10% of cases. No precise cause has been identified. Over-the-counter medications are sufficient in treating the rising in temperature, not requiring any additional therapy. Almost all the time, the fever regressed spontaneously within 3 days post-RFA. If rising in temperature persist, blood exams and imaging test (US, CT scan, MRI) are suggested.

21.2.3.3 Nodule Rupture

Nodule rupture is a quite rare complication. During thyroid RFA, the RF needle can disrupt the thyroid capsule and thyroid nodule capsule, generating a leakage of thyroid material into the neck muscle fascia (Fig. 21.3). This spill does not occur immediately after RFA but requires 1–5 months to appear and give symptoms. A red and painful lump arises when the content of the nodule has spread through the muscle plan to the subcutaneous tissue between skin and thyroid gland. Patients report sudden neck swelling and pain at the RFA site [8, 13]. Even if nodule rupture is often considered as a "major complication," it heals spontaneously in 2–4 months. However, patients can complain a lot about pain and compressive and cosmetic symptoms. To avoid nodule rupture, few strategies have been proposed. When moving backward the needle performing RFA, it is important not heat up the needle's entry point into the nodule or the thyroid. In fact, when immersed in ablating tissue, it is not easy to perfectly see the tip of the RF needle. When going back, approaching the nodule capsule at the entrance of the needle, the tip of the needle can be not sufficiently good visualized at ultrasound, heating and destroying the capsule, creating a bridge. Then, when the nodule physiologically liquefies after RFA, the liquid goes through the bridge, spreading to surrounding tissues. To avoid this complication, it can be useful to maintain a safety space of 2–4 mm form the needle entry point through capsule and the tip of the needle when active, to be sure to not interrupt the barrier. Other proposed mechanism of nodule rupture may be delayed bleeding caused by micro-vessel leakage within the nodule. Sonography and/or computed tomography (CT) could help diagnose this complication, which is visualized as the breakdown of the thyroid capsule and the formation of a new mass located between intra- and extra-thyroidal lesions at the RF site [4]. In literature, one case requiring

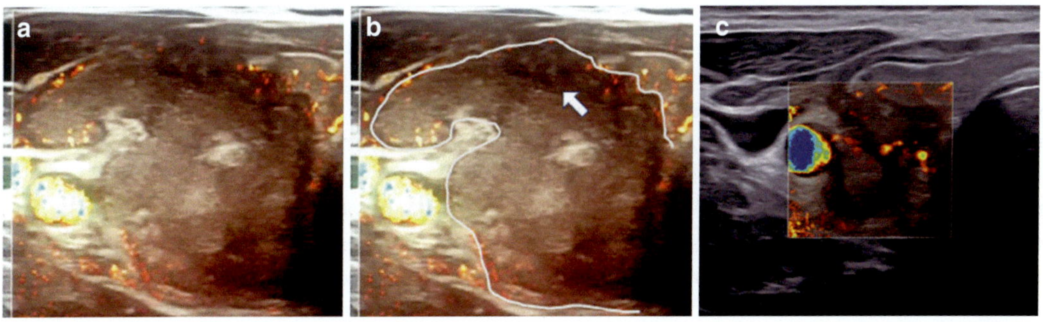

Fig. 21.3 (**a**, **b**) Thyroid capsule disruption indicated by the arrow in the image **b**, leakage of thyroid material through the muscle plan to the subcutaneous tissue between skin and thyroid gland. (**c**) Improvement of leakage of thyroid material into the neck after 3 months from drainage

surgery for cellulitis and anterior neck and abscess formation is described, while three patients ultimately underwent incision and drainage due to worsening clinical signs [13]. No specific nodule characteristics were predictive of nodule rupture; however, bigger size nodules requiring a longer ablating time with higher power can be at risk. In our center, nodule rupture occurred in 1 patient who underwent RFA in ambulatory setting, while no patient who underwent RFA in operating room setting have had nodule rupture, probably due to general sedation that allows physician to operate without movement interferences, then better visualizing the active tip in the delicate phases of the intervention. Oral methylprednisolone 16 mg/day course after RFA for 15–25 days with a stepdown approach, plus lansoprazole 30 mg/day during oral methylprednisolone administration reduces the incidence of this side effect. There is no established management protocol for nodule rupture. Patients should be managed conservatively, including over-the-counter anti-inflammatory and analgesics drugs. Antibiotics can be used if necessary. The drainage of melted tissue can aid in accelerating recovery and provide immediate relief for patients from pain and skin tension caused by swelling. Following drainage, the administration of broad-spectrum antibiotics can decrease the likelihood of infection or abscess formation. While some authors caution against invasive procedures such as drainage or aspiration due to potential infection risks, skilled operators performing these procedures in sterile conditions can minimize such risks.

21.2.3.4 Nodule Colliquation

Colliquation or pseudocystic transformation can occur few weeks after the procedure. Patients complain about pain and sudden swelling, similarly to nodule rupture. Differently from nodule rupture, the colliquated material stays into the nodule capsule, generating in case compressive or cosmetic symptoms. Oral methylprednisolone 16 mg/day course after RFA for 15–25 days with a stepdown approach, plus lansoprazole 30 mg/day during oral methylprednisolone administration reduces the incidence of this side effect. US could be useful for diagnosing pseudocystic transformation, but we should note that the normal sonographic appearance of thyroid nodules post-PFA, such as marked hypoechogenicity, heterogeneity, and irregular margins, may be misleading [7, 8, 12]. No specific nodule characteristics were predictive of nodule rupture; however, bigger size nodules requiring a longer ablating time with higher power can be at risk. Certain authors consider nodule rupture as a further complication of nodule colliquation, occurring when there is a disruption in the capsule of a colliquated nodule.

21.2.3.5 Thyroid Dysfunction

No clear data exist between RF ablation and post-intervention hypothyroidism. Very rarely, in patients with pre-treatment high level of serum antithyroid peroxidase antibody (anti-TPOAb), transient subclinical hypothyroidism can occur.

No clear data exist between RF ablation and post-intervention hyperthyroidism as well. In our experience, 1 month after ablation, clinical overt hyperthyroidism developed in two patients with negative TPOAb and TgAb levels. It was associated with a transient TRAb peak (68 and 82 U/L at month 1, respectively) without any change in TPOAb and TgAb levels. The first hyperthyroid patient received methimazole (5–10 mg/day) therapy for 1 year; after methimazole withdrawal, TSH, thyroid hormone, and TRAb levels remained normal during the 3-year follow-up period. The second hyperthyroid patient received radioiodine therapy, became hypothyroid at 6 months, and was put on thyroxine replacement therapy. There have been only a few reported cases on this matter [14].

21.2.4 Other

There are other theoretical possible complications of RF ablation that have not previously been reported. For example, esophageal injury, a life-threatening complication, may be prevented by maintaining a safety margin between the esophagus and the tip of the RF electrode. In addition, patients should be asked to swallow cold water during the ablation of a conceptual unit adjacent to the esophagus. Since RF current passes through the heart during thyroid RF ablation, heart attacks and arrhythmias may be possible complications.

21.3 Discussion

Our thorough examination encompasses an array of both minor and major complications that have been reported after undergoing thyroid RFA, as well as their corresponding management strategies. Some of the commonly cited complications include voice changes, pain, swelling, and temporary hoarseness, among others. However, it is essential to note that these complications are generally mild and usually resolve within a few weeks after the procedure (Table 21.1).

In terms of the potential management of complications, several measures may be employed to alleviate any discomfort or side effects, such as pain medications, ice packs, and voice rest. In rare cases, more significant complications, such as infection or bleeding, may require further medical intervention.

Despite the possibility of complications, RFA has been demonstrated in numerous studies to be a safe and effective treatment option for thyroid nodules, with excellent long-term results. RFA has a high success rate in reducing nodule size,

Table 21.1 Summary of side effects and complications of thyroid RFA

Side effect/complication	Incidence	Signs or symptoms	Prevention
Intra-operative			
Intense pain	2–17.5%	Localized at the entrance point of the needle or diffusely in the anterior part of the neck. Pain can radiate around the neck	Local anesthesia with lidocaine 2%
Intranodular and Pericapsular bleeding	7.5 and 2.5%	Most of the time hemorrhages are asymptomatic. Rapidly expanding hypoechoic or anechoic signal at ultrasound	Stop medications associated with hemorrhage risk. Immediate ablation soon after needle insertion. Mild pressure after needle removal
Vasovagal reaction	2%	Bradycardia hypotension Bronchospasm vomiting Defecation	Stop the procedure until the complete recovery. Atropine administration could be precious for severe reactions
Intense cough	5%	Intense cough	Powering off and repositioning of the needle
Immediate post-operative			
Swelling	10%	At ultrasound, amount of edema surrounding thyroid parenchyma	Intravenous methylprednisolone during procedure
Cutaneous burn	<1%	Skin redness and mild pain	Ice pack soon after RFA
Laryngeal dysfunction	5%	Voice change and hoarseness	Hydrodissection
Brachial plexus injury	<1%	Numbness and decreased sensation in fingers	Hydrodissection
Horner's syndrome	<1%	Ptosis, miosis, anhidrosis	Hydrodissection
Periprocedural and delayed			
Fever	5–10%	Fever	None
Nodule rupture	<1%	Sudden neck swelling and pain	Not heat up the needle's entry point. Methylprednisolone after RFA
Nodule colliquation	<1%	Sudden neck swelling and pain	Methylprednisolone after RFA

improving thyroid function, and enhancing patient quality of life. Therefore, the benefits of RFA far outweigh the potential risks, making it an ideal treatment option for thyroid nodules. Patients should discuss the potential risks and benefits of RFA with their healthcare provider to determine if this treatment option is appropriate for their individual needs.

References

1. Kim JH, Baek JH, Lim HK, Ahn HS, Baek SM, Choi YJ, et al.; Guideline Committee for the Korean Society of Thyroid Radiology (KSThR) and Korean Society of Radiology. 2017 thyroid radiofrequency ablation guideline: Korean Society of Thyroid Radiology. Korean J Radiol. 2018;19(4):632–655. https://doi.org/10.3348/kjr.2018.19.4.632.
2. Lewis CA, Allen TE, Burke DR, Cardella JF, Citron SJ, Cole PE, Drooz AT, Drucker EA, Haskal ZJ, Martin LG, Van Moore A, Neithamer CD, Oglevie SB, Rholl KS, Roberts AC, Sacks D, Sanchez O, Venbrux A, Bakal CW. Quality improvement guidelines for central venous access. The standards of Practice Committee of the Society of Cardiovascular & Interventional Radiology. J Vasc Interv Radiol. 1997;8(3):475–9.
3. Cesareo R, Palermo A, Pasqualini V, Cianni R, Gaspa G, Manfrini S, et al. Radiofrequency ablation for the management of thyroid nodules: a critical appraisal of the literature. Clin Endocrinol (Oxf). 2017;87(6):639–48. https://doi.org/10.1111/cen.13422.
4. Wang JF, Wu T, Hu KP, Xu W, Zheng BW, Tong G, Yao ZC, Liu B, Ren J. Complications following radiofrequency ablation of benign thyroid nodules: a systematic review. Chin Med J (Engl). 2017;130(11):1361–70. https://doi.org/10.4103/0366-6999.206347.
5. Laeseke PF, Sampson LA, Brace CL, Winter TC 3rd, Fine JP, Lee FT Jr. Unintended thermal injuries from radiofrequency ablation: protection with 5% dextrose in water. AJR Am J Roentgenol. 2006;186(5 Suppl):S249–54. https://doi.org/10.2214/AJR.04.1240.
6. Sacks D, McClenny TE, Cardella JF, Lewis CA. Society of Interventional Radiology clinical practice guidelines. J Vasc Interv Radiol. 2003;14(9 Pt 2):S199–202. https://doi.org/10.1097/01.rvi.0000094584.83406.3e.
7. Valcavi R, Novizio R. Side effects rates comparison in thyroid radiofrequency ablation between ambulatory setting and operating room setting. Thyroid. 2021;31(Suppl. 1):A127.
8. Valcavi R, Tsamatropoulos P. Health-related quality of life after percutaneous radiofrequency ablation of cold, solid, benign thyroid nodules: a 2-year follow-up study in 40 patients. Endocr Pract. 2015;21(8):887–96. https://doi.org/10.4158/EP15676.OR.
9. Aysan E, Idiz UO, Akbulut H, Elmas L. Single-session radiofrequency ablation on benign thyroid nodules: a prospective single center study: radiofrequency ablation on thyroid. Langenbecks Arch Surg. 2016;401(3):357.
10. Bernardi S, Lanzilotti V, Papa G, Panizzo N, Dobrinja C, Fabris B, et al. Full-thickness skin burn caused by radiofrequency ablation of a benign thyroid nodule. Thyroid. 2016;26(1):183–4. https://doi.org/10.1089/thy.2015.0453.
11. Li XL, Xu HX, Lu F, Yue WW, Sun LP, Bo XW, et al. Treatment efficacy and safety of ultrasound-guided percutaneous bipolar radiofrequency ablation for benign thyroid nodules. Br J Radiol. 2016;89(1059):20150858. https://doi.org/10.1259/bjr.20150858.
12. Baek JH, Lee JH, Sung JY, Bae JI, Kim KT, Sim J, et al; Korean Society of Thyroid Radiology. Complications encountered in the treatment of benign thyroid nodules with US-guided radiofrequency ablation: a multicenter study. Radiology. 2012;262(1):335–342. https://doi.org/10.1148/radiol.11110416.
13. Shin JH, Jung SL, Baek JH, Kim JH. Rupture of benign thyroid tumors after radio-frequency ablation. AJNR Am J Neuroradiol. 2011;32(11):2165–9. https://doi.org/10.3174/ajnr.A2661.
14. McAninch EA, Desai K, McCowen KC, Orloff LA. Hyperthyroidism due to Graves disease after radiofrequency ablation. JCEM Case Rep. 2023;1(3):luad056. https://doi.org/10.1210/jcemcr/luad056.

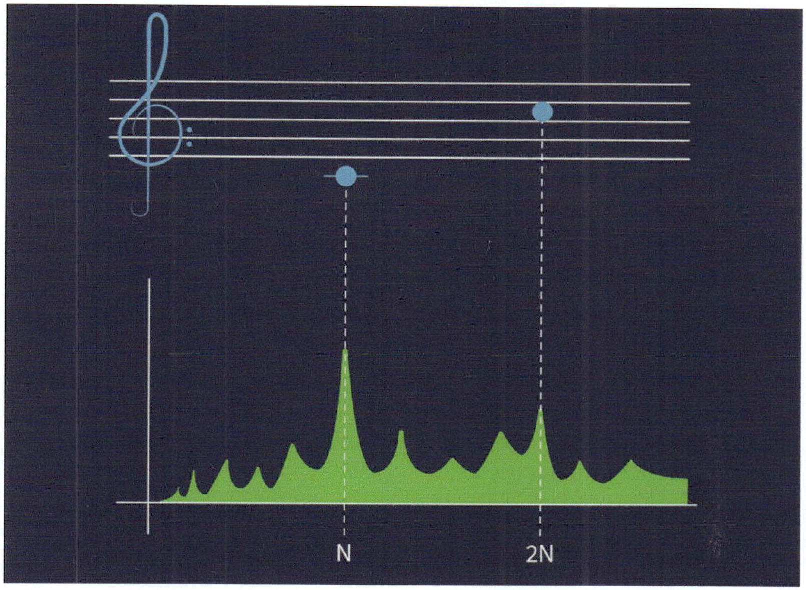

Fig. 22.2 The second harmonic has a frequency that is twice the fundamental frequency and corresponds to a superior octave

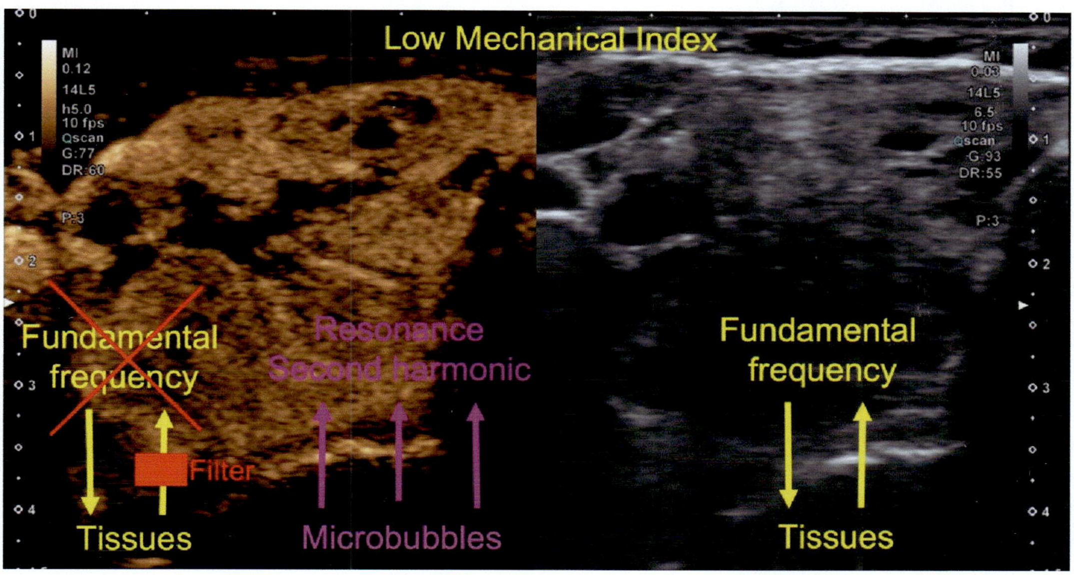

Fig. 22.3 Display on the CEUS mode screen

22.2 Practical Concepts

When intravenous contrast is prepared, a white fluid filled with millions of microbubbles is obtained (Fig. 22.4). To prepare the contrast, the entire contents of a vial must be mixed with 4.8 cc. of a saline solution that is inside a syringe. Inside the vial is a gas (sulfuric hexafluoride) and a lyophilizate of palmitic acid and phospholipids. The vial adapter must be securely connected to the syringe before puncturing the vial to prevent gas from escaping. Shake for 20 seconds until the white lyophilizate is dissolved. Fortunately, technical improvements in ultrasound devices, by adjusting the acoustic power values, allow us to reduce the dose. Before, the full dose was administered, but now half the dose (2.4 cc.) is enough. It is preferable to administer the contrast immediately after it has been mixed but it is also possible to delay the administration by a few minutes, up to an hour, but before administering the contrast must be mixed again slowly.

We administer this contrast intravenously. The nurse assists in placing the intravenous access. To prevent bubbles from breaking, it is better to use a large catheter. The administration must be rapid, continuous and without greatly increasing the pressure inside the syringe. In the end, it is fine to administer 10 cc. of saline to push the contrast.

Ultrasound contrast has only an intravascular distribution. The gas that fills the bubbles (sulfuric hexafluoride) is eliminated by the lungs 11 min later. The bubble stabilizers (phospholipids and palmitic acid) are metabolized by the liver.

Although adverse reactions to the contrast have been described, these are very rare [8–12].

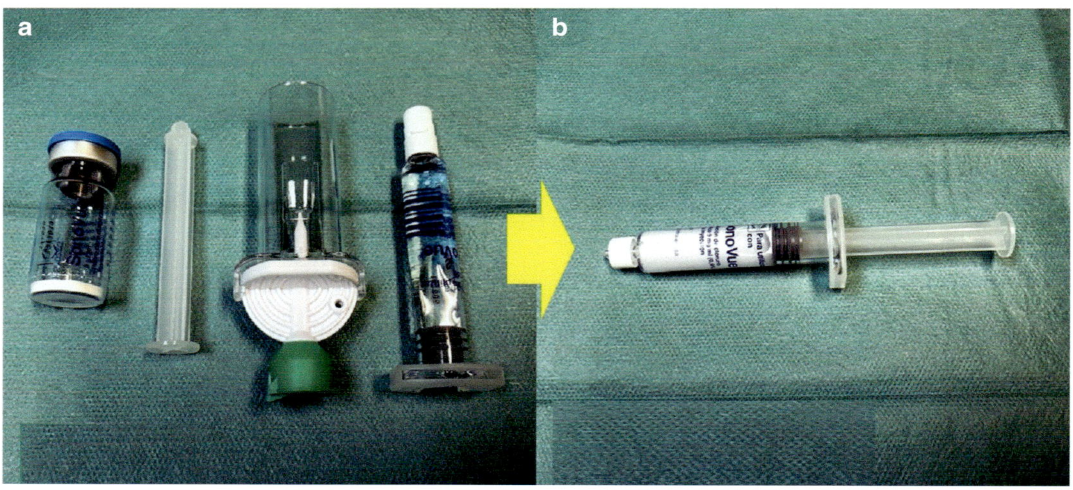

Fig. 22.4 (**a**) To prepare the contrast, you need the vial with the gas and the lyophilized inside, the syringe, the plunger, and an adapter to mix. (**b**) A white fluid filled with millions of microbubbles is obtained

22.3 Clinical Applications

The thyroid gland has a high blood flow in relation to its low weight, which favors contrast studies of this gland. Its weight is approximately 20 g, and the percentage it receives from the heart rate is 1.56% [13]. This means that the blood flow in relation to its weight is one of the highest in the body (500 mL/100 g/min), similar to the adrenal gland (508 mL/100 g/min), and much higher than the kidney (396 mL/100 g/min), which is one of the most vascularized organs [14]. This characteristic makes the thyroid gland particularly susceptible to being studied with contrast and could also explain why many thyroid nodules can bleed internally in stressful situations [15].

The goal of minimally invasive treatments is to induce coagulative necrosis, and the coagulation of vessels results in ischemia. Therefore, it makes perfect sense to study the effect of these percutaneous treatments with CEUS, which allows us to assess microvascularization and evaluate the effectiveness of the procedure [16–18]. That is why it is convenient to administer contrast before and after the procedure to be able to compare the changes produced by the ablation. In a poorly vascularized lesion, the use of contrast will be of little use in assessing the effectiveness of the treatment. One drawback is the artifact produced by the water vapor generated during radiofrequency or microwave thermoablation [19]. The hyperechogenicities produced by alcohol are also a limitation for CEUS immediately after alcoholization. For this reason, it would be advisable to wait for the water vapor to dissipate before performing the post-ablation CEUS control. However, it is not recommended to wait too long with the ablation needle inside the nodule in case re-treatment of any undertreated area is needed, as detected by CEUS. It should be noted that hyperechogenicities from water vapor bubbles or alcohol can be distinguished from microbubbles in intravenous contrast. Water vapor bubbles produce a static artifact, while microbubbles display dynamic and changing small hyperechogenicities. Since the temperature achieved with microwaves is higher, the water vapor generated remains longer and takes longer to condense again, which likely limits the immediate post-ablation CEUS study in the case of microwave treatment.

The clinical use of CEUS basically focuses on the treatment of benign thyroid nodules. However, it is also a valuable tool that can aid in the evaluation of the treatment of papillary microcarcinomas, laterocervical nodes, local recurrences, parathyroid adenomas, and parathyroid carcinomas.

22.3.1 Benign Thyroid Nodules

Many benign thyroid nodules are isoechoic or hyperechoic. When a radiofrequency treatment is carried out, the echogenicity of the nodule is reduced. The reduction in echogenicity becomes noticeable when the temperature increases just before the appearance of water vapor, that is, below 100 °C, and this change can be observed in some cases during radiofrequency ablation. This change in echogenicity helps us distinguish treated areas from undertreated areas. Additionally, we have Doppler systems that are much more sensitive to small vessel flow, aiding in distinguishing viable vascularized areas from those that have been treated and necrosed. Under normal conditions, the use of CEUS is not strictly necessary thanks to the differences in echogenicity that exist in B-mode between the treated and the untreated area, and subsequent controls with CEUS should not be performed. Necrotic tissue, hypoechoic and heterogeneous, with echogenic paths of carbonization, correlates with areas of greater hardness on elastography.

Ruan et al. [20]. adapted the ACR TI-RADS by incorporating CEUS which allows for risk stratification of malignancy. CEUS features include enhancement direction (scattered or centripetal/centrifugal), peak intensity (iso, hyper, or hypo-enhancement), presence of ring enhancement, and solid composition. The area under the receiver operating characteristic curve, biopsy yield of malignancy, and unnecessary biopsy rate of CEUS TI-RADS were 0.93, 66%, and 34%, respectively.

There are benign nodules that are heterogeneous or have a spongy pattern, and in these two cases, it becomes more difficult to distinguish viable tissue from necrotic tissue after treatment using only with B-mode and color Doppler. In addition, we are increasingly using alcohol to treat nodules with a significant cystic component, exceeding 20%, which will later be definitively treated with radiofrequency. In such cases, especially for nodules with multi-septate and multi-trabeculated cystic nodules, the "moving-shot" technique can be employed during the alcoholization (Fig. 22.5). This technique involves aspirating and injecting alcohol along the withdrawal path of the needle. During alcoholization, the alcohol accentuates the heterogeneity of the nodule because its distribution and the effects are more unevenly spread out. The heterogeneity observed with B-mode after alcoholization makes it challenging to accurately determine the degree of effectiveness. In these cases, the use of CEUS is of great help as it allows us to better assess the treatment's effectiveness and distinguish viable tissue from necrotic tissue.

In the first published series, there was a 75% improvement in hyperthyroidism in the hyperfunctioning thyroid nodules treated with radiofrequency [21, 22]. To further increase this percentage, it is crucial to ensure complete ablation in hyperfunctioning nodules, and CEUS can be instrumental in ensure complete ablation in hyperfunctioning nodules, and CEUS can be instrumental in achieving this goal (Fig. 22.6).

Using CEUS immediately after treatment and before removing the needle can help identify the areas that still show vascularization and perfusion, which need to be further treated. To minimize the presence of undertreated triangles (Fig. 22.7) that represent viable subcortical tissue, it is advisable to ensure that during treatment, when the ablation needle is in the subcortical region of the nodule, it remains as extended as possible to maximize the radius of the ablation ball. During the moving shot, it is better to think about making a cone of heat than a cylinder.

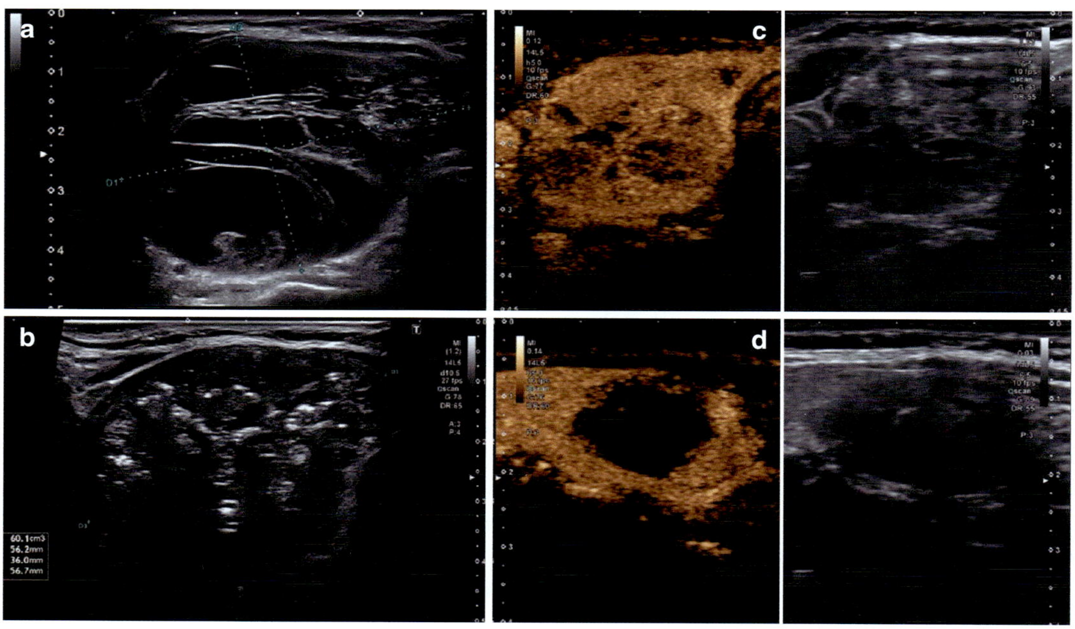

Fig. 22.5 Large cystic nodule in a 71-year-old woman patient treated with alcoholization using the moving shot technique twice and finally with a radiofrequency ablation. (**a**) Initial B-mode scan of this 77.8 cc cystic nodule in which multiple thin septa are visible. (**b**) B-mode immediately after alcoholization, showing hyperechogenicities distributed throughout the nodule. (**c**) CEUS scan taken 25 months after the two alcoholizations, demonstrating a nearly complete reduction of the cystic component and a volume of 28.2 cc with a VRR of 64%. Consequently, we decided to proceed with radiofrequency ablation. (**d**) CEUS scan 30 months after the first alcoholization reveals a volume of 5.2 cc with a cumulative VRR of 93%. In this sagittal section, we can observe viable tissue that continues to retain the contrast in its lower pole, necessitating further monitoring

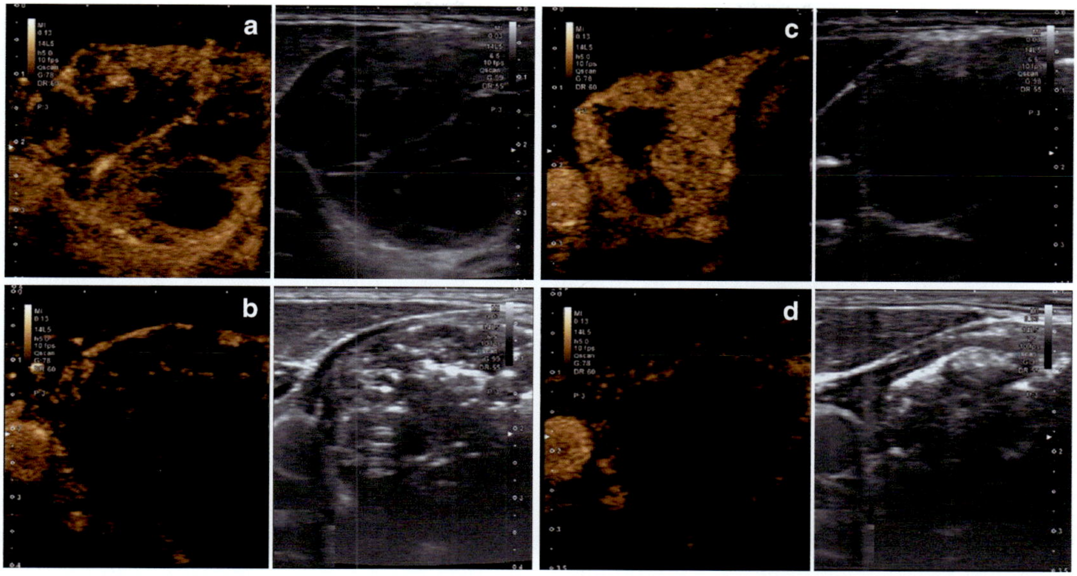

Fig. 22.6 Hyperfunctioning multiseptated cystic nodule in a 29-year-old male patient (TSH = 0.068 mU/L) treated with alcoholization using the moving shot technique and 2 months later with radiofrequency ablation. (**a**) Initial CEUS image prior to alcoholization. (**b**) CEUS image immediately after alcoholization using the moving shot technique, demonstrating an absence of contrast uptake. (**c**) CEUS image taken 2 months after alcoholization, revealing an area of central necrosis, lack of cystic component, significant reduction in the nodule's volume (7.4 cc, VRR = 73%), and a normalization of hyperthyroidism (TSH = 2.467 mU/L). (**d**) CEUS image taken immediately after radiofrequency ablation, displaying an absence of contrast uptake

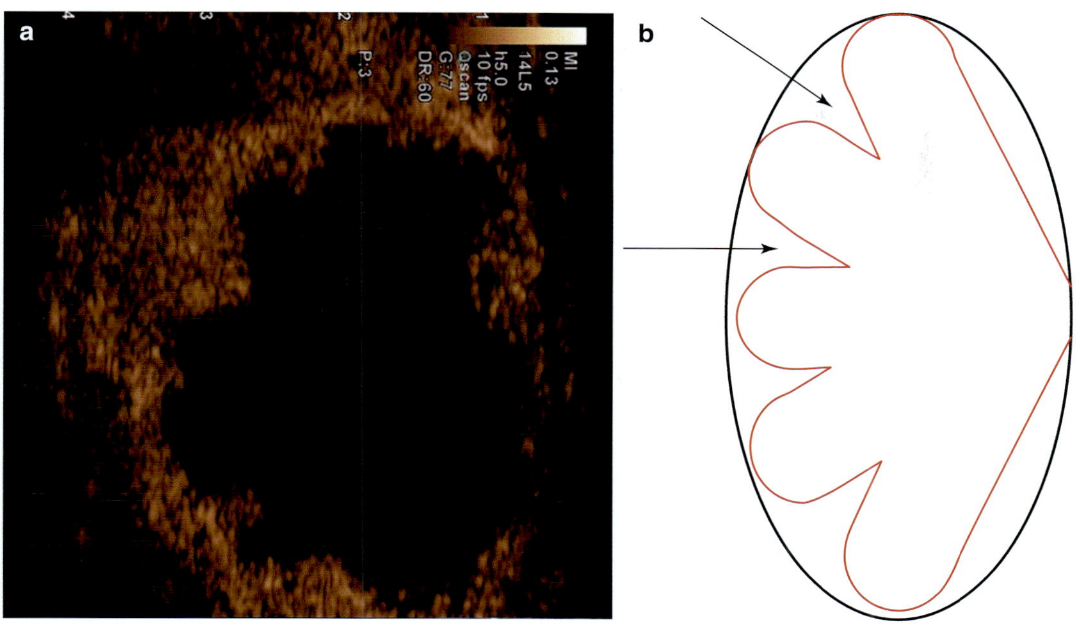

Fig. 22.7 (**a**) CEUS performed 4 days after radiofrequency ablation of a nodule in the region of the isthmus, conducted with spatial limitations due to pain during the moving shot technique. The patient, a 45-year-old female, experienced pain and fever 4 days after the treatment. The CEUS image reveals a noticeable irregularity at the interface between the viable and the non-viable zones, characterized by a triangular morphology. (**b**) Highlighting one of the drawbacks of the moving shot technique, namely the triangular shape of the non-ablated areas

The goal of radiofrequency ablation of thyroid nodules is to treat most of the nodule with minimal risk of capsule rupture or injury to adjacent tissues. For this reason, there will always be a peripheral portion of viable tissue surrounding the central necrotic portion. This necrotic portion will gradually be reabsorbed over time until it even disappears [23].

Elastography is useful in monitoring thyroid nodules, especially in evaluating the central necrotic portion, as it loses elasticity and becomes harder due to increased fibrotic components, carbonization, or dehydration, and may even present dystrophic calcifications.

The applications of CEUS in radiofrequency ablation of thyroid nodules focus on the baseline study before treatment, the assessment of viable tissue that can be ablated during the procedure, the evaluation of the volume percentage of viable tissue in relation to the total nodule during follow-up, and the assessment of the possibility of regrowth [17].

Color Doppler is not as sensitive as CEUS in detecting areas of slow-flow vascularization. CEUS also allows the assessment of tissue perfusion [24, 25]. In recent years, there has been an increase in articles on the usefulness of Superb Microvascular Imaging (SMI) for assessing the microvascularization of thyroid nodules, showing similar sensitivity to CEUS in detecting viable tissue after treatment [26, 27], although they seem to detect different parameters; SMI detects larger-diameter microvessels, while CEUS detects smaller-diameter microvessels [26].

Cao et al. [28] studied the enhancement pattern of thyroid nodules prior to the procedure. In the arterial phase, 53.23% of them exhibited hyperenhancement, while 46.77% showed isoenhancement compared to the rest of the parenchyma. A subset of the nodules displayed a ring enhancement with varying thickness.

Greater vascularization of the nodule has been associated with lower treatment efficacy due to heat dispersion during ablation, resulting in a lower percentage of volume reduction and a higher risk of regrowth [29, 30].

22.3.1.1 Follow-Up Study and Possibility of Regrowth

The reduction in the size of thyroid nodules after radiofrequency ablation is similar in most studies [31–35]. For example, Baek et al. [35] reported a reduction between 33 and 58% at 1 month and 51 and 85% at 6 months, and Jeong et al. [34] reported reductions of 58.2%, 74.4%, and 84.8% at 1 month, 3 months, and 6 months, respectively.

The final volume of the nodule, once almost all the central necrotic tissue has been reabsorbed, depends mainly on the viable tissue left during the radiofrequency ablation procedure. As shown in the diagram in Fig. 22.8, the final volume is proportional to the thickness of the untreated subcapsular layer at baseline.

Most studies detect long-term regrowth [23, 34, 36, 37], with a risk of regrowth of 20–30% [36, 38]. During the first years, most nodules decrease in size due to the reduction of the central necrotic component, which masks the potential regrowth of the peripheral viable component. Sim et al. [39] conclude that the growth of the viable portion of the nodule occurs up to a year before an increase in the nodule's overall diameter. In another article by the group of Sim et al. [40]), they establish the quantitative index IAR (initial ablation ratio) 1 month after radiofrequency ablation (volume of viable tissue/total nodule volume), with a higher likelihood of therapeutic success if the index exceeds 70%. Zhu et al. reached a similar conclusion with a cutoff point of 75% [41].

One possible solution for detecting regrowth is the use of CEUS, which can detect the actual viable component and provide a volumetric assessment [39]. In the studies published to date, CEUS has not shown greater efficacy than B-mode ultrasound in detecting viable peripheral tissue and differentiating it from central necrotic tissue. However, it has allowed for greater reproducibility and inter-observer/intra-observer agreement compared to B-mode ultrasound alone [16], especially in cases where the echogenicity of central necrotic tissue and

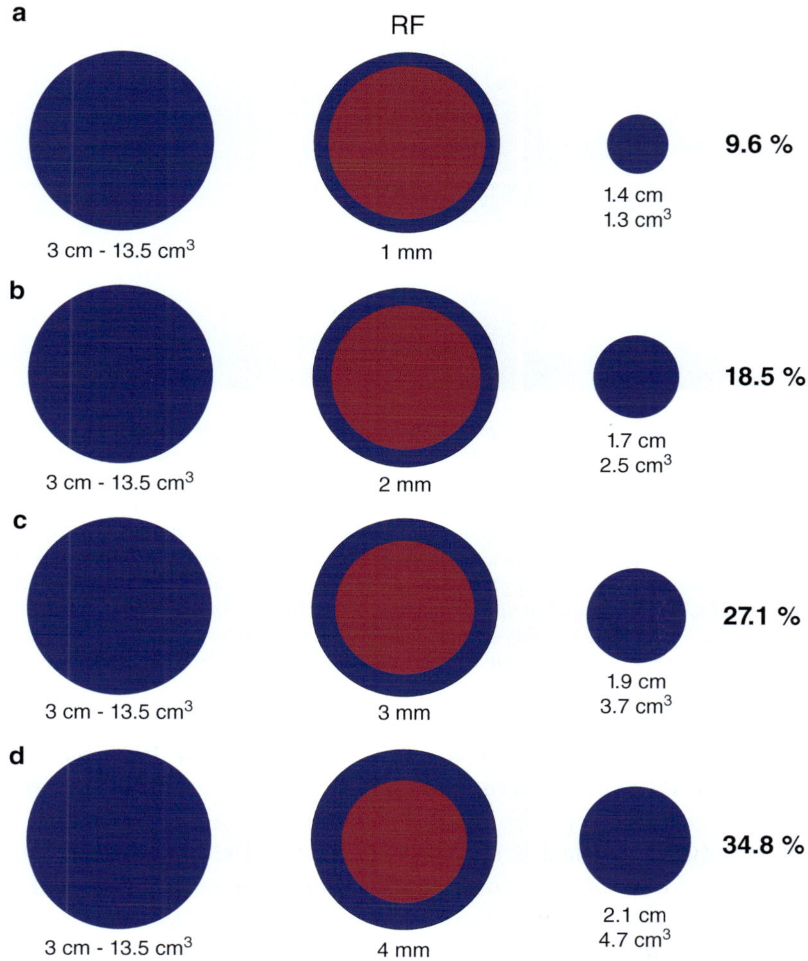

Fig. 22.8 This diagram illustrates the significance of ensuring that nodule tissue at the periphery is not left untreated. This factor plays a crucial role in determining the volume of the remaining nodule after the necrotic tissue has been absorbed, particularly in cases where there is no regrowth of viable residual tissue

peripheral viable tissue is not very different. Yan et al. [42] agree with this higher inter-observer/intra-observer agreement offered by CEUS compared to B-mode ultrasound in defining ablated necrotic tissue, especially in the first few months after ablation, while it is lower in the long term (12 months). They also conclude that B-mode ultrasound overestimates ablated necrotic tissue compared to CEUS, especially in nodules with a baseline volume greater than 10 mL compared to those smaller than 10 mL.

22.3.2 Thyroid Carcinomas

Radiofrequency ablation of papillary thyroid microcarcinomas is a viable, safe, and effective therapeutic alternative for those patients with surgical risk or who do not wish to undergo surgery [43, 44]. The utility of CEUS lies in its performance before and immediately after the procedure to verify that the lesion is contained within the ablation ball, (Fig. 22.9) also in the subsequent follow-up to assess the presence of residual tumors and the risk of recurrence.

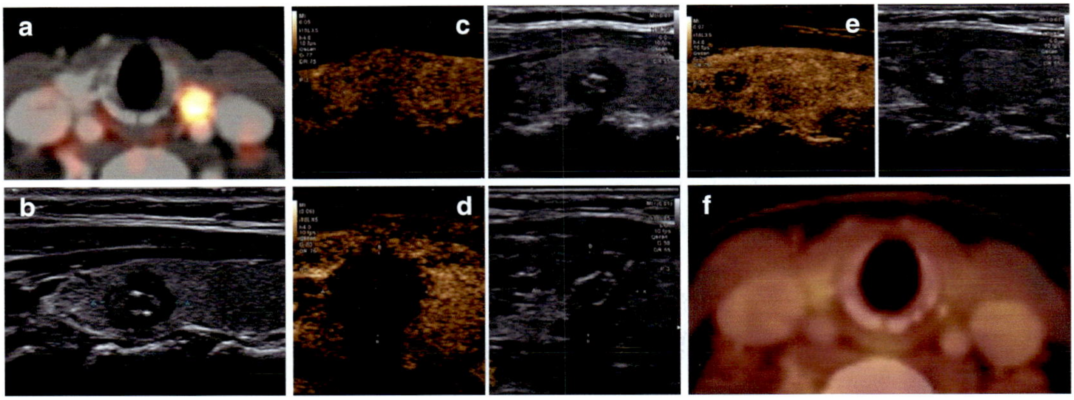

Fig. 22.9 A 50-year-old female patient diagnosed with breast cancer and liver metastases that exhibited positive response to chemotherapy and immunotherapy, with the exception of two metastatic sites. These two sites were addressed through radiofrequency treatment. Subsequently, the patient has remained without evidence of disease. (**a**) The only focus of glucose uptake identified in the PET-CT was a minor left apical thyroid nodule. (**b**) A sagittal sonographic cross-section displays this hypoechoic nodule with a central annular calcification, Bethesda V cytology was confirmed. (**c**) CEUS illustrates its isoechoic nature in relation to the rest of the thyroid parenchyma. (**d**) CEUS immediately after radiofrequency ablation confirms the precise containment of the papillary microcarcinoma by the thermal ablation zone. (**e**) Three months following ablation, CEUS reveals a reduction in the ablation zone's size with a residual avascular area containing a central calcification remains. (**f**) PET-CT scan indicates a complete absence of glucose uptake throughout the patient's body

22.3.3 Metastatic Lymph Nodes and Local Recurrences

Radiofrequency ablation is a safe and effective alternative for the treatment of metastatic lymph nodes. Most studies use this procedure in patients with thyroid carcinoma metastases [45]. CEUS is performed before radiofrequency ablation in several of these studies and also used for follow-up to assess the presence of residual tumors or recurrence. Dong et al. [45] demonstrated complete ablation of all 20 studied metastatic lymph nodes using CEUS, with complete or over 80% reduction in 9 cases and between 50 and 80% reduction in 9 other cases studied. Similar results were obtained by Guang et al. [46], who studied 54 metastatic lymph nodes and observed a progressive reduction in size during follow-up, with complete disappearance in 61% and the presence of scar in 39% at their last 24-month control. In Fig. 22.10, we can see the utility of using CEUS in the immediate control after radiofrequency ablation of a metastatic laterocervical node.

22.3.4 Parathyroid Adenomas and Carcinomas

The use of CEUS in the differential diagnosis between parathyroid adenoma and parathyroid hyperplasia has been studied [47, 48]. It was observed that hyperplastic lesions showed rapid and homogeneous enhancement, while parathyroid adenomas exhibited peripheral enhancement with central washout, along with higher values of "wash-in" and "wash-out."

Similarly, another utility of CEUS in the management of parathyroid adenomas is pre-surgical or prebiopsy detection [49, 50]. In some cases, it has shown a higher sensitivity than conventional ultrasound [51, 52].

There are few published articles regarding the usefulness of CEUS in assessing the percentage of ablation of parathyroid lesions after treatment or its utility in the long-term follow-up of parathyroid lesions treated with radiofrequency. Jiang et al. [53] used CEUS as a complement to percutaneous laser ablation in 21 patients, observing

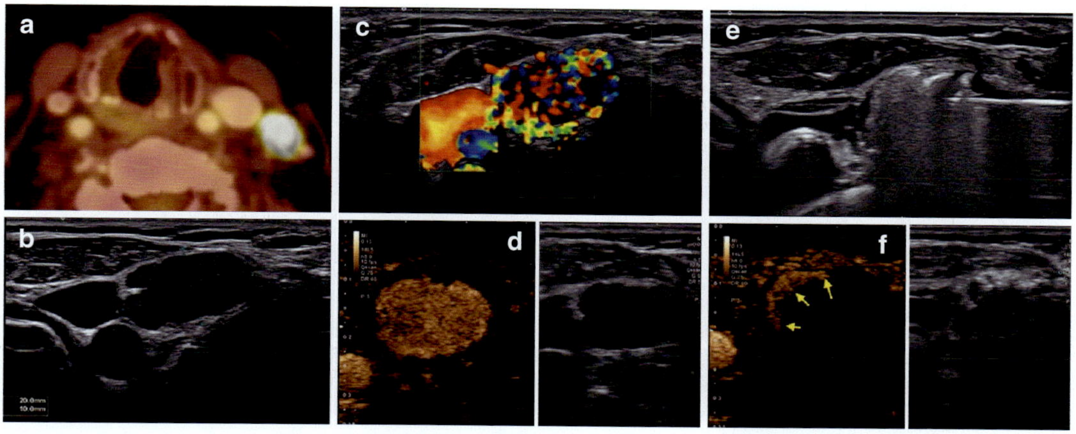

Fig. 22.10 A 74-year-old woman diagnosed with papillary thyroid carcinoma since 2003, with multiple recurrences and subsequent lymphadenectomies. Four new lymph nodes were identified, and the decision was made to address them through radiofrequency ablation. (**a**) PET-CT scan indicates one of the four lymph nodes with detectable glucose uptake. (**b**) Ultrasound section of this lymph node. (**c**) Color Doppler reveals a noticeable diffuse signal within. (**d**) CEUS highlights significant contrast uptake during the arterial phase. (**e**) Radiofrequency ablation in progress. (**f**) CEUS image captured immediately after treatment, indicating persisting activity (as denoted by yellow arrows) prompting the decision for additional treatment at the same time

complete ablation (absence of contrast enhancement) immediately after the procedure in all of them and therapeutic success (normalization of PTH and calcium levels at 12 months) in 81% of cases, with a 48% reduction in tumor size.

In Fig. 22.11, we can see the usefulness of using CEUS in the management of the treatment of a parathyroid carcinoma.

22.3.5 Future Developments

For effective follow-up of thyroid nodule treatments, it is easy to envision in the not-too-distant future, we will have the capability to perform volumetric acquisitions with contrast that can be analyzed using artificial intelligence. These analyses will automatically provide us with information about the volume of the nodule, the volume of necrosis produced, and the ratio between necrotic tissue and viable tissue that remains vascularized. Automated analyses will allow us to determine if there is real regrowth of viable residual tissue or if the volume remains stable as the necrotic part is reabsorbed. However, distinguishing between the persistence of viable tissue and the regrowth of viable tissue can be challenging. This is due to the reduction of necrotic tissue and the effective decrease in nodule volume, which results in an apparent increase in the thickness of viable tissue as the necrotic component involutes. The paradox is that, as the total volume of the treated nodule decreases, three things can happen: the tissue volume of the undertreated nodule can increase progressively, remain the same, or decrease.

Thanks to innate immunity, it must be borne in mind that conceptually, when there is a burn, immediate hyperemia occurs, which paradoxically can favor the regrowth of viable tissue. On the other hand, when we introduce alcohol, there may be a transient vasoconstriction phenomenon. Similarly, the ability of the organism to reabsorb necrotic material, thanks to the phagocytic mononuclear system, is decisive in the rate of reduction of necrosis. Conversely, the genetic characteristics of the treated nodule will also play a crucial role in determining which nodules will have an easier time regrowing or not. Additionally, we must consider the acquired immunological

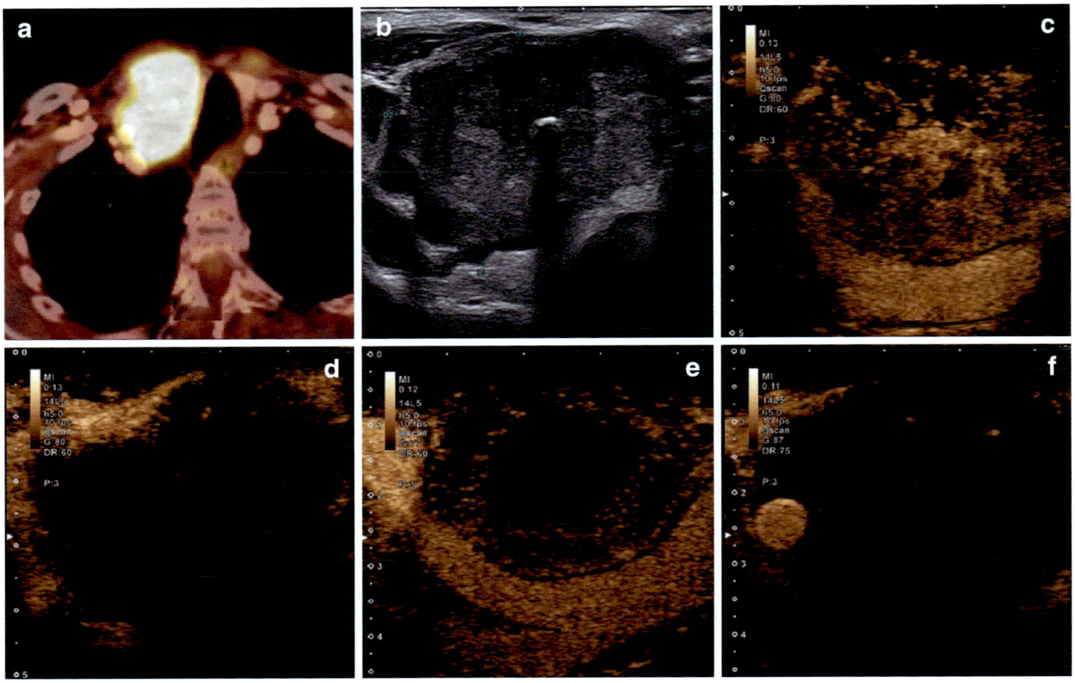

Fig. 22.11 Parathyroid carcinoma diagnosed in a 93-year-old woman with severe hyperparathyroidism and a right laterocervical mass. Upon admission to our hospital, she was in a terminal stage, experiencing complete paralysis, and deemed unsuitable for surgery. The decision was made to pursue radiofrequency ablation. (**a**) PET-CT scan reveals a single glucose uptake within the mass at the right cervicothoracic junction. (**b**) Solid mass with central calcification. (**c**) CEUS examination exhibited low perfusion, heterogeneity, and rapid washout characteristics. (**d**) Immediate post-radiofrequency ablation CEUS confirms complete ablation. (**e**) Three months later, CEUS confirms recurrence prompting a repeat treatment decision. (**f**) Subsequent CEUS following a second radiofrequency treatment demonstrates complete ablation. This patient experienced a third recurrence, which was successfully managed with another round of treatment. Unfortunately, lung metastases emerged. Nevertheless, the patient gained an additional 8 months of life, during which she enjoyed a notably high quality of life

response, which can be directed to the nodule itself or to the thyroid gland after these minimally invasive procedures. Whatever the case, the study of all these little-studied and little-known phenomena can be explained and corroborated thanks to a detailed study of the microvascularization with volumetric acquisition using contrast for the treated thyroid nodules.

Acknowledgments Carolina Alemany Botelho (Figs. 22.1 and 22.2) and Aitor Rodriguez Martinez (Fig. 22.8).

References

1. Carovac A, Smajlovic F, Junuzovic D. Application of ultrasound in medicine. Acta Inform Med. 2011;19:168. https://doi.org/10.5455/aim.2011.19.168-171.
2. Gramiak S. Echocardiography of the aortic root. Invest Radiol. 1968;3:301–88.
3. Feinstein SB, Cheirif J, Ten Cate FJ, Silverman PR, Heidenreich PA, Dick C, et al. Safety and efficacy of a new transpulmonary ultrasound contrast agent: initial multicenter clinical results. J Am Coll Cardiol. 1990;16:316–24. https://doi.org/10.1016/0735-1097(90)90580-I.

4. Appis AW, Tracy MJ, Feinstein SB. Update on the safety and efficacy of commercial ultrasound contrast agents in cardiac applications. Echo Res Pract. 2015;2:R55–62. https://doi.org/10.1530/ERP-15-0018.
5. Dietrich C, Averkiou M, Nielsen M, Barr R, Burns P, Calliada F, et al. How to perform contrast-enhanced ultrasound (CEUS). Ultrasound Int Open. 2018;4:E2–15. https://doi.org/10.1055/s-0043-123931.
6. Shapiro RS, Wagreich J, Parsons RB, Stancato-Pasik A, Yeh HC, Lao R. Tissue harmonic imaging sonography: evaluation of image quality compared with conventional sonography. Am J Roentgenol. 1998;171:1203–6. https://doi.org/10.2214/ajr.171.5.9798848.
7. van Neer PLMJ, Danilouchkine MG, Verweij MD, Demi L, Voormolen MM, van der Steen AFW, et al. Comparison of fundamental, second harmonic, and superharmonic imaging: a simulation study. J Acoust Soc Am. 2011;130:3148–57. https://doi.org/10.1121/1.3643815.
8. Ntoulia A, Anupindi SA, Back SJ, Didier RA, Hwang M, Johnson AM, et al. Contrast-enhanced ultrasound: a comprehensive review of safety in children. Pediatr Radiol. 2021;51:2161–80. https://doi.org/10.1007/s00247-021-05223-4.
9. Yusuf GT, Sellars ME, Deganello A, Cosgrove DO, Sidhu PS. Retrospective analysis of the safety and cost implications of pediatric contrast-enhanced ultrasound at a single center. Am J Roentgenol. 2017;208:446–52. https://doi.org/10.2214/AJR.16.16700.
10. Sidhu P, Cantisani V, Dietrich C, Gilja O, Saftoiu A, Bartels E, et al. The EFSUMB guidelines and recommendations for the clinical practice of contrast-enhanced ultrasound (CEUS) in non-hepatic applications: update 2017 (long version). Ultraschall Med. 2018;39:e2–44. https://doi.org/10.1055/a-0586-1107.
11. Piscaglia F, Bolondi L. The safety of Sonovue® in abdominal applications: retrospective analysis of 23188 investigations. Ultrasound Med Biol. 2006;32:1369–75. https://doi.org/10.1016/j.ultrasmedbio.2006.05.031.
12. Main ML. Ultrasound contrast agent safety. JACC Cardiovasc Imaging. 2009;2:1057–9. https://doi.org/10.1016/j.jcmg.2009.05.008.
13. Maravall FJ, Gómez-Arnáiz N, Gumá A, Abós R, Soler J, Gómez JM. Reference values of thyroid volume in a healthy, non-iodine-deficient Spanish population. Horm Metab Res. 2004;36:645–9. https://doi.org/10.1055/s-2004-825901.
14. Cowles AL, Borgstedt HH, Gillies AJ. Tissue weights and rates of blood flow in man for the prediction of anesthetic uptake and distribution. Anesthesiology. 1971;35:523–6. https://doi.org/10.1097/00000542-197111000-00013.
15. Ren J, Baek JH, Chung SR, Choi YJ, Jung CK, Lee JH. Degenerating thyroid nodules: ultrasound diagnosis, clinical significance, and management. Korean J Radiol. 2019;20:947. https://doi.org/10.3348/kjr.2018.0599.
16. Schiaffino S, Serpi F, Rossi D, Ferrara V, Buonomenna C, Alì M, et al. Reproducibility of ablated volume measurement is higher with contrast-enhanced ultrasound than with B-mode ultrasound after benign thyroid nodule radiofrequency ablation—a preliminary study. J Clin Med. 2020;9:1504. https://doi.org/10.3390/jcm9051504.
17. Zhao C-K, Xu H-X, Lu F, Sun L-P, He Y-P, Guo L-H, et al. Factors associated with initial incomplete ablation for benign thyroid nodules after radiofrequency ablation: first results of CEUS evaluation. Clin Hemorheol Microcirc. 2017;65:393–405. https://doi.org/10.3233/CH-16208.
18. Yan L, Li X, Xiao J, Li Y, Zhu Y, He H, et al. Contrast-enhanced ultrasound is a reliable and reproducible assessment of necrotic ablated volume after radiofrequency ablation for benign thyroid nodules: a retrospective study. Int J Hyperthermia. 2022;39:40–7. https://doi.org/10.1080/02656736.2021.1991009.
19. Bansal S, Gui J, Merrill C, Wong JK, Burak KW, Wilson SR. Contrast-enhanced US in local ablative therapy and secondary surveillance for hepatocellular carcinoma. Radiographics. 2019;39:1302–22. https://doi.org/10.1148/rg.2019180205.
20. Ruan J, Xu X, Cai Y, Zeng H, Luo M, Zhang W, et al. A practical CEUS thyroid reporting system for thyroid nodules. Radiology. 2022;305:149–59. https://doi.org/10.1148/radiol.212319.
21. Cervelli R, Mazzeo S, Boni G, Boccuzzi A, Bianchi F, Brozzi F, et al. Comparison between radioiodine therapy and single-session radiofrequency ablation of autonomously functioning thyroid nodules: a retrospective study. Clin Endocrinol (Oxf). 2019;90:608–16. https://doi.org/10.1111/cen.13938.
22. De Boer H, Bom W, Veendrick P, Bom E, Van Borren M, Joosten F. Hyperactive thyroid nodules treated by radiofrequency ablation: a Dutch single-centre experience. Neth J Med. 2020;78:64–70.
23. Sim JS, Baek JH. Long-term outcomes of thermal ablation for benign thyroid nodules: the issue of regrowth. Int J Endocrinol. 2021;2021:1–7. https://doi.org/10.1155/2021/9922509.
24. Yeh C-K, Kang S-T. Ultrasound microbubble contrast agents for diagnostic and therapeutic applications: current status and future design. Biomed J. 2012;35:125. https://doi.org/10.4103/2319-4170.106159.
25. Alvarez-Sánchez M-V. Contrast-enhanced harmonic endoscopic ultrasound imaging: basic principles, present situation and future perspectives. World J Gastroenterol. 2014;20:15549. https://doi.org/10.3748/wjg.v20.i42.15549.
26. Liu W, Zhou P, Zhao Y, Tian S, Wu X. Superb microvascular imaging compared with contrast-enhanced ultrasound for assessing laser ablation treatment of benign thyroid nodules. Biomed Res Int. 2018;2018:1–8. https://doi.org/10.1155/2018/1025657.

27. Lan Y, Li N, Song Q, Zhang M, Luo Y, Zhang Y. Correlation and agreement between superb micro-vascular imaging and contrast-enhanced ultrasound for assessing radiofrequency ablation treatment of thyroid nodules: a preliminary study. BMC Med Imaging. 2021;21:175. https://doi.org/10.1186/s12880-021-00697-y.
28. Cao J, Fan P, Wang F, Shi S, Liu L, Yan Z, et al. Application of contrast-enhanced ultrasound in minimally invasive ablation of benign thyroid nodules. J Interv Med. 2022;5:32–6. https://doi.org/10.1016/j.jimed.2021.12.008.
29. Baek JH. Factors related to the recurrence of benign thyroid nodules after thermal ablation. Int J Hyperth. 2017;33:1–2. https://doi.org/10.1080/02656736.2017.1364791.
30. Offi C, Garberoglio S, Antonelli G, Esposito MG, Brancaccio U, Misso C, et al. The ablation of thyroid nodule's afferent arteries before radiofrequency ablation: preliminary data. Front Endocrinol (Lausanne). 2021;11:565000. https://doi.org/10.3389/fendo.2020.565000.
31. Baek JH, Kim YS, Lee D, Huh JY, Lee JH. Benign predominantly solid thyroid nodules: prospective study of efficacy of sonographically guided radiofrequency ablation versus control condition. Am J Roentgenol. 2010;194:1137–42. https://doi.org/10.2214/AJR.09.3372.
32. Faggiano A, Ramundo V, Assanti A, Fonderico F, Machia C, Misso C, et al. Thyroid nodules treated with percutaneous radiofrequency thermal ablation: a comparative study. J Clin Endocrinol Metab. 2012;97:4439–45. https://doi.org/10.1210/jc.2012-2251.
33. Jeong WK, Baek JH, Rhim H, Kim YS, Kwak MS, Jeong HJ, et al. Radiofrequency ablation of benign thyroid nodules: safety and imaging follow-up in 236 patients. Eur Radiol. 2008;18:1244–50. https://doi.org/10.1007/s00330-008-0880-6.
34. Lim HK, Lee JH, Ha EJ, Sung JY, Kim JK, Baek JH. Radiofrequency ablation of benign non-functioning thyroid nodules: 4-year follow-up results for 111 patients. Eur Radiol. 2013;23:1044–9. https://doi.org/10.1007/s00330-012-2671-3.
35. Shin JH, Baek JH, Ha EJ, Lee JH. Radiofrequency ablation of thyroid nodules: basic principles and clinical application. Int J Endocrinol. 2012;2012:1–7. https://doi.org/10.1155/2012/919650.
36. Bernardi S, Giudici F, Cesareo R, Antonelli G, Cavallaro M, Deandrea M, et al. Five-year results of radiofrequency and laser ablation of benign thyroid nodules: a multicenter study from the Italian minimally invasive treatments of the thyroid group. Thyroid. 2020;30:1759–70. https://doi.org/10.1089/thy.2020.0202.
37. Deandrea M, Trimboli P, Garino F, Mormile A, Magliona G, Ramunni MJ, et al. Long-term efficacy of a single session of RFA for benign thyroid nodules: a longitudinal 5-year observational study. J Clin Endocrinol Metab. 2019;104:3751–6. https://doi.org/10.1210/jc.2018-02808.
38. Papini E, Rago T, Gambelunghe G, Valcavi R, Bizzarri G, Vitti P, et al. Long-term efficacy of ultrasound-guided laser ablation for benign solid thyroid nodules. Results of a three-year multicenter prospective randomized trial. J Clin Endocrinol Metab. 2014;99:3653–9. https://doi.org/10.1210/jc.2014-1826.
39. Sim JS, Baek JH, Lee J, Cho W, Jung S II. Radiofrequency ablation of benign thyroid nodules: depicting early sign of regrowth by calculating vital volume. Int J Hyperthermia. 2017;33:1–6. https://doi.org/10.1080/02656736.2017.1309083.
40. Sim JS, Baek JH, Cho W. Initial ablation ratio: quantitative value predicting the therapeutic success of thyroid radiofrequency ablation. Thyroid. 2018;28:1443–9. https://doi.org/10.1089/thy.2018.0180.
41. Zhu Y, Jiao Z, Zhu L, Xie F, Song Q, Yan L, et al. A new perspective for predicting the therapeutic success of RFA in solid BTNs: quantitative initial RFA ratio by contrast-enhanced ultrasound. Front Endocrinol (Lausanne). 2022;13:1–9. https://doi.org/10.3389/fendo.2022.904459.
42. Yan L, Luo Y, Xiao J, Lin L. Non-enhanced ultrasound is not a satisfactory modality for measuring necrotic ablated volume after radiofrequency ablation of benign thyroid nodules: a comparison with contrast-enhanced ultrasound. Eur Radiol. 2021;31:3226–36. https://doi.org/10.1007/s00330-020-07398-0.
43. Lin Y, Wu ZR, Shi YP, Ding M, Tang XY, He Y, et al. Radiofrequency ablation of unifocal papillary thyroid microcarcinoma with BRAF V600E mutation. J Clin Endocrinol Metab. 2023;108(11):e1298–305. https://doi.org/10.1210/clinem/dgad269.
44. Zhang M, Luo Y, Zhang Y, Tang J. Efficacy and safety of ultrasound-guided radiofrequency ablation for treating low-risk papillary thyroid microcarcinoma: a prospective study. Thyroid. 2016;26:1581–7. https://doi.org/10.1089/thy.2015.0471.
45. Wang L, Ge M, Xu D, Chen L, Qian C, Shi K, et al. Ultrasonography-guided percutaneous radiofrequency ablation for cervical lymph node metastasis from thyroid carcinoma. J Cancer Res Ther. 2014;10:144. https://doi.org/10.4103/0973-1482.145844.
46. Guang Y, Luo Y, Zhang Y, Zhang M, Li N, Zhang Y, et al. Efficacy and safety of percutaneous ultrasound guided radiofrequency ablation for treating cervical metastatic lymph nodes from papillary thyroid carcinoma. J Cancer Res Clin Oncol. 2017;143:1555–62. https://doi.org/10.1007/s00432-017-2386-6.
47. Pavlovics S, Radzina M, Niciporuka R, Ratniece M, Mikelsone M, Tauvena E, et al. Contrast-enhanced ultrasound qualitative and quantitative characteristics of parathyroid gland lesions. Medicina (Kaunas). 2021;58:2. https://doi.org/10.3390/medicina58010002.
48. Agha A, Hornung M, Stroszczynski C, Schlitt HJ, Jung EM. Highly efficient localization of pathologi-

cal glands in primary hyperparathyroidism using contrast-enhanced ultrasonography (CEUS) in comparison with conventional ultrasonography. J Clin Endocrinol Metab. 2013;98:2019–25. https://doi.org/10.1210/jc.2013-1007.
49. Navarro SM, Malhi H, Deurdulian C, Grant E. Localization of parathyroid adenoma using contrast-enhanced sonography. J Ultrasound Med. 2019;38:259–60. https://doi.org/10.1002/jum.14672.
50. Piccin O, D'Alessio P, Serra C, Felicani C, Vicennati V, Repaci A, et al. The diagnostic value of contrast-enhanced ultrasound for localization of parathyroid lesions in primary hyperparathyroidism. J Ultrasound Med. 2023;42:91–8.
51. Hornung M, Jung EM, Stroszczynski C, Schlitt HJ, Agha A. Contrast-enhanced ultrasonography (CEUS) using early dynamic in microcirculation for localization of pathological parathyroid glands: first-line or complimentary diagnostic modality? Clin Hemorheol Microcirc. 2011;49:83–90. https://doi.org/10.3233/CH-2011-1459.
52. Lerner A, Grant EG, Acharya J, Chambers TN, Maceri DR, Cen SY, et al. Utility of contrast-enhanced ultrasound and 4-dimensional computed tomography for preoperative detection and localization of parathyroid adenomas compared with surgical results. J Ultrasound Med. 2022;41:2295–306. https://doi.org/10.1002/jum.15916.
53. Jiang T, Chen F, Zhou X, Hu Y, Zhao Q. Percutaneous ultrasound-guided laser ablation with contrast-enhanced ultrasonography for hyperfunctioning parathyroid adenoma: a preliminary case series. Int J Endocrinol. 2015;2015:1–6. https://doi.org/10.1155/2015/673604.

23 Metastatic Thyroid Tumor Thermal Ablation

Antonio Rahal Junior

23.1 Introduction

Thyroid pathologies are highly prevalent in the global population, with an estimated one-third of individuals over 40 years of age experiencing some form of dysfunction in the "body gland of balance." Among the thyroid alterations manifest in imaging studies, notable instances include those primarily affecting the glandular parenchyma. Parenchymal heterogeneity, varying in degree, is a common feature in thyroiditis, intensifying with the severity of the inflammatory process. Additionally, the presence of nodules stemming from diverse etiologies is observed [1, 2].

Most thyroid nodules are benign and do not disrupt hormonal function, often remaining asymptomatic. Nevertheless, these benign nodules can induce symptoms, particularly those associated with local growth. Such symptoms may encompass tracheal compression, esophageal compression leading to dysphagia, the sensation of a foreign object, cosmetic effects ranging from mild to moderate, growth toward the mediastinum resulting in "thoracic or diving" goiters, and compression of mediastinal structures. Autonomous toxic nodules can also arise, manifesting symptoms of hyperthyroidism to varying degrees [1].

Over the past 15 years, specific medical centers worldwide have begun to focus on benign nodules for ablative therapies, initially targeting non-autonomous or non-toxic nodules and later expanding to toxic nodules, particularly favoring smaller nodules. Initially, chemical ablation using absolute ethanol (PEI) was employed, followed by interstitial laser ablation (ILA). These minimally invasive treatments have been directed at confirmed benign thyroid nodules, especially those in the thyroids of patients with normal hormonal levels, as an alternative to thyroidectomy, yielding highly satisfactory outcomes [3, 4].

The advancement of these methodologies, under the notable guidance of esteemed South Korean medical groups like the team led by Baek et al., saw the introduction of ultrasound-guided radiofrequency thermal ablation (RFA) with remarkable outcomes. Many scientific publications emerged during this period, showcasing significant success in the minimally invasive treatment of thyroid nodules, mainly through RFA. The procedure is typically carried out via trans-isthmic access, focusing strongly on the "Moving-shot" technique. Several articles featuring impressive case series have illustrated volumetric reductions of up to approximately 90%, 95%, and even complete nodular disappearance in select cases within 12 months post-treatment [5–8].

A. R. Junior (✉)
Department of Interventional Radiology, University of Sao Paulo, Sao Paulo, Brazil

Thyroid Imaging and Intervention Center, Hospital Israelita Albert Einstein, Sao Paulo, Brazil

R. Valcavi et al. (eds.), *Thyroid Ablation*, https://doi.org/10.1007/978-3-031-88229-6_23

In a multicenter study conducted in 2013 involving American, South Korean, and Italian physicians, notable figures such as Gharib, Hegedus, Pacella, Baek, and Papini [3] highlighted the benefits, safety, and efficacy of chemical alcohol ablation (PEI) for recurrent post-puncture thyroid cysts. The study also underscored the effectiveness of interstitial laser ablation (ILA) and radiofrequency ablation (RFA) for symptomatic solid nodules in patients with normal thyroid function and those with altered function. Microwave thermal ablation (MWA) and high-intensity focused ultrasound (HIFU) were identified in this multicenter study, published nearly a decade ago, as emerging and promising modalities.

Presently, MWA is extensively utilized for ablating both benign and malignant nodules, with a substantial body of literature indicating comparable outcomes between RFA and MWA. Notably, the application of thermo ablation in recurrent thyroid cancer within the cervical region was already mentioned in this study, showing promising results. Long-term follow-up assessments have demonstrated the enduring effectiveness of ablative treatments for benign nodules, with a minimal "regrowth" rate observed after 60 months of monitoring (below 10%).

Significant advancements were also observed in treating autonomous, confirmed benign nodules, particularly in the subset of "single toxic" nodules in Plummer disease, with volumes reaching up to 12.0 cc. The primary objectives in these cases included substantial volumetric reduction and the normalization of TSH levels, typically achieved within the initial 60 days following treatment [5, 6].

The remarkable success of RFA in treating benign thyroid nodules prompted leading medical groups worldwide to explore new frontiers by targeting primary malignant lesions. Specifically, lesions with a maximum diameter of approximately 1.0 cm, well-positioned within the gland parenchyma, and exhibiting low aggressiveness on cytopathological or histopathological evaluation were the focus. These lesions are commonly referred to as PTMCs (Papillary Thyroid Microcarcinomas).

According to recent data from the American Cancer Society, thyroid cancer ranks as the most prevalent endocrine malignancy, with an estimated 42,720 new cases projected for 2023 in the United States (12,540 in men and 31,180 in women, with a male-to-female ratio of around 1:3). Approximately 2120 deaths are anticipated to be associated with thyroid cancer this year (970 in men and 1150 in women). A crucial aspect in comprehending the current landscape of the increasing application of ablative therapies in thyroid cancer is the emergence and implementation of criteria for active surveillance in the management of thyroid cancer.

Initially suggested by Akira Miyauchi in 1993, active surveillance gradually gained recognition and endorsement from the ATA (American Thyroid Association) and different experts on this subject from 2015 onwards. In the same year, the ATA officially approved active surveillance as a viable therapeutic option in carefully chosen cases [9]. The ATA established criteria for active surveillance of PTMCs in selected situations.

Table 23.1 shows the characteristics that are prerequisites for a microcarcinoma to qualify for active surveillance, which also render the nodule suitable for thermo ablation. Radiofrequency ablation (RFA) and microwave ablation (MW) are the primary techniques currently employed by the most prominent and seasoned medical groups worldwide for the treatment of these papillary thyroid microcarcinomas (PTMCs).

Table 23.2 shows situations where active surveillance may not be ideal but is still a viable consideration, such as in cases of multifocal microcarcinomas and other specific characteristics, thermal ablation should be approached cautiously. While thermal ablation may yield slightly inferior results compared to the ablation of PTMCs meeting the criteria outlined in Table 23.1, the existing medical literature and the expertise of leading specialists consistently regard the outcomes of thermal ablation in this group as highly favorable, with resolution rates typically exceeding 90%.

Table 23.3 delineates instances where active surveillance is deemed inappropriate. Noteworthy among these criteria is the expansion of the nod-

Table 23.1 Ideal candidates for active surveillance

Candidates for observation	Tumor/neck US characteristics	Patient characteristics	Medical team characteristics
Ideal	– Solitary thyroid nodule – Well-defined margins – Surrounded by ≥2 mm normal thyroid parenchyma – Absence of extrathyroidal extension – Previous US documenting stability – Absence of lymph node metastasis – Absence of distant metastasis	– Older patients (>60 years) – Willing to accept an active surveillance approach – Aware of that a surgical intervention may be necessary in the future – Willing to participate in follow-up plans – Supportive significant others	– Experienced multidisciplinary management team – High-quality neck ultrasonography – Prospective data collection – Tracking/reminder – Program to ensure proper follow-up

Table 23.2 Appropriate candidates for active surveillance

Candidates for observation	Tumor/neck US characteristics	Patient characteristics	Medical team characteristics
Appropriate	– Multifocal papillary microcarcinomas – Subcapsular locations not adjacent to the RLN without evidence of extrathyroidal extension ill-defined margins – Background ultrasonographic findings that will make follow-up difficult (thyroiditis, non-specific lymphadenopathy, and multiple other benign-appearing thyroid nodules) FDG avid PTMC	– Middle-aged patients (18–59 years) – Strong family history of papillary thyroid cancer child-bearing potential	– Experienced endocrinologist or thyroid surgeon – Neck ultrasonography routinely available

RLN recurrent laryngeal nerve

Table 23.3 Inappropriate candidates for active surveillance

Candidates for observation	Tumor/neck US characteristics	Patient characteristics	Medical team characteristics
Inappropriate	– Evidence of aggressive cytology on FNAB (rare) – Subcapsular locations adjacent to the RLN – Evidence of extrathyroidal extension – Clinical evidence of invasion of the RLN or trachea (rare) – N1 disease at the initial evaluation or identified during follow-up – M1 disease (rare) – Documented increase in size of ≥3 mm in a confirmed papillary thyroid cancer tumor	– Young patients (<18 years) – Unlikely to be compliant with follow-up plans – Not willing to accept an observation approach	– Reliable neck ultrasonography not available – Little experience with thyroid cancer management

FNAB fine needle aspiration biopsy

ule beyond 3 mm in its longest axis, a parameter that does not preclude ablation as long as it remains within 1.0 cm (10 mm) of the maximum external diameter. Moreover, younger patients present an advantageous profile for ablation, particularly when considering preserving their quality of life by maintaining intact thyroid hormonal function. These two characteristics exemplify instances where the criteria for recommending thermal ablation diverge from those requisite for active surveillance.

Carcinomas exhibiting the characteristics delineated in Table 23.1 qualify for an immediate non-surgical approach for newly diagnosed PTMCs, with the option of active surveillance over 5 years involving serial annual assessments. Conversely, malignant nodules displaying the attributes outlined in Table 23.2 are not deemed ideal candidates for active surveillance; nonetheless, surveillance may be contemplated in specific circumstances. In the event of noteworthy tumor growth or the emergence of locoregional and/or distant metastases during this period, thyroidectomy would be the recommended course of action.

On the other hand, cancers manifesting the features specified in Table 23.3 are not deemed suitable for active surveillance [2, 9, 10]. Consequently, leading medical institutions specializing in thyroid therapies have initiated the application of radiofrequency thermal ablation (RFA) in selected cases of small papillary carcinomas (PTMCs), initially focusing on patients at elevated surgical risk, those with comorbidities, or individuals for whom the surgical approach is contraindicated.

The outcomes stemming from adopting thermal ablative therapies have shown increasing promise, encompassing factors such as lesion eradication, cost-effectiveness, expedited recovery, complications mitigation, and, crucially, preservation of hormonal function. Notably, the application of thermal ablative interventions in the context of selected PTMCs has yielded results that are on par with those observed in patients undergoing thyroidectomy, whether total or partial. The growing body of literature featuring extended post-ablation follow-up periods exceeding 72 months is becoming more prevalente [7, 11, 12].

The introduction of radiofrequency thermal ablation for treating thyroid nodules has undoubtedly represented a significant paradigm shift in medical practice. It is both rational and desirable to incorporate thermal ablative therapies into the array of therapeutic options for symptomatic benign nodules, toxic nodules, and selected PTMCs, thereby creating a comprehensive treatment "menu" that includes surgery, each technique with its distinctive characteristics [13, 14].

However, delving into the focal point of this chapter, a prevalent scenario encountered among cancer patients undergoing surgical treatment for thyroid cancer is the presence of lymph node metastases identified post-operatively. In light of this, could thermal ablation also serve as a viable therapeutic option in this context, offering an alternative to additional surgical interventions that can be disfiguring, fraught with potential complications, and challenging in terms of surgical re-approach?

23.2 Lymph Node Metastases in Thyroid Cancer

In cases of cervical recurrences of well-differentiated thyroid carcinomas, the conventional approach typically involves a new surgical intervention. Studies suggest that the risk of cervical recurrence in thyroid carcinoma varies, ranging from approximately 15.4% for early-stage cancers (stage I) to around 66.7% for more advanced cases (stage IV) [1, 15].

While thyroid gland resection surgery remains the established standard for treating malignancies, each subsequent surgical procedure presents escalating technical challenges due to the scarring of the surgical site, heightened fibrosis, risks associated with general anesthesia, potential for new scars or revisiting existing scars, and the complexities often encountered in locating and excising non-adjacent metastatic lymph nodes. Consequently, considering minimally invasive techniques to address such lesions becomes increasingly favorable, offering benefits such as avoiding incisions, physical scarring that can be limiting, general anesthesia, and facilitating a prompt return to normal activities [4, 16–18].

In the context of cervical recurrences of thyroid cancer, particularly in lymph nodes accessible via percutaneous means, percutaneous ablation emerges as a viable and advantageous option—initial iterations of percutaneous ablation techniques centered on chemical ablation utilizing absolute ethanol (PEI). However, the application and efficacy of PEI relative to radiofrequency thermal ablation are constrained by the challenges posed by ethanol dispersion in solid tissues, which is less predictable and controllable compared to radiofrequency thermal ablation. While PEI continues to play a role in thyroid ablation, demonstrating excellent efficacy in predominantly cystic, benign nodules and serving as the preferred choice for many in such cases, radiofrequency thermal ablation exhibits clear superiority in treating solid lesions, as corroborated by various published studies.

The 10-year relative survival rates for patients diagnosed with well-differentiated and moderately differentiated papillary and follicular carcinomas stand at 1.0 and 0.99, respectively, with approximately 97% of patients undergoing surgical interventions. In these cases, the initial cure rate following surgery and radioiodine therapy reaches 90%. However, the cure rate for patients treated at stage V of the disease ranges from 7 to 26.1% [4, 16, 18, 19].

Mortality rates observed over an average follow-up period of 11.3 years vary, with rates at 1.7% for stage I, 15.8% for stage II, 30% for stage III, and 60.9% for stage IV [1, 4, 19, 20]. The literature still needs more consistency regarding the treatment and efficacy of surgical interventions and I-131 radioiodine therapy for these locoregional metastases, highlighting the complexity of this situation that necessitates careful attention and individualized decision-making based on specific case characteristics [4, 16, 19].

The application of radiofrequency thermal ablation in treating metastatic cervical lymph nodes and recurrent malignant lesions in the surgical bed was first reported in 2001. Ablative therapy was initially chosen for cases involving high surgical risk or scenarios where surgery was not a viable option. It is worth noting that despite the high prevalence of this condition, relatively few reports have addressed the use of thermo ablation for metastatic lesions since 2001. Some publications merely mention reports, while others discuss small series, and a few rare articles touch upon a limited number of cases, typically at most 30–40 cases (Table 23.4).

A recent meta-analysis by Tang et al. focused on evaluating studies related to thermal ablation for lymph node metastases in papillary thyroid carcinoma. Notably, even among Asians, who possess substantial experience with this therapeutic modality, there is a scarcity of studies featuring a substantial cohort of patients with cervical metastases treated through ablation. Regarding the number of lymph nodes treated across multiple sessions, the literature references varying quantities, such as $N = 10$ in 5 patients and up to $N = 71$ in 45 patients. However, as of now, extensive series have yet to be reported in the available literature [21]. An important observation highlighted in this meta-analysis is the power settings and procedure time when targeting metastatic lymph nodes rather than thyroid nodules. Typically, the power levels selected for lymph node ablation procedures vary widely, ranging from very low values, such as 4 or 5 W, up to 40 W. Most of the studies included in the analysis utilize power settings between 20 and 30 W, which are notably lower than the power levels employed for thyroid nodules. In cases involving thyroid nodules, power settings can reach 40, 50 W, or even higher, depending on the exposure of the active tip of the probe. It is worth noting that modern probes are equipped with adjustable active tips, enhancing the treatment of thyroids with nodules of various sizes (Table 23.5).

Despite small, the available literature on this subject is quite encouraging, with results that place the choice of thermo ablation as a real alternative to be listed, with high accuracy, few and rare complications, and association with the quality of life of treated patients [4, 15, 22, 23].

Surgery to approach cervical metastases is, even today, the gold standard treatment, but thermo ablation has been increasingly used, mentioned, and considered as a therapeutic option [8, 24, 25].

Table 23.4 Mean characteristics of the studies involving patients who underwent thermal ablation for lymph node metastases in papillary thyroid carcinoma

Authors	Year	Location	Study design	Period	No. of patients (F/M)	Age	No. of lymph nodes	Follow-up time (month)
MWA								
Han et al.	2020	China	Retrospective	2015.6–2020.1	37 (20/17)	43.58 ± 13.77	98	11.09 ± 9.21
Zhou et al.	2018	China	Retrospective	2017.1–2018.4	14 (11/3)	45.1 ± 12.1	21	8.4 ± 4.1
Teng et al.	2018	China	Retrospective	2014.5–2015.6	11 (8/3)	40.36 ± 10.52	24	30.5 ± 8.7
Cao et al.	2020	China	Retrospective	2015.11–2018.11	14 (11/3)	46.9 ± 11.9	38	23.6 ± 9.3
Yue et al.	2015	China	Prospective	2010.10–2013.3	17 (14/3)	54.1 ± 13.6	23	13.1 ± 6
RFA								
Bake et al.	2011	Korea	Retrospective	2004.12–2018.6	10 (6/4)	43.2 ± 18	12	23 ± 5.5
Lim et al.	2014	Korea	Retrospective	2008.9–2012.4	39 (25/14)	52.8 ± 16.7	61	26.4 ± 13.7
Wang et al.	2014	China	Retrospective	2013.1–2014.8	8 (7/1)	43.6 ± 9.3	20	9.4 ± 5.1
Yan et al.	2021	Italy	Retrospective	2014.12–2018.3	5 (3/2)	15.6 ± 2.97	10	52 ± 21.4
Guang et al.	2017	China	Retrospective	2013.7–2014.8	33 (22/11)	43.7 ± 10.7	54	21 ± 4
Guang et al.	2018	China	Retrospective	2013.7–2014.8	45 (29/16)	41.5 ± 11.4	71	23 ± 5
LA								
Offi et al.	2021	Italy	Retrospective	2019.6–2020.12	10 (5/5)	40.2 ± 17.98	10	6
Papini et al.	2012	Italy	Prospective	2009.1–2010.12	5 (4/1)	53.6 ± 18.3	8	12
Mauri et al.	2016	Italy	Retrospective	2010.9–2013.12	24 (13/11)	62.3 ± 13.2	46	30 ± 11
Mauri et al.	2013	Italy	Prospective	2010.9–2012.4	15 (7/8)	62 ± 14	24	12
Guo et al.	2019	China	Retrospective	2016.6–2017.9	8 (5/3)	39 ± 11.6	18	12.8 ± 2.1
Zhang et al.	2017	China	Prospective	2014.1–2015.3	17 (14/3)	43.94 ± 10.5	21	17.86 ± 4.7

F/M female/male, *MWA* microwave ablation, *RFA* radiofrequency ablation, *LA* laser ablation
Adapted from [21]

Table 23.5 Procedural characteristics of the studies involving patients who underwent thermal ablation for lymph node metastases in papillary thyroid carcinoma

Authors	Year	Power (W) (range)	Ablation time (s) (range)
MWA			
Han et al.	2020	20 (mean)	206.55 (mean)
Zhou et al.	2018	35–40	30–190
Teng et al.	2018	20 (mean)	12–174
Cao et al.	2020	30 (mean)	10–685
Yue et al.	2015	40 (mean)	NA
RFA			
Bake et al.	2011	10–40	60–900
Lim et al.	2014	10–50	33–1200
Wang et al.	2014	20–35	30–360
Yan et al.	2021	3–6	98–263
Guang et al.	2017	3–5	25–447
Guang et al.	2018	3–5	25–479
LA			
Offi et al.	2021	3–4	270–420
Papini et al.	2012	NA	NA
Mauri et al.	2016	3–4	NA
Mauri et al.	2013	NA	NA
Guo et al.	2019	3–3.5	NA
Zhang et al.	2017	NA	NA

Adapted from [21]

23.3 Technical Details Associated with Thermal Ablation of Lymph Node Metastases

23.3.1 Anatomy

Lymph nodes of the head and neck are approximately 300 in number. About 30% of the total lymph nodes in the human body are in this topography. Regarding their distribution, cervical lymph nodes are divided according to a topographical reference.

They are classified into five levels (Fig. 23.1):

Level I: Corresponds to the areas of the submandibular (IA) and submental (IB) triangles.

Level II: Anterior to the internal jugular vein, superior.

Level III: Anterior to the internal jugular vein, median.

Level IV: Anterior to the internal jugular vein, inferior.

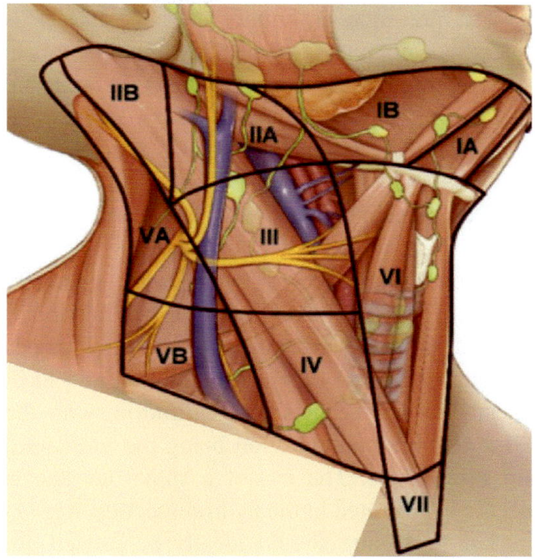

Fig. 23.1 Cervical lymph node levels

Level V: Lymph nodes in the topography of accessory nerve path, located in the posterior cervical region.

Level VI: Paratracheal and pre-tracheal, perithyroid and pre-cricoid lymph nodes.

Figure 23.1 shows the cervical lymph node levels with greater spatial clarity. Unlike what occurs in approach to thyroid nodules, in which "trans-isthmic" approach is preferable, in most cases in which we treat metastatic cervical lymph nodes by thermo ablation, the lateral approach is preferable, in most cases. As we can see, lymph nodes in more inferior topographies, such as levels IV and VII, as well as central, more caudal nodes, are technically more difficult to approach due to US-GUIDANCE, but not impossible. A careful assessment of cervical profile, whether shorter or longer, as well as a precise pre-procedure ultrasound assessment is mandatory.

Traditionally, it is assumed that carcinomas metastasize preferentially via the lymphatic route, while sarcomatous tumors do so via the hematogenous route. Most lesions metastasize to ipsilateral lymph nodes. More central lesions can, more frequently, produce bilateral lesions.

The presence of lymph node metastases is unequivocally one of the most essential factors in determining the survival of patients with thyroid cancer.

23.3.2 Materials

Ablation of cervical lymph nodes generally requires the same materials used in the ablation of thyroid nodules. We usually select 10 mL syringes for the instillation of glucose solution and local anesthetic and needles for infiltration, with the 30 × 0.7 mm configuration being the most used for infiltrations. The use of a spinal anesthesia needle is indicated in the hydrodissection stage.

The procedure should ideally be carried out under antisepsis and with protective fields. The option for antibiotic prophylaxis is individual, respecting group-by-group options. This author particularly appreciates the use.

Given the delicacy and training required by the procedure, the most recommended ablation probes are 0.5 cm and 0.7 cm active tips.

23.3.2.1 Technique and Access

The "Moving shot" technique has become an excellent method for treating thyroid gland nodules. In this technique, we move the ablation probe under close and precise visualization of the ultrasound transducer with the generator turned on, delivering heat.

Regarding the treatment of metastatic lymph nodes and focal lesions, however, this technique can sometimes be replaced by "Multiple shot"; that is, we do not use the classic movement of the probe in most lesions since it is of lesions often much smaller than thyroid nodules, significantly smaller than benign nodules eligible for ablation, and also due to the absence of adjacent thyroid parenchymal tissue, which can protect adjacent areas from the "owen effect" promoted at the surgical site.

Regarding access, given the erratic and often more lateralized distribution of metastatic lymph nodes, trans-isthmic access is often not used, or is used less in these cases. The lateral neck approach, usually with probe insertion lateral to the sternocleidomastoid muscle, is the most used, facilitating a precise approach and a shorter path to metastasis [26].

It is also important to mention the generator power used. Due to the reduced dimensions of the target lymph nodes and the different tissue response to thermal ablation in relation to other lesions, we usually choose to start with lower power than that used in benign nodules and progress, if necessary. In the cases of radiofrequency ablations, we usually start with 20 or 30 W.

An equally relevant factor in the thermal ablation of cervical metastatic lymph nodes is hydrodissection in terms of optimizing as much as possible the technical elements of protection for the most delicate structures, such as the recurrent laryngeal nerves associated with hoarseness in cases of injury, and of the vagal branches that border the common carotid arteries, thus avoiding complications such as the dreaded Horner's syndrome [27]. Hydrodissection in lymph node ablation differs substantially from that performed in treating thyroid nodules. Hydrodissection is essential and mandatory. However, excess fluid can excessively compress the target lymph node and sometimes make it impossible to visualize, especially when in a less favorable topography and with reduced dimensions (less than 1.0 cm).

23.4 Clinical Cases

23.4.1 Case #1

A 58-year-old male patient who underwent total thyroidectomy for a T1b N2 M0 papillary carcinoma, measuring 1.4 cm in the longest axis, with multiple microcalcifications, localized in the upper third of the right thyroid lobe, and also with another malignant nodule measuring 0.7 cm at the isthmus/left lobe transition (Figs. 23.2, 23.3, 23.4, and 23.5).

At initial imaging diagnosis, he presented two metastatic lymph nodes at level III on the right.

T0—Underwent total thyroidectomy with anterior lymph node resection.

2 years after thyroidectomy—First lymph node recurrence detected, levels VI and III on the

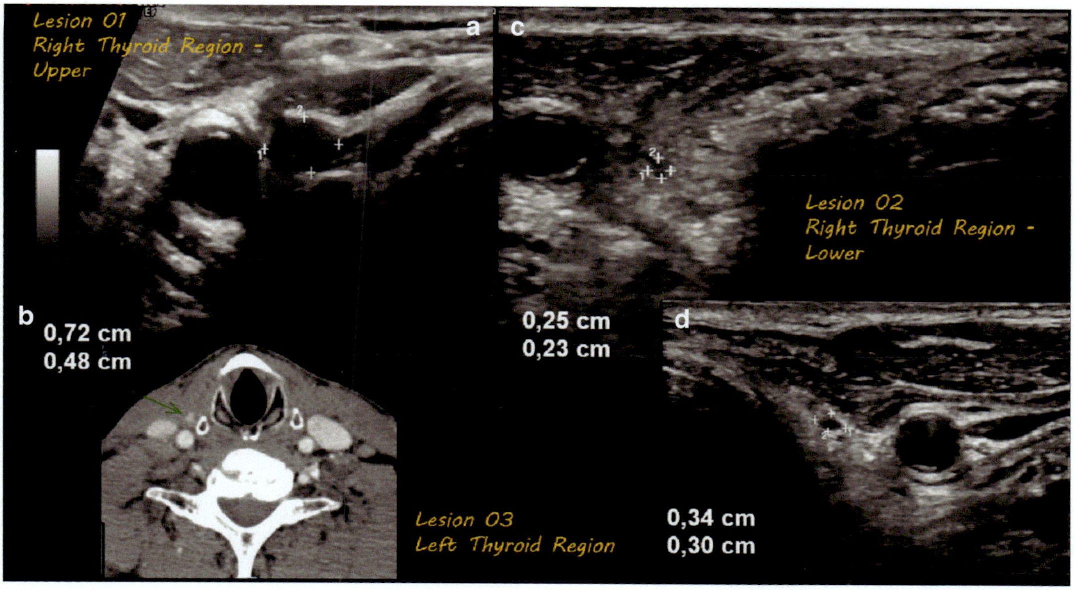

Fig. 23.2 (**a**) We can see the largest recurrence in the right thyroid bed in the upper left corner. Note the proximity to the medial aspect of the right common carotid artery. (**b**) We see the same lesion in a computed tomography image, axial section, with appreciable enhancement by iodinated contrast, showing that it is a well-vascularized lesion, which is an excellent marker in post-ablation follow-up. (**c**) We see the second metastatic lesion from the right thyroid pocket, significantly smaller than the ipsilateral lesion. (**d**) In the lower right quadrant, the third metastatic lesion from the left thyroid pocket

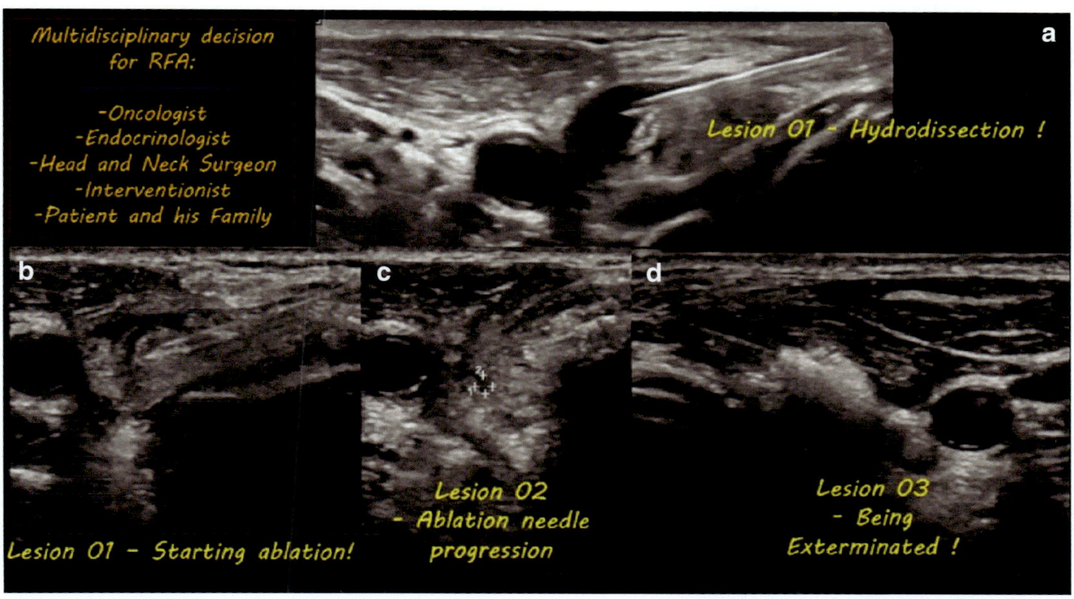

Fig. 23.3 (**a**) The spinal anesthesia needle is precisely positioned anterior to the larger lesion on the right side, performing anterior and lateral hydrodissection. We note that the target lesion is already reasonably far from the common carotid artery. (**b**) We notice the radiofrequency "probe" introduced in the middle of the larger lesion on the right side, starting the RFA. (**c** and **d**) An ablation "probe" was inserted into the lesion in the left thyroid region, which was already in the middle of the procedure. Note the large amount of gas bubbles originating from the ablation. Any inadvertent movement can cause us to lose our sense of reference in relation to the lesion, given its small size

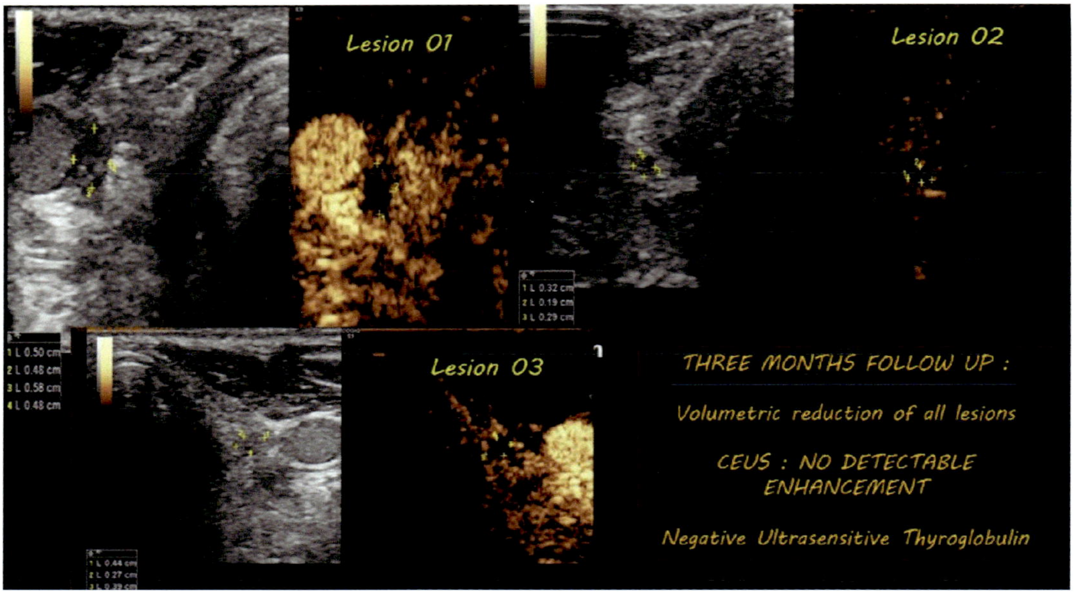

Fig. 23.4 The images above are part of the 3-month follow-up after ablative therapy. At this time, we chose to carry out control not only using B-mode US and Doppler, but also using microbubble contrast (CEUS—Contrast Enhanced Ultrasound), a useful tool once we deal with previously well-vascularized lesions. Note that none of the three lesions treated present, at the therapeutic site, appreciable enhancement by ultrasound contrast. It is important to point out that the areas evident in mode B correspond not only to the lesions, but to the lesions together with their safety margins, which was only possible due to the hydrodissection carried out previously

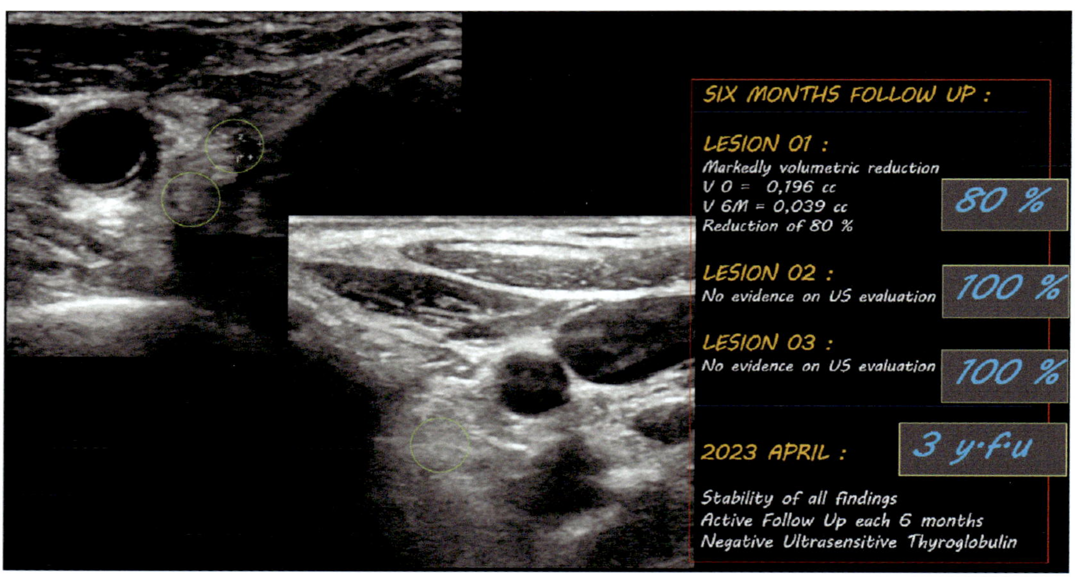

Fig. 23.5 Image control 6 months post-ablation. We noticed that the largest lesion presented an estimated volumetric reduction of 80% (previously with a volume of 0.196 cc and, in this control, with a volume of 0.039 cc). The remaining lesions disappeared (100% volumetric reduction). After 3 years of treatment, the patient remains without other suspicious lesions, asymptomatic, and with undetectable thyroglobulin

right. He underwent new surgery, with selective lymph node dissection.

5 years after thyroidectomy—Second recurrence (THIRD SURGERY). An extended lymph node resection.

8 years after thyroidectomy—Third recurrence. During a routine follow-up examination, three other cervical lymph nodes were identified with suspicious characteristics on ultrasound evaluation, all positive for metastatic malignancy on FNAB.

23.4.2 Case #2

Female patient, 24 years old.

T0—Underwent total thyroidectomy for a single papillary carcinoma, T1b N0 M0 on imaging and cytopathological diagnosis, with a cancer measuring 1.2 cm in the longest axis in the lower third of the right thyroid lobe (Figs. 23.6, 23.7, 23.8, and 23.9).

1.5 years after thyroidectomy—1 lymph node was detected on the right with confirmation of metastatic malignancy. The patient underwent enlarged lymph node resection on the right.

4 years after thyroidectomy—2 lymph nodes were detected on the right, confirming metastatic malignancy. The patient underwent a new lymphadenectomy.

8 years after thyroidectomy—Two new metastatic lymph nodes were detected, both at level IV on the right. Both lymph nodes showed a significant volumetric increase in the 6-month interval between diagnosis and ablative therapy. At the time of ablative treatment, they presented 1.9 cm and 1.3 cm in the longest axis, respectively, the largest and smallest lesion at level IV on the right.

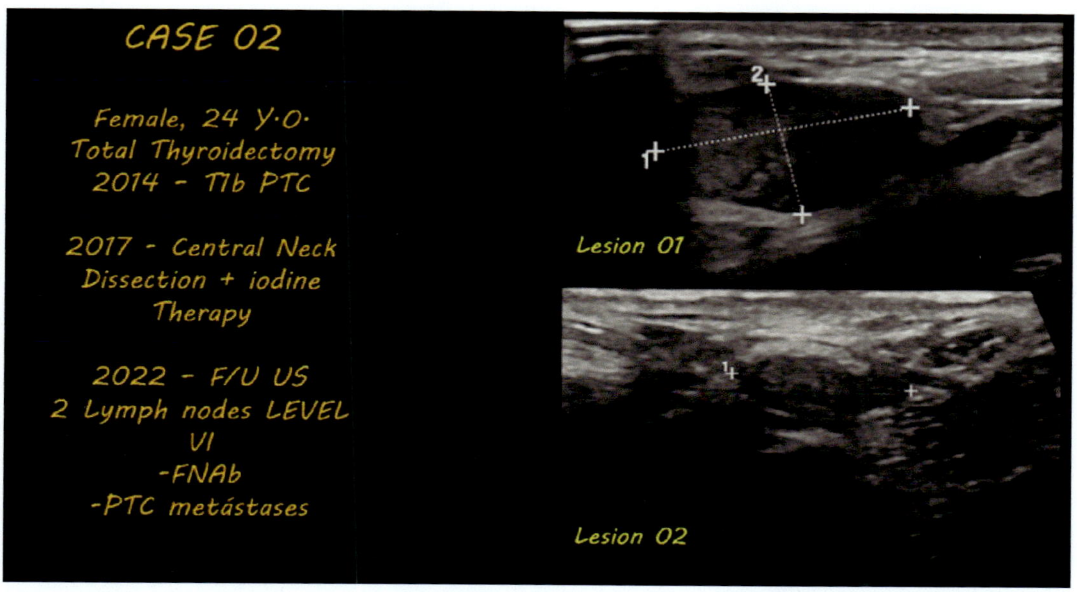

Fig. 23.6 Above, we observe two metastatic lymph nodes at level IV on the right, the largest measuring 1.9 cm on the longest axis, while the smallest measures 1.3 cm on the longest axis. These lymph nodes exhibit a globular shape with hilar suppression, cortical thickening, and the presence of intervening microcalcifications, which is a very typical appearance of thyroid carcinoma metastases

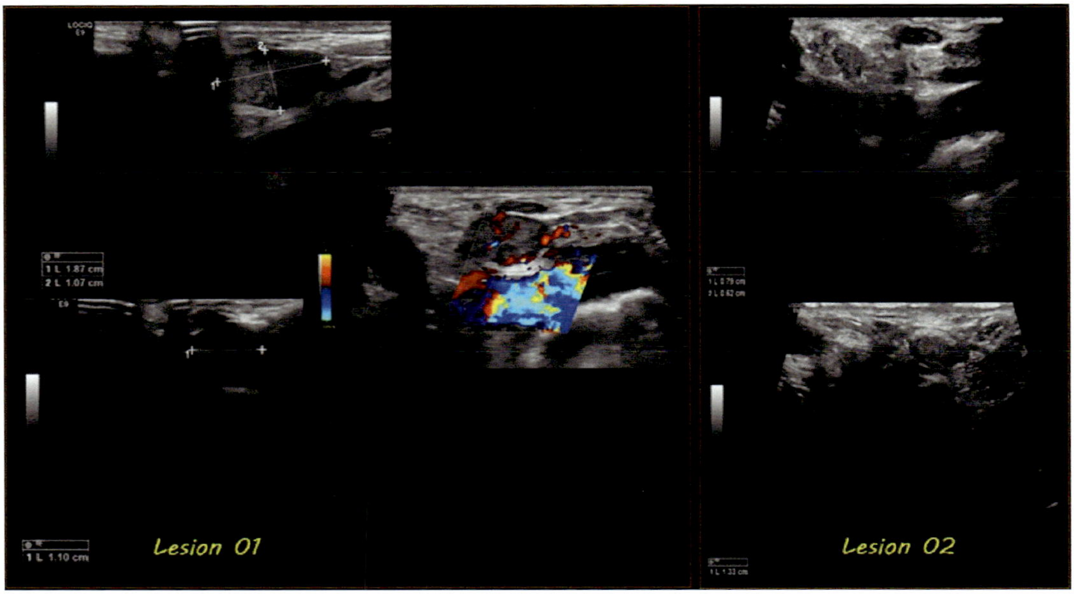

Fig. 23.7 Above, in addition to the measurements of the lymph nodes in the three axes, a central image with color Doppler also shows that these are well-vascularized metastases, which serves as a marker for the "END-POINT" of the ablation and for control ultrasound imaging

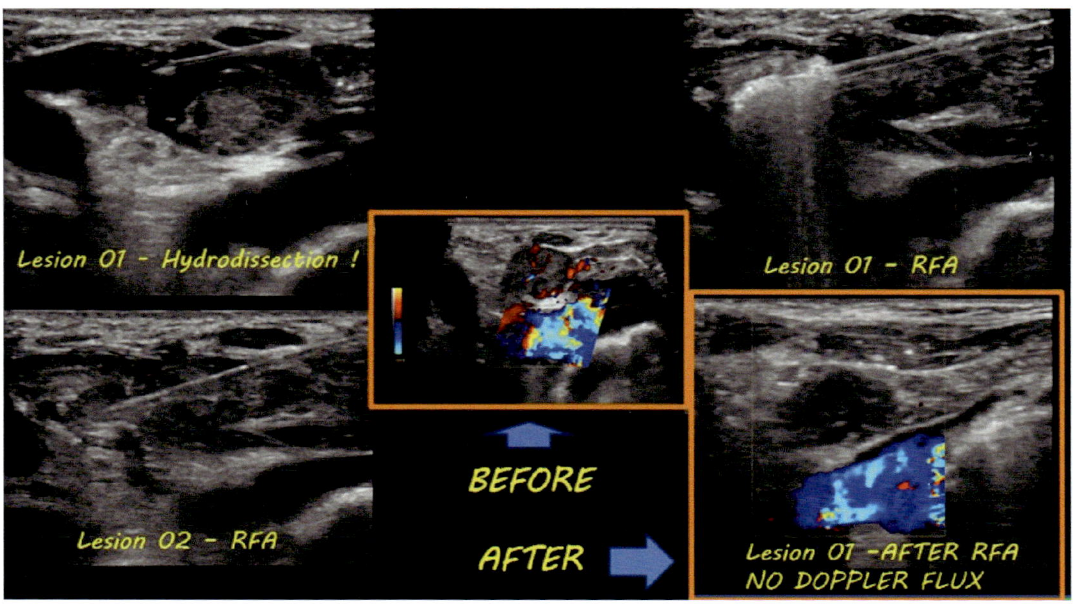

Fig. 23.8 In this image, we can see the generous hydrodissection carried out pre-ablation in the upper left corner. It was possible as it was a larger lesion. In the lower left corner, the ablation probe is positioned inside the largest lesion, in its central axis. In the upper right corner, we see the ablation in progress, with gas bubbles obscuring the ablative bed. In the lower right image, we see the largest treated lesion, completely without flow, which is the exact "END-POINT" of the ablation. We also noted, after the treated lesion, the proximity to the ipsilateral subclavian artery, which appears preserved and patent

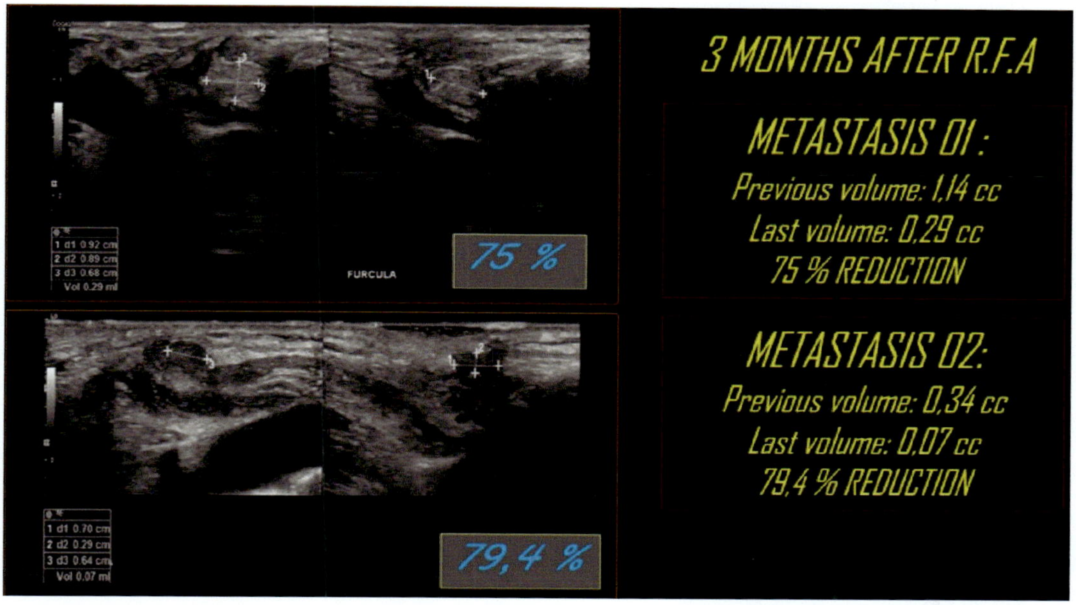

Fig. 23.9 After 3 months after ablative therapy, we observed no complications, and volumetric reductions were estimated at 75% for the larger lesion and 79.4% for the smaller lesion

23.4.3 Case #3

Male patient, 33 years old.

T0—Underwent total thyroidectomy for a single papillary carcinoma, T1a N0 M0 on imaging and cytopathological diagnosis in the middle third of the left thyroid lobe. Wide neck dissection was performed on the left (Figs. 23.10, 23.11, and 23.12).

1 year after thyroidectomy—1 lymph node was detected on the left, level III, globose, with microcalcifications and hilar suppression, measuring around 1.8 cm in the longest axis. The lymph above the node appeared, posteriorly bordering the left common carotid artery.

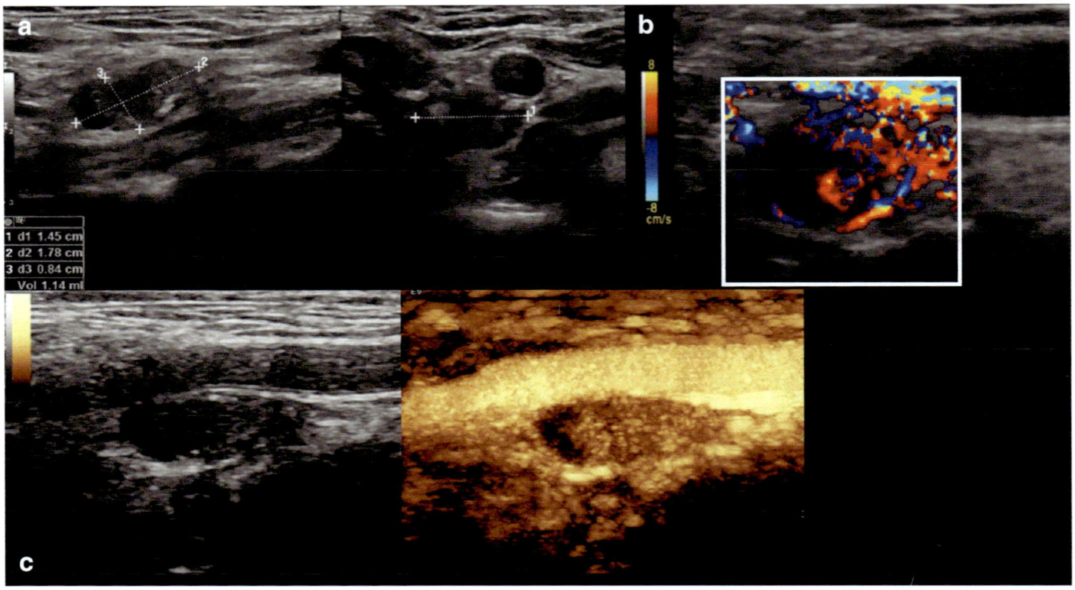

Fig. 23.10 Above, we can see, in the upper left image (**a**), the metastatic lymph node measuring approximately 1.8 cm in the longest axis, globose, calcified, with hilar suppression and slightly irregular contours. The lesion was posteriorly adjacent to the Left Common Carotid Artery (LCCA). Images **b** and **c** demonstrate the color Doppler evaluation, with exuberant flow on mapping, and the pre-procedure evaluation with CEUS, also demonstrating a well-vascularized lesion

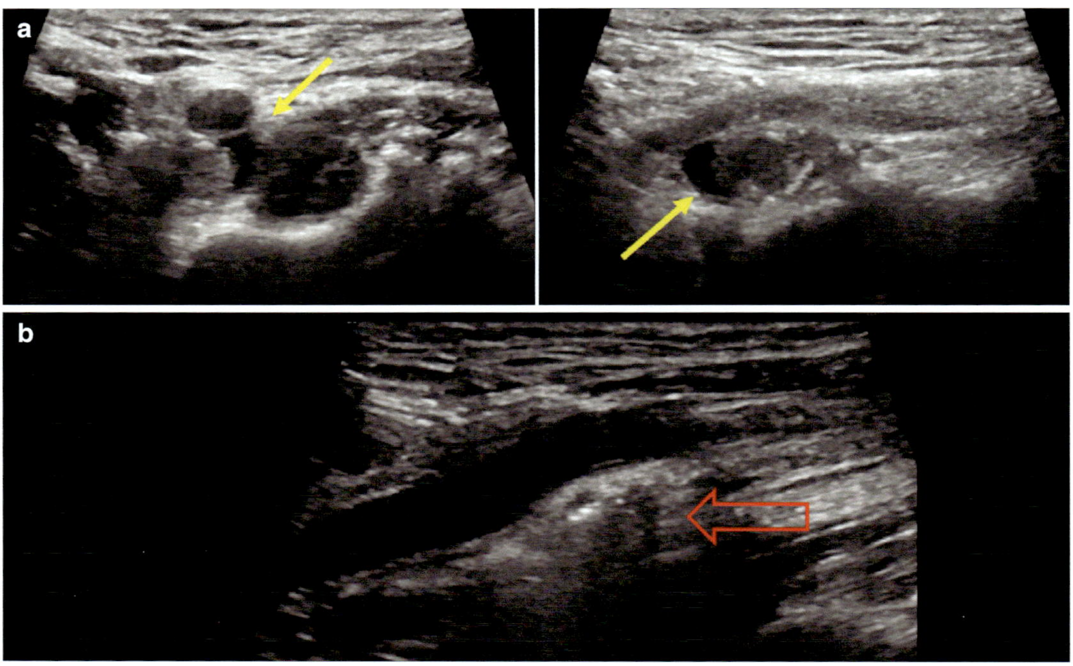

Fig. 23.11 In image **a**, we see the hydrodissection blades in the upper image. We achieved a reasonable separation on the lateral aspects, but we could not move the lymph node much further away from the LCCA. In image **b**, lower, we observe the immediate post-ablation "status," with gas bubbles occupying the ablation bed

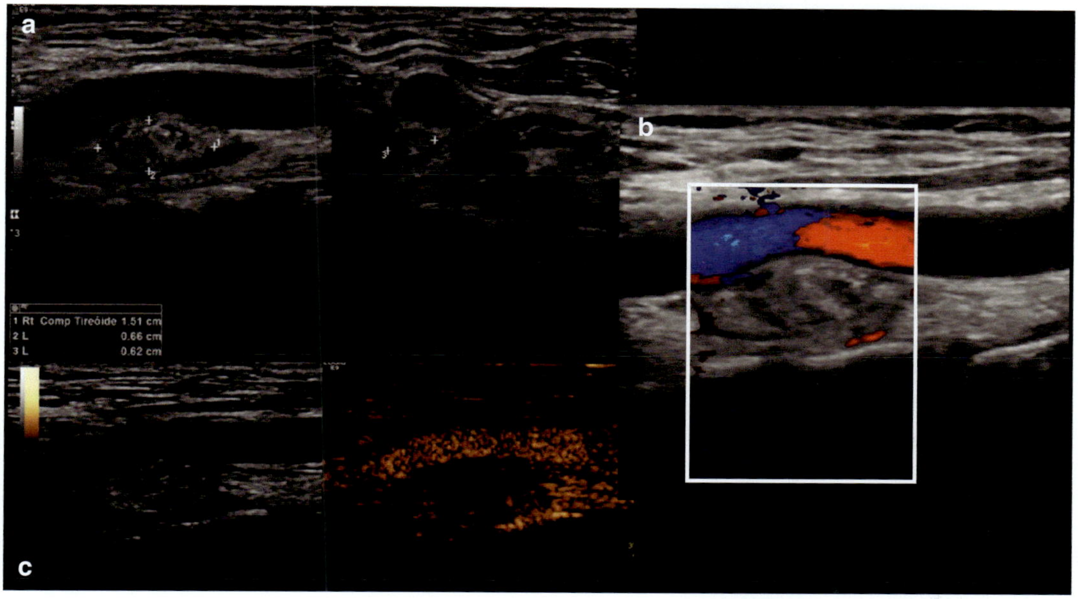

Fig. 23.12 Forty days after treatment, we observed a marked volumetric reduction in the treated lymph node, with a current volume of 0.28 cc (before it measured 1.14 cc—72% reduction) (**a**). Likewise, in image **b**, the absence of flow on color Doppler mapping is clear, as is the absence of enhancement on CEUS. Six months after ablative treatment, the patient has undetectable thyroglobulin, confirming the effectiveness of the treatment and without any symptoms (**c**)

23.5 Final Considerations

Thermal ablation applied to thyroid nodules, initially dedicated to symptomatic benign nodules and, currently, increasingly applied in the context of selected papillary carcinomas smaller than 1.0 cm (PTMCs), has been breaking paradigms regarding the treatment of thyroid nodules. In well-indicated cases, it provides preservation of the glandular parenchyma through a minimally invasive technique.

Regarding the application of thermal ablation in post-thyroidectomy cervical lymph node metastases, although surgical resection is still considered the gold standard treatment, it is increasingly considered in specific cases, especially in patients who have already undergone more than one surgical treatment. It could be an option to be offered to patients. Effective and safe, fast, without the need for general anesthesia, with discharge in a few hours, and early return to usual activities, in addition to providing treatment with excellent cost-effectiveness compared to the overall cost of surgery, ablation has a growing present and a promising future.

It is essential to point out the need for adequate training/specialization for doctors who wish to begin working in this area, even due to the unequivocal greater technical difficulty and precision of ablation in lymph node metastases compared to the technique in large benign nodules. The technique is different, as is the access and specific details in most cases.

As with all ablative treatments applied to the thyroid field, an adequate indication is the main key to successful treatment. New publications, with greater follow-ups and larger series, will certainly add a lot to the knowledge of the technique and may attract more enthusiasts. Perhaps, in the future, it will position itself as a more robust therapeutic alternative, effectively alongside conventional surgery.

References

1. Tarver T. Cancer facts & figures 2012. American Cancer Society (ACS): Atlanta: American Cancer Society, 2012. 66 p., pdf. http://www.cancer.org/Research/CancerFactsFigures/CancerFactsFigures/cancer-facts-figures-2012. J Consum Health Internet. 2012;16(3):366–367. https://doi.org/10.1080/15398285.2012.701177.
2. Eleanor W, Venessa T, Matti G. Patients electing active surveillance for low-risk papillary thyroid cancer have lower baseline anxiety. Clin Thyroidol. 2023;35(7):290–2.
3. Gharib H, Hegedüs L, Pacella CM, Baek JH, Papini E. Clinical review: nonsurgical, image-guided, minimally invasive therapy for thyroid nodules. J Clin Endocrinol Metab. 2013;98(10):3949–57. https://doi.org/10.1210/jc.2013-1806.
4. Lewis BD, Hay ID, Charboneau JW, McIver B, Reading CC, Goellner JR. Percutaneous ethanol injection for treatment of cervical lymph node metastases in patients with papillary thyroid carcinoma. AJR Am J Roentgenol. 2002;178(3):699–704. https://doi.org/10.2214/ajr.178.3.1780699.
5. Baek JH, Jeong HJ, Kim YS, Kwak MS, Lee D. Radiofrequency ablation for an autonomously functioning thyroid nodule. Thyroid. 2008;18(6):675–6. https://doi.org/10.1089/thy.2007.0274.
6. Jeong WK, Baek JH, Rhim H, Kim YS, Kwak MS, Jeong HJ, et al. Radiofrequency ablation of benign thyroid nodules: safety and imaging follow-up in 236 patients. Eur Radiol. 2008;18(6):1244–50. https://doi.org/10.1007/s00330-008-0880-6.
7. Choi Y, Jung SL. Efficacy and safety of thermal ablation techniques for the treatment of primary papillary thyroid microcarcinoma: a systematic review and meta-analysis. Thyroid. 2020;30(5):720–31. https://doi.org/10.1089/thy.2019.0707.
8. Monchik JM, Donatini G, Iannuccilli J, Dupuy DE. Radiofrequency ablation and percutaneous ethanol injection treatment for recurrent local and distant well-differentiated thyroid carcinoma. Ann Surg. 2006;244(2):296–304. https://doi.org/10.1097/01.sla.0000217685.85467.2d.
9. Ito Y, Miyauchi A. Active surveillance of low-risk papillary thyroid microcarcinomas. Gland Surg. 2020;9(5):1663–73. https://doi.org/10.21037/gs-2019-catp-03.
10. Kim JK, Kwon H, Lim W, Moon BI, Paik NS. Active surveillance of papillary thyroid cancer: past, present, and future. Ewha Med J. 2021;44(2):37–40.
11. Ntelis S, Linos D. Efficacy and safety of radiofrequency ablation in the treatment of low-risk papillary thyroid carcinoma: a review. Hormones (Athens). 2021;20(2):269–77. https://doi.org/10.1007/s42000-021-00283-5.
12. Lan Y, Luo Y, Zhang M, Jin Z, Xiao J, Yan L, et al. Quality of life in papillary thyroid microcarcinoma patients undergoing radiofrequency ablation or surgery: a comparative study. Front Endocrinol (Lausanne). 2020;11:249. https://doi.org/10.3389/fendo.2020.00249.
13. Rahal Junior A, Falsarella PM, Mendes GF, Hidal JT, Andreoni DM, Lúcio JFF, et al. Percutaneous laser ablation of benign thyroid nodules: a one year follow-up study. Einstein (Sao Paulo). 2018;16(4):eAO4279. https://doi.org/10.31744/einstein_journal/2018AO4279.
14. Russ G, Ben Hamou A, Poirée S, Ghander C, Ménégaux F, Leenhardt L, Buffet C. Learning curve for radiofrequency ablation of benign thyroid nodules. Int J Hyperthermia. 2021;38(1):55–64. https://doi.org/10.1080/02656736.2021.1871974.
15. Guenette JP, Monchik JM, Dupuy DE. Image-guided ablation of postsurgical locoregional recurrence of biopsy-proven well-differentiated thyroid carcinoma. J Vasc Interv Radiol. 2013;24(5):672–9. https://doi.org/10.1016/j.jvir.2013.02.001.
16. Loh KC, Greenspan FS, Gee L, Miller TR, Yeo PP. Pathological tumor-node-metastasis (pTNM) staging for papillary and follicular thyroid carcinomas: a retrospective analysis of 700 patients. J Clin Endocrinol Metab. 1997;82(11):3553–62. https://doi.org/10.1210/jcem.82.11.4373.
17. Alesina PF, Rolfs T, Hommeltenberg S, Hinrichs J, Meier B, Mohmand W, et al. Intraoperative neuromonitoring does not reduce the incidence of recurrent laryngeal nerve palsy in thyroid reoperations: results of a retrospective comparative analysis. World J Surg. 2012;36(6):1348–53. https://doi.org/10.1007/s00268-012-1548-6.
18. Esnaola NF, Cantor SB, Sherman SI, Lee JE, Evans DB. Optimal treatment strategy in patients with papillary thyroid cancer: a decision analysis. Surgery. 2001;130(6):921–30. https://doi.org/10.1067/msy.2001.118370.
19. Farahati J, Reiners C, Stuschke M, Müller SP, Stüben G, Sauerwein W, et al. Differentiated thyroid cancer. Impact of adjuvant external radiotherapy in patients with perithyroidal tumor infiltration (stage pT4). Cancer. 1996;77(1):172–80. https://doi.org/10.1002/(SICI)1097-0142(19960101)77:1<172::AID-CNCR28>3.0.CO;2-1.
20. Rondeau G, Fish S, Hann LE, Fagin JA, Tuttle RM. Ultrasonographically detected small thyroid bed nodules identified after total thyroidectomy for differentiated thyroid cancer seldom show clinically significant structural progression. Thyroid. 2011;21(8):845–53. https://doi.org/10.1089/thy.2011.0011.
21. Tang W, Tang X, Jiang D, Zhang X, Wang R, Niu X, et al. Safety and efficacy of thermal ablation for cervical metastatic lymph nodes in papillary thyroid carcinoma: a systematic review and meta-analysis. Front Endocrinol (Lausanne). 2022;13:967044. https://doi.org/10.3389/fendo.2022.967044.

22. Volpi E, Rahal A. Thermal ablation therapies: a reasonable alternative for patients with lymph node metastases of recurrent papillary thyroid cancer. Clin Thyroidol. 2023;35(2):64–6.
23. Rubino C, de Vathaire F, Dottorini ME, Hall P, Schvartz C, Couette JE, et al. Second primary malignancies in thyroid cancer patients. Br J Cancer. 2003;89(9):1638–44. https://doi.org/10.1038/sj.bjc.6601319.
24. Park KW, Shin JH, Han BK, Ko EY, Chung JH. Inoperable symptomatic recurrent thyroid cancers: preliminary result of radiofrequency ablation. Ann Surg Oncol. 2011;18(9):2564–8. https://doi.org/10.1245/s10434-011-1619-1.
25. Zhao Q, Tian G, Kong D, Jiang T. Meta-analysis of radiofrequency ablation for treating the local recurrence of thyroid cancers. J Endocrinol Invest. 2016;39(8):909–16. https://doi.org/10.1007/s40618-016-0450-8.
26. Wang W, Zhang Z, Zhao Y, Xue W, Xia F, Li X. Management of lateral multiple-level metastasis in N1b papillary thyroid microcarcinoma. Front Oncol. 2020;10:1586. https://doi.org/10.3389/fonc.2020.01586.
27. Souza KP, Rahal A Jr, Volpi EM, Falsarella PM, Hidal JT, Andreoni DM, Francisco-Neto MJ, Queiroz MRG, Garcia RG. Hydrodissection and programmed stop sedation in 100% of benign thyroid nodules treated with radiofrequency ablation. Eur J Radiol. 2020;133:109354. https://doi.org/10.1016/j.ejrad.2020.109354.

24 Intrathoracic Goiter RFA

Turtulici Giovanni and Orlandi Davide

24.1 Introduction

Thyroid nodules are abnormal growths of tissue within the thyroid gland, which is located in the front of the neck. These nodules can be solid or cystic and often develop without causing obvious symptoms. However, in some cases, they can cause issues such as pain, difficulty swallowing, or changes in voice. Most thyroid nodules are benign, but it is crucial to exclude the possibility of thyroid cancer through accurate diagnostic tests and cytological/histological biopsies [1].

Traditional treatment options for thyroid nodules include:

24.1.1 Watchful Waiting

If the nodules are small, asymptomatic, and do not show signs of malignancy, the physician may recommend periodic monitoring without treatment.

24.1.2 Hormone Therapy

For nodules associated with thyroid function problems, hormonal medications may be prescribed to control their growth.

T. Giovanni (✉) · O. Davide
Department of Radiology, Ospedale Evangelico Internazionale, Genoa, Italy

24.1.3 Radioactive Iodine Therapy

This treatment is primarily used for thyroid cancer.

24.1.4 Surgical Removal

In cases where nodules have a cytological/histological diagnosis of malignancy, grow rapidly, or cause significant symptoms, such as tracheal compression that sometimes narrows significantly in elderly individuals, surgical removal of the thyroid or part of it is often recommended. In these situations, surgery was traditionally considered the only possible option. However, it presents risks, including scarring, post-operative complications such as recurrent nerve injury, and the need to take thyroid hormones for life after full thyroid removal. Additionally, not all patients are ideal candidates for surgery, particularly those with pre-existing medical conditions or frailty [2].

Today, with the advent of reducible percutaneous treatments [3–8], it is possible to reduce nodules volume using thermal (laser, radiofrequency, and cryoablation) or ultrasonic (HIFU) percutaneous techniques to eliminate associated symptoms, thus representing a valid alternative.

These minimally invasive procedures have been developed to offer an alternative to traditional surgery and involve the prior preparation of the patient, who undergoes a detailed

R. Valcavi et al. (eds.), *Thyroid Ablation*, https://doi.org/10.1007/978-3-031-88229-6_24

evaluation of the thyroid through ultrasound and/or other imaging tests to confirm the presence and size of the nodules.

Subsequently, local anesthesia is administered to ensure the patient's comfort during the procedure.

During the ablation, the physician uses ultrasound to guide the ablation needle to the thyroid nodule, ensuring excellent precision in delivering the treatment, during which the use of thermal energy destroys the interior of the nodular tissue, significantly reducing its size (Figs. 24.1 and 24.2).

Since radiofrequency ablation is minimally invasive, most patients can return to their normal daily activities within a few hours or days after the procedure.

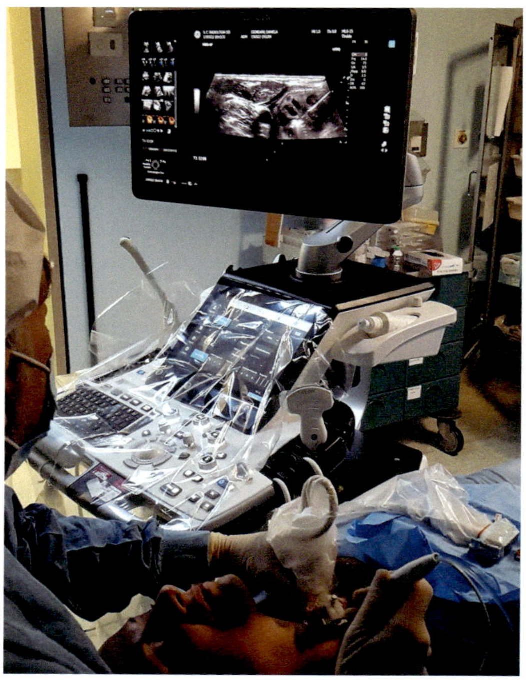

Fig. 24.1 Surgery room setup for RF ablation of a thyroid nodule. Note the needle guide mounted on the ultrasound probe, the RF needle with electromagnetic position sensors, and the electromagnetic generator. On the ultrasound screen, the operator can see the thyroid nodule and have a real-time tracking of the needle tip

In the case of giant nodules and goiters with a retrojugular and substernal attitude, it is not always easy to perform a proper ultrasound guidance of the treatment while respecting the margins and avoiding damage to the anatomical structures that run in the lower neck lodge [5, 9–11].

To this end, both surgical and percutaneous ablation treatment planning for thyroid goiters with substernal development require a prior computed tomography (CT) scan to assess the correct anatomical relationships with the neck and mediastinal structures [9, 11].

When opting for percutaneous ablation treatment for thyroid goiters with substernal development, it is necessary to use specific techniques that allow the procedure to be safely completed. To this end, several operators have adopted specific techniques, ranging from the simple use of low-frequency convex probes that allow better visualization of deep soft tissues; ablative techniques performed in two stages (3–6 months apart) such as the iceberg technique described by Rahal in 2023 [12]; and finally, the use of technologically advanced equipment such as fusion imaging and virtual tracking, which allow monitoring the path of the needle even in situations where ultrasound does not provide adequate imaging [13, 14].

In our opinion, even using low-frequency convex probes with lateral trapezoidal vision, it is not always possible to safely perform this treatment because it is not always possible to monitor the margins of the nodule with absolute certainty, avoiding thermal damage to adjacent structures (vascular nerve bundle, esophagus, and trachea) [10, 15, 16].

Regarding the iceberg technique, it must be considered that, although it provides good results in a significant percentage of patients, it involves a significant increase in costs (ablation scheduled in two different stages with the consequent need to use two different ablation needles) and also the elevation of the nodule after the first treatment is not always sufficient to allow a subsequent com-

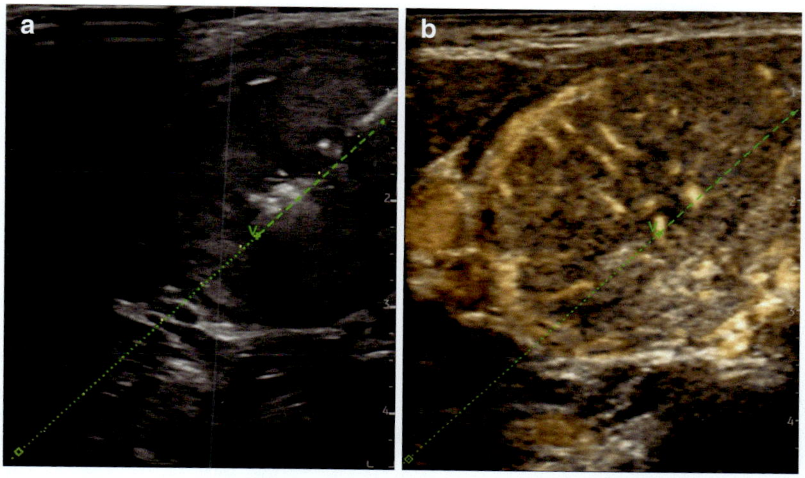

Fig. 24.2 Transverse ultrasound (US) image indicating radiofrequency (RF) ablation performed with the "moving shot" technique using a 18-gauge, 150 mm, fixed RF electrode (STARmed, Korea). (**a**) RF ablation. The virtual track is displayed in green. The RF electrode active tip is graphically displayed as a green cross near the "V" and is partially hided by gas bubbles produced in the ablation process. (**b**) Corresponding microvascular nodule imaging obtained using a 6–15 MHz ML-6-15 linear probe, GE Healthcare, USA

plete ablation of the more caudal nodular portion.

Following these considerations, it would be desirable to fuse information from different imaging modalities, combining the panoramic views and the elevated anatomical detail of CT with the ease of use and high availability of ultrasound. Nowadays, this is possible using newer fusion imaging techniques as recently described by Orlandi et al. in 2022 [11].

In this published series, the combination of US-CT fusion imaging with virtual needle tracking (VT) systems allowed a thorough visualization of the whole nodule and improved monitoring of RF electrode tip during the ablation, reducing inaccurate RF electrode placements due to poor needle visualization, gas bubbles produced by the ablation, and radiofrequency artifacts. The use of such devices also enables RF electrode placements with an out-of-plane approach that may be required in some cases (Fig. 24.3). Moreover, despite the potential higher risk of percutaneous ablation of substernal nodules presented in this series, thanks to the increased safety given by the combination of fusion imaging and virtual tracking, it showed a low adverse event rate without any major complication.

In conclusion, as recently stated by an international multidisciplinary consensus [17], minimally invasive percutaneous ablation and related ultrasound-guided ablation technologies should be considered a safe and valuable treatment options for thyroid nodules, also in challenging conditions such as substernal goiters.

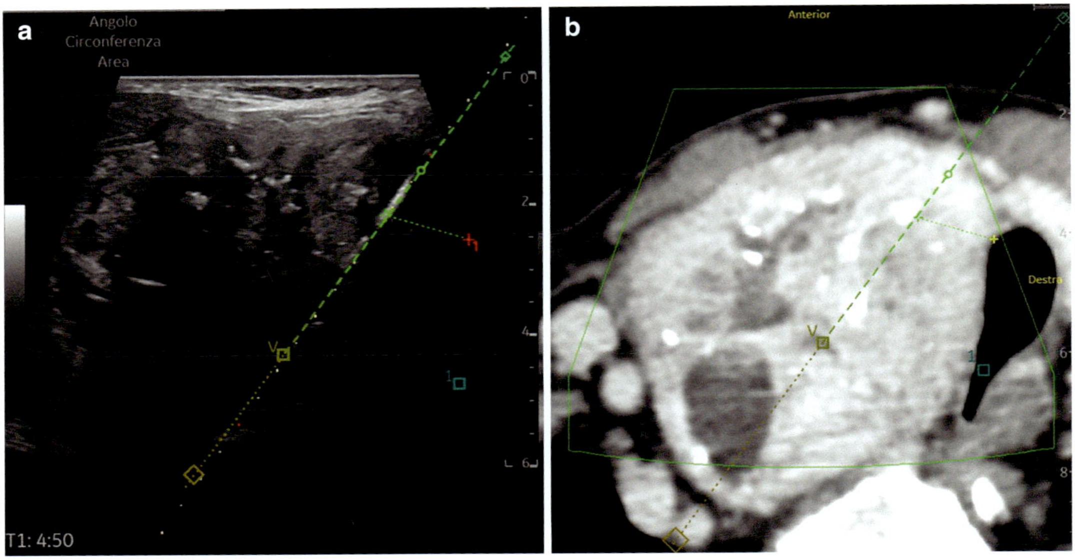

Fig. 24.3 US image (**a**) and corresponding CT scan (**b**) of radiofrequency (RF) ablation of a large thyroid nodule that dislocates laterally the trachea. Note the accuracy point at the lateral margin of the trachea used to synchronize US with TC images

References

1. Gharib H, Papini E, Garber JR, Duick DS, Harrell RM, Hegedüs L, et al. American association of Clinical Endocrinologists, American college of endocrinology, and Associazione Medici Endocrinologi medical guidelines for clinical practice for the diagnosis and management of thyroid nodules—2016 update. Endocr Pract. 2016;22(5):622–39. https://doi.org/10.4158/EP161208.GL.
2. Brenet E, Dubernard X, Mérol JC, Louges MA, Labrousse M, Makeieff M. Assessment and management of cervico-mediastinal goiter. Eur Ann Otorhinolaryngol Head Neck Dis. 2017;134(6):409–13. https://doi.org/10.1016/j.anorl.2017.06.001.
3. Felício JS, Conceição AM, Santos FM, Sato MM, Bastos Fde A, Braga de Souza AC, et al. Ultrasound-guided laser thermal ablation for treatment of benign thyroid nodules. Endocr Pract. 2004;10(3):276–83. https://doi.org/10.4158/EP.10.3.276.
4. Pacella CM, Mauri G, Achille G, Barbaro D, Bizzarri G, De Feo P, et al. Outcomes and risk factors for complications of laser ablation for thyroid nodules: a multicenter study on 1531 patients. J Clin Endocrinol Metab. 2015;100(10):3903–10. https://doi.org/10.1210/jc.2015-1964.
5. Baek JH, Lee JH, Valcavi R, Pacella CM, Rhim H, Na DG. Thermal ablation for benign thyroid nodules: radiofrequency and laser. Korean J Radiol. 2011;12(5):525–40. https://doi.org/10.3348/kjr.2011.12.5.525.
6. Papini E, Monpeyssen H, Frasoldati A, Hegedüs L. 2020 European thyroid association clinical practice guideline for the use of image-guided ablation in benign thyroid nodules. Eur Thyroid J. 2020;9(4):172–85. https://doi.org/10.1159/000508484.
7. Lang BH, Wu ALH. High intensity focused ultrasound (HIFU) ablation of benign thyroid nodules—a systematic review. J Ther Ultrasound. 2017;5:11. https://doi.org/10.1186/s40349-017-0091-1.
8. Cheng Z, Liang P. Advances in ultrasound-guided thermal ablation for symptomatic benign thyroid nodules. Adv Clin Exp Med. 2020;29(9):1123–9. https://doi.org/10.17219/acem/125433.
9. Mauri G, Monfardini L, Della Vigna P, Montano F, Bonomo G, Buccimazza G, et al. Real-time US-CT fusion imaging for guidance of thermal ablation in of renal tumors invisible or poorly visible with US: results in 97 cases. Int J Hyperth. 2021;38(1):771–6. https://doi.org/10.1080/02656736.2021.1923837.
10. Baek JH, Lee JH, Sung JY, Bae JI, Kim KT, Sim J, et al. Complications encountered in the treatment of benign thyroid nodules with us-guided radiofrequency ablation: a multicenter study. Radiology. 2012;262(1):335–42. https://doi.org/10.1148/radiol.11110416.
11. Orlandi D, Viglino U, Dedone G, Leale G, Caruso P, Mauri G, et al. US-CT fusion-guided percutaneous radiofrequency ablation of large substernal benign thyroid nodules. Int J Hyperth. 2022;39(1):847–54. https://doi.org/10.1080/02656736.2022.2091167.
12. Junior AR, Volpi EM, Schmid BP, Falsarella PM, Garcia RG. The iceberg technique: an innovative

approach for radiofrequency ablation of diving thyroid nodules. Diagn Interv Radiol. 2023;29(4):628–31. https://doi.org/10.4274/dir.2022.221467.
13. Turtulici G, Orlandi D, Corazza A, Sartoris R, Derchi LE, Silvestri E, et al. Percutaneous radiofrequency ablation of benign thyroid nodules assisted by a virtual needle tracking system. Ultrasound Med Biol. 2014;40(7):1447–52. https://doi.org/10.1016/j.ultrasmedbio.2014.02.017.
14. Mauri G, Gennaro N, de Beni S, Ierace T, Goldberg SN, Rodari M, et al. Real-time US-18 FDG-PET/CT image fusion for guidance of thermal ablation of 18 FDG-PET-positive liver metastases: the added value of contrast enhancement-enhanced ultrasound CT computed tomography 18 FDG-PET 18 fluorodeoxyglucose positron emission tomography MRI magnetic resonance imaging PET positron emission tomography. Cardiovasc Intervent Radiol. 2019;42(1):60–8. https://doi.org/10.1007/s00270-018-2082-1.
15. Ju Ha E, Hwan Baek J, Hyun Lee J, Kim JK, Shong YK. Clinical significance of vagus nerve variation in radiofrequency ablation of thyroid nodules. Eur Radiol. 2011;21(10):2151–7. https://doi.org/10.1007/s00330-011-2167-6.
16. Park JK, Jeong SY, Lee J-H, Lim GC, Chang JW. Variations in the course of the cervical Vagus nerve on thyroid ultrasonography. AJNR Am J Neuroradiol. 2011;32(7):1178–81. https://doi.org/10.3174/ajnr.A2476.
17. Orloff LA, Noel JE, Stack BC Jr, Russell MD, Angelos P, Baek JH, et al. Radiofrequency ablation and related ultrasound-guided ablation technologies for treatment of benign and malignant thyroid disease: an international multidisciplinary consensus statement of the American Head and Neck Society Endocrine Surgery Section with the Asia Pacific Society of Thyroid Surgery, Associazione Medici Endocrinologi, British Association of Endocrine and Thyroid Surgeons, European Thyroid Association, Italian Society of Endocrine Surgery Units, Korean Society of Thyroid Radiology, Latin American Thyroid Society, and Thyroid Nodules Therapies Association. Head Neck. 2022;44(3):633–60. https://doi.org/10.1002/hed.26960.

25 Patient Follow-Up After Thermal Ablation

Mary Elizabeth Cunnane, Marika D. Russell, and Lisa A. Orloff

25.1 Introduction

Thermal ablation of benign thyroid nodules results in a gradual decrease in the size of the nodule over the course of a year or more. During this time, patients require ongoing follow-up to monitor the response to treatment. This should include assessment for complications, evaluation of treatment efficacy, and consideration of further intervention to achieve therapeutic goals. In this chapter, we will discuss factors to evaluate during follow-up, features which predict long-term success and different approaches to retreatment.

There are multiple published guidelines on thermal ablation [1–6] (see Table 25.1), and most guidelines set the first follow-up appointment at 1–3 months, followed by 6-month and 1-year appointments. All recommend clinical and ultrasonographic evaluation, and many also recommend biochemical evaluation.

M. E. Cunnane (✉)
Department of Radiology, Massachusetts Eye and Ear, Boston, MA, USA
e-mail: marybeth_cunnane@meei.harvard.edu

M. D. Russell
Department of Otolaryngology-Head & Neck Surgery, Massachusetts Eye and Ear, Boston, MA, USA
e-mail: mrussell20@meei.harvard.edu

L. A. Orloff
Department of Otolaryngology-Head & Neck Surgery, Stanford University School of Medicine, Stanford, CA, USA
e-mail: Lorloff@standford.edu

R. Valcavi et al. (eds.), *Thyroid Ablation*, https://doi.org/10.1007/978-3-031-88229-6_25

Table 25.1 Summary of follow-up recommendations in published guidelines on radiofrequency ablation of benign non-functioning thyroid nodules

Author	Timing of follow-up in first year	Timing of follow-up after first year	Components of clinical follow-up	Radiographic follow-up	Laboratory tests	Metric of volume change
Kim 2018 [1]	Not specified	Not specified	Symptom score, cosmetic score	US	TSH, T3, T4	VRR
Dobnig 2020 [2]	3, 12 months	1–2 years	ENT exam of vocal cord status at 3 months	US	TSH, fT3, fT4, TPOAB, TGAB	None specified
Papini 2020 [3]	3, 6, 12 months	1–2 years	Not specified	US	At least TSH	None specified
Ha, 2021 [4]	1, 6, 12 months	Every 6–12 months	Symptom score, cosmetic score	US	None	VRR
Orloff 2022 [5]	3, 6, 12 months	Long term f/u recommended; timing not specified	Symptom score, cosmetic score	US (CT or MRI considered at 12 months if necessary based on location/size)	TSH at 3–6 and 12 months	VRR
Sinclair 2023 [6]	1–3, 6, 12 months	Not specified	Documented laryngeal exam if contralateral procedure planned	US	At 1 month for patients with hypo- or hyperthyroid symptoms	VRR

25.2 Clinical Exam

Clinical follow-up should include a review of systems with particular attention to an update in the symptoms for which the patient originally sought out thyroid ablation. Clinical examination of the patient, including a detailed history, should evaluate for change in voice, particularly at the first follow-up visit. If there are any changes in vocal quality, laryngoscopy should be performed for assessment of vocal fold mobility. In addition, if there are plans for future treatment of a contralateral nodule, laryngoscopy is prudent as vocal fold paresis can be occult on assessment of voice [7]. At the time of clinical follow-up, symptom scores (1–10 on a visual analog scale) and cosmetic scores (1, no palpable mass; 2, invisible palpable mass; 3, mass visible to experienced clinician; 4, easily visible mass) allow quantitative tracking of clinical progress [8]. A validated thyroid ablation-specific quality of life survey is not yet available but development of such an instrument has been proposed.

Nodule rupture is a rare complication of thermal ablation which can present between 2 weeks and 3 months or more following ablation. Patients typically present with neck pain and a bulging mass (Fig. 25.1). Ultrasound shows abnormal soft tissue extending from the nodule into the extrathyroidal space, most commonly into the anterior strap muscles [9, 10] (Fig. 25.2). Fistulization through the skin can occur (Fig. 25.3). These patients are often treated with analgesics and observation and sometimes antibiotics, though typically the fluid collections are culture negative [11]. Rarely, aspiration or incisional drainage may be necessary to resolve the inflammatory change [9] (Fig. 25.4).

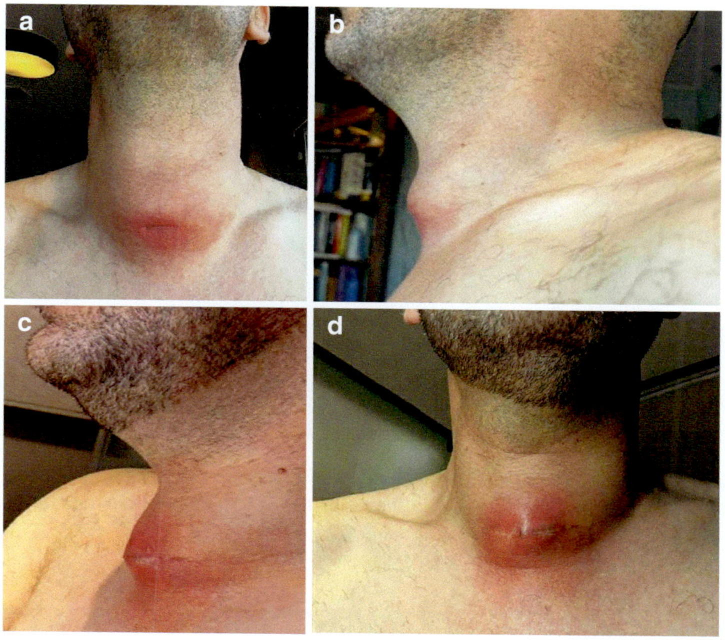

Fig. 25.1 Early presentation of nodule rupture: (**a**) A 50-year-old male who had undergone prior contralateral thyroid lobectomy underwent RFA of a 6.3 × 3.2 × 6.4 cm solid benign nodule. He presented on postoperative day 20. (**a**) Clinical photo in AP view demonstrates skin erythema surrounding the needle entry site, within the prior thyroidectomy scar. (**b**) Lateral clinical photo shows bulging of the nodule and overlying erythema. (**c**) AP view on postoperative day 31 and (**d**) lateral view on postoperative day 31 show progressive erythema and bulging

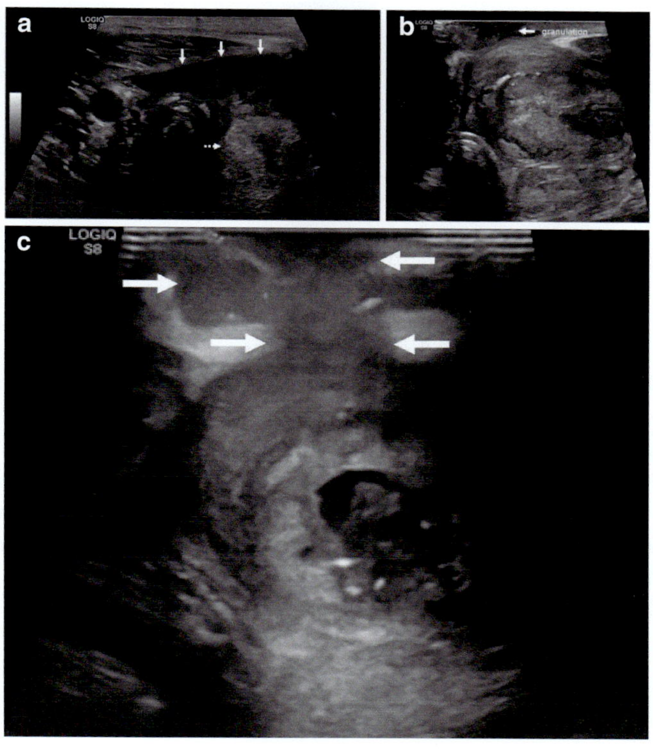

Fig. 25.2 Ultrasound of nodule rupture: (**a**) transverse image demonstrates left thyroid nodule (dotted arrow), the patient is status-post right hemithyroidectomy. Hypoechoic soft tissue (solid arrows) extends from the left nodule anteriorly into the extrathyroidal space, including strap muscles. (**b** and **c**) Transverse US images performed later in the course demonstrate hypoechoic granulation tissue which has extended to the skin (arrows)

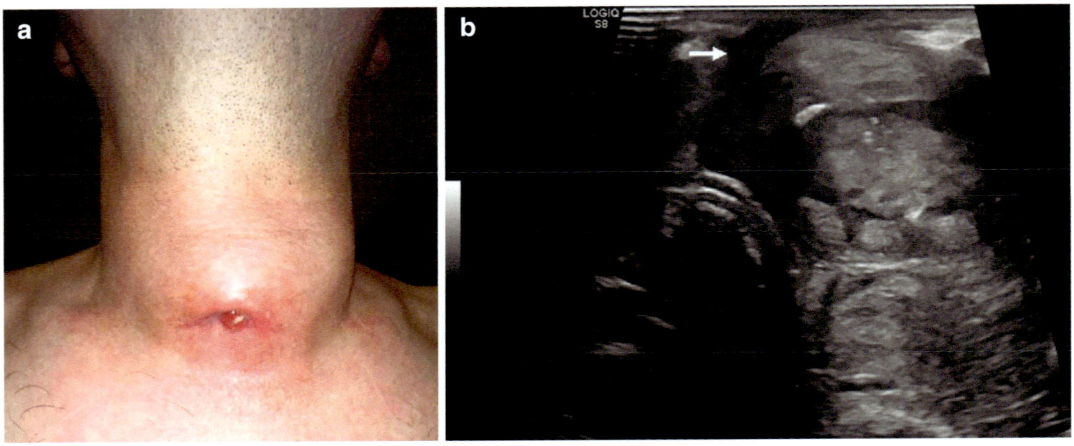

Fig. 25.3 Fistulization through skin: (**a**) clinical photograph demonstrates a fistula through the skin within the hemithyroidectomy scar as well as some granulation tissue at the skin surface. (**b**) Ultrasound also demonstrates the fistula as a hypoechoic tract (*arrows*)

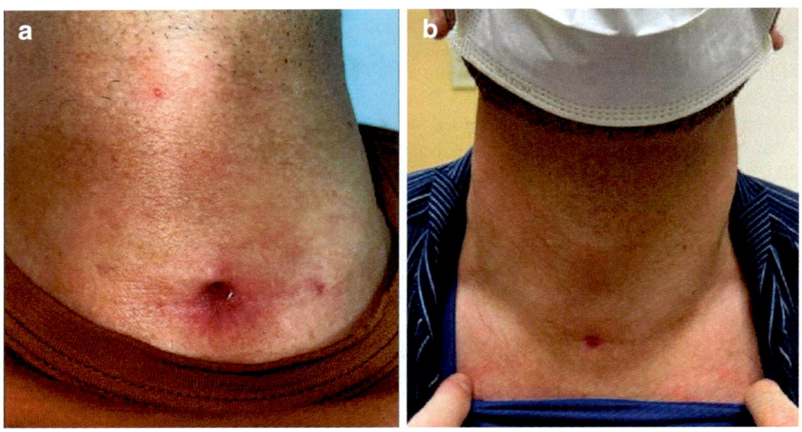

Fig. 25.4 (**a**) Clinical photograph demonstrates a sealed fistula tract with residual granulation tissue. (**b**) Clinical photograph 1 year post-procedure demonstrates a healed/epithelialized fistula. Ultimate VRR was 71%

25.3 Biochemical Evaluation

While alterations in thyroid function are uncommon following thermal ablation for non-functioning thyroid nodules, both hypothyroidism and hyperthyroidism can occur [12–14]. Many guidelines recommend at least a serum TSH in follow-up. If biochemical evaluation is not performed, the practitioner should be alert for signs and symptoms of thyroid dysfunction at the clinical exam. Patients with autonomously functioning thyroid nodules should have more thorough biochemical evaluation and be managed by an endocrinologist. Since these patients have often been prescribed thionamides, and a main goal of ablation is to restore normal thyroid function, follow-up is important for titration and potential weaning off thionamide therapy.

25.4 Ultrasound Evaluation

Ultrasound (US) is recommended at all follow-up time points with measurement of the nodule and calculation of the volume reduction ratio (VRR) [(initial volume-final volume)/initial volume] x 100. A meta-analysis of long-term follow-up of patients treated by thermal ablation demonstrated VRRs of 54.7% after 6 months, 62.8% after 12 months, 62.1% after 24 months, 62.7% after 36 months, and 76.9% at last follow-up [15]. This suggests that most nodule shrinkage occurs in the first year, plateaus from 12 to 36 months and then some nodules may experience additional shrinkage after 36 months. It is important to note, however, that many of the studies included in this meta-analysis treated patients with multiple sessions of thermal ablation.

The sonographic appearance of thyroid nodules after thermal ablation tends to significantly differ from their pre-ablation appearance and often will appear more concerning on follow-up imaging due to new hypoechoic foci, more lobulated borders, and an overall decrease in echogenicity [6] (Fig. 25.5). If ultrasound is not performed by the treating physician or if the patient assumes care with a new provider, the history of thermal ablation of a cytologically benign nodule should be communicated in order to avoid US interpretation and reporting which confuses or alarms the patient and/or confounds the new treatment team.

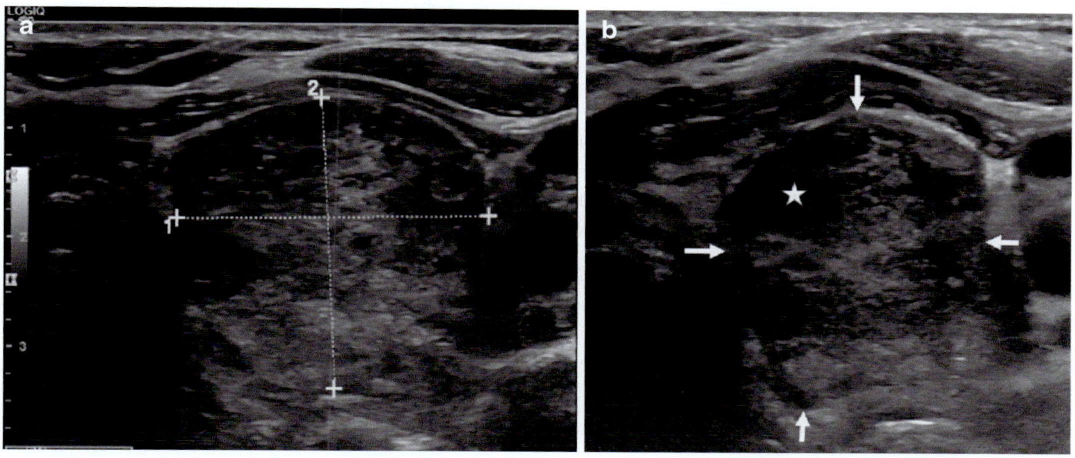

Fig. 25.5 (**a**) Initial US prior to treatment demonstrates a solid nodule which is minimally heterogeneous and as wide as tall. (**b**) Follow-up US after RFA demonstrates a nodule which is more heterogeneous in echotexture, has a taller than wide appearance (*arrows*), and contains a portion which is markedly hypoechoic (*star*). The nodule demonstrates features which would be concerning without the knowledge of prior thermal ablation

25.5 Evaluation of Efficacy and Need for Retreatment

The majority of guidelines recommend tracking VRR in follow-up after thermal ablation. However, additional measurements may allow better prediction of the success of treatment or earlier recognition of patients for whom retreatment should be considered (Table 25.2). After thermal ablation, total nodule volume is composed of the ablated volume in the center of the nodule (Va) and the untreated or vital volume at the periphery of the nodule (Vv). In other words, Vt = Va + Vv. On the day of ablation, the margin between ablated and non-ablated tissue may be obscured by edema or hemorrhage. For best accuracy, Vt is measured prior to RFA, whereas Va is measured at the first follow-up exam [16] (Fig. 25.6). Contrast-enhanced US has been proposed to measure the Va at the conclusion of the RFA procedure, as the vital portions of a nodule will demonstrate vascularity, while the ablated central portion will not [17].

Table 25.2 Measurements used to evaluate thyroid nodules before and after thermal ablation

Volume of a nodule	$\frac{\pi \bullet \text{length} \bullet \text{width} \bullet \text{height}}{6}$
Volume Reduction Ratio (VRR)	$\frac{\text{initial volume} - \text{final volume}}{\text{initial volume}} \times 100$
Initial Ablation Ratio (IAR)	$\frac{\text{Va}(\text{ablated volume})}{\text{Vt}(\text{total volume})}$
Vital volume	Vital volume = total volume − ablated volume

Knowledge of the ablated volume (Va) allows calculation of the initial ablation ratio (IAR), which is Va/Vt [16]. IAR may then be used to predict the success of ablation. If IAR is greater than or equal to 50%, then the nodule will shrink by at least 50% by the end of the first year [18]. IAR >73% also predicts volume reduction at 5 years and identifies patients who will not likely need retreatment during that time [18].

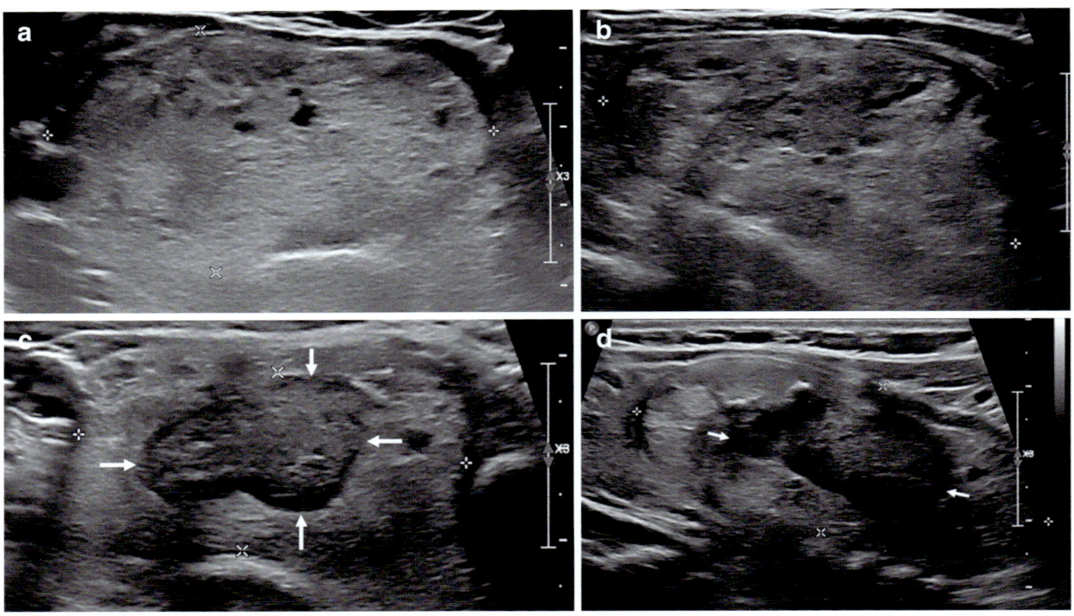

Fig. 25.6 (**a**) Transverse and (**b**) sagittal images prior to RFA allow measurement of Vt. (**c**) Transverse and (**d**) sagittal ultrasound at the 3-month follow-up allow measurement of Va which is the hypoechoic nodule within the center of the total nodule (*arrows*). Vital volume can then be calculated as Vt = Va + Vv

Many different criteria have been used to determine which patients to retreat and when to retreat them. One option is treating patients who experience nodule regrowth. The most common definition of regrowth is a 50% growth over the minimum previously demonstrated nodule volume. Using this definition, studies by both Bernardi and Kim demonstrate that nodule regrowth occurred in about 28% of patients followed for multiple years [19, 20].

Regrowth typically occurs because the untreated portion of tissue at the periphery of a nodule or the vital volume (Vv) increases over time. In the first year of treatment, as long as the ablated volume (Va) decreases in size more than the Vv increases, the total volume of the nodule itself will not demonstrate regrowth. Some authors have therefore advocated for the use of vital volume regrowth (>50% increase in Vv) as a means of early identification of nodules which will require retreatment, as increase in vital volume occurs about a year prior to nodule regrowth [21]. Similarly, initial IAR <70% and increased vascularity on US can identify growing nodules before they have increased by 50% in total volume [20].

Approaches in which nodule growth is identified early and aggressively retreated can result in higher overall VRR. While overall volume reductions after RFA average around 70%, in Lim's study of RFA treatment of 123 nodules in 111 patients, 93.4% volume reduction was obtained at 4 years. However, 58% of patients in this series were retreated, with 34% treated between three and seven times. This approach may be less feasible in practices in which patients are self-pay or third-party payers are reluctant to pay for thermal ablation treatments.

While aggressive retreatment may yield larger volume reductions, it is notable that recurrence of compressive symptoms is less prevalent than objective regrowth as measured by US, and tends to occur later in follow-up. In Bernardi's series, only 26% of patients with documented regrowth had recurrence of their symptoms [19]. In Kim's series, patients who experienced nodule regrowth did so at an average of 2 years post RFA, whereas symptom progression occurred 5 years after RFA [20]. On the other hand, Yan et al. demonstrated that patients who were retreated based on an increase in vital volume rather than clinical symptoms showed greater improvement in symptom and cosmetic scores in follow-up [22].

Ultimately retreatment should be based on shared decision-making between the patient and the physician. Table 25.3 summarizes indications for retreatment in recent society guidelines for thermal ablation. Patients with larger nodules or nodules close to structures such as the danger triangle are more likely to need retreatment due to the difficulties of initial complete ablation and they can be warned of this possibility before treatment or early in follow-up. On the other hand, compressive symptoms are relieved in some patients even with less than 50% VRR, and ultimately, patient satisfaction regarding compressive or cosmetic symptoms may render retreatment unnecessary.

In many series, patients with nodule regrowth are treated with repeat ablation, often without a new biopsy. In Bernardi's series, the patients who demonstrated regrowth were also offered surgery. Of the patients who opted for surgery, 16/46 or 35% had non-benign pathology, despite having had two benign FNAs prior to treatment [19]. The authors suggested that volume decrease of less than 20% at the end of the first year of

Table 25.3 Summary of indications for retreatment in guidelines on radiofrequency ablation of benign thyroid nodules

	Indication for retreatment
Papini 2020 [3]	Demonstration of regrowth in untreated areas New FNA suggested before retreatment
Ha, 2021 [4]	Marginal regrowth <50% volume reduction Incomplete resolution or relapse of symptoms/cosmetic appearance No repeat cytology suggested
Sinclair 2023 [6]	<30% reduction in growth at 6 months Regrowth in untreated peripheral areas Persistent or new compressive symptoms Can consider FNA

FNA fine needle aspiration

follow-up was a factor that might predict non-benign pathology. The occurrence of malignancy in patients who were carefully evaluated demonstrates the importance of continued follow-up in this patient population.

References

1. Kim JH, Baek JH, Lim HK, Ahn HS, Baek SM, Choi YJ, et al. 2017 thyroid radiofrequency ablation guideline: Korean Society of Thyroid Radiology. Korean J Radiol. 2018;19(4):632–55. https://doi.org/10.3348/kjr.2018.19.4.632.
2. Dobnig H, Zechmann W, Hermann M, Lehner M, Heute D, Mirzaei S, et al. Radiofrequency ablation of thyroid nodules: "good clinical practice recommendations" for Austria: an interdisciplinary statement from the following professional associations: Austrian Thyroid Association (OSDG), Austrian Society for Nuclear Medicine and Molecular Imaging (OGNMB), Austrian Society for Endocrinology and Metabolism (OGES), Surgical Endocrinology Working Group (ACE) of the Austrian Surgical Society (OEGCH). Wien Med Wochenschr. 2020;170(1–2):6–14. https://doi.org/10.1007/s10354-019-0682-2.
3. Papini E, Monpeyssen H, Frasoldati A, Hegedus L. 2020 European thyroid association clinical practice guideline for the use of image-guided ablation in benign thyroid nodules. Eur Thyroid J. 2020;9(4):172–85. https://doi.org/10.1159/000508484.
4. Ha EJ, Baek JH, Che Y, Chou YH, Fukunari N, Kim JH, et al. Radiofrequency ablation of benign thyroid nodules: recommendations from the Asian conference on tumor ablation task force—secondary publication. J Med Ultrasound. 2021;29(2):77–83. https://doi.org/10.4103/JMU.JMU_178_20.
5. Orloff LA, Noel JE, Stack BC Jr, Russell MD, Angelos P, Baek JH, et al. Radiofrequency ablation and related ultrasound-guided ablation technologies for treatment of benign and malignant thyroid disease: an international multidisciplinary consensus statement of the American Head and Neck Society Endocrine Surgery Section with the Asia Pacific Society of Thyroid Surgery, Associazione Medici Endocrinologi, British Association of Endocrine and Thyroid Surgeons, European thyroid association, Italian Society of Endocrine Surgery Units, Korean Society of Thyroid Radiology, Latin American Thyroid Society, and Thyroid Nodules Therapies Association. Head Neck. 2022;44(3):633–60. https://doi.org/10.1002/hed.26960.
6. Sinclair CF, Baek JH, Hands KE, Hodak SP, Huber TC, Hussain I, et al. General principles for the safe performance, training, and adoption of ablation techniques for benign thyroid nodules: an American Thyroid Association statement. Thyroid. 2023;33(10):1150–70. https://doi.org/10.1089/thy.2023.0281.
7. Hanna BC, Brooker DS. A preliminary study of simple voice assessment in a routine clinical setting to predict vocal cord paralysis after thyroid or parathyroid surgery. Clin Otolaryngol. 2008;33(1):63–6. https://doi.org/10.1111/j.1749-4486.2007.01592.x.
8. Baek JH, Kim YS, Lee D, Huh JY, Lee JH. Benign predominantly solid thyroid nodules: prospective study of efficacy of sonographically guided radiofrequency ablation versus control condition. AJR Am J Roentgenol. 2010;194(4):1137–42. https://doi.org/10.2214/AJR.09.3372.
9. Chung SR, Baek JH, Sung JY, Ryu JH, Jung SL. Revisiting rupture of benign thyroid nodules after radiofrequency ablation: various types and imaging features. Endocrinol Metab (Seoul). 2019;34(4):415–21. https://doi.org/10.3803/EnM.2019.34.4.415.
10. Austerlitz JMD, Noel JE, Orloff LA. Thyroid nodule rupture following radiofrequency ablation for benign thyroid nodules. JAMA Otolaryngol Head Neck Surg. 2024;150:651. https://doi.org/10.1001/jamaoto.2024.1400.
11. Ferraro T, Sajid S, Hodak SP, Baldwin CK. Thyroid nodule rupture after radiofrequency ablation: case report and literature review. Front Endocrinol (Lausanne). 2024;15:1355383. https://doi.org/10.3389/fendo.2024.1355383.
12. Wang N, Zheng B, Wu T, Tan L, Lian Y, Ma Y, et al. Thyroid dysfunction following radiofrequency ablation for benign thyroid nodules: more likely to occur within one-week and in high-risk population. Int J Hyperth. 2021;38(1):1060–8. https://doi.org/10.1080/02656736.2021.1950849.
13. McAninch EA, Desai K, McCowen KC, Orloff LA. Hyperthyroidism due to graves disease after radiofrequency ablation. JCEM Case Rep. 2023;1(3):luad056. https://doi.org/10.1210/jcemcr/luad056.
14. Baek JH, Lee JH, Sung JY, Bae JI, Kim KT, Sim J, et al. Complications encountered in the treatment of benign thyroid nodules with US-guided radiofrequency ablation: a multicenter study. Radiology. 2012;262(1):335–42. https://doi.org/10.1148/radiol.11110416.
15. Cho SJ, Baek JH, Chung SR, Choi YJ, Lee JH. Long-term results of thermal ablation of benign thyroid nodules: a systematic review and meta-analysis. Endocrinol Metab (Seoul). 2020;35(2):339–50. https://doi.org/10.3803/EnM.2020.35.2.339.
16. Sim JS, Baek JH, Cho W. Initial ablation ratio: quantitative value predicting the therapeutic success of thyroid radiofrequency ablation. Thyroid. 2018;28(11):1443–9. https://doi.org/10.1089/thy.2018.0180.
17. Zhu Y, Jiao Z, Zhu L, Xie F, Song Q, Yan L, et al. A new perspective for predicting the therapeutic success of RFA in solid BTNs: quantitative initial RFA ratio

by contrast-enhanced ultrasound. Front Endocrinol (Lausanne). 2022;13:904459. https://doi.org/10.3389/fendo.2022.904459.

18. Bernardi S, Cavallaro M, Colombin G, Giudici F, Zuolo G, Zdjelar A, et al. Initial ablation ratio predicts volume reduction and retreatment after 5 years from radiofrequency ablation of benign thyroid nodules. Front Endocrinol (Lausanne). 2020;11:582550. https://doi.org/10.3389/fendo.2020.582550.
19. Bernardi S, Giudici F, Cesareo R, Antonelli G, Cavallaro M, Deandrea M, et al. Five-year results of radiofrequency and laser ablation of benign thyroid nodules: a multicenter study from the Italian minimally invasive treatments of the thyroid group. Thyroid. 2020;30(12):1759–70. https://doi.org/10.1089/thy.2020.0202.
20. Kim HJ, Baek JH, Cho W, Sim JS. Long-term follow-up of the radiofrequency ablation of benign thyroid nodules: the value of additional treatment. Ultrasonography. 2022;41(4):661–9. https://doi.org/10.14366/usg.21231.
21. Sim JS, Baek JH, Lee J, Cho W, Jung SI. Radiofrequency ablation of benign thyroid nodules: depicting early sign of regrowth by calculating vital volume. Int J Hyperth. 2017;33(8):905–10. https://doi.org/10.1080/02656736.2017.1309083.
22. Yan L, Luo Y, Zhang M, Xiao J. Vital volume increase versus clinical evaluation as the indication of additional radiofrequency ablation for benign thyroid nodule: a single center retrospective study. Int J Hyperth. 2020;37(1):777–85. https://doi.org/10.1080/02656736.2020.1778197.

Global Guidelines for RFA

26

Julia E. Noel, Marika D. Russell, Tejas S. Athni,
Louise Davies, and Gregory W. Randolph

26.1 Introduction

Over recent years, there has been growing global interest in utilizing minimally invasive thermal ablation techniques to treat a variety of thyroid pathologies. Radiofrequency ablation (RFA) of the thyroid was first performed in 2002, and since 2006 there has been a growing body of evidence informing its use [1]. As RFA is performed by multiple disciplines (endocrinologists, radiologists, and surgeons), there is need to define and standardize optimal application and dissemination of this emerging technology. Many groups across the globe have published guidelines or statements to inform best practices. This chapter reviews the available guidelines, consensus statements, and position statements, summarizing key concepts and recommendations across all phases of care.

26.2 Overview of Available Guidelines

Globally, several guidelines and statements on performance of RFA have been developed, and these are summarized in Table 26.1. Most are multidisciplinary in nature and are endorsed by one or more professional societies. A recent consensus statement by the American Head and Neck Society—Endocrine Section (AHNS-ES) [2] represents a multidisciplinary and international collaborative effort endorsed by nine distinct medical or surgical societies. Overall, this cohort of publications encompasses varied methodological approaches, and groups have varied in how they handle the degrees of evidence to support their recommendations. For example, the methodological approach for consensus statements published by Mauri et al. [3] and Papini

J. E. Noel (✉)
Division of Otolaryngology Head & Neck Surgery, Santa Clara Valley Medical Center, Santa Clara, CA, USA

Department of Otolaryngology-Head & Neck Surgery, Stanford University School of Medicine, Stanford, CA, USA
e-mail: jnoel@stanford.edu

M. D. Russell · T. S. Athni
Division of Thyroid and Parathyroid Endocrine Surgery, Department of Otolaryngology-Head and Neck Surgery, Massachusetts Eye and Ear Infirmary, Harvard Medical School, Boston, MA, USA
e-mail: mrussell20@meei.harvard.edu; tathni@hms.harvard.edu

L. Davies
Department of Surgery, Geisel School of Medicine at Dartmouth, Hanover, NH, USA
e-mail: Louise.Davies@dartmouth.edu

G. W. Randolph
Division of Thyroid and Parathyroid Surgery, Department of Otolaryngology, Massachusetts Eye and Ear, Harvard Medical School, Boston, MA, USA

Division of Surgical Oncology, Endocrine Surgery Service, Department of Surgery, Massachusetts General Hospital, Harvard Medical School, Boston, MA, USA
e-mail: Gregory_Randolph@meei.harvard.edu

R. Valcavi et al. (eds.), *Thyroid Ablation*, https://doi.org/10.1007/978-3-031-88229-6_26

Table 26.1 Global radiofrequency ablation guidelines and statements

Publication	Year	Document type	Society(ies) or groups of origin/endorsement	Specialty(ies) represented	Methodology
Hamou et al.	2022	Consensus statement	French Society of Endocrinology (SFE), French Association of Endocrine Surgery (AFCE) and French Society of Nuclear Medicine (SFMN)	Endocrinology Radiology Surgery	Unstated
Orloff et al.	2021	Consensus statement	American Head and Neck Society—Endocrine Section (AHNS-ES), Asia Pacific Society of Thyroid Surgery (APTS), Associazione Medici Endocrinologi (AME), British Association of Endocrine and Thyroid Surgeons (BAETS), European Thyroid Association (ETA), Italian Society of Endocrine Surgery Units (SIUEC), Korean Society of Thyroid Radiology (KSThR), Latin American Thyroid Society (LATS), and Thyroid Nodules Therapies Association (TNT)	Endocrinology Radiology Surgery	Modified Delphi method
Ha et al.	2021	Task force recommendations	Asian Conference on Tumor Ablation Task Force	Radiology Surgery	Modified Delphi method
Mauri et al.	2021	Clinical guideline	The European Thyroid Association (ETA) and the Cardiovascular and Interventional Radiological Society of Europe (CIRSE)	Endocrinology Radiology Surgery	The Grading of Recommendations, Assessment, Development, and Evaluation (GRADE) system
Papini et al.	2020	Clinical guideline	European Thyroid Association (ETA)	Endocrinology	The Grading of Recommendations, Assessment, Development, and Evaluation (GRADE) system
Dobnig et al.	2020	Consensus statement	Austrian Thyroid Association (ÖSDG), Austrian Society for Nuclear Medicine and Molecular Imaging (OGNMB), Austrian Society for Endocrinology and Metabolism (ÖGES), Surgical Endocrinology Working Group (ACE) of the Austrian Surgical Society (OEGCH)	Endocrinology Radiology Surgery	Unstated

(continued)

Table 26.1 (continued)

Publication	Year	Document type	Society(ies) or groups of origin/endorsement	Specialty(ies) represented	Methodology
Feldkamp et al.	2020	Consensus statement	Thyroid Section (German Society for Endocrinology), the Thyroid Working Committee (German Society for Nuclear Medicine), and the German Association of Endocrine Surgeons (CAEK) for the German Society of General and Visceral Surgery (DGAV)	Endocrinology Radiology Surgery	Grading of Recommendations, Assessment, Development, and Evaluation (GRADE) system
Papini et al.	2019	Consensus statement	Italian Minimally Invasive Treatments of the Thyroid (MITT) Group	Endocrinology Pathology Radiology Surgery	Modified Delphi Method
Xu et al.	2019	Consensus statement	Thyroid Tumor Ablation Experts Group of Chinese Medical Doctor Association	Endocrinology Pathology Radiology Surgery	Unstated
Kim et al.	2018	Clinic guideline	Korean Society of Thyroid Radiology (KSThR)	Radiology	Internally developed level of evidence and recommendation grading system; modified Delphi method
National Institute for Health and Care Excellence (NICE)	2016	Guidance document	Healthcare Improvement Scotland	–	Unstated
Garberoglio et al.	2015	Position statement	Societa' Italiana di Ultrasonologia in Medicina e Biologia (SIUMB), Societa' Italiana di Endocrinologia (SIE), Associazione Medici Endocrinologi (AME), Societa` Italiana di Radiologia Medica (SIRM), Club delle Unita` di Endocrinochirurgia Italiane (Club delle UEC), Societa` Italiana di Chirurgia (SIC), Associazione Italiana di Medicina Nucleare (AIMN)	Endocrinology Radiology Surgery	In Accordance with NIH Consensus Development Program

et al. [4] contains great detail, including specifying how levels of evidence were determined, whereas the publications by Hamou et al. [5], Dobnig et al. [6], and Xu et al. [7] provide fewer details. Nearly all address RFA for benign disease, with some addressing treatment for both benign and malignant conditions. Only one guideline [3] is dedicated exclusively to the application of RFA in treatment of thyroid malignancy.

26.3 Selection and Candidacy

26.3.1 Benign Nodules

Appropriate patient selection is a key for successful application of RFA. Benign nodules causing compressive symptoms (i.e., dysphagia, foreign body sensation, discomfort, and cough) or cosmetic disturbance are uniformly considered appropriate for treatment with RFA [2, 4–13]. The minimum size for treatment remains an area of debate. A threshold of 2 cm with continued growth was suggested in an early Italian position statement [10] and later echoed by the Korean Society of Thyroid Radiology (KSThR) guidelines [8], the European Thyroid Association (ETA) guidelines [4], and the AHNS-ES clinical consensus statement [2]. It is recognized that symptomatology may be impacted by body habitus, as nodules may be more prominent in individuals with thin necks [2, 4, 8]. Additionally, the location of the nodule may impact the size at which it becomes symptomatic. Nodules located in the isthmus may become problematic at a smaller size and would be appropriate for treatment [2, 4, 8]. The ETA guidelines and German consensus statement recommend against treatment of asymptomatic nodules [4, 12], whereas a consensus statement published by the French Society of Endocrinology (SFE), French Association of Endocrine Surgery (AFCE), and French Society of Nuclear Medicine (SFMN) advocates for treatment of asymptomatic nodules >4 cm cm which are exhibiting significant growth [5]. An upper limit of size appropriate for treatment is not defined, though it is noted that additional treatment sessions may be necessary in larger nodules [9]. Additionally, thyroid nodules with retrosternal extension or extension into the tubercle of Zuckerkandl can be difficult to access and may require multiple treatment sessions [9].

26.3.2 Autonomously Functioning Nodules

Hyperfunctioning nodules may be considered for RFA, though TSH normalization occurs with less frequency or predictability than with RAI or surgery [2]. For this reason, RFA is uniformly recommended in each guideline that addresses it as a second-line alternative in patients for whom first line options are not suitable [2, 4, 5, 8, 9, 13]. As efficacy is associated with a reduction in nodule volume of 80% or greater, RFA is best suited for patients with small (≤3 cm) nodules. Importantly, Graves' disease and toxic multinodular goiter are not appropriate for treatment with RFA because of the diffuse nature of these pathologies [2, 4].

26.3.3 Malignancy

Adoption of RFA for treatment of thyroid malignancy is nascent and lacking uniformity. Few guidelines explicitly address this topic, and indications for treatment are still evolving. The KSThR guidelines and AHNS-ES consensus statement endorse treatment of recurrent malignancy for patients who decline surgery or for whom surgical treatment poses significant surgical risk. Treatment of recurrent nodal disease is described as favorable when limited to fewer than three or four nodes with tumor diameters smaller than 1.5–2 cm [2, 8]. Importantly, treatment intent, whether curative or palliative, should be determined and discussed with the patient by the treating team [2]. While surgery remains the first line of treatment of primary tumors, both the KSThR and AHNS-ES documents acknowledge evolving indications for RFA treatment of papillary thyroid microcarcinoma (PTMC) [2, 8]. Guidance from multiple groups suggests that

PTMC selected for RFA treatment should be of a non-aggressive subtype, unifocal and confined to the thyroid gland without capsular abutment, extrathyroidal extension, lymph node metastases, or a high-risk molecular signature [2, 3, 5]. Along with PTMC and recurrent disease, unresectable thyroid cancer and distant metastatic disease such as lung and bone metastases are considered appropriate indications for palliative treatment, though data remains limited in these areas [2, 3]. The AHNS-ES suggests that RFA may be considered for palliative treatment in locally advanced disease if it is anticipated to reduce symptom burden [2].

26.3.4 Indeterminate Cytology

At present, RFA is not advised for treatment of nodules with indeterminate cytology (Bethesda III or IV) [2, 3, 5, 8]. Unlike surgery, treatment with RFA does not facilitate exclusion of malignancy. Lack of complete radiographic disappearance with treatment and potential confounding of future attempts to obtain a cytologic diagnosis may lead to management dilemmas [2, 8]. While molecular testing may allow increased assurance of benignity, such commercial testing platforms are not widely available.

26.4 Pre-procedural Evaluation

26.4.1 Benign Nodules

Published guidance uniformly acknowledges pre-procedural ultrasound (US) as a critical step in the evaluation of thyroid nodules being considered for RFA [2, 4, 6, 8, 9] (Fig. 26.1). US facilitates characterization of nodule location, size, solid component, internal vascularity, and relationship to surrounding structures, including the vagus nerve, the trachea, and the expected location of the recurrent laryngeal nerve [2, 6, 8]. It is important to assess for the presence of high-risk US features and to avoid treatment of nodules with suspicious features, so as to not confound the diagnosis and treatment of a malignancy [2, 8]. Nodules should be measured in three dimensions to facilitate calculation of a volume reduction ratio (VRR) with treatment. Cross-sectional imaging is advised by some to better evaluate nodules suspected of intrathoracic extension in order to determine candidacy for treatment [2, 4, 8, 9].

Confirmation of benignity with two US-guided fine needle aspiration (FNA) or core biopsies is generally recommended [2, 4, 8, 9, 13]; however, there is agreement that nodules with US characteristics highly suggestive of benignity (such as spongiform appearance) are eligible for treatment with a single FNA or core biopsy [2, 4, 8, 9, 13]. There is lack of a uniform directive regarding the need for cytologic confirmation of benignity in treatment of autonomously functioning nodules. The KSThR guidelines suggest that a single biopsy confirming benignity is appropriate [8], whereas the AHNS-ES consensus statement indicates FNA of autonomously functioning nodules is not a prerequisite [2] and the SFE-AFCE-SFMN consensus statement suggests that the decision of whether to obtain a biopsy may be left to the discretion of the treating team [5].

There is a nearly uniform recommendation for obtaining thyroid function studies prior to treatment for both non-functioning and autonomously functioning nodules [2, 4–9]. Guidance for additional laboratory testing is more heterogeneous. Some recommend routinely obtaining coagulation studies [5–9]. Autoantibodies (anti-thyroid peroxidase and anti-thyroglobulin antibodies) are advised by some [5, 6, 8, 9]. Calcitonin screening to rule out medullary cancer is recommended by many European societies [4–6, 12], reflecting regional practice patterns.

Measurement of symptom and cosmetic scores before (and after) treatment is recommended by several groups [2, 6, 8, 9, 12]. The majority of these groups advise using a 1–10 visual analog scale for symptoms (as assessed by the patient) and a 4-point grading scale for cosmetic impact, designated by the clinician as (1) no palpable mass; (2) no cosmetic problem but a palpable mass; (3) cosmetic problem only during swallowing; and (4) nodule readily visible [2, 6, 8, 9].

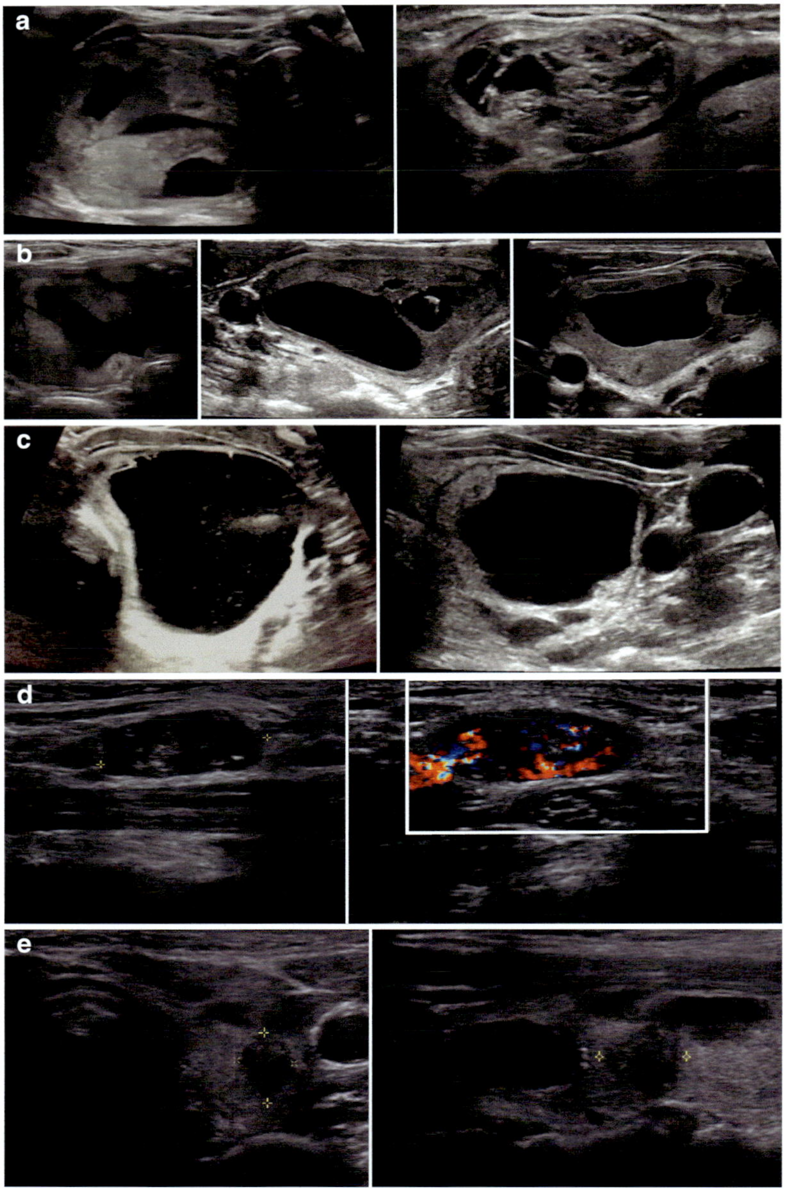

Fig. 26.1 Ultrasonographic examples and recommended ablative techniques. Sonographic patterns of candidate lesions for ablation. (**a**) Examples of benign nodules with primarily solid or spongiform patterns that would be amenable to radiofrequency ablation. (**b**) Examples of mixed solid and cystic nodules with a significant cystic component best addressed with a combination of ethanol ablation (EA) for the cystic portion and RFA for the solid portion. (**c**) Examples of entirely or nearly entirely cystic nodules likely to be sufficiently reduced by ethanol ablation (EA) alone. (**d**) Examples of isolated recurrent papillary thyroid carcinoma in lateral neck lymph nodes, amenable to RFA. (**e**) Example of a unifocal papillary thyroid microcarcinoma without adverse features or radiographic evidence of metastatic disease, amenable to RFA. (*Reprinted with permission from Orloff LA, Noel JE, Stack BC Jr,* et al. *Radiofrequency ablation and related ultrasound-guided ablation technologies for treatment of benign and malignant thyroid disease: An international multidisciplinary consensus statement of the American Head and Neck Society Endocrine Surgery Section with the Asia Pacific Society of Thyroid Surgery, Associazione Medici Endocrinologi, British Association of Endocrine and Thyroid Surgeons, European Thyroid Association, Italian Society of Endocrine Surgery Units, Korean Society of Thyroid Radiology, Latin American Thyroid Society, and Thyroid Nodules Therapies Association. Head Neck. 2022 Mar;44*(3)*:633–660. Copyright ©2021, John Wiley and Sons, Inc.*)

There is general agreement that it is the responsibility of the treating clinician to set clear treatment expectations and that the following items should be discussed during the informed consent process: (1) expected decrease in nodule size with potential for regrowth or need for additional treatment; (2) possibility of pain or discomfort during the procedure, including pain extending to the ears, jaw, or back; (3) potential complications; and (4) alternative management options [2, 4–8, 12]. Additional emphasis is placed importance of long-term follow-up [4] and awareness that alterations in tissue may confound future US assessment [12].

26.4.2 Malignancy

As with benign nodules, pre-procedural US is considered critical for characterization of tumor dimensions, location, vascularity, and solid proportion (Fig. 26.1). Importantly relationships to surrounding structures should be assessed to facilitate safe performance of RFA [2, 8]. In particular, it is advised that distance to the thyroid capsule and the likely location of the recurrent laryngeal nerve and the trachea be noted [5]. Additionally, US examination should screen for macroscopic extrathyroidal extension and suspicious lymph nodes, both of which would preclude RFA treatment of primary PTMC under existing guidance [2, 5, 8]. There is limited guidance on the utilization of cross-sectional imaging in treatment of malignancy. The KSThR recommends CT of the neck to identify any recurrent disease not detected on US [8]; the AHNS-ES guidelines suggest that for patients judged to be at risk for distant metastatic disease, cross-sectional and/or functional imaging to detect distant metastases may help inform treatment intent [2]. It is recommended that tumor recurrence be confirmed by US-guided FNA, thyroglobulin (Tg) rinse or core needle biopsy prior to treatment with RFA [2, 3, 8]. In addition to TSH measurement, laboratory evaluation should include measurement of Tg and Tg antibodies (TgAb) [2]. A rapid increase in serum Tg levels may be seen during the 48 h following RFA treatment of malignancy; after this, Tg reaches its nadir and may be used to determine treatment efficacy [2, 3], although at present there is no guidance defining successful treatment outcomes. Similarly, preoperative serum calcitonin level may be used as a marker for assessing treatment impact in medullary thyroid cancer, though guidance in this area is also lacking [3].

26.5 General Considerations

Patient factors and comorbidities should be evaluated when determining candidacy for RFA. There is general agreement among the published guidelines that patients should be assessed for a history of bleeding/clotting disorders, pregnancy status, and presence of a pacemaker [2, 4, 6, 8]. Though not considered absolute contraindications to RFA, pregnancy or the presence of a pacemaker should prompt use of a bipolar treatment probe (if available) to contain spread of electrical current during the procedure [2, 5, 8, 9].

Guidance is less clear with respect to absolute contraindications for RFA. Some groups [2, 7] suggest that benign nodules which are retrosternal are contraindicated for treatment, whereas the Asian Conference on Tumor Ablation Task Force [9] suggests that this finding does not preclude treatment but may require additional treatment sessions. Additional contraindications that have been suggested include the presence of contralateral vocal fold paralysis (VFP), presence of a severe blood clotting disorder, and major organ dysfunction [7]. As previously noted, Graves' disease, toxic multinodular goiter, indeterminate cytology, and aggressive subtypes of PTMC are considered unsuitable for treatment [3, 4, 7, 12].

Discontinuation of anticoagulation therapy to minimize procedural bleeding risk is specifically addressed by some groups, and when addressed, the recommendations are consistent. Anti-platelet medications such as aspirin or clopidogrel should be stopped 7–10 days prior to the procedure. Similarly, warfarin should be held 3–5 days and heparin stopped 4–6 h before the procedure. Direct oral anticoagulants, including dabigatran, rivaroxaban, apixaban, and edoxaban are held for 24–36 h pre-procedure [2, 8, 9].

Recommendations for pre-procedural laryngeal examination with fiberoptic laryngoscopy are not uniform. The German consensus statement and Austrian workgroup indicate that pre-procedural laryngoscopy is mandatory [6, 12]. However, a recommendation for routine pre-procedural laryngeal examination did not meet consensus in the AHNS-ES statement. The ETA suggests that laryngeal examination is warranted in patients with hoarseness, previous thyroid surgery, or when nodules are located close to the airway or expected course of the recurrent laryngeal nerve. The Asian Conference on Tumor Ablation Task Force suggests against routine laryngoscopic examination but suggests its necessity in patients with suspected vocal cord paralysis. These authors also suggest US evaluation of the larynx can be effective for the patients with no history of hoarseness.

26.6 Technique

The majority of groups recommend that ablation be performed under local anesthesia. Perithyroidal anesthesia is infiltrated between the thyroid capsule, where sensory nerves lie, and the strap musculature [2, 4, 7–9]. Austrian guidelines describe that a few centers use intravenous analgesics or sedatives but acknowledge that this is rarely necessary [6]. General anesthesia is not recommended [8, 9]. It precludes detection and potential avoidance of major complications such as recurrent laryngeal nerve or tracheal injury, and minor injuries like skin burn. The AHNS-ES consensus statement suggests that an oral anxiolytic may be given prior to the procedure to maximize comfort and tolerance while not interfering with patient responsiveness [2].

In regard to peri-procedural monitoring, there is relatively limited and somewhat varied guidance. The ETA advocates monitoring of vital signs only for patients receiving conscious sedation, while Austrian guidelines state that ECG, blood pressure, and pO2 should be monitored in all patients throughout the RFA procedure [4, 6]. Expert consensus workshop findings from China also advocate for close monitoring of heart rate, rhythm, oxygen saturation, and respiratory rate [7]. Consensus from the AHNS-ES suggests vital signs be taken immediately prior to and following RFA, but that, similar to the ETA, continuous monitoring is not required unless conscious sedation is being administered [2]. Other guidelines and consensus statements do not specifically address the monitoring of vital signs peri-procedurally.

In the technical execution of thermal ablation, there is universal recommendation for the use of the transisthmic approach, wherein the electrode is introduced via the isthmus and directed laterally though the target nodule so as to allow for continuous US monitoring and to ensure stability of the probe with movement [2, 4, 6–11]. There may be select situations in which a lateral approach is required for optimal access [7]. For large lesions, particularly benign thyroid nodules, the moving shot technique, as originally described by Na et al. in the 2012 KSThR consensus statement [14], is unanimously recommended [2–11, 13]. Few societies specifically address technique differences in ablating malignant lesions, but Xu et al. write that a fixed ablation strategy may be appropriate for small lesions, such as PTMC or cervical nodal recurrences [7]. Their recommendation also emphasizes the importance of ensuring the ablation area extends slightly beyond the borders of a malignant lesion so as to achieve local cure [7]. Regardless of approach or pathology, continuous US monitoring of ablation progress is mandatory to prevent thermal injury to adjacent critical structures.

Hydrodissection is a more advanced strategy in thermal ablation [15–17]. The AHNS-ES and Asian Conference on Tumor Ablation Task Force both propose it as a potentially useful technique in all settings to create additional distance between the target lesion and vital structures [2, 9]. The KSThR recommends this step as a component of the standard approach in the ablation of a recurrent metastatic lesion [8]. All three organizations advocate use of 5% dextrose in water (D5W) to minimize conduction and provide a thermal barrier [2, 8, 9].

26.7 Post-procedural Evaluation

Post-procedural management can be divided into the acute phase and the more extended follow-up period. Ultrasonographic evaluation of the treated area is necessary to identify early complications as well as to evaluate the completeness of the ablation in the target lesion [2, 4, 5, 7, 8]. There is agreement that the immediate post-procedural US includes assessment of the completeness of ablation, wherein the entirety of the nodule has ideally taken on a hypoechoic and heterogenous appearance with echogenic areas scattered throughout [2, 4, 8]. Use of Doppler is also important to visualize nodule vascularization and target any remaining viable areas for optimal outcome [2, 4, 5, 8]. While all societies agree that US is the best imaging modality for both immediate and extended follow-up, the Italian consensus statement and Chinese expert consensus workshop recommend contrast-enhanced US (CEUS) be considered as a primary imaging modality [7, 13]. Other statements mention this as an option but acknowledge the barriers to application in practice and leave adoption to the discretion of the operator [2, 4, 8, 9]. Several authors have noted that the assessment of small vessel vascularity and remnant viable nodular tissue is superior with CEUS vs. B-mode US, which can highlight the need for additional intervention [18–20]. The ability to determine vital area in follow-up to predict nodular regrowth is also improved and less subjective [20–22].

For benign nodules, the follow-up period typically involves an early (1–3 months), intermediate (~6 months), and late (~12 months) assessment. Beyond the first year, the ETA and Austrian Working Group suggest that routine US monitoring on a 1–2 year basis is warranted to assess for growth or structural change [4]. The Asian Conference on Tumor Ablation Task Force recommends more frequent assessment every 6–12 months depending on treatment success and nodule status [9]. At each follow-up, a combination of radiographic, biochemical, and symptomatic data points is obtained. Via US, the treated nodule is assessed to determine current dimensions and volume and and identify un- or under-treated areas with remnant vascularity [2, 5–9, 13]. Thyroid function tests are typically obtained during the early to intermediate follow-up range [2, 4–6, 8] and are considered unnecessary for non-functional nodules beyond 1 year [4]. The Austrian Working Group additionally recommends obtaining TPOAb and TGAb levels for, at minimum, the early follow-up appointment [23]. Of note, recent study has suggested that immediate post-procedure hypothyroidism might occur in up to 36% of patients undergoing RFA, particularly those with elevated anti-thyroid antibodies [24]. However, this is typically transient with levels returned to baseline by 1 month [24]. Numerous studies have demonstrated that the long-term risk of thyroid dysfunction after RFA is exceedingly low in all patients [11, 25–28]. Finally, many organizations recommend an assessment of cosmetic and/or symptoms scores at each follow-up visit consistent with the preoperative evaluation [2, 8, 9, 11].

In autonomously functioning nodules, thyroid function testing is a key component of each follow-up evaluation after RFA given the unknown kinetics of change and durability of cure [2, 5, 8, 9]. Relatively few groups address repeat imaging in AFTN, with some stating that consideration be given to repeating thyroid scintigraphy [2, 8, 9]. The Austrian Working Group advocates that scintigraphy be performed at the 3-month follow-up visit [6].

Published guidance regarding the post-procedural follow-up after RFA for primary thyroid cancer is currently limited. Though evidence suggests that thermal ablation might be an effective and safe therapeutic intervention, particularly for PTMC [3, 27, 29–32], its role relative to active surveillance and surgery has yet to be clearly described. Ultrasound remains the dominant post-procedural examination following RFA for primary thyroid malignancy [8]. As with benign lesions, the dimensions of the target lesion are assessed, as is the presence of any remnant vascularity [7, 8]. A comprehensive evaluation for cervical lymphadenopathy as well as the presence of new thyroid lesions is carefully documented. Cross-sectional imaging of the neck with CT can be considered as a complementary modality [8].

Biochemical evaluation for tumor disappearance or recurrence in this context can be challenging as the majority of the normal thyroid parenchyma remains, and there is currently no recommendation regarding the utility of Tg and TgAb in the post-ablative setting. While prior studies have described a potential role for FNA or CNB after RFA to confirm complete tumor disappearance [33–35], KSThR guidelines suggest repeat histologic evaluation be reserved for tumors unresponsive to or increasing in size after ablation [8].

Following ablation of cervical recurrences of well-differentiated thyroid cancer, US is again fundamental to evaluation. An early (1–2 months), intermediate (6 months), and late (12 months) follow-up schedule is suggested, as with benign nodules, wherein volume reduction, tumor dimensions, and residual vascularity are assessed [2, 8]. US includes a comprehensive cervical examination, and cross-sectional imaging is selectively indicated for visualization of newly developed tumors or remnants that are not readily visible on US [2, 8]. It is expected that the enhancement of a tumor disappears after a complete ablation, and thus may be more clear to assess tumor response than with US [36, 37]. Thyroid function testing is performed, and, as with surgery, Tg and TgAb are assessed at each follow-up to evaluate therapeutic response and monitor for regrowth or new recurrence [2, 3, 8].

Laryngeal following RFA is a subject of much debate and is worth separately highlighting. The German consensus statement recommendations and Austrian Working Group guidelines agree that laryngoscopy is a mandatory component of the post-ablative assessment [6, 12]. AHNS-ES recommendations indicate that a subjective voice assessment first be performed, and laryngoscopy or laryngeal US be pursued in case of any change or concern [2]. The SFE-AFCE-SFMN consensus also advocates subjective voice assessment and additionally recommends that laryngeal US be included in the routine immediate post-procedural evaluation [5]. The AHNS-ES is the only organization to address bilateral ablation and states that confirmation of intact vocal fold motion is necessary before proceeding on the contralateral side [2].

26.8 Practice Implementation

As RFA and other thermal ablative techniques gain acceptance and increased adoption, there is a need for published recommendations regarding pathways to proficiency and competent practice. The first component of responsible implementation is widely recognized to be expertise in thyroid and neck ultrasound for both diagnostic and interventional purposes. The SFE-AFCE-SFMN consensus statement recommends that the operator has experience in FNAB/CNB, cyst aspiration and removal, and percutaneous ethanol injection [5]. Austrian guidelines include a requirement for 40 documented transisthmic interventions, including five alcohol ablations, as a prerequisite for training in RFA [6]. A desirable but not mandatory addition is the ability to perform "work shadowing" in an endocrine surgical center [6]. The AHNS-ES recommends advanced training in and facility with cervical US as well as proficiency with US-guided FNAB, ideally via transisthmic approach, prior to specific training in thermal ablation [2].

Didactic education in RFA is obtained via formal courses or workshops with ability to practice on phantom models [2, 6]. Observation of cases performed by an experienced colleague and proctoring of initial cases is also considered best practice by the Austrian RFA Working Group and the AHNS-ES [2, 6]. It is worth highlighting that the Austrian RFA Working Group is the only organization to propose formal and standardized training and quality assurance in RFA. In addition to the above, this more specifically includes attendance at eight to ten RFA procedures performed by a colleague who has carried out 100 RFAs, 1 day of training for assisting personnel, and four proctored on-site RFA cases [6]. As noted, the technical details of the procedure can be difficult to communicate in larger courses and new operators benefit significantly from one-on-one teaching. The Austrian RFA Working Group will provide certification to physicians completing this training, and subsequent participation in the outlined quality control program is expected, wherein standard documentation of cases and outcomes is performed and submitted to the Working Group at regular intervals [6].

A final consideration in the implementation of RFA in practice is the availability of follow-up and support. German consensus strongly recommends that RFA be performed in an institution capable of treating complications of thermal ablation [12]. The ETA/CIRSE and AHNS Endocrine Section suggests that the operator be a member of an integrated multidisciplinary team that can both evaluate patients for appropriate candidacy and will take responsibility for longitudinal follow-up care [2, 3]. The Austrian RFA Working Group also includes readily available connection to an endocrine surgery center as a requirement for quality assurance in RFA performance [6]. Overall, consensus is that optimal care is delivered in the setting where all phases of procedural evaluation, execution, and follow-up can be fluidly coordinated.

26.9 Summary

RFA for thyroid lesions is receiving increasing interest around the globe. Several organizations have published guidelines or consensus statements to promote adoption of best practices across a multidisciplinary environment. This chapter addresses key concepts and recommendations across all phases of care, highlighting areas where guidance is discrepant or lacking. As further adoption and study is undertaken, we are likely to see continued evolution of clinical guidance.

References

1. Kuo JH, McManus C, Lee JA. Analyzing the adoption of radiofrequency ablation of thyroid nodules using the diffusion of innovations theory: understanding where we are in the United States? Ultrasonography. 2022;41(1):25–33. https://doi.org/10.14366/usg.21117.
2. Orloff LA, Noel JE, Stack BCJ, Russell MD, Angelos P, Baek JH, et al. Radiofrequency ablation and related ultrasound-guided ablation technologies for treatment of benign and malignant thyroid disease: an international multidisciplinary consensus statement of the American Head and Neck Society Endocrine Surgery Section with the Asia Pacific Society of Thyroid Surgery, Associazione Medici Endocrinologi, British Association of Endocrine and Thyroid Surgeons, European Thyroid Association, Italian Society of Endocrine Surgery Units, Korean Society of Thyroid Radiology, Latin American Thyroid Society, and Thyroid Nodules Therapies Association. Head Neck. 2022;44(3):633–60. https://doi.org/10.1002/hed.26960.
3. Mauri G, Hegedus L, Bandula S, Cazzato RL, Czarniecka A, Dudeck O, et al. European thyroid association and cardiovascular and interventional radiological Society of Europe 2021 clinical practice guideline for the use of minimally invasive treatments in malignant thyroid lesions. Eur Thyroid J. 2021;10(3):185–97. https://doi.org/10.1159/000516469.
4. Papini E, Monpeyssen H, Frasoldati A, Hegedüs L. 2020 European thyroid association clinical practice guideline for the use of image-guided ablation in benign thyroid nodules. Eur Thyroid J. 2020;9(4):172–85. https://doi.org/10.1159/000508484.
5. Ben Hamou A, Ghanassia E, Muller A, Ladsous M, Paladino NC, Brunaud L, et al. SFE-AFCE-SFMN 2022 consensus on the management of thyroid nodules: thermal ablation. Ann Endocrinol (Paris). 2022;83(6):423–30. https://doi.org/10.1016/j.ando.2022.10.011.
6. Dobnig H, Zechmann W, Hermann M, Lehner M, Heute D, Mirzaei S, et al. Radiofrequency ablation of thyroid nodules: "good clinical practice recommendations" for Austria: an interdisciplinary statement from the following professional associations: Austrian Thyroid Association (ÖSDG), Austrian Society for Nuclear Medicine and M. Wien Med Wochenschr. 2020;170(1–2):6–14. https://doi.org/10.1007/s10354-019-0682-2.
7. Xu D, Ge M, Yang A, Cheng R, Sun H, Wang H, et al. Expert consensus workshop report: guidelines for thermal ablation of thyroid tumors (2019 edition). J Cancer Res Ther. 2020;16(5):960–6. https://doi.org/10.4103/jcrt.JCRT_558_19.
8. Kim JH, Baek JH, Lim HK, Ahn HS, Baek SM, Choi YJ, et al. 2017 thyroid radiofrequency ablation guideline: Korean Society of Thyroid Radiology. Korean J Radiol. 2018;19(4):632–55. https://doi.org/10.3348/kjr.2018.19.4.632.
9. Ha EJ, Baek JH, Che Y, Chou YH, Fukunari N, Kim JH, et al. Radiofrequency ablation of benign thyroid nodules: recommendations from the Asian conference on tumor ablation task force. Ultrasonography. 2021;40(1):75–82. https://doi.org/10.14366/usg.20112.
10. Garberoglio R, Aliberti C, Appetecchia M, Attard M, Boccuzzi G, Boraso F, et al. Radiofrequency ablation for thyroid nodules: which indications? The first Italian opinion statement. J Ultrasound. 2015;18(4):423–30. https://doi.org/10.1007/s40477-015-0169-y.
11. Thyroid disease: assessment and management. London: National Institute for Health and Care Excellence (NICE); 2019.

12. Feldkamp J, Grünwald F, Luster M, Lorenz K, Vorländer C, Führer D. Non-surgical and non-radioiodine techniques for ablation of benign thyroid nodules: consensus statement and recommendation *. Exp Clin Endocrinol Diabetes. 2020;128(10):687–92. https://doi.org/10.1055/a-1075-2025.
13. Papini E, Pacella CM, Solbiati LA, Achille G, Barbaro D, Bernardi S, et al. Minimally-invasive treatments for benign thyroid nodules: a Delphi-based consensus statement from the Italian minimally-invasive treatments of the thyroid (MITT) group. Int J Hyperth. 2019;36(1):376–82. https://doi.org/10.1080/02656736.2019.1575482.
14. Na DG, Lee JH, Jung SL, Kim JH, Sung JY, Shin JH, et al. Radiofrequency ablation of benign thyroid nodules and recurrent thyroid cancers: consensus statement and recommendations. Korean J Radiol. 2012;13(2):117–25. https://doi.org/10.3348/kjr.2012.13.2.117.
15. Laeseke PF, Sampson LA, Brace CL, Winter TC, Fine JP, Lee FT. Unintended thermal injuries from radiofrequency ablation: protection with 5% dextrose in water. AJR Am J Roentgenol. 2006;186(5 Suppl):S249–54. https://doi.org/10.2214/AJR.04.1240.
16. Laeseke PF, Sampson LA, Winter TC 3rd, Lee FT Jr. Use of dextrose 5% in water instead of saline to protect against inadvertent radiofrequency injuries. AJR Am J Roentgenol. 2005;184(3):1026–7. https://doi.org/10.2214/ajr.184.3.01841026.
17. Xiaoyin T, Ping L, Dan C, Min D, Jiachang C, Tao W, et al. Risk assessment and hydrodissection technique for radiofrequency ablation of thyroid benign nodules. J Cancer. 2018;9(17):3058–66. https://doi.org/10.7150/jca.26060.
18. Yao Z, Wu T, Zheng B, Tan L, Lian Y, Liu B, et al. A novel strategy for single-session ultrasound-guided radiofrequency ablation of large benign thyroid nodules: a pilot cohort study. Front Endocrinol (Lausanne). 2020;11:560508. https://doi.org/10.3389/fendo.2020.560508.
19. Yan L, Li XY, Xiao J, Li YY, Zhu Y, He H, et al. Contrast-enhanced ultrasound is a reliable and reproducible assessment of necrotic ablated volume after radiofrequency ablation for benign thyroid nodules: a retrospective study. Int J Hyperth. 2022;39(1):40–7. https://doi.org/10.1080/02656736.2021.1991009.
20. Zhao CK, Xu HX, Lu F, Sun LP, He YP, Guo LH, et al. Factors associated with initial incomplete ablation for benign thyroid nodules after radiofrequency ablation: first results of CEUS evaluation. Clin Hemorheol Microcirc. 2017;65(4):393–405. https://doi.org/10.3233/CH-16208.
21. Yan L, Luo Y, Xie F, Zhang M, Xiao J. Residual vital ratio: predicting regrowth after radiofrequency ablation for benign thyroid nodules. Int J Hyperth. 2020;37(1):1139–48. https://doi.org/10.1080/02656736.2020.1825835.
22. Schiaffino S, Serpi F, Rossi D, Ferrara V, Buonomenna C, Alì M, et al. Reproducibility of ablated volume measurement is higher with contrast-enhanced ultrasound than with b-mode ultrasound after benign thyroid nodule radiofrequency ablation—a preliminary study. J Clin Med. 2020;9(5):1504. https://doi.org/10.3390/jcm9051504.
23. Lee M, Baek JH, Suh CH, Chung SR, Choi YJ, Lee JH, et al. Clinical practice guidelines for radiofrequency ablation of benign thyroid nodules: a systematic review. Ultrasonography. 2021;40(2):256–64. https://doi.org/10.14366/usg.20015.
24. Wang N, Zheng B, Wu T, Tan L, Lian Y, Ma Y, et al. Thyroid dysfunction following radiofrequency ablation for benign thyroid nodules: more likely to occur within one-week and in high-risk population. Int J Hyperth. 2021;38(1):1060–8. https://doi.org/10.1080/02656736.2021.1950849.
25. Kim C, Lee JH, Choi YJ, Kim WB, Sung TY, Baek JH. Complications encountered in ultrasonography-guided radiofrequency ablation of benign thyroid nodules and recurrent thyroid cancers. Eur Radiol. 2017;27(8):3128–37. https://doi.org/10.1007/s00330-016-4690-y.
26. Jung SL, Baek JH, Lee JH, Shong YK, Sung JY, Kim KS, et al. Efficacy and safety of radiofrequency ablation for benign thyroid nodules: a prospective multicenter study. Korean J Radiol. 2018;19(1):167–74. https://doi.org/10.3348/kjr.2018.19.1.167.
27. Monpeyssen H, Alamri A, Ben HA. Long-term results of ultrasound-guided radiofrequency ablation of benign thyroid nodules: state of the art and future perspectives—a systematic review. Front Endocrinol (Lausanne). 2021;12:622996. https://doi.org/10.3389/fendo.2021.622996.
28. Lim JY, Kuo JH. Thyroid nodule radiofrequency ablation: complications and clinical follow up. Tech Vasc Interv Radiol. 2022;25(2):100824. https://doi.org/10.1016/j.tvir.2022.100824.
29. Choi Y, Jung SL. Efficacy and safety of thermal ablation techniques for the treatment of primary papillary thyroid microcarcinoma: a systematic review and meta-analysis. Thyroid. 2020;30(5):720–31. https://doi.org/10.1089/thy.2019.0707.
30. Yan L, Lan Y, Xiao J, Lin L, Jiang B, Luo Y. Long-term outcomes of radiofrequency ablation for unifocal low-risk papillary thyroid microcarcinoma: a large cohort study of 414 patients. Eur Radiol. 2021;31(2):685–94. https://doi.org/10.1007/s00330-020-07128-6.
31. Wu R, Luo Y, Tang J, Yang M, Li J, Zhang Y, et al. Ultrasound-guided radiofrequency ablation for papillary thyroid microcarcinoma: a retrospective analysis of 198 patients. Int J Hyperth. 2020;37(1):168–74. https://doi.org/10.1080/02656736.2019.1708480.
32. Lim HK, Cho SJ, Baek JH, Lee KD, Son CW, Son JM, et al. US-guided radiofrequency ablation for low-risk papillary thyroid microcarcinoma: efficacy and safety in a large population. Korean J Radiol. 2019;20(12):1653–61. https://doi.org/10.3348/kjr.2019.0192.
33. Kim JH, Yoo WS, Park YJ, Park DJ, Yun TJ, Choi SH, et al. Efficacy and safety of radiofrequency ablation for treatment of locally recurrent thyroid cancers

smaller than 2 cm. Radiology. 2015;276(3):909–18. https://doi.org/10.1148/radiol.15140079.
34. Chu KF, Dupuy DE. Thermal ablation of tumours: biological mechanisms and advances in therapy. Nat Rev Cancer. 2014;14(3):199–208. https://doi.org/10.1038/nrc3672.
35. Yan L, Luo Y, Zhang Y, Zhu Y, Xiao J, Lan Y, et al. The clinical application of core-needle biopsy after radiofrequency ablation for low-risk papillary thyroid microcarcinoma: a large cohort of 202 patients study. J Cancer. 2020;11(18):5257–63. https://doi.org/10.7150/jca.42673.
36. Papini E, Bizzarri G, Bianchini A, Valle D, Misischi I, Guglielmi R, et al. Percutaneous ultrasound-guided laser ablation is effective for treating selected nodal metastases in papillary thyroid cancer. J Clin Endocrinol Metab. 2013;98(1):E92–7. https://doi.org/10.1210/jc.2012-2991.
37. Zhang L, Zhou W, Zhan W, Peng Y, Jiang S, Xu S. Percutaneous laser ablation of Unifocal papillary thyroid microcarcinoma: utility of conventional ultrasound and contrast-enhanced ultrasound in assessing local therapeutic response. World J Surg. 2018;42(8):2476–84. https://doi.org/10.1007/s00268-018-4500-6.

27 Future Directions of Thyroid Ultrasound-Guided Ablation

Jennifer H. Kuo and Roberto Valcavi

27.1 Introduction

There are many advantages offered by ultrasound-guided thermal ablation techniques for the management of thyroid nodules. The lure of highly effective, minimally invasive treatments that can be performed in an outpatient setting without the use of general anesthesia avoids an operation and neck scar, allows for patients to optimize their chances of not needing thyroid hormone replacement, and explains why the popularity of these techniques has grown exponentially in the last few decades. As physicians continue to explore additional clinical settings where these techniques prove to be safe, alternative surgical options to surgery, these thermal ablative techniques will undoubtedly continue to revolutionize the algorithms that we use to treat benign, as well as, malignant thyroid disease for the next few years. The future of non-operative, interventional techniques and their increasing role in the management of thyroid disease certainly looks bright, but consideration of the medical advances coming down the line suggests that the future may not solely be a "hot" one.

Traditional thermal approaches to ablation include all of the different forms of energy discussed in this handbook thus farradiofrequency, microwave, and laser techniques that are generally performed percutaneously, with high-intensity focused ultrasound (the only non-percutaneous technique). Although all highly efficacious, they are not without their limitations. These techniques, especially radiofrequency ablation, are prone to heat sink effects caused by blood flow that can diminish the effectiveness of treatment and prolong procedure times. There is also lack of predictability of ablation margins and thermal spread that limit their use and increase the chance of damage to nearby sensitive structures, such as nerves, the trachea, or the esophagus. Some of these techniques also rely heavily on physician expertise and judgment for successful outcomes (Table 27.1). As we continue our drive to discover and optimize less invasive but more effective procedures, other technologies may offer solutions to the inadequacies of thermal ablation.

J. H. Kuo (✉)
The Columbia Thyroid Center, Section of Endocrine Surgery, Columbia University, New York, NY, USA
e-mail: jhk2029@cumc.columbia.edu

R. Valcavi
Department of Endocrinology, The Endocrine & Thyroid Clinic, Reggio Emilia, Italy

R. Valcavi et al. (eds.), *Thyroid Ablation*, https://doi.org/10.1007/978-3-031-88229-6_27

Table 27.1 Characteristics of different ablation techniques

	Ablation technique	Ablation effect	Ablation function	Advantages	Limitations
Laser ablation	Application of light energy	Tissue hyperthermia	Coagulation necrosis	Easier learning curve due to fixed application	Longer procedure time, smaller ablation zone
Radiofrequency ablation	Application of a high-frequency oscillating electric field	Resistive heating surrounding the electrode tip and tissue hyperthermia	Coagulation necrosis	Most widely studied regarding safety and efficacy	Heat sink effect, tissue charring
Microwave ablation	Application of propagating electromagnetic energy	Tissue hyperthermia by dielectric hysteresis	Coagulation necrosis	Larger, more efficient tumor ablation volume; less heat effect and tissue charring	Potential greater risk for thermal injury
Cryoablation	Application of liquid nitrogen or argon gas	Crystal formation and osmotic shock	Protein denaturation	Larger tumor ablation volume	Longer procedural time due to freeze-thaw cycle; higher hemorrhage risk due to lack of tissue cauterization; variable damage in margin zones and injury to adjacent structures
Irreversible electroporation	Application of electric pulses	Irreversible cell membrane disruption	Cellular apoptosis	Less procedural time and more precise treatment margins due to non-thermal electric characteristic	High electric current requires general anesthesia and adequate neuromuscular blockade; contraindicated in cardiac arrhythmias
Histotripsy	Application of high-pressure sonographic waves	Cellular disruption	Tissue homogenization	More precise treatment margins with less risk of injury to adjacent structures	Clinical efficacy has yet to be established

27.2 Cryoablation

In contrast to thermal ablative technique that uses extreme heat to cause cellular destruction, cryoablation is a percutaneous ablation technique that uses extreme low temperatures for tumor destruction ("Cryo" from Greek meaning extreme cold or frost) [1, 2]. Cytotoxic cell destruction occurs through formation of intracellular ice crystals below temperatures −40 °C. Cryoablation can be performed by means of some gas as argon and liquified nitrogen gas. These gases pass through cryoprobes and expands into a gaseous state at the end of the probe to create temperatures as low as −196 °C for liquid nitrogen and −120 °C for argon (Joule–Thomson effect). Usually, the procedure is constituted by three steps: freezing–thawing and freezing. Newer systems use a thawing phase that follows this freezing phase, replacing the liquified gas with helium or internal heating of the needle. Systems that use liquid nitrogen do not require a heating phase. The repeated process of freezing–thawing–freezing results in an effective and complete ablation, typically with a circumferential margin of 1 cm around the tumor [1]. In addition to the physical damage of the cellular membrane by ice formation, cellular death by cryoablation is accomplished through other mechanisms including initiation of cellular stress responses (kill switch activation) and necrosis and apoptosis cascade, vascular stasis during thawing process, and likely activation of immune responses (Fig. 27.1) [3].

Similar to thermal ablative procedures, cryoablation has shown to reduce complications, costs, and recovery time [4, 5], but it has distinct advantages over other modes of ablation in that it can be monitored with imaging during the procedure, has greater control of the shape of the ablation zone, and mitigates pain. It has excellent cure rates for small tumors, but does appear to have less efficacy for tumors >2 cm, with higher rate complications and recurrence with larger volume disease [6]. Cryoablation is currently used to treat benign and malignant tumors of the liver, prostate, kidney, lung, breast, and bone, as well as non-tumor heart diseases.

Although thermal energies have dominated thyroid tumor ablation, cryoablation has also been used. Hamed et al. published their series of 40 patients with benign thyroid nodules who were treated with cryoablation [7]. At 6 months post-ablation, the thyroid nodules demonstrated a VRR of 25.0% (IQR: 4.2–50.0%), without any change in thyroid function tests. It has also been used to successfully treat metastatic bone lesions from thyroid cancer [8].

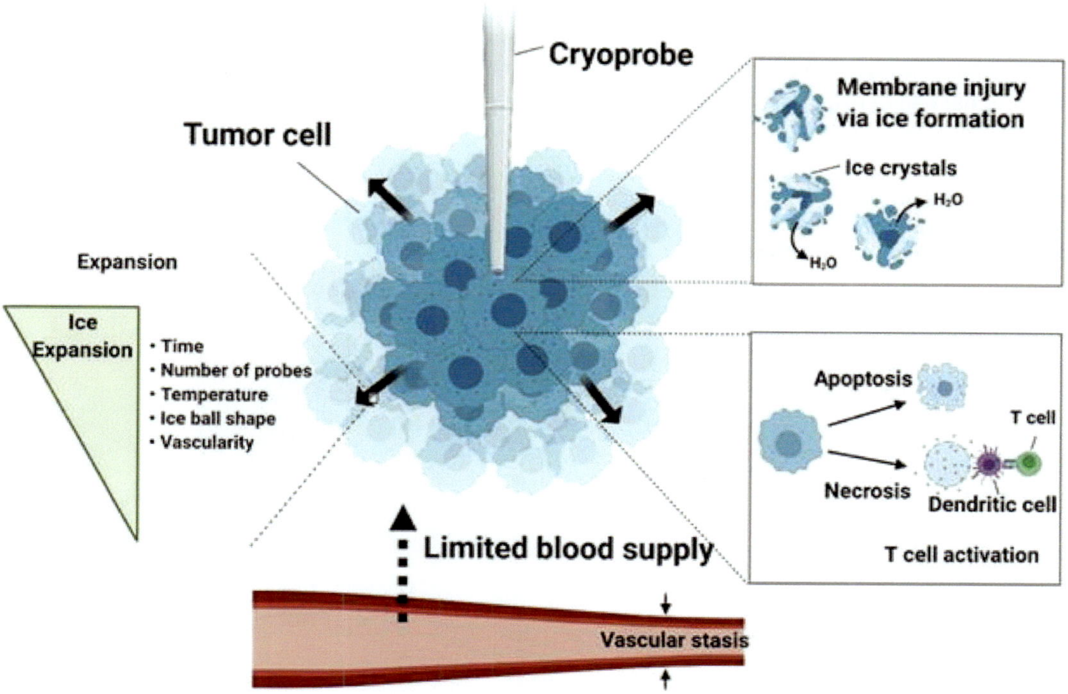

Fig. 27.1 Cryoablation (Kwak et al., Theranostics 2022)

27.3 Irreversible Electroporation

Irreversible electroporation (IRE) is a non-thermal tumor ablation modality [9, 10] that delivers ultra-short high-voltage electrical impulses through specific needles. The resultant strong external electric field causes permeable nanoscale pores to form in the cell membrane, or electroporation [11–14]. Irreversible electroporation can be induced if the intensity of the electric field exceeds a particular threshold (Fig. 27.2) [15] or by long pulses applications. Once the nanopores remain permanently open, the membrane loses its physiological function and leads to cell apoptosis and the clearing away of cell debris by the host immune system [10–12]. IRE has a distinct advantage over thermal ablative techniques and cryoablation because of the lack of exposure to extreme heat or cold that helps to minimize potential damage to surrounding healthy tissue. IRE preserves vital structures as veins, arteries, nerves, and ducts. This happens because the electric field is not affecting the protein structures. Numerous clinical studies have demonstrated its efficacy as an alternative approach to the treatment of tumors in sensitive areas of the body [16].

Theoretically, IRE can be used to treat all solid tumors; however, the application of IRE has thus far generally been limited to tumors of the liver, pancreas, prostate, and kidneys. Nonetheless, several studies have demonstrated the feasibility and safety of IRE in treating locally advanced cancers in critical areas [13, 15, 17, 18], including the thyroid gland, but its use in treating these types of cancers has not been widespread. Systemic adverse effects are rare, and damage caused to adjacent areas has been within acceptable limits.

IRE does have several limitations. The electrical current used can cause significant muscle contractions that can displace the location of the probes, induce muscle damage, pain and in severe cases, and can cause rhabdomyolysis and acute kidney damage. Therefore, patients must receive general anesthesia and undergo complete muscle relaxation prior to the administration of IRE [11]. The electric current can also cause life-threatening arrhythmias and significant elevations in systolic blood pressures (20–30 mmHg on average), though it tends to be self-limited with blood pressure returning to baseline at the end of the procedure. On this basis Hepato-Pancreatic-Biliary (HPB) IRE

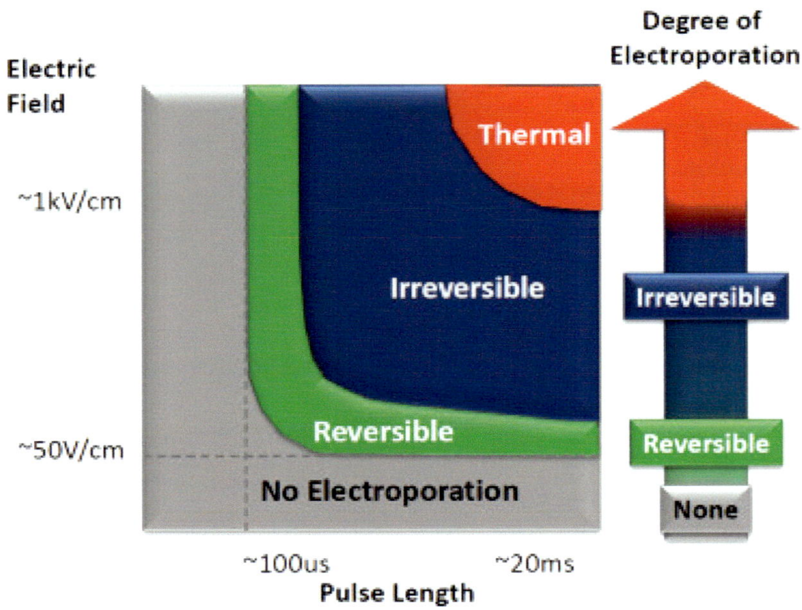

Fig. 27.2 Electroporation (Hsiao et al., Journal of Medical Ultrasound 2017)

procedures must be synchronized with heart synchro devices. Newer, high-frequency IRE systems that do not cause muscle contraction would produce less pain and not require general anesthesia, but have yet to be studied specifically for the treatment of thyroid nodules. Thus absolute contraindications for IRE include patients who are unable to tolerate general anesthesia, patients presenting with cardiovascular comorbidities, such as cardiac arrhythmia, coronary artery disease, or recent myocardial infarction, and patients with a history of poorly controlled hypertension, and patients with metallic implants, such as a pacemaker or intraluminal stent, as the metal in these devices would provide an alternate path for the electric current due to its lower electrical resistance.

Complications associated with IRE ablation are often related to effects of electrical pulses and can include cardiovascular problems, pneumothorax, and severe muscle contractions. Electroporation can cause cellular leakage of electrolytes, with elevations in serum potassium and chloride, a very similar phenomenon to tumor lysis syndrome following chemotherapy and relieved by adequate hydration. This is most problematic in patients with impaired renal function or who undergo a large ablation area. Similar to thermal ablative techniques, local complications at the insertion site (bleeding, infection) can also occur [13]. However, post-procedural pain has been noted less frequently for IRE treatment than for thermal ablation techniques, such as RFA and MWA. In most situations, these effects are mild and can be relieved by oral medications [13].

27.4 Histotripsy

Histotripsy is a novel modality of non-invasive tumor ablation that uses overlapping high-pressure ultrasound pulses to disrupt cellular architecture. Focused ultrasound waves create precise regions of extreme pressure changes at a point of convergence that ultimately results in acoustic cavitation and is able to mechanically homogenize tissue that results in a liquefied homogenate that is gradually reabsorbed [19–21]. In contrast to high-frequency ultrasound (HIFU), histotripsy avoids any generation of heat and risk of thermal spread and injury, by separating the microsecond-length ultrasound pulses by milliseconds off-time or longer.

As a newer technology, the clinical efficacy of histotripsy for various tumors is currently being investigated in clinical trials.

27.5 Summary

The introduction and adoption of minimally invasive thermal ablative techniques are quickly changing the way we think about and manage thyroid diseases, offering patients many desired advantages compared to surgical options of management. Although highly effective, they are nonetheless, limited by the risk of thermal spread and injury to adjacent, critical structures, and their susceptibility to the heat sink effect. There are, however, newer, non-thermal, ablative techniques that are emerging as potential alternatives that could potentially avoid these pitfalls. Their role in the management of thyroid diseases has yet to be investigated thoroughly, but certainly serve as a promise for continued evolution and advances for the field of interventional ablative techniques.

References

1. Aarts BM, Klompenhouwer EG, Rice SL, Imani F, Baetens T, Bex A, et al. Cryoablation and immunotherapy: an overview of evidence on its synergy. Insights Imaging. 2019;10(1):53. https://doi.org/10.1186/s13244-019-0727-5.
2. Cazzato RL, Garnon J, Ramamurthy N, Koch G, Tsoumakidou G, Caudrelier J, et al. Percutaneous image-guided cryoablation: current applications and results in the oncologic field. Med Oncol. 2016;33(12):1–16. https://doi.org/10.1007/s12032-016-0848-3.
3. Baust JG, Snyder KK, Santucci KL, Robilotto AT, Van Buskirk RG, Baust JM. Cryoablation: physical and molecular basis with putative immunological consequences. Int J Hyperth. 2019;36(SUP1):10. https://doi.org/10.1080/02656736.2019.1647355.

4. Solomon SB, Silverman SG. Imaging in interventional oncology. Radiology. 2010;257:624–40. https://doi.org/10.1148/radiol.10081490.
5. Link RE, Permpongkosol S, Gupta A, Jarrett TW, Solomon SB, Kavoussi LR. Cost analysis of open, laparoscopic, and percutaneous treatment options for nephron-sparing surgery. J Endourol. 2006;20(10):782–9. https://doi.org/10.1089/end.2006.20.782.
6. Kwak K, Yu B, Lewandowski RJ, Kim D-H. Recent progress in cryoablation cancer therapy and nanoparticles mediated cryoablation. Theranostics. 2022;2022(5):2175–204. https://doi.org/10.7150/thno.67530.
7. Hamed M, Mansour S, Halawa M, Bahaaeldin A, Ibrahim N, Ghoneim A. Cryoablation of goiter irrespective of thyroid profile. Thyroid Res Pract. 2019;16(1):6. https://doi.org/10.4103/trp.trp_54_18.
8. Autrusseau PA, Schneegans O, Koch G, Weiss J, Caudrelier J, Dalili D, et al. Safety and efficacy of percutaneous Cryoablation of Extraspinal thyroid cancer bone metastases with curative intent: single-center experience with a median follow-up of more than 5 years. J Vasc Interv Radiol. 2022;33(7):797–804. https://doi.org/10.1016/j.jvir.2022.03.016.
9. Davalos RV, Mir LM, Rubinsky B. Tissue ablation with irreversible electroporation. Ann Biomed Eng. 2005;33(2):223–31. https://doi.org/10.1007/s10439-005-8981-8.
10. Wagstaff PGK, Buijs M, van den Bos W, de Bruin DM, Zondervan PJ, de la Rosette JJMCH, et al. Irreversible electroporation: state of the art. Onco Targets Ther. 2016;9:2437–46. https://doi.org/10.2147/OTT.S88086.
11. Hong S, Calzetti D, Dopita MA, Blair WP, Whitmore BC, Balick B, et al. Large-scale shock-ionized and photoionized gas in M83: the impact of star formation. Astrophys J. 2011;731(1):45. https://doi.org/10.48550/arXiv.1102.2444.
12. Pavšelj N, Préat V, Miklavčič D. A numerical model of skin electropermeabilization based on in vivo experiments. Ann Biomed Eng. 2007;35(12):2138–44. https://doi.org/10.1007/s10439-007-9378-7.
13. Scheffer HJ, Nielsen K, De Jong MC, Van Tilborg AAJM, Vieveen JM, Bouwman A, et al. Irreversible electroporation for nonthermal tumor ablation in the clinical setting: a systematic review of safety and efficacy. J Vasc Interv Radiol. 2014;25(7):997–1011. https://doi.org/10.1016/j.jvir.2014.01.028.
14. Jiang C, Davalos RV, Bischof JC. A review of basic to clinical studies of irreversible electroporation therapy. IEEE Trans Biomed Eng. 2015;62(1):4–20. https://doi.org/10.1109/TBME.2014.2367543.
15. Narayanan G, Froud T, Suthar R, Barbery K. Irreversible electroporation of hepatic malignancy. Semin Intervent Radiol. 2013;30(1):67–73. https://doi.org/10.1055/s-0033-1333655.
16. Narayanan G. Irreversible electroporation. Semin Intervent Radiol. 2015;32(4):349–55. https://doi.org/10.1055/s-0035-1564706.
17. Martin RCG, McFarland K, Ellis S, Velanovich V. Irreversible electroporation therapy in the management of locally advanced pancreatic adenocarcinoma. J Am Coll Surg. 2012;215(3):361–9. https://doi.org/10.1016/j.jamcollsurg.2012.05.021.
18. Murray KS, Ehdaie B, Musser J, Mashni J, Srimathveeravalli G, Durack JC, et al. Pilot study to assess safety and clinical outcomes of irreversible electroporation for partial gland ablation in men with prostate cancer. J Urol. 2016;196(3):883–90. https://doi.org/10.1016/j.juro.2016.02.2986.
19. Bhatia SS, Arya R, Narayanan G. Niche applications of irreversible electroporation. Tech Vasc Interv Radiol. 2015;18(3):170–5. https://doi.org/10.1053/j.tvir.2015.06.008.
20. Silk M, Tahour D, Srimathveeravalli G, Solomon SB, Thornton RH. The state of irreversible electroporation in interventional oncology. Semin Intervent Radiol. 2014;31(2):111–7. https://doi.org/10.1055/s-0034-1373785.
21. Bower M, Sherwood L, Li Y, Martin R. Irreversible electroporation of the pancreas: definitive local therapy without systemic effects. J Surg Oncol. 2011;104(1):22–8. https://doi.org/10.1055/s-0034-1373785.

Index

R. Valcavi et al. (eds.), *Thyroid Ablation*, https://doi.org/10.1007/978-3-031-88229-6

U

V

Z